# Your Pregnancy and Childbirth

## Month to Month

*Revised Sixth Edition*

The American College of
Obstetricians and Gynecologists

*Women's Health Care Physicians*

*Your Pregnancy and Childbirth: Month to Month,* Revised Sixth Edition, was developed by a panel of experts working in consultation with staff of the American College of Obstetricians and Gynecologists (ACOG):

**Editorial Task Force Members**

Patrice Weiss, MD, *Chair*
Ann Brown, CNM, MSN
Bonnie J. Dattel, MD
Kacey Eichelberger, MD
Brian M. Mercer, MD
Patrick S. Ramsey, MD
Nancy C. Rose, MD
Dane M. Shipp, MD

**ACOG Staff**

Christopher M. Zahn, MD, *Vice President, Practice Activities*
Deirdre W. Allen, *Senior Director, Publications*
Yvonne C. Dorsey, *Director of Production*
Kathleen Scogna, *Director, Patient Education*
Veronica Valderrama, *Managing Editor, Professional Publications*
Lara Bonner, *Editor, Patient Education*

*The contributions of the following people are gratefully acknowledged:*

Glenda Fauntleroy, *Writer*
Naylor Design, Inc., *Book Design*
Dragonfly Media Group, *Illustration*
John Yanson, *Illustration*
Lightbox Visual Communications, Inc., *Illustration*

**Library of Congress Cataloging-in-Publication Data**

Names: American College of Obstetricians and Gynecologists. Women's Health Care Physicians.
Title: Your pregnancy and childbirth : month to month / The American College of Obstetricians and Gynecologists, Women's Health Care Physicians.
Other titles: ACOG guide to planning for pregnancy, birth, and beyond
Description: Revised sixth edition. | Washington, DC : American College of Obstetricians and Gynecologists Washington, DC, 2016. | Revision of: ACOG guide to planning for pregnancy, birth, and beyond. 1990.
Identifiers: LCCN 2016012684 | ISBN 9781934984598
Subjects: LCSH: Pregnancy--Popular works. | Childbirth--Popular works.
Classification: LCC RG525 .A26 2016 | DDC 618.2--dc23 LC record available at http://lccn.loc.gov/2016012684

*Your Pregnancy and Childbirth: Month to Month* sets forth current information and opinions on subjects related to women's health and reproduction. The information does not dictate an exclusive course of treatment or procedure to be followed and should not be construed as excluding other acceptable methods of practice. Variations, taking into account the needs of the individual patient, resources, and limitations unique to the institution or type of practice, may be appropriate. The mention of a product, device, or drug in this publication does not constitute or guarantee endorsement of the quality or value of such product, device, or drug or of the claims made for it by the manufacturer.

2345/0987

# Contents

PREFACE   xvii

 **Pregnancy Month by Month   1**

**CHAPTER 1:  Getting Ready for Pregnancy   3**

The Preconception Visit   3
*Infections and Immunizations • Your Family Health History • Preconception Carrier Screening • Preexisting Health Conditions • Medications and Supplements • Past Pregnancies*

A Healthy Lifestyle   10
*Eat Right • Get Regular Exercise • Take Folic Acid • Reach and Maintain a Healthy Weight • Quit Using Unhealthy Substances • Keep Your Environment Safe*

Getting Pregnant   15
*The Menstrual Cycle • When Are You Most Fertile? • Fertility Awareness • Stopping Birth Control*

RESOURCES   21

Illustrations of Prenatal Development   22

**CHAPTER 2: MONTHS 1 AND 2 (WEEKS 1–8)   33**

YOUR GROWING BABY   33

YOUR PREGNANCY   37

Your Changing Body   37
*Hormones • Signs and Symptoms of Pregnancy • Pregnancy Tests • Your Due Date*

Discomforts and How to Manage Them   41
*Morning Sickness • Fatigue*

Nutrition   44
*Focus on Folic Acid • Prenatal Multivitamin Supplements • Weight Gain*

Exercise   46
*Pregnancy Changes That Can Affect Your Exercise Routine • Starting an Exercise Program During Pregnancy • Activities to Avoid • Exercise of the Month: Kegel Exercises*

Healthy Decisions   50
*Things to Avoid During Pregnancy • What Do I Do About Medications? • Choosing a Health Care Provider for Your Pregnancy • When to Spread the News*

Other Considerations   58
*A Safe Workplace • Tips for Working During Early Pregnancy*

Prenatal Care Visits   59

Special Concerns   60
*Miscarriage • Ectopic Pregnancy*

ASK THE EXPERTS   61
*Caffeine and Pregnancy • Douching During Pregnancy*

RESOURCES   62

## CHAPTER 3: MONTH 3 (WEEKS 9–12)   65

YOUR GROWING BABY   65

YOUR PREGNANCY   67

Your Changing Body   67

Discomforts and How to Manage Them   67
*Nausea • Fatigue and Sleep Problems • Acne • Breast Changes • Constipation*

Nutrition   71
*Weight Gain • Sugar and Sugar Substitutes • Focus on Iron*

Exercise   72
*Exercise of the Month: 4-Point Kneeling • Get Moving*

Healthy Decisions   73
*Vaginal Birth After Cesarean Delivery • Prenatal Genetic Screening and Diagnosis*

Other Considerations   76
*Emotional Changes • Skin Changes • Getting Sick*

Prenatal Care Visits   78
*Ultrasound Exam • Pelvic Exam • Lab Tests • Genetic Testing*

Special Concerns   83
*Sexually Transmitted Infections • Intimate Partner Violence*

ASK THE EXPERTS   85
*Saunas and Hot Tubs • Cats and Toxoplasmosis • Using Hair Dye*

RESOURCES   86

## CHAPTER 4: MONTH 4 (WEEKS 13–16)   89

YOUR GROWING BABY   89

YOUR PREGNANCY   91

Your Changing Body   91

Discomforts and How to Manage Them   91
*Lower Abdominal Pain • Mouth and Dental Changes • Strange Dreams • Excessive Salivation • Spider Veins*

Nutrition   93
*Weight Gain • Focus on High- and Low-Glycemic Foods • Food Cravings*

Exercise   95
*Walking: A Great Way to Stay Motivated • Exercise of the Month: Seated Ball Balance*

Healthy Decisions   96
*Your Workplace Rights • Pregnancy Discrimination Act • Occupational Safety and Health Act • Family and Medical Leave Act • Birth Places*

Other Considerations   99
*Financial Issues • Health Insurance*

Prenatal Care Visits   101
*Tests • Exams*

Special Concerns   101
*Urinary Tract Infections • Vaginal Discharge • Pregnancy-Related Stress*

**ASK THE EXPERTS   104**
*Surgery While Pregnant • Dental X-Rays • Allergy Medication*

**RESOURCES**   105

## CHAPTER 5: MONTH 5 (WEEKS 17–20)   107

**YOUR GROWING BABY   107**

**YOUR PREGNANCY   109**

Your Changing Body   109

Discomforts and How to Manage Them   109
*Congestion and Nosebleeds • Lower Back Pain • Dizziness • Forgetfulness*

Nutrition   111
*Fish Precautions During Pregnancy • Focus on Omega-3 Fatty Acids • Healthy Snacking • Weight Gain*

Exercise   113
*Alternative Exercises • Exercise of the Month: Ball Wall Squat • Tips for Safe and Healthy Exercise*

Healthy Decisions   115
*Knowing the Baby's Sex • Choosing Your Baby's Physician*

Other Considerations   116
*Travel During Pregnancy • By Car • By Plane • By Ship • Sleeping Positions*

Prenatal Care Visits   122

Special Concerns   123
*Prenatal Lead Exposure • Assessment of Your Baby's Movement*

**ASK THE EXPERTS   126**
*Sushi Safety • Getting a Massage*

**RESOURCES**   127

## CHAPTER 6: MONTH 6 (WEEKS 21–24)   129

**YOUR GROWING BABY   129**

**YOUR PREGNANCY   131**

Your Changing Body   131

Discomforts and How to Manage Them   131
*Heartburn • Hot Flashes • Aches and Pains*

Nutrition   132
*Focus on B Vitamins and Choline • Salt and Monosodium Glutamate • Avoiding Food Poisoning • Weight Gain*

Exercise   135
*Loss of Balance • Exercise of the Month: Ball Shoulder Stretch*

Healthy Decisions   136
*Labor and Delivery: Things to Start Thinking About • Labor and Delivery in Water • Cesarean Delivery on Request*

Other Considerations    138
*Early Preterm Birth • Body Image • Sex • Involving Your Other Children in Your Pregnancy*

Prenatal Care Visits    141

Special Concerns    141
*Preterm Labor • Preeclampsia • Fast or Racing Heartbeat • Keepsake Ultrasound Photos*

ASK THE EXPERTS    144
*Chickenpox • Back Labor*

RESOURCES    144

## CHAPTER 7: MONTH 7 (WEEKS 25–28)    147

### YOUR GROWING BABY    147

### YOUR PREGNANCY    149

Your Changing Body    149

Discomforts and How to Manage Them    149
*Lower Back Pain • Pelvic Bone Pain • Constipation • Braxton Hicks Contractions*

Nutrition    151
*Weight Gain • Focus on Water and Fiber*

Exercise    153
*Swimming • Exercise of the Month: Seated Side Stretch*

Healthy Decisions    153
*Doulas • Birth Plan • Cord Blood Banking*

Other Considerations    159
*Depression, Anxiety, and Stress • Safe Sleep Position*

Prenatal Care Visits    164

Special Concerns    165
*Preterm Labor • Vaginal Bleeding • Amniotic Fluid Problems*

ASK THE EXPERTS    166
*Birth Control After the Baby Is Born • Why Breastfeeding Is Best • Vitamin D Deficiency*

RESOURCES    168

## CHAPTER 8: MONTH 8 (WEEKS 29–32)    171

### YOUR GROWING BABY    171

### YOUR PREGNANCY    173

Your Changing Body    173

Discomforts and How to Manage Them    173
*Shortness of Breath • Hemorrhoids • Varicose Veins and Leg Swelling • Leg Cramps • Fatigue • Itchy Skin*

Nutrition    175
*Focus on Calcium*

Exercise    176
*Relaxation Techniques • Exercise of the Month: Kneeling Heel Touch*

Healthy Decisions    177
*Circumcision for Boys • Child Care • Getting Ready for Delivery*

Other Considerations    180
*Childbirth Preparation Methods • Hospital Tour • Pain Relief During Labor • Bed Rest*

Prenatal Care Visits    182

Special Concerns    183
*Preterm Labor • Premature Rupture of Membranes*

**ASK THE EXPERTS**   184
*Signs or Symptoms That Cause Concern • Delayed Cord Clamping • Lactose Intolerance*
**RESOURCES**   185

## CHAPTER 9: MONTH 9 (WEEKS 33–36)   187
**YOUR GROWING BABY**   187
**YOUR PREGNANCY**   189
Your Changing Body   189
Discomforts and How to Manage Them   189
*Frequent Urination • Prelabor (Braxton Hicks) Contractions • Trouble Sleeping • Leg Swelling and Pain • Pelvic Pressure • Numbness of Legs and Feet*
Nutrition   191
*Focus on Vitamin C*
Exercise   191
*Exercise of the Month: Standing Back Bend*
Healthy Decisions   192
*Positions for Labor and Childbirth • Your Baby's Hospital Stay • Packing for the Hospital • Feeding Your Baby*
Other Considerations   196
*Preparing Your Home for the Baby • Buying a Car Seat*
Prenatal Care Visits   199
*Group B Streptococci Screening • Other Screening Tests*
Special Concerns   201
*Preeclampsia • Breech Presentation*
**ASK THE EXPERTS**   202
*Pedicures • Breastfeeding Right After Birth • Inverted Nipples and Breastfeeding*
**RESOURCES**   202

## CHAPTER 10: MONTH 10 (WEEKS 37–40)   205
**YOUR GROWING BABY**   205
**YOUR PREGNANCY**   207
Your Changing Body   207
Discomforts and How to Manage Them   207
*Frequent Urination • Snoring*
Nutrition   208
*Focus on Docosahexaenoic Acid • What to Eat if You Think You Are Going Into Labor*
Exercise   210
*Exercise of the Month: Paced Breathing*
Healthy Decisions   211
*Delivery Before 39 Weeks • When to Go to the Hospital • Children in the Delivery Room*
Other Considerations   212
*Knowing When You're in Labor • Having Sex • Nesting*
Prenatal Care Visits   214
Special Concerns   214
*Signs of Preeclampsia • Rupture of Membranes • Changes in the Baby's Movement • Vaginal Spotting • Late-Term and Postterm Pregnancy • Old Wives' Tales*

**ASK THE EXPERTS  218**
*Episiotomy • Operative Vaginal Delivery*

**RESOURCES  218**

---

**II  Labor, Delivery, and Postpartum Care  221**

**CHAPTER 11: PAIN RELIEF DURING CHILDBIRTH  223**

Medications for Pain Relief  223
*System Analgesics • Local Anesthesia • Regional Analgesia and Regional Anesthesia • General Anesthesia*

Childbirth Preparation Methods  227

Pain Relief Techniques  229
*Positions • Warm Baths and Showers • Walking*

Continuous Labor Support  232

**RESOURCES  232**

**CHAPTER 12: LABOR INDUCTION  235**

Reasons for Labor Induction  235

When Is Labor Not Induced?  237

How Induction Is Done  237
*Ripening the Cervix • Stripping the Amniotic Membranes • Amniotomy • Oxytocin*

Risks  239

If Your Labor Is Going to Be Induced  240

**RESOURCES  240**

**CHAPTER 13: LABOR AND DELIVERY  243**

Common Terms  243

Stages of Childbirth  244
*Stage 1: Early Labor • Stage 1: Active Labor • Transition to Stage 2 • Stage 2: Pushing and Delivery • Stage 3: Delivery of the Placenta*

After the Baby Is Born  253

**RESOURCES  253**

**CHAPTER 14: OPERATIVE DELIVERY AND BREECH PRESENTATION  255**

Operative Vaginal Delivery  255
*Types of Operative Vaginal Delivery • Risks*

Breech Presentation  257
*The Baby's Position • Turning the Baby • Options for Delivery*

**RESOURCES  261**

**CHAPTER 15: CESAREAN DELIVERY AND VAGINAL BIRTH AFTER CESAREAN DELIVERY  263**

Why You May Need a Cesarean Delivery  263

What Happens During a Cesarean Delivery   265
*Anesthesia • Preparing You for Surgery • Making the Incisions • Delivering the Baby • Afterbirth and Closing the Incisions*

Risks   268

Recovery   268

Back at Home   269

Vaginal Birth After Cesarean Delivery   269
*Is It Right for You? • Benefits • Risks • Best Chances for Success • Be Prepared for Changes*

**RESOURCES   272**

## CHAPTER 16: THE POSTPARTUM PERIOD   275

Right After the Baby Is Born   275
*Your Baby's Apgar Score • Your Baby's First Breath • Maintaining the Baby's Temperature • Getting to Know Your Baby • What Happens to Your Baby Next*

Postpartum: The First Week   280
*Bleeding • Uterine Contractions • Perineal Pain • Painful Urination • Abdomen • Hemorrhoids • Bowel Problems*

Postpartum: Weeks 2–12   286
*Your Changing Body • Postpartum Danger Signs • Postpartum Sadness and Depression • Exercise • Nutrition • Lifestyle Changes*

Life With Your New Baby   292

Postpartum Check-Up   292

Sex After Childbirth   293

Birth Control   295
*Intrauterine Devices • Implant • Injection • Combined Hormonal Methods • Progestin-Only Pills • Barrier Methods • Lactational Amenorrhea Method • Emergency Contraception*

Permanent Birth Control   304
*Female Sterilization • Male Sterilization*

Returning to Work   308

**RESOURCES   309**

 **Nutrition   311**

## CHAPTER 17: NUTRITION DURING PREGNANCY   313

Balancing Your Diet   314
*Protein • Carbohydrates • Fats*

Planning Healthy Meals   316

The Five Food Groups   316

Key Vitamins and Minerals   318
*Folic Acid • Iron • Calcium • Vitamin D*

Putting It All Together   320

Weight Gain During Pregnancy   321

Special Concerns   322
*Fish and Shellfish • Caffeine • Vegetarian Diets • Lactose Intolerance • Celiac Disease • Food Safety*

**RESOURCES   326**

## CHAPTER 18: BREASTFEEDING AND FORMULA-FEEDING YOUR BABY   329

The Benefits of Breastfeeding   329

Who Should Not Breastfeed   331

Deciding to Breastfeed   332
*After the Baby Is Born • Get the Baby Latched On • Check the Baby's Technique • Watch Your Baby, Not the Clock • Nurse on Demand • Give a Vitamin D Supplement*

Breastfeeding Challenges   338
*Sore Nipples • Engorgement • Delayed Milk Production • Low Milk Supply • Inverted or Flat Nipples • Blocked Ducts • Mastitis*

Common Questions About Breastfeeding   342
*How long should I breastfeed my baby? • What is "exclusive" breastfeeding? • Is my baby getting enough milk? • What should I eat and how much? • Now that I'm no longer pregnant, is it OK for me to smoke cigarettes and drink alcohol again? • Can I give my baby a pacifier? • I'm expecting twins. Can I breastfeed them? • I've had breast surgery. Can I still breastfeed? • I've heard about human milk banks. What are they? • What do I need to know about taking medications while breastfeeding?*

Going Back to Work   349
*Tell Your Employer • Expressing Breast Milk*

Choosing to Formula-Feed   353
*Picking a Formula • Bottles • The Challenges*

Final Thoughts on Feeding Your Baby   356

RESOURCES   356

 ## IV   Special Considerations   359

## CHAPTER 19: MULTIPLES: WHEN IT'S TWINS, TRIPLETS, OR MORE   361

Making Multiples   361
*Fraternal or Identical Twins? • Three or More Babies*

How to Know When It's More Than One Baby   364

Risks   364
*Preterm Birth • Chorionicity and Amnionicity • Gestational Diabetes Mellitus • High Blood Pressure and Preeclampsia • Growth Problems*

What to Expect   369
*Nutritional Considerations • Weight Gain • Exercise • Prenatal Genetic Screening and Diagnosis • Monitoring • Bed Rest and Hospitalization*

Delivery   372

Getting Ready   373

RESOURCES   374

## CHAPTER 20: OBESITY AND EATING DISORDERS   377

Obesity and Pregnancy   377
*Defining Obesity • Risks of Obesity During Pregnancy • Risks of Obesity During Childbirth • Managing Obesity During Pregnancy • Losing Weight After Pregnancy*

Eating Disorders and Pregnancy   384
*Types of Eating Disorders • How Eating Disorders Can Harm You and Your Baby • Getting Help • If You Have a History of Eating Disorders*

RESOURCES   386

**CHAPTER 21: REDUCING RISKS OF BIRTH DEFECTS   389**

Teratogens and Pregnancy   392

What Is an Exposure History?   392

Medications   394
*Prescription Medications • Over-the-Counter Medications*

Alcohol   397

Environmental Toxins   398
*Toxins in the Workplace • Avoiding Known Environmental Toxins*

Other Potential Hazards   401
*X-Rays • Elevated Core Body Temperature*

If You Have Questions   402

RESOURCES   402

 **Medical Problems During Pregnancy   405**

**CHAPTER 22: HYPERTENSION AND PREECLAMPSIA   407**

Blood Pressure   407

Chronic Hypertension   408
*Risks • Treatment*

Gestational Hypertension   410

Preeclampsia   411
*Risks • Signs and Symptoms • Diagnosis • Treatment*

Prevention   414
*Preconception Care • Aspirin Therapy*

RESOURCES   415

**CHAPTER 23: DIABETES MELLITUS   417**

Gestational Diabetes Mellitus   417
*Risk Factors • How Gestational Diabetes Can Affect You and Your Baby • Testing for Gestational Diabetes • Controlling Gestational Diabetes • Specials Tests • Labor and Delivery • Care After Pregnancy*

Pregestational Diabetes Mellitus   422
*Risks to Your Pregnancy • Preconception Care • Controlling Your Diabetes During Pregnancy • Special Tests • Labor and Delivery • Care After Pregnancy*

RESOURCES   427

**CHAPTER 24: OTHER CHRONIC CONDITIONS   429**

Heart Disease   429

Kidney Disease   430

Asthma   431

Thyroid Disease   433

Digestive Diseases   434
*Inflammatory Bowel Disease • Irritable Bowel Syndrome • Celiac Disease*

Other Autoimmune Diseases   436
*Antiphospholipid Syndrome • Lupus • Multiple Sclerosis • Rheumatoid Arthritis*

Thrombophilias   438

Von Willebrand Disease   440

Seizure Disorders   440

Mental Illness   442

Physical Disability   443

RESOURCES   444

 **Testing   447**

**CHAPTER 25: SCREENING AND DIAGNOSTIC TESTING FOR GENETIC DISORDERS   449**

Genes and Chromosomes   450

Inherited Disorders   452
*Autosomal Dominant Disorders • Autosomal Recessive Disorders • Sex-Linked Disorders • Multifactorial Disorders*

Chromosomal Disorders   455
*Aneuploidy • Structural Chromosomal Disorders*

Assessing Your Risk   457

Types of Tests for Genetic Disorders   459

Deciding Whether to Be Tested   461

Carrier Screening   462
*Results • Timing • Important Considerations • If You or Your Partner Is a Carrier*

Screening Tests for Aneuploidy and Neural Tube Defects   465
*First-Trimester Screening • Second-Trimester Screening • Integrated and Sequential Screening • Results • If Screening Test Results Show an Increased Risk*

Diagnostic Tests   468
*Amniocentesis • Chorionic Villus Sampling • Preimplantation Genetic Diagnosis • How the Cells Are Analyzed • If Your Baby Has a Disorder*

RESOURCES   472

**CHAPTER 26: TESTING TO MONITOR FETAL WELL-BEING   475**

Why Testing May Be Done   475

Interpreting Test Results   477

When Tests Are Done   477

Types of Special Tests   478
*Fetal Movement Counts • Ultrasound Exam • Nonstress Test • Biophysical Profile • Modified Biophysical Profile • Contraction Stress Test*

RESOURCES   483

 **Complications During Pregnancy and Childbirth   485**

**CHAPTER 27: PRETERM LABOR, PREMATURE RUPTURE OF MEMBRANES, AND PRETERM BIRTH   487**

Preterm Labor   487
*Risk Factors • Diagnosis • Management • Prevention*

Premature Rupture of Membranes   491
*Risk Factors • Diagnosis • Management*

Preterm Birth   493
*Neonatal Intensive Care • Surfactant Replacement Therapy • Resuscitation and Breathing Support • Making Difficult Decisions*
Caring for a Preterm Baby   495
**RESOURCES   496**

**CHAPTER 28: BLOOD TYPE INCOMPATIBILITY   499**
Rh Incompatibility   499
*How It Affects Your Baby • How Sensitization Can Occur • Prevention • Treatment if Antibodies Develop*
ABO Incompatibility   503
*How It Affects Your Baby • Treatment*
**RESOURCES   504**

**CHAPTER 29: PLACENTAL PROBLEMS   507**
Placenta Previa   507
*Types • Signs and Symptoms • Diagnosis • Treatment*
Placental Abruption   510
*Types • Signs and Symptoms • Treatment*
Placenta Accreta   511
*Types • Signs and Symptoms • Diagnosis • Treatment*
**RESOURCES   513**

**CHAPTER 30: PROTECTING YOURSELF FROM INFECTIONS   515**
What Happens During an Infection   515
Immunizations and Pregnancy   516
Vaccine-Preventable Diseases   518
*Influenza • Pertussis • Tetanus and Diphtheria • Varicella • Hepatitis Infections • Human Papillomavirus • Measles, Mumps, and Rubella • Meningococcal Meningitis • Pneumococcal Pneumonia*
Other Infections   526
*Group B Streptococci • Urinary Tract Infections • Sexually Transmitted Infections • Hepatitis C Infection • Tuberculosis • Bacterial Vaginosis • Listeriosis • Cytomegalovirus • Toxoplasmosis • Parvovirus*
**RESOURCES   538**

**CHAPTER 31: GROWTH PROBLEMS   541**
Fetal Growth Restriction   541
*Causes • Diagnosis • Management • Prevention*
Macrosomia   544
*Diagnosis • Complications*
**RESOURCES   546**

**CHAPTER 32: PROBLEMS DURING LABOR AND DELIVERY   549**
Abnormal Labor   549
*Causes • Risks • Assessment • Management*
Shoulder Dystocia   551
Umbilical Cord Compression   553
*Risk Factors • Signs and Symptoms • Management*

Umbilical Cord Prolapse    553
*Risk Factors • Signs and Symptoms • Management*
Postpartum Hemorrhage    555
*Risk Factors • Management*
Endometritis    556
*Risk Factors • Signs and Symptoms • Management*
RESOURCES    557

## VIII  Pregnancy Loss    559

### CHAPTER 33: EARLY PREGNANCY LOSS: MISCARRIAGE, ECTOPIC PREGNANCY, AND GESTATIONAL TROPHOBLASTIC DISEASE    561

Miscarriage    561
*Causes • Signs and Symptoms • Diagnosis • Treatment • Recovery • Trying Again*
Ectopic Pregnancy    565
*Risk Factors • Signs and Symptoms • Diagnosis • Treatment*
Gestational Trophoblastic Disease    568
*Signs, Symptoms, and Diagnosis • Treatment*
Coping With the Loss    569
RESOURCES    570

### CHAPTER 34: LATE PREGNANCY LOSS: STILLBIRTH    573

How Stillbirth Is Diagnosed    573
What Went Wrong?    574
Tests and Evaluations    574
Grieving    575
The Stages of Grief    575
*Shock, Numbness, and Disbelief • Searching and Yearning • Anger or Rage • Depression and Loneliness • Acceptance*
You and Your Partner    578
Seeking Support    578
Another Pregnancy    579
The Future    579
RESOURCES    580

## IX  Looking Ahead    583

### CHAPTER 35: HAVING ANOTHER BABY: WHAT TO EXPECT THE SECOND TIME AROUND    585

Planning Another Baby    585
*How Long Should You Wait? • Is Your Body Ready?*
You're Pregnant Already    587
*How Will It Be Different? • Possible Problems*
Telling Your Other Children    589
RESOURCES    591

GLOSSARY    593
APPENDIX A: BODY MASS INDEX CHART    614
APPENDIX B: HEALTH QUESTIONS FOR YOUR FIRST PRENATAL VISIT    617
INDEX    623

# Preface

Pregnancy is a life-changing experience, and it's crucial that you have the best information available about this important life event. *Your Pregnancy and Childbirth: Month to Month* is written by experts at the American College of Obstetricians and Gynecologists (the College)—the preeminent authority on women's health. For more than 50 years, this distinguished group of more than 52,000 leading health care professionals has provided leadership and guidance on all aspects of women's health. *Your Pregnancy and Childbirth* draws on this vast body of knowledge and experience to provide a pregnancy resource that you can trust. Great effort has gone into this book to make sure that the information is presented in a reassuring, straightforward, and easy-to-understand way. We also advocate a collaborative approach to pregnancy care. We don't want to tell you what to do; instead, *Your Pregnancy and Childbirth* encourages you to be informed about your pregnancy and empowers you to work with your health care provider as an active participant and decision maker during one of the most fulfilling times in your life.

The book is designed with your concerns in mind. The first half of the book is a detailed, month-to-month prenatal guide that takes you through the developmental milestones that your baby will reach that month, the changes taking place in your body, advice on exercise and nutrition appropriate for that particular month, a description of the month's prenatal visit, and a discussion of issues and decisions that you may want to think about at that point in your pregnancy. The second half of the book includes sections on labor, delivery, and the postpartum period, from the first few days up to

6 weeks and beyond; nutrition and feeding your baby; common medical conditions that can affect pregnancy; and pregnancy complications. Up-to-date information is offered on the topics of most concern to pregnant women, such as weight gain during pregnancy, how to handle labor, breastfeeding tips for working moms, and the various tests that are used to monitor the baby's well-being. The book also addresses how to navigate the medical care side of pregnancy and gives suggestions about choosing a health care provider for your pregnancy (and for your baby) and planning your birth experience.

This revised sixth edition contains the latest breastfeeding recommendations published by the College in February 2016; new exercises to do during pregnancy; and updated resources. The following content was included in the original sixth edition in response to reader feedback:

- A separate chapter on cesarean delivery and vaginal birth after cesarean delivery that presents the latest thinking from the College about how to have a safe and successful vaginal birth after cesarean delivery (see Chapter 15, "Cesarean Delivery and Vaginal Birth After Cesarean Delivery")

- The most current information about your options for preconception and prenatal genetic testing and a timeline that clarifies when and how genetic testing is done and what the various tests can tell you about your risk of having a child with a genetic disorder (see Chapter 25, "Screening and Diagnostic Testing for Genetic Disorders")

- Answers to your questions about potential environmental hazards—what do we know about what causes birth defects, and are there any steps a mom-to-be can take to lower the risk of having a baby with a birth defect? (See Chapter 21, "Reducing Risks of Birth Defects")

- Straightforward discussion on pain relief during labor that includes medication options as well as options that do not involve medications (see Chapter 11, "Pain Relief During Childbirth")

One of the many things that sets this book apart from other pregnancy books is the use of illustrations throughout the text. The book includes a full-color section that shows fetal development and the changes that take place in the mother's body. Other illustrations show you various positions to use for breastfeeding, what genes are, and the events that happen during each stage of labor, to name a few.

Despite the many changes to this book over the years, what has not changed is the College's commitment to providing a complete, factual guide to pregnancy and childbirth. We sincerely hope that *Your Pregnancy and Childbirth* becomes a trusted resource and a comforting presence that you can turn to throughout your pregnancy.

# Part I
# Pregnancy Month by Month

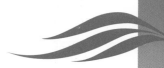

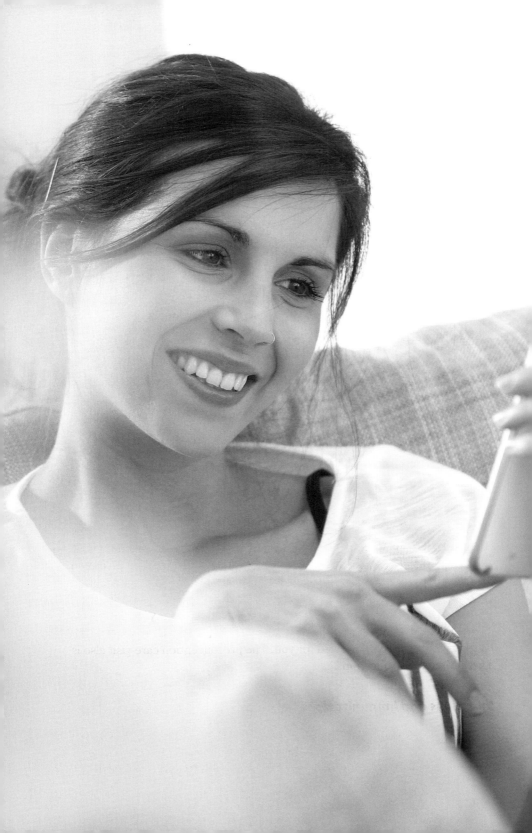

# Chapter 1

# Getting Ready for Pregnancy

Congratulations! You've decided to have a baby. Welcome to the first part of a journey that will transform your life forever. But before you try to get pregnant, there are some important things you need to do to give yourself the best chance of having a healthy pregnancy and a healthy baby.

By planning ahead and making needed changes before you become pregnant, you are more likely to be prepared. That is why ***preconception care*** is so important.

## The Preconception Visit

A preconception care checkup is the first step in planning a healthy pregnancy. The goal of this checkup is to find things that could affect your pregnancy. Identifying these factors before you become pregnant gives you time to make any necessary changes in your health. During a preconception care visit, your health care provider will ask about your diet and lifestyle, your medical and family history, medications you take, and any past pregnancies. You'll review your immunizations to be sure that you have all of the vaccines that are recommended for you. The preconception care visit also is a great time to ask questions.

### Infections and Immunizations

Certain infections during pregnancy can cause ***birth defects*** or illness in a ***fetus***. Some also can cause pregnancy complications. Many infections can be prevented with proper immunization. You should get all of the vaccines recommended for your age group before you try to get pregnant (see the "Resources" section in this chapter for more information).

Some vaccines, known as live attenuated vaccines, should not be given during pregnancy. These vaccines are made from live *viruses* that have been weakened so they do not cause disease. They pose a very small risk to the fetus if given during pregnancy. Live vaccines include the ***measles–mumps–rubella (MMR) vaccine***, the flu nasal spray vaccine (but not the flu shot), and the ***chickenpox (varicella)*** vaccine. If you need the MMR vaccine or the varicella vaccine, get these immunizations at least 1 month before becoming pregnant. During this time, keep using birth control. If you are planning a trip to a country where you might come into contact with diseases that are not common in the United States, you may need additional immunizations before you become pregnant.

Other vaccines contain inactivated or killed versions of the germs that cause disease. For example, the flu shot is made from killed flu viruses. The pneumonia vaccine is made with parts of the ***bacteria*** that cause pneumonia. Others, such as the ***tetanus toxoid, reduced diphtheria toxoid, and acellular pertussis (Tdap) vaccine***, are made with the inactivated ***toxin*** made by the disease-causing organisms. None of these things can cause the disease itself when given as a vaccine. These vaccines are safe to get during pregnancy.

It is especially important for pregnant women to get a flu shot. A pregnant woman who gets the flu is at high risk of serious complications for her and her fetus. The flu shot helps protect her and her unborn baby from the flu and its complications. Another important vaccine for pregnant women is the Tdap vaccine. It's now recommended that all pregnant women receive a dose of this vaccine during the third ***trimester*** of each pregnancy to protect their infants against ***pertussis*** (whooping cough).

Other infections that can be harmful during pregnancy are those passed on by sexual contact. These are called ***sexually transmitted infections (STIs)***. These infections can affect your ability to become pregnant and can infect and harm your baby if you already are pregnant. The following are the most common STIs:

- *Chlamydia*
- *Gonorrhea*
- *Genital herpes*
- *Human papillomavirus*
- *Trichomoniasis*
- *Hepatitis B virus*
- *Syphilis*
- *Human immunodeficiency virus (HIV)*

Using a male or female condom regularly will decrease your risk of getting an STI. A woman who is not using these forms of birth control (for instance, if she is trying to become pregnant) is at higher risk of getting an STI if she has sex with more than one partner or if her partner has sex with someone else. STIs such as herpes, HIV, and hepatitis B have no known cures. Many STIs have no symptoms in the early stages.

Getting tested for STIs before pregnancy gives you and your partner the opportunity to be treated promptly and avoid potential complications that many of these infections may cause during pregnancy. Preconception testing for the following STIs is recommended:

- You should be tested for chlamydia if you are aged 25 years or younger or if you are older than 25 years with risk factors (for example, you have a new sex partner or have multiple sex partners).

- You should be tested for gonorrhea if you are aged 25 years or younger and you have certain risk factors—you've had a previous case of gonorrhea or another STI, you have new or multiple sex partners and have not used condoms consistently, you live in an area where gonorrhea rates are high, or your lifestyle puts you at risk.

- All women should be tested for HIV. Knowing your HIV status allows you to make important decisions about whether to become pregnant and to familiarize yourself with treatment options that may make it less likely that you will pass the infection on to your baby.

### Your Family Health History

Some health conditions occur more often in certain families or ethnic groups. These conditions are called genetic or inherited disorders. If a close relative has one of these medical conditions, you or your baby could be at greater risk of having it, too. During your preconception visit, your health care provider may ask you to complete a family history questionnaire (see "Resources" in this chapter). This form helps identify whether you and your partner are at risk of having a child with an inherited medical condition. It asks for information such as your and your family's medical history, your race and ethnicity, and any problems that you had in past pregnancies.

In some situations, your health care provider may recommend that you and your partner undergo genetic counseling. A ***genetic counselor*** is a specially trained health care professional who can help couples understand their chances of having a baby with an inherited disorder. Genetic counseling involves taking a detailed family history and sometimes doing physical exams and lab tests.

## Preconception Carrier Screening

For some disorders, *carrier* screening may be available (see Table 1-1). This *screening test* allows you and your partner to find out if you are carriers of certain *genetic disorders*, even if you do not have any signs or symptoms. Carrier screening involves testing a sample of blood or saliva.

Carrier screening has traditionally been recommended for people who are at higher risk of certain genetic disorders because of their family history, ethnicity, or race:

- People of Eastern European Jewish descent (Ashkenazi Jews) are offered screening for **Tay–Sachs disease, Canavan disease, familial dysautonomia,** and **cystic fibrosis**. Individuals can ask about screening for other disorders. Carrier screening is available for **mucolipidosis IV, Niemann– Pick disease type A, Fanconi anemia group C, Bloom syndrome**, and **Gaucher disease.**

- Individuals of French Canadian and Cajun descent are offered screening for Tay–Sachs disease.

- Individuals of African, African American, and African Caribbean descent are offered carrier screening for **sickle cell disease** and for the blood disorders beta-**thalassemia** and alpha-thalassemia.

### Table 1-1 Some Genetic Disorders for Which Carrier Screening Tests Are Available*

| Disorder | What it Means | Who is at Risk? | Comments |
|---|---|---|---|
| Cystic fibrosis | Causes problems with digestion and breathing. Symptoms appear in childhood, sometimes right after birth. Some people have milder symptoms than others. Over time the problems tend to become worse and harder to treat. | White individuals of Northern European descent | Carrier screening is offered to all women. |
| Sickle cell disease | Red blood cells have a crescent or "sickle" shape rather than the normal doughnut shape. The sickle cells can get caught in the blood vessels and prevent oxygen from reaching organs and tissues. | African Americans or individuals of African descent, Greeks, Italians (particularly Sicilians), Turks, Arabs, Southern Iranians, and Asian Indians | Carrier screening should be offered to people of African, Mediterranean, and Southeast Asian descent. |

**Table 1-1 Some Genetic Disorders for Which Carrier Screening Tests Are Available,** *continued*

| Disorder | What it Means | Who is at Risk? | Comments |
|---|---|---|---|
| Thalassemias | Several types of blood disorders that cause anemia; some types are more severe than others and can cause early death if not treated. | Depends on the type of disorder; individuals who are of Mediterranean, African, and Southeast Asian descent | Carrier screening should be offered to people of Mediterranean, African, and Southeast Asian descent. |
| Tay–Sachs disease | Causes severe intellectual disability, blindness, and seizures. Symptoms first occur at about 6 months of age. Death usually occurs by age 5 years. | Individuals of Ashkenazi Jewish, French Canadian, and Cajun descent | Carrier screening is recommended for individuals of Ashkenazi Jewish, French Canadian, and Cajun descent. |
| Fragile X syndrome | Causes varying degrees of intellectual disability or learning disabilities and behavioral or emotional problems. Affects males and females, but males usually are affected more severely. | Males and females | Carrier screening is recommended for those who have a family history of fragile X-related disorders, unexplained intellectual disability or developmental delay, autism, or premature ovarian insufficiency (a condition in which the ovaries stop working before age 40 years). |
| Hemophilia | A disorder caused by the lack of a substance in the blood that helps it clot. Affected individuals are treated with factors that help the blood clot to help prevent excessive bleeding. | Males | Women with a family history of hemophilia may request carrier screening. |
| Spinal muscular atrophy (SMA) | Causes breakdown of the muscles and overall weakness; in one type (type 1), death occurs by age 2 years. | | Genetic counseling and carrier screening should be offered to those with a family history of SMA or SMA-like disease. |

*The tests that are available and who they should be offered to frequently change as a result of new research.*

- Individuals of Southeast Asian descent are offered screening for beta-thalassemia and alpha-thalassemia.

- Individuals of Mediterranean descent are offered screening for beta-thalassemia.

In recent years, it has become increasingly difficult to assign an individual to one particular ethnic group or race. Carrier testing based on ethnicity or race may not be as useful as it was in the past. For this reason, all individuals are offered carrier screening for cystic fibrosis, which is one of the most common genetic disorders. Many health care providers now offer **expanded carrier screening**, in which an individual is offered many different screening tests using a single sample. If you are interested in this type of screening, talk to your health care provider or genetic counselor. For more information about carrier screening, see Chapter 25, "Screening and Diagnostic Testing for Genetic Disorders."

You can have carrier screening before pregnancy or during pregnancy. If you had carrier testing in a previous pregnancy, testing does not have to be repeated. If it is done before pregnancy, you have a broader range of options and more time to make decisions. You may decide not to have children, or you may decide to adopt. You may want to explore the option of **assisted reproductive technology**. You also can find out whether prenatal genetic testing is available for the condition you're concerned about. Once you are pregnant, there are **diagnostic tests** that can tell whether a fetus has certain genetic disorders. It usually takes a long time to get the results of these tests. The pregnancy may be fairly advanced before the results are known. Because of this, your options are more limited.

## Preexisting Health Conditions

Your health care provider will ask about the diseases that you have had in the past and any chronic (long-lasting) conditions that you may have now. Some medical conditions—such as **diabetes mellitus**, **high blood pressure**, **depression**, and **seizure disorders**—can cause problems during pregnancy. Some may increase the risk of problems for the baby, such as birth defects. Others may increase the risk of health problems for you. Having one of these conditions does not mean that you cannot have a healthy pregnancy or baby. However, proper management before pregnancy may reduce pregnancy-related risks.

If you have a medical condition, your health care provider will discuss with you the changes that you may need to make in order to bring your condition under control before you try to get pregnant. For example, women with diabetes usually are advised to keep their **glucose** levels in the normal range for some time before they become pregnant (if it is not already in the normal range). The first 8 weeks of pregnancy is the time when major fetal organ systems develop. If you are having trouble with glucose control, it is best to make the necessary changes in your medication, diet, and exercise program to bring your levels into the healthy range before you become pregnant.

Even if a health problem is well managed, the demands of pregnancy can cause it to worsen. To keep such conditions in check, you may need to make lifestyle changes, see your health care provider more often, or get other special care during pregnancy.

## Medications and Supplements

Some medications, including over-the-counter medications and herbal supplements, can be harmful to a fetus and should not be taken while you are pregnant. For example, *isotretinoin* is a prescription medication used to treat severe acne. It can cause severe birth defects if used during pregnancy. Even common nutritional supplements could be harmful. Some multivitamin supplements contain high levels of vitamin A, which has been shown to cause severe birth defects if taken in large doses during pregnancy. If you are taking two or three multivitamin supplements daily, you could potentially expose your fetus to harmful levels of vitamin A.

For other medications, there may not be enough information available to determine whether they are harmful during pregnancy. Studies of a drug may have been performed only on animals or studies may be incomplete.

The preconception period is the ideal time to evaluate all of the medications, alternative remedies (such as herbal supplements), and vitamin supplements that you take with your health care provider to determine their safety during pregnancy. Tell your health care provider about all of the medications you are taking. Better yet, take the bottles along with you to your preconception care checkup. You may need to stop using a certain medication or switch to another before you try to get pregnant. Do not stop taking a prescription medication, however, until you have talked with your health care provider. Although some medications may increase the risk of birth defects, the benefits of continuing to take the medication during pregnancy may outweigh the risks to your baby.

## Past Pregnancies

During your preconception care checkup, your health care provider will review your obstetric history. You will be asked about any previous pregnancies and any problems you have had. Some problems may increase the risk of having the same problem in a later pregnancy. These problems include **pre-term** birth, high blood pressure, **preeclampsia**, and **gestational diabetes mellitus**. Getting proper care before and during pregnancy may decrease the chances of these problems happening again.

Women who have had a **miscarriage** or **stillbirth** often fear that it will happen again. Most women who experience a pregnancy loss go on to have normal pregnancies and healthy babies. It is important, however, to allow enough time for physical and emotional healing before trying to get pregnant again.

## A Healthy Lifestyle

The weeks and months before you become pregnant are the best time to take a close look at your lifestyle and take any necessary steps to be healthier. These steps include eating right, getting regular exercise, reaching and maintaining a healthy weight, quitting the use of unhealthy substances, and keeping your environment safe.

### Eat Right

A healthy diet is important at all times in your life, but it is especially so when you are preparing to become pregnant and during your pregnancy. The food you eat is the main source of **nutrients** and energy for you and your baby. As the baby grows and places new demands on your body, you will need more **calories** and nutrients. But simply doubling up on the amount that you eat—or "eating for two"—is no longer recommended as a healthy nutritional strategy for pregnancy. Experts now stress the importance of eating healthy, nutrient-rich foods; gaining an appropriate amount of weight; and staying active to maximize your chances of having a healthy pregnancy and a healthy baby. Putting these things into practice before you become pregnant ensures that you and your baby will get the best possible start.

Before your preconception visit, you may want to think about any special dietary needs that you have and make a note to discuss them with your health care provider. Some of the questions you can ask yourself include the following:

- Are you a vegetarian? If so, do you eat dairy products?
- Do you have any food allergies?
- Do you have trouble digesting milk and other dairy products?

* Do you ever fast?
* Do you have celiac disease?

If you are new to eating in a healthy way, or if you just want help planning a healthy diet, a great place to start is the U.S. Department of Agriculture's "MyPlate" food-planning guide at www.choosemyplate.gov. The MyPlate web site helps everyone from dieters to children to pregnant women learn how to make healthy food choices at every meal. MyPlate makes it easy to remember the key principles of a healthy diet:

* Make one half of your plate fruits and vegetables. The other half should be grains and protein foods.

* Vary your proteins. Protein foods include meat, fish, beans and peas, nuts and seeds, and eggs.

* Eat a small amount of dairy foods, such as milk, cheese, or yogurt, at each meal. Drink 1% milk instead of full-fat milk.

* Try to make at least one half of the grains you eat whole grains. Whole grains contain the entire grain kernel, as opposed to refined grains, which have been processed to remove certain parts that provide *dietary fiber*. Whole-grain foods include brown rice, bulgur, and oatmeal. Whole grains also are used as ingredients in breads and pastas. Read the labels on these foods carefully.

* Limit your intake of fats, oils, sugars, and salty foods.

## Get Regular Exercise

Good health at any time in your life involves getting plenty of exercise—and that includes during pregnancy. Experts recommend that most pregnant women get at least 30 minutes of moderate exercise on most, if not all, days of the week. The type and amount of exercise that you can do safely during pregnancy depends on your health and how active you were before you were pregnant.

It is best to have an exercise routine in place before getting pregnant. If you are just starting out, good exercises to begin with are those you probably have done before—walking, swimming, or bicycling. Brisk walking is an easy and inexpensive way to be physically active. It also is a good way to lose weight. If you are not used to a lot of exercise, discuss safety guidelines with your health care provider ahead of time and take it slow at first.

## Take Folic Acid

Taking a *folic acid* (also known as folate) supplement is crucial before and during pregnancy. Research confirms that getting 400 micrograms (0.4 mg) of this B vitamin for at least 1 month before pregnancy and during pregnancy decreases the risk of having a baby with birth defects of the brain and spine called **neural tube defects**. Although folic acid is found in many foods and is added to breads, pastas, and cereals, it may be difficult to get the recommended 400 micrograms per day from food alone. For this reason, women capable of becoming pregnant should take a supplement containing 400 micrograms of folic acid every day. You can get the recommended amount in a folic acid supplement or by taking a prenatal vitamin that contains the recommended amount.

## Reach and Maintain a Healthy Weight

To stay healthy, you should keep your weight at the level that is best for your height. Your **body mass index (BMI)** is a number calculated from height and weight that is used to determine whether you are underweight, normal weight, overweight, or obese. You can find out your BMI by using an online calculator at web sites such as www.nhlbi.nih.gov/health/educational/lose_wt/BMI/ or use the BMI chart provided in Appendix A.

Having a BMI of less than 18.5 is underweight; 18.5–24.9 is normal; and 25–29.9 is overweight. A person with a BMI of 30 or higher is obese. Being underweight or overweight can cause problems during pregnancy, so the goal is to reach the normal range.

If you are underweight, you should try to gain weight by taking in more calories each day than you use up. Add healthy high-calorie snacks to your daily meal plan. Some good choices are nuts, granola bars, meal replacement shakes, fruit smoothies, and yogurt.

Overweight and obese women should lose weight by cutting back on the number of daily calories they consume and becoming more physically active. Two easy ways to cut calories are to avoid sugary drinks and foods that are high in fat and to pay attention to the amount of food you eat. Portion control is key.

Exercise burns calories and helps you lose weight. Most people who have lost weight and kept it off get 60–90 minutes of moderate-intensity activity on most days of the week. A moderate-intensity activity is one in which you can carry on a conversation, but you cannot sing. Brisk walking and raking leaves are examples of moderate-intensity activities. You may be able to reduce the minutes you exercise by adding vigorous activity. A vigorous activity is one that raises your heart rate and that makes it difficult to talk. Examples are jogging or running, jumping rope, or swimming laps. You do not have to do all of the recommended minutes at once. For instance, you can do 20–30 minutes of exercise three times a day.

Make sure you get your health care provider's approval before starting an exercise program if you are overweight or obese. It also may be a good idea to consult a physical trainer at your local gym or health club for help with an exercise program.

For some people, it may be hard to lose weight through diet and exercise alone. If you have a BMI of 30 or greater, or a BMI of at least 27 with certain medical conditions, such as diabetes or heart disease, medications may be able to help you lose weight. These medications should be combined with a healthy eating plan and regular physical activity.

**Bariatric surgery**, or weight-loss surgery, may be an option for people who are very obese (a BMI of 40 or greater) or who have a BMI between 35 and 39 and also have major health problems caused by **obesity**. Bariatric surgery can result in significant weight loss. This may decrease the risk of the serious health problems associated with obesity. See Chapter 20, "Obesity and Eating Disorders," for more information about this option.

### Quit Using Unhealthy Substances

Smoking, drinking alcohol, and using other unhealthy substances during pregnancy can have serious, long-lasting effects for your baby, such as birth defects, a lower-than-average birth weight, and premature birth. Substance abuse includes using illegal drugs (such as heroin, cocaine, methamphetamine, and marijuana) as well as using prescription medications, such as oxycodone, for nonmedical reasons.

When should you stop using these substances? It is best to quit smoking completely before pregnancy. Experts recommend that you completely avoid alcohol while trying to become pregnant and throughout your pregnancy. You should stop using other harmful substances before you become pregnant as well. If you need help stopping these behaviors, tell your health care provider. He or she often can suggest ways to get through the early stages or put you in touch with addiction treatment counselors and programs. For quitting smoking, the National Cancer Institute's Smoking Quitline (1-877-44U-QUIT or 1-877-448-7848) is a great place to start your journey to being a nonsmoker.

Your partner also should give up these harmful substances. Many studies have shown that smoking and using drugs also can lower his fertility and damage his **sperm** (see box "Tips for Future Dads"). Living with someone who smokes means that you are likely to breathe in harmful amounts of secondhand smoke. Secondhand smoke contains chemicals that are harmful to both your health and that of your growing baby. Being around secondhand smoke while you are pregnant has been linked to a higher risk of **sudden infant death syndrome** and to having a smaller-than-average baby. If your partner or coworkers are not willing to quit, ask them to smoke outside, and do not allow anyone to smoke in your car or your home.

## Tips for Future Dads

When a couple decides to have a baby, a lot of attention is given to the mother-to-be. The role of the future father, however, is just as important. Male partners who are preparing to enter fatherhood should be aware of a few things to make sure they are as healthy as possible for their new responsibilities:

- Get healthier, too—Join your partner in eating healthier and exercising every day. For instance, she'll have to cut back on caffeine and junk food, so make it easier on her by cutting back as well.

- STIs—Get tested and treated for any STIs. Continue to protect yourself and your partner from STIs when she becomes pregnant. While a woman is pregnant, she and the unborn baby have no protection against these diseases. If she becomes infected with an STI while pregnant, the results could be very serious, even life threatening, for her and the baby.

- Give up smoking and substance use—Cigarette smoking and alcohol and illegal drug use can decrease the number of sperm a man produces (your sperm count) and how well the sperm moves. Secondhand smoke is also dangerous for pregnant women.

- Check your fertility—For about 40% of couples that have difficulty getting pregnant, the problem can be traced to male problems, such as low sperm count. Male infertility has many possible causes, including disease, certain medications, and steroid use. If you have difficulty getting pregnant, visit a urologist for a fertility test.

- Be supportive—Trying to get pregnant or going through a pregnancy can be an emotional rollercoaster. When the time comes, try to make it to at least some of your partner's many **prenatal care** appointments, and ask questions. Let her know you're enjoying seeing her belly grow. Be a strong shoulder to lean on if she has difficult days.

## Keep Your Environment Safe

Chemicals are all around us—in the air, water, soil, the food we eat, and products we use. Before you become pregnant and during your pregnancy, you may be exposed to these agents at work, at home, or in your community.

A few chemicals are known to have harmful effects on a developing fetus. The effects of many chemicals on pregnancy are not known. Some substances found in the home or the workplace may make it harder for you to get pregnant.

Take a close look at your home and workplace. Women who work in farming, factories, dry cleaners, electronics, or printing or who have hobbies such as painting or pottery glazing should be sure to talk about possible harmful agents with their health care providers.

## Getting Pregnant

Knowing how pregnancy happens will help you find out when you are most fertile—that is, when you are most likely to get pregnant. To have a better chance of getting pregnant, sex has to happen around the time of *ovulation*.

## The Menstrual Cycle

The changes that occur during the menstrual cycle are caused by changing levels of *hormones* called *estrogen* and *progesterone*. Each month, hormones signal your *uterus* to build up a blood-rich lining called the *endometrium*. These hormones also send a signal to an *egg* to ripen in a follicle—tiny, fluid-filled clusters of *cells* in your *ovaries*. When the egg is ready, it is released from the ovary and moves into a *fallopian tube*, one of a pair of tubes that connects the ovaries to the uterus. This process is called ovulation. Signs that you may be ovulating include a cramp in your lower abdomen or back. You also may notice some breast tenderness, an increase in vaginal discharge, or an increase in sexual desire around the time an egg is released.

The average menstrual cycle lasts about 28 days, counting from the first day of one period (day 1) to the first day of the next. Cycles ranging from as few as 21 days to as many as 35 days are normal.

In an average 28-day menstrual cycle, ovulation occurs on day 14. The number of days from ovulation to the start of the menstrual period is the most consistent time period in a menstrual cycle. This time period is 14 days in a menstrual cycle of 28 days.

If pregnancy does not occur, your body absorbs the egg and the hormone levels decrease. This decrease signals the lining of the uterus to shed. The shedding is your monthly menstrual period.

## The Menstrual Cycle

### Day 1

The first day of your menstrual period is considered day 1 of your menstrual cycle.

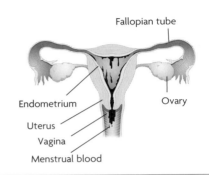

Fallopian tube

Endometrium

Ovary

Uterus

Vagina

Menstrual blood

### Day 5

Estrogen levels start to increase. Estrogen causes the endometrium (the lining of the uterus) to grow and thicken.

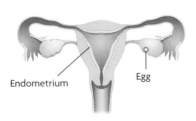

Endometrium

Egg

### Day 14

An egg is released from the ovary and moves into one of the two fallopian tubes (ovulation). After ovulation, progesterone levels begin to increase, while estrogen levels decrease.

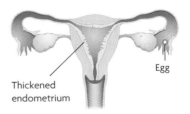

Thickened endometrium

Egg

### Day 28

If the egg is not fertilized, progesterone and estrogen levels decrease, and the endometrium is shed during menstruation.

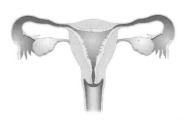

## When Are You Most Fertile?

For pregnancy to occur, sperm must be present in the fallopian tubes and must join with an egg. When a man climaxes during sex and ejaculates, millions of sperm are deposited in a woman's **vagina**. After ejaculation, the sperm move through the **cervix** into the uterus and fallopian tubes. Sperm can live inside a woman's body for 3 days and sometimes up to 5 days. An egg's life span is much shorter—just 12–24 hours. Therefore, pregnancy can occur if an egg is already present in the fallopian tubes when you have sex, or it can occur if you ovulate within a day or two after you have sex. This means that you are fertile anywhere from 5 days before ovulation until 1 day after ovulation.

## Fertility Awareness

There is no foolproof way to calculate your fertile days. There are, however, a number of methods that can help you predict when these days occur in your menstrual cycle. A variety of smart phone apps also are available to help you keep track of your fertility. Many of these apps incorporate one or more of the fertility awareness-based methods discussed below.

**Chart your cycle.** An easy way to spot your fertile days is to keep a menstrual calendar to figure out how long your cycles tend to last. If your cycle is between

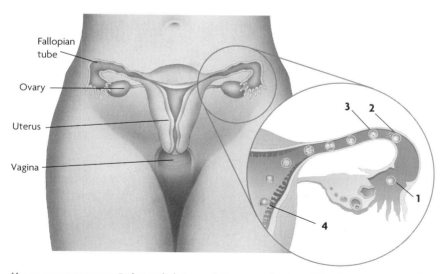

**How pregnancy occurs.** Each month during ovulation, an egg is released (1) and moves into one of the fallopian tubes. If a woman has sex around this time, and an egg and sperm meet in the fallopian tube (2), the two may join. If they join (3), the fertilized egg then moves through the fallopian tube into the uterus and attaches there to grow during pregnancy (4).

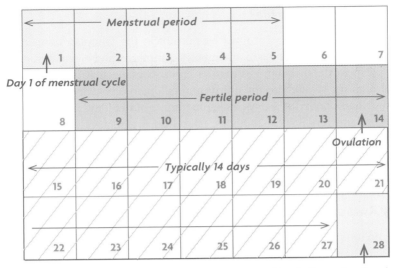

**Fertility and ovulation.** Ovulation typically occurs 11–14 days before the start of the next menstrual cycle (day 1 of the next menstrual period). In an average 28-day menstrual cycle, ovulation occurs on day 14. The fertile period is considered to be 2–3 days before ovulation until 12–24 hours after ovulation.

26 days and 32 days long, day 8 through day 19 are the days when you are most likely to become pregnant. To promote pregnancy, you should try to have intercourse between day 8 and day 19 either every day or every other day.

**Use an ovulation predictor kit.** These are sold over the counter at drug stores or pharmacies and test the level of *luteinizing hormone* in your urine. When your levels rise, it means that one of your ovaries is about to release an egg.

**Monitor your cervical mucus.** Noticing changes in your cervical mucus can help you recognize when ovulation nears. This method involves checking the mucus at the opening of the vagina each time you urinate and assessing it for changes starting with the first day after menstrual bleeding has stopped.

Just before ovulation, the amount of mucus made by the cervix increases, and the mucus becomes thin and slippery. The last day this thin and slippery mucus is present is called the Peak Day. Ovulation occurs within 24 to 48 hours of the Peak Day. Just after ovulation, the amount of mucus decreases, and it becomes thicker and less noticeable. To promote pregnancy, you should time intercourse to occur every day or every other day when cervical mucus is present.

## Keeping a Menstrual Calendar

When you are thinking of becoming pregnant, you may want to keep track of your menstrual cycle. By charting your menstrual periods on a calendar for a few months, you can spot patterns in your cycle (how many days your menstrual periods last, for instance, and whether your cycle is typically 25 days or 30 days long). You also may be able to pinpoint the days that you are most fertile. To use the calendar, simply circle the days that you menstruate each month. If you can, chart your cycle for a few months and bring the calendar along with you to your preconception care checkup. Smartphone apps also are available to help you chart your cycle.

| | | | | | | | | | | | | | | | | | | | | | | | | | | | | | | |
|---|---|---|---|---|---|---|---|---|---|---|---|---|---|---|---|---|---|---|---|---|---|---|---|---|---|---|---|---|---|---|
| Jan. | 1 | 2 | 3 | 4 | 5 | 6 | 7 | 8 | 9 | 10 | 11 | 12 | 13 | 14 | 15 | 16 | 17 | 18 | 19 | 20 | 21 | 22 | 23 | 24 | 25 | 26 | 27 | 28 | 29 | 30 | 31 |
| Feb. | 1 | 2 | 3 | 4 | 5 | 6 | 7 | 8 | 9 | 10 | 11 | 12 | 13 | 14 | 15 | 16 | 17 | 18 | 19 | 20 | 21 | 22 | 23 | 24 | 25 | 26 | 27 | 28 | 29 | | |
| March | 1 | 2 | 3 | 4 | 5 | 6 | 7 | 8 | 9 | 10 | 11 | 12 | 13 | 14 | 15 | 16 | 17 | 18 | 19 | 20 | 21 | 22 | 23 | 24 | 25 | 26 | 27 | 28 | 29 | 30 | 31 |
| April | 1 | 2 | 3 | 4 | 5 | 6 | 7 | 8 | 9 | 10 | 11 | 12 | 13 | 14 | 15 | 16 | 17 | 18 | 19 | 20 | 21 | 22 | 23 | 24 | 25 | 26 | 27 | 28 | 29 | 30 | |
| May | 1 | 2 | 3 | 4 | 5 | 6 | 7 | 8 | 9 | 10 | 11 | 12 | 13 | 14 | 15 | 16 | 17 | 18 | 19 | 20 | 21 | 22 | 23 | 24 | 25 | 26 | 27 | 28 | 29 | 30 | 31 |
| June | 1 | 2 | 3 | 4 | 5 | 6 | 7 | 8 | 9 | 10 | 11 | 12 | 13 | 14 | 15 | 16 | 17 | 18 | 19 | 20 | 21 | 22 | 23 | 24 | 25 | 26 | 27 | 28 | 29 | 30 | |
| July | 1 | 2 | 3 | 4 | 5 | 6 | 7 | 8 | 9 | 10 | 11 | 12 | 13 | 14 | 15 | 16 | 17 | 18 | 19 | 20 | 21 | 22 | 23 | 24 | 25 | 26 | 27 | 28 | 29 | 30 | 31 |
| Aug. | 1 | 2 | 3 | 4 | 5 | 6 | 7 | 8 | 9 | 10 | 11 | 12 | 13 | 14 | 15 | 16 | 17 | 18 | 19 | 20 | 21 | 22 | 23 | 24 | 25 | 26 | 27 | 28 | 29 | 30 | 31 |
| Sept. | 1 | 2 | 3 | 4 | 5 | 6 | 7 | 8 | 9 | 10 | 11 | 12 | 13 | 14 | 15 | 16 | 17 | 18 | 19 | 20 | 21 | 22 | 23 | 24 | 25 | 26 | 27 | 28 | 29 | 30 | |
| Oct. | 1 | 2 | 3 | 4 | 5 | 6 | 7 | 8 | 9 | 10 | 11 | 12 | 13 | 14 | 15 | 16 | 17 | 18 | 19 | 20 | 21 | 22 | 23 | 24 | 25 | 26 | 27 | 28 | 29 | 30 | 31 |
| Nov. | 1 | 2 | 3 | 4 | 5 | 6 | 7 | 8 | 9 | 10 | 11 | 12 | 13 | 14 | 15 | 16 | 17 | 18 | 19 | 20 | 21 | 22 | 23 | 24 | 25 | 26 | 27 | 28 | 29 | 30 | |
| Dec. | 1 | 2 | 3 | 4 | 5 | 6 | 7 | 8 | 9 | 10 | 11 | 12 | 13 | 14 | 15 | 16 | 17 | 18 | 19 | 20 | 21 | 22 | 23 | 24 | 25 | 26 | 27 | 28 | 29 | 30 | 31 |

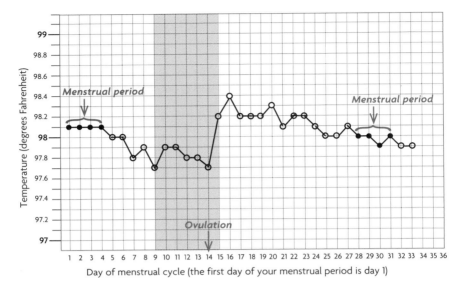

**Sample basal body temperature chart.** Keeping a basal body temperature chart for several months may help you predict when you will ovulate. Body temperature rises 24–48 hours after ovulation and stays high for at least 3 days.

**Track your temperature.** Most women's **basal body temperature** increases slightly—about one half of a degree—after they ovulate. To use this method, take your temperature at the same time every morning before you get out of bed. You'll need a thermometer that measures by tenths of degrees. Chart the temperature on a graph that also shows the days you menstruate. Your temperature will go up 24–48 hours after you ovulate.

By itself, tracking your temperature is not a good way to time intercourse to promote pregnancy. It shows only when ovulation has occurred, not when it is going to occur. Combining methods may work best. For example, a cervical mucus method can be used to find out when your fertile time begins, and the temperature method can be used to find out when your fertile time ends.

## Stopping Birth Control

You can start trying to conceive right after stopping hormonal birth control. There is no increased risk of pregnancy problems if you become pregnant soon after stopping these methods. With most hormonal methods, such as birth control pills, the patch, and the hormonal **intrauterine device (IUD)**, ovulation can occur within 2 weeks of stopping. This also is true for the copper IUD. If you use the birth control injection, however, it may take up to 10 months or longer to resume normal ovulation.

If you become pregnant while using a hormonal birth control method, do not worry. It does not increase the risk of birth defects as once believed. However, once you know that you are pregnant, you should stop using your method immediately. Rarely, pregnancy may occur with the IUD. If it does, the IUD should be removed if it is possible to do so without surgery.

# RESOURCES

The following resources offer more information about some of the topics discussed in this chapter:

**Immunization & Pregnancy**
Centers for Disease Control and Prevention (CDC)
www.cdc.gov/vaccines/pubs/downloads/f_preg_chart.pdf
*Easy-to-read chart that shows the immunizations that you should have before, during, and after pregnancy.*

**Immunization for Women: Pregnancy**
Immunization for Women
www.immunizationforwomen.org/patients/Pregnancy/pregnancy.php
*Page devoted to immunizations and women's health that details the immunizations that women need before and during pregnancy.*

**Know Your Family Health History**
Talk Health History Campaign
www.talkhealthhistory.org
*Offers tools and resources on collecting and sharing family health history with health care providers and relatives.*

**My Family Health Portrait Tool**
National Institutes of Health/Department of Health and Human Services
https://familyhistory.hhs.gov/FHH/html/index.html
*Helps you create a personalized family health history report. Generates a drawing of your family tree and a health history chart based on the information you enter.*

**Preconception Health and Health Care**
Centers for Disease Control and Prevention (CDC)
www.cdc.gov/preconception
*Trusted site with tips for women who are planning a pregnancy and men who will become future fathers. Also includes information on making a "reproductive life plan"—a worksheet for how to achieve the goals for having or not having children.*

The following full-color illustrations show fetal development and the changes that occur in a woman's body throughout pregnancy. Seeing them all together gives an idea of how a woman's body adjusts to accommodate the growth of a baby. These illustrations also are found in each month-to-month chapter.

**Mother and baby: Weeks 1–8.**

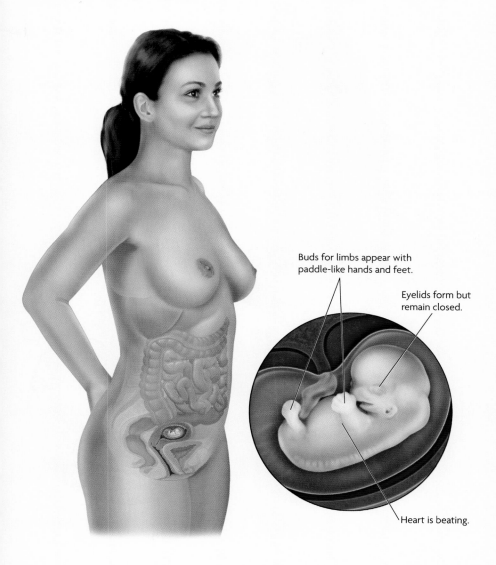

Buds for limbs appear with paddle-like hands and feet.

Eyelids form but remain closed.

Heart is beating.

The first 8 weeks of pregnancy are a time of rapid growth for your baby. At the end of 8 weeks, most of the organ systems have begun to form. The baby is about ½ inch long and weighs about ¼ ounce.

## Mother and baby: Weeks 9–12.

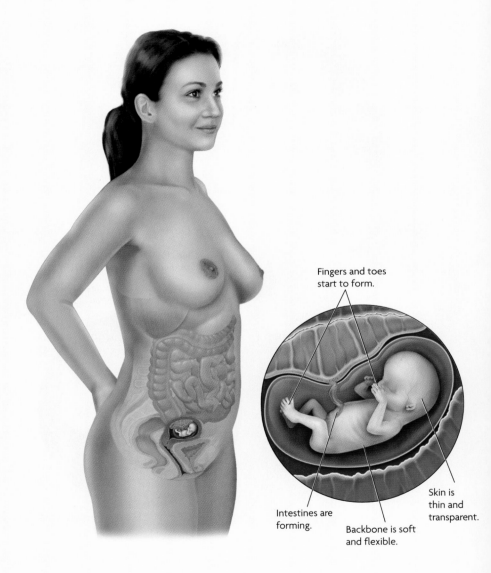

Fingers and toes start to form.

Skin is thin and transparent.

Intestines are forming.

Backbone is soft and flexible.

At this point, the baby weighs about ½ ounce and is about 2 inches long.

**Mother and baby: Weeks 13–16.**

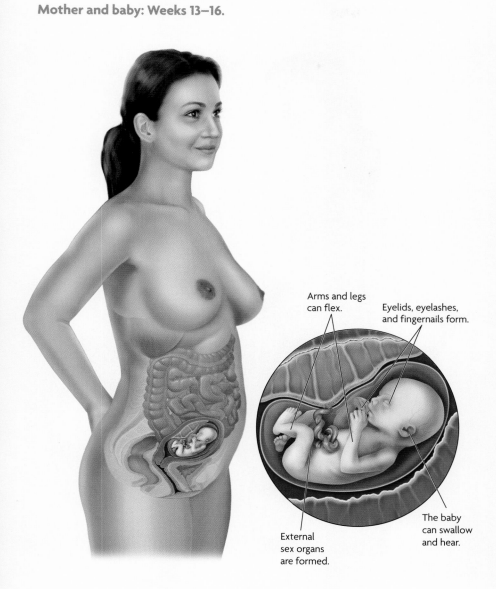

Arms and legs can flex.

Eyelids, eyelashes, and fingernails form.

External sex organs are formed.

The baby can swallow and hear.

The baby weighs about 5 ounces and is now about 5 inches long.

## Mother and baby: Weeks 17–20.

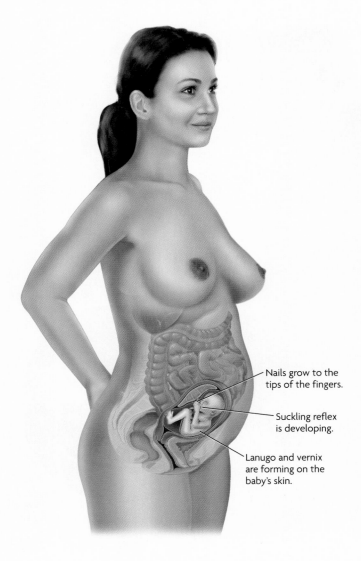

Nails grow to the tips of the fingers.

Suckling reflex is developing.

Lanugo and vernix are forming on the baby's skin.

The baby may weigh close to 1 pound and is about 10 inches long. You may be able to feel your baby move this month.

**Mother and baby: Weeks 21–24.**

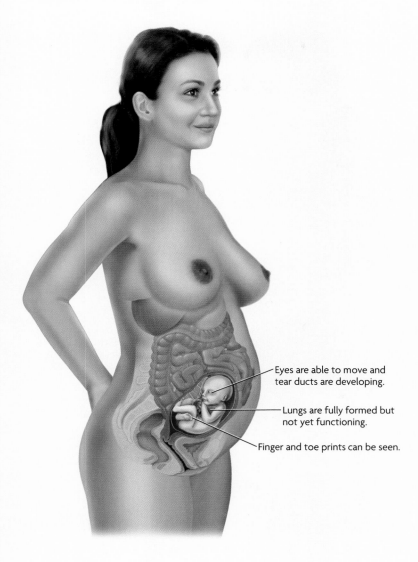

Eyes are able to move and tear ducts are developing.

Lungs are fully formed but not yet functioning.

Finger and toe prints can be seen.

By the end of this month, the baby weighs just more than 1 pound and is almost 12 inches long.

## Mother and baby: Weeks 25–28.

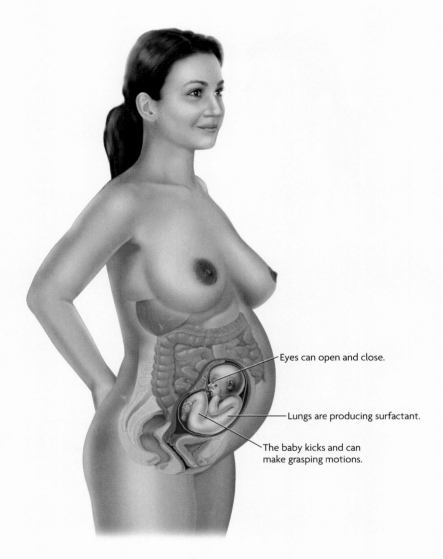

Eyes can open and close.

Lungs are producing surfactant.

The baby kicks and can make grasping motions.

By the end of this month, the baby weighs approximately 2 ½ pounds and is about 14 inches long.

## Mother and baby: Weeks 29–32.

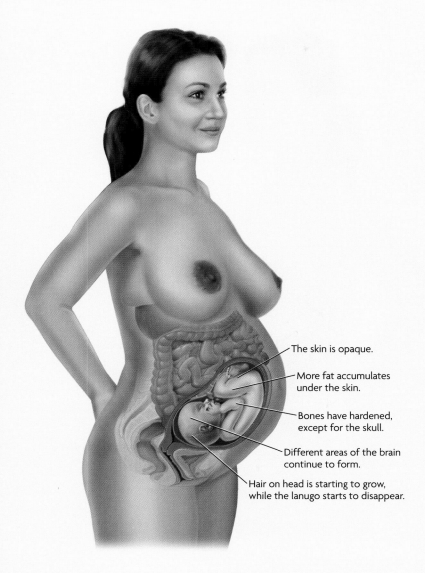

The skin is opaque.

More fat accumulates under the skin.

Bones have hardened, except for the skull.

Different areas of the brain continue to form.

Hair on head is starting to grow, while the lanugo starts to disappear.

By the end of this month, the baby weighs between 4½ pounds and 5 pounds and is about 18 inches long.

## Mother and baby: Weeks 33–36.

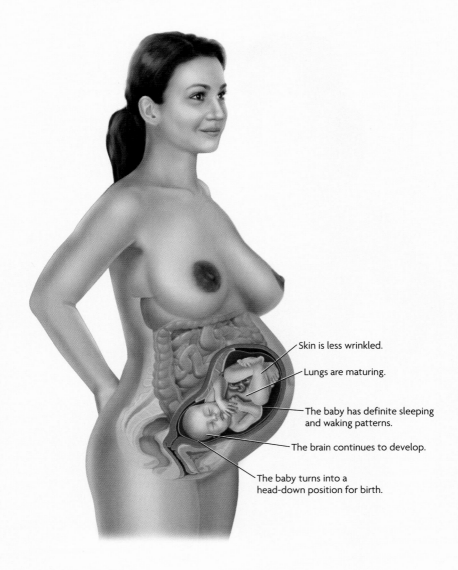

Skin is less wrinkled.

Lungs are maturing.

The baby has definite sleeping and waking patterns.

The brain continues to develop.

The baby turns into a head-down position for birth.

By the end of this month, the baby weighs 6–7 pounds and is almost 20 inches long.

## Mother and baby: Weeks 37–40.

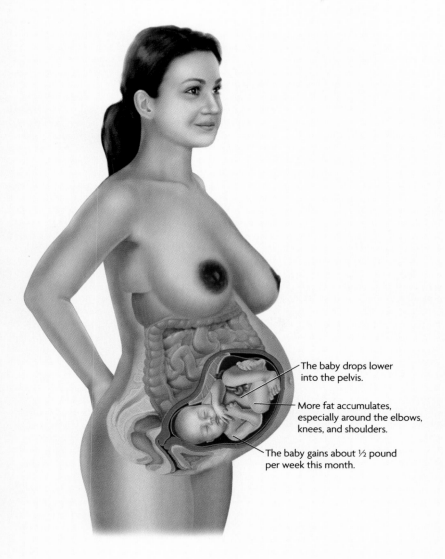

The baby drops lower into the pelvis.

More fat accumulates, especially around the elbows, knees, and shoulders.

The baby gains about ½ pound per week this month.

Most babies are now about 7½ pounds and are 20 inches long. The baby is now ready to be born.

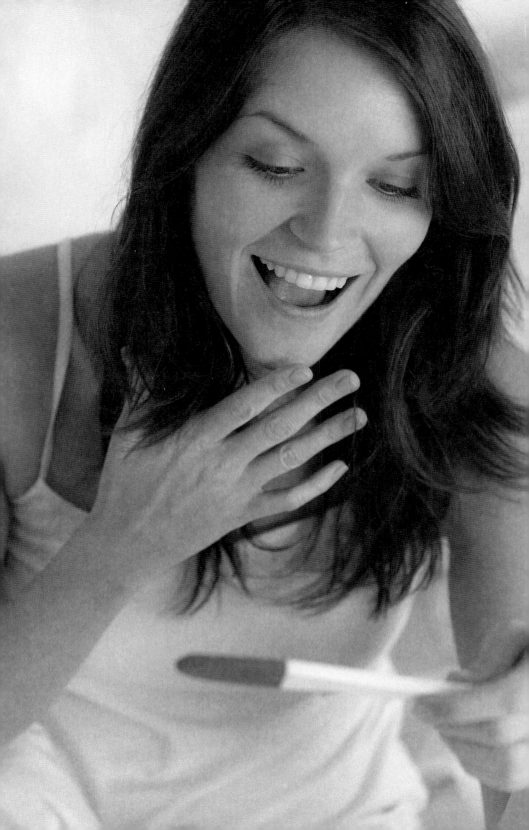

# Chapter 2

# Months 1 and 2

### (Weeks 1–8)

---

## YOUR GROWING BABY

### Week 1

**Fertilization,** the union of an **egg** and a **sperm**, is the first step in a complex series of events that lead to pregnancy. When the egg and sperm unite, they form a single **cell** called a zygote. Fertilization takes place in the woman's **fallopian tube**. After fertilization, the zygote divides, forming two cells. These cells then divide, forming four cells, and then eight cells, and so on. At the same time, the mass of dividing cells moves down the fallopian tube toward the **uterus**.

### Week 2

Approximately 8–9 days after fertilization, the rapidly dividing cluster of cells, now called a **blastocyst**, enters the uterus. The blastocyst has started to make an important pregnancy **hormone** called **human chorionic gonadotropin (hCG)**. The **endometrium**, or uterine lining, has prepared itself for potential pregnancy. The blastocyst burrows deep into the uterine lining in a process called implantation.

### Week 3

Once the blastocyst has implanted in the uterine lining, the levels of hCG produced by the blastocyst rapidly increase. The hCG hormone signals your **ovaries** to stop releasing eggs and triggers your body to produce more of the hormones **estrogen** and **progesterone**. The increased levels of these hormones stop your menstrual period and start the growth of the **placenta**.

33

## Week 4

Some of the cells of the blastocyst develop into the **embryo**, and other cells start to form the placenta. Once fully formed, the placenta functions as the life support system for the baby. It also provides a pathway for harmful substances that may enter your body, such as drugs and **viruses**, to reach the baby. As the placenta takes shape, small finger-like projections grow out of it. In these projections, called **chorionic villi**, blood vessels form. The tips of these vessels burrow into the uterine wall. **Oxygen**, **nutrients**, and hormones from the pregnant woman's blood supply are transferred across these blood vessels to reach the baby, and waste products from the baby are transferred to the woman for removal. On the side of the placenta nearest the baby, the **umbilical cord** forms. This tube-like structure is attached to the baby in the center of the belly. After birth, this cord is cut. The remnants become the baby's navel.

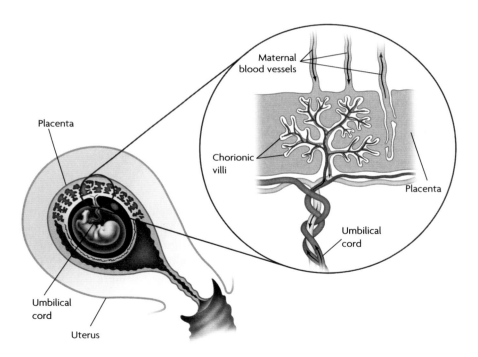

**The placenta.** The placenta connects the baby to the wall of the uterus. Finger-like projections, called chorionic villi, contain blood vessels that allow the exchange of nutrients, oxygen, and waste products between the mother's blood supply and the developing baby. The umbilical cord bridges the connection between the mother's bloodstream and the baby and is attached to the baby in the center of the belly.

## Week 5

The neural tube, from which the brain, spinal cord, and backbone will form, is completing its development. Balls of cells called somites start to appear along the neural tube. They eventually will develop into the bones of the spine and muscles of the back. Other major organs, such as the heart and lungs, are developing during this period. Although the heart is not yet fully formed, it has started to beat. Also present are the **amniotic sac**, which contains the baby during the pregnancy, and **amniotic fluid**, which cushions the baby as it grows.

At this stage, the baby looks like a curled tube and is about ¼ of an inch long—about the size of a pumpkin seed. Arm and leg buds appear. The long tube that will become your baby's digestive tract has taken shape.

## Week 6

Your baby's heart is beating approximately 105 times per minute, and it is possible to see and hear the heart beating if you have an **ultrasound exam**. The nose, mouth, and ears are beginning to form, and webbed fingers and toes are poking out from your baby's hands and feet. The inner ear begins to develop.

## Week 7

Bones are forming but won't begin to harden for a few weeks. Fingers and toes are present. Your baby's external genitals are starting to develop. Eyelids form but remain closed.

## Week 8

At 8 weeks, your baby is about ½ of an inch long. By the end of the second month, all major organs and body systems have begun to develop. Breathing tubes extend from the throat to the developing lungs. In the brain, nerve cells are branching out to connect with one another. Up until the eighth week of development, the baby is known as an embryo. This week marks the end of the embryonic phase of development. After the end of week 8, the baby is called a **fetus**.

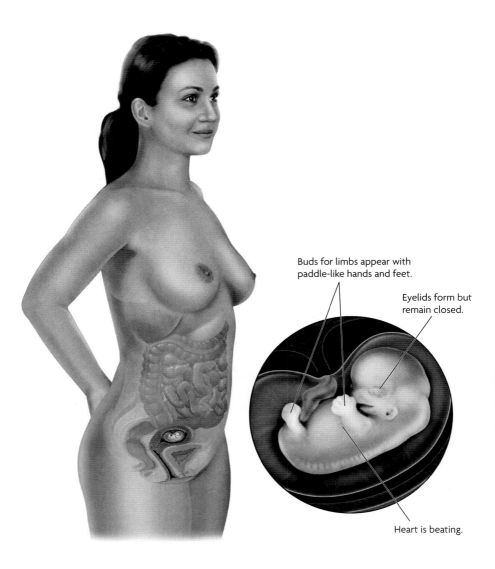

Buds for limbs appear with paddle-like hands and feet.

Eyelids form but remain closed.

Heart is beating.

**Mother and baby: Weeks 1–8.** The first 8 weeks of pregnancy are a time of rapid growth for your baby. At the end of week 8, most of the organ systems have begun to form.

# YOUR PREGNANCY

## Your Changing Body

By the end of week 2, you probably don't know that you are pregnant. You may notice a little spotting. Known as implantation bleeding, this spotting can occur when the fertilized egg becomes attached to the lining of the uterus. The spotting is very light, and not all women have it. Some women mistake it for menstrual bleeding. Implantation bleeding is normal and usually doesn't signal a problem.

Many signs and symptoms of pregnancy are thought to be caused by changing hormone levels. Some women are not aware of the early signs and symptoms, while others notice the sometimes subtle changes right away.

### Hormones

Hormones are the chemical messengers that orchestrate the body's functions. The following hormones play a leading role in reproduction, pregnancy, and birth:

- Estrogen and progesterone—Initially produced by the ovaries, these hormones trigger the lining of the uterus to thicken during each menstrual cycle and to be shed if pregnancy doesn't occur. After an egg is fertilized, an increase in estrogen and progesterone levels prevents the ovaries from releasing any eggs for the duration of the pregnancy.

- **Follicle-stimulating hormone (FSH)** and **luteinizing hormone (LH)**—These hormones are made by the pituitary gland, a small organ at the base of the brain. Follicle-stimulating hormone causes an egg to ripen in one of the ovaries. Luteinizing hormone triggers the egg's release.

- **Gonadotropin-releasing hormone (GnRH)**—This hormone is made in a part of the brain called the hypothalamus. It signals the pituitary gland to produce FSH and LH.

- Human chorionic gonadotropin (hCG)—Made by certain cells from the fertilized and dividing egg, hCG spurs increased estrogen and progesterone production during pregnancy. This is the hormone that is detected by pregnancy tests.

## *Signs and Symptoms of Pregnancy*

Could you be pregnant? Most likely you will not have symptoms until about the time you've missed your menstrual period or even about 1 week or 2 weeks later. Some women notice symptoms earlier than others.

A missed menstrual period is the most obvious sign of pregnancy. If your menstrual cycles are regular and your menstrual period does not arrive on time, you may suspect that you are pregnant long before you notice any signs or symptoms. Here are the six most common signs and symptoms:

1. Tender, swollen breasts—One of the early signs of pregnancy is sensitive, sore breasts caused by increasing levels of hormones. The soreness may feel like a more intense version of how your breasts feel before your menstrual period. The pain and discomfort should decrease after the first few weeks as your body adjusts to the hormonal changes.

2. Frequent urination—Soon after you become pregnant, you may find yourself rushing to the bathroom all the time. During pregnancy, the amount of blood in your body increases, which leads to extra fluid being processed by your **kidneys** and ending up in your **bladder**. This symptom usually continues as your pregnancy progresses and your growing baby puts more pressure on your bladder.

3. Nausea or vomiting—Most women do not experience a queasy stomach and vomiting until about 1 month after becoming pregnant. However, some women start to feel nausea a bit earlier, and some women never experience nausea or vomiting.

4. Fatigue—Fatigue is a common symptom of early pregnancy. No one knows for sure what causes early-pregnancy fatigue, but rapidly increasing levels of the hormone progesterone may be contributing to your sleepiness. You should start to feel more energetic once you enter your second **trimester**. Fatigue usually returns late in pregnancy when you're carrying around a lot more weight and some of the common discomforts of pregnancy make it more difficult to get a good night's sleep.

5. Moodiness—You may notice that your emotions are up one moment and down the next. Having mood swings during this time is normal.

6. Bloating—Hormonal changes in early pregnancy may leave you feeling bloated, similar to the feeling some women have just before their menstrual periods start. The bloating may cause your clothes to fit tighter around the waistline, even early on when your uterus is still quite small.

## Pregnancy Tests

If you've missed your menstrual period and are experiencing some of the previously mentioned symptoms, it's time to take a pregnancy test or see your health care provider. There are several brands of home pregnancy tests you can buy. All of them are easy to use and can be done in the privacy of your own home. Results are ready in a few minutes.

With home pregnancy tests, you urinate on a stick that detects the presence of hCG in your urine. The blastocyst (the dividing fertilized egg at about 6–7 days after fertilization) starts to produce hCG as it moves down the fallopian tube towards the uterus. After the blastocyst implants in the uterus, production of hCG increases rapidly. Depending on the brand, home pregnancy tests are able to detect 20 mIU/mL, 50 mIU/mL, or 100 mIU/mL of hCG in the urine. It's important to read the label on the test because not all tests can detect the same level of hCG. In general, the lower the level of hCG that the test is able to detect, the better the test is at accurately identifying pregnancy in a woman.

Many home pregnancy tests claim to be approximately 99% accurate in detecting pregnancy on the first day after your missed menstrual period. However, in research studies of these tests, it was found that most brands of tests do not consistently detect pregnancy that early. A false-negative result is a negative result that occurs when you are actually pregnant. Most false-negative results are caused by taking the test too early, when there is not enough hCG in the urine. If you get a negative result and you have some pregnancy symptoms, you may want to retake the test when your menstrual period is at least 1 week late. Also, make sure that you follow the directions for taking the test exactly as indicated. Doing so may yield more accurate results. For example, most tests advise you to take the test with the first urine of the day, when hCG levels are highest.

Home pregnancy tests also can give a false-positive result. This means that your test result is positive even though you are not pregnant. The most common reasons for a false-positive home pregnancy test result are not following the test's directions or reading the results incorrectly.

If you have a positive home pregnancy test result or if your result is negative and you really want to be sure, you can see your health care provider to have a blood test and a physical exam. The blood test for pregnancy is more sensitive than most urine tests for two reasons: 1) it can detect hCG levels of 5–10 mIU/mL, and 2) more hCG is present in the blood than in the urine. These two factors allow the blood test to detect pregnancy 6–10 days after ovulation, which for many women is even before the menstrual period is missed.

## Your Due Date

Health care providers are more likely to refer to weeks and days of pregnancy rather than months. A normal pregnancy lasts about 40 weeks from the date of the first day of your **last menstrual period (LMP)**. Weeks of pregnancy sometimes are divided into days. For example, "36 and 3/7" means "36 weeks and 3 days of pregnancy."

Weeks of pregnancy are divided into three **trimesters**. Each trimester lasts about 12–13 weeks (or about 3 months):

• First trimester: 0 weeks to 13 and 6/7 weeks (months 1–3)
• Second trimester: 14 and 0/7 weeks to 27 and 6/7 weeks (months 4–7)
• Third trimester: 28 and 0/7 weeks to 40 and 6/7 weeks (months 7–9)

The day your baby is due is called the **estimated due date (EDD)** (see box "Estimating Your Due Date"). The EDD is used to determine the baby's **gestational age** throughout pregnancy. Although only approximately 1 in 20 women give birth on their exact due dates, the EDD is useful for a number of reasons. It is used as a guide for checking the baby's growth as your pregnancy progresses and affects the timing of certain prenatal tests for **birth defects**. It also can affect management decisions if you have signs and symptoms of **preterm** labor.

Your due date is calculated from the first day of your LMP. However, some women may be uncertain about the date of their LMP. Factors such as a recent pregnancy, using hormonal birth control, or breastfeeding can make it more difficult to ascertain when your last period started. For this reason, an ultrasound exam may be done to calculate the EDD (see "Prenatal Care Visits" later in this chapter). If you had **in vitro fertilization**, the EDD is set by the age of the embryo and the date that the embryo is transferred to the uterus.

You may notice that, according to the LMP dating method, your last menstrual period is included even though you were not actually pregnant yet.

## Estimating Your Due Date

1. Take the date that your last normal menstrual period started.
2. Add 7 days.
3. Count back 3 months.

**Example:** The first day of your last menstrual period was January 1. Add 7 days to get January 8. Then count back 3 months. Your due date is October 8.

Pregnancy is assumed to occur 2 weeks after the first day of your last menstrual period. Therefore, an extra 2 weeks is counted at the beginning of your pregnancy when you aren't actually pregnant. Many women are surprised to learn that pregnancy "officially" lasts 10 months (40 weeks)—not 9 months—because of these extra weeks. Also, this dating technique is based on a 28-day cycle, which does not apply to all women. It's important to realize that the EDD gives only a rough idea of when your baby will be born. Most women go into labor within approximately 2 weeks of their due dates—either before or after.

## Discomforts and How to Manage Them

The signs and symptoms of early pregnancy are mere annoyances for some women; for others, they can be severe. It's not possible to predict which women will have more severe symptoms. A woman may have different symptoms during each of her pregnancies. Whether they are mild or severe, there are ways to manage these discomforts safely and effectively.

### Morning Sickness

Morning sickness is not just a feeling that happens before noon. The nausea and vomiting that define morning sickness can strike at any time of day—morning, afternoon, or night—and may last all day long. Between 70% and 85% of pregnant women experience morning sickness during their first trimester. The nausea usually starts between week 4 and week 9 of pregnancy. It tends to get worse over the next month or so. Most women who experience nausea and vomiting usually feel complete relief by approximately 16 weeks of pregnancy. For some women, however, nausea and vomiting continue for several weeks or months. And for a few women, morning sickness lasts throughout the entire pregnancy.

No one knows for sure what causes the nausea and vomiting, but the increasing levels of hormones during pregnancy may play a role. Hormonal changes may heighten your sense of smell and make you much more sensitive to certain odors. These changes also can cause your sense of taste to be "off"—you may have a sour or bitter taste in your mouth, and nothing may taste good to you.

If you have morning sickness, there are a few things that you can try to help make it more bearable and to ensure that you are getting enough nutrients and fluids:

• Take a multivitamin—Taking a multivitamin supplement before and during pregnancy may reduce the risk of having severe morning sickness.

- Keep snacks by the bed—Try eating dry toast or crackers in the morning before you get out of bed to avoid moving around on an empty stomach.

- Drink fluids—Your body needs more water in these early months, so aim to drink fluids often during the day. Not drinking can lead to dehydration (loss of fluids in the body), which can make nausea worse. If you are having trouble drinking water because of a bad taste in your mouth, try chewing gum or eating hard candies.

- Avoid smells that bother you—Foods or odors that may never have bothered you before may now trigger nausea. Do your best to stay away from them. Use a fan when cooking. Have someone else empty the trash.

- Eat small and often—Make sure your stomach is never empty by eating five or six small meals each day.

- Try bland foods —The "BRATT" diet (bananas, rice, applesauce, toast, and tea) is low in fat and easy to digest. If these foods don't appeal to you, try others that do. The goal is to find foods that you can eat and that stay down. If you can, try to add a protein food at each meal. Good, nonmeat sources of protein are dairy foods (milk, ice cream, yogurt), nuts and seeds (including nut butters), and protein powders and shakes.

- Try ginger—Ginger ale made with real ginger, ginger tea made from fresh grated ginger, ginger capsules, and ginger candies can help settle your queasy stomach.

If you have a lot of vomiting, be aware that it can cause some of your tooth enamel to wear away. This happens because your stomach contains a lot of acid. Rinsing your mouth with a teaspoon of baking soda dissolved in a cup of water may help neutralize the acid and protect your teeth.

If you try these remedies and they don't work, your health care provider may recommend medication. A combination of vitamin $B_6$ with or without another medication called doxylamine usually is recommended first. If this does not work, other medications then may be tried.

Up to 2% of women who have morning sickness have a severe form called *hyperemesis gravidarum*. No one knows what causes this condition. It has been suggested that women carrying more than one baby (twins, triplets, or more) are more likely to have severe nausea and vomiting than women carrying a single baby. Hyperemesis gravidarum can be a serious condition if it is not treated promptly. Call your health care provider if you have any of the following signs or symptoms:

- You have not been able to keep any food or fluids down for 24 hours or more.

- Your lips, mouth, and skin are very dry.

- You are urinating less often (less than three times a day), you are not producing much urine, or your urine is dark and has an odor.

- You are not gaining weight or have lost 5 or more pounds over a 1-week to 2-week period.

Your health care provider most likely will examine you to rule out other causes of your symptoms. If hyperemesis gravidarum is diagnosed, you may be given medication to help control your nausea and vomiting. If you have a severe case of hyperemesis gravidarum, you may need to receive fluids intravenously.

If you don't have morning sickness, it's not a cause for worry. About 15% of women do not have nausea or vomiting during pregnancy.

## Fatigue

During your first trimester, you probably will feel totally exhausted and wiped out. You may find it hard just to get out of bed in the morning. This is normal. Being pregnant puts a strain on your entire body, which can make you feel very tired. Your body is supporting a developing new life. Your hormone levels have increased and your **metabolism** is running high and burning energy, even while you sleep. Women may experience even more fatigue during subsequent pregnancies than during their first pregnancy because of the need to take care of other children as well as other demands on their time.

To help alleviate fatigue, listen to the signals your body is sending you. Slow down and get the rest you need. Try going to bed earlier than usual or take a 15-minute nap during lunchtime. Don't forget that during these first couple of months, getting enough rest is important—more important than finishing everything on your "to do" list. So, if need be, let some things go undone until you have the energy to do them, or enlist some help from your partner, friends, or family members. A healthy diet and exercise also may help boost your energy.

Fatigue usually begins to go away after the first trimester. By your fourth month, most of your energy will come back. However, many women begin to feel tired again in the last months of pregnancy.

## ⤳ Nutrition

For some women, pregnancy is a planned event. They've been exercising, eating healthy foods, and taking vitamins for months beforehand. For others, pregnancy is a surprise. Many women need to make lifestyle changes after they become pregnant. Although it's best to make these changes before pregnancy, it's also OK to adjust your lifestyle when you first find out you're pregnant.

Chapter 17, "Nutrition During Pregnancy," provides comprehensive information about planning a healthy pregnancy diet. One of the most important things you need to do in early pregnancy (and, ideally, before pregnancy) is make sure that you are getting enough *folic acid*, a vitamin that helps reduce the risk of certain birth defects.

### Focus on Folic Acid

Folic acid, also known as folate, is a B vitamin. At least 1 month before pregnancy and during pregnancy, you should get at least 400 micrograms (0.4 mg) of folic acid daily in order to reduce the risk of **neural tube defects**, such as **spina bifida** and **anencephaly**. It's recommended that all women of childbearing age take a vitamin supplement containing 400 micrograms of folic acid daily. Neural tube defects occur when the coverings of the spinal cord do not close completely early in prenatal development. If you have had a previous child with one of these defects or if you have certain health conditions (such as **sickle cell disease**), it is recommended that you take 10 times this amount—4 mg daily—as a separate vitamin supplement at least 1 month before pregnancy and for the first 3 months of pregnancy. You and your health care provider can discuss whether you need this amount of folic acid based on your health history.

Current dietary guidelines recommend that women get 600 micrograms of folic acid while they are pregnant. Although folic acid is found in many foods and also is added as a supplement to breads, cereals, and pastas, it is difficult to get the recommended amount from diet alone. To ensure that you are getting enough folic acid, you can take a prenatal vitamin supplement containing the recommended amount. Prenatal multivitamin supplements usually contain 600–800 micrograms of folic acid, so if you were taking a prenatal multivitamin before pregnancy, you don't need to take an extra daily folic acid supplement during pregnancy.

## Prenatal Multivitamin Supplements

The recommended dietary allowances for some vitamins and nutrients increase during pregnancy. It's a good idea to start taking a prenatal multivitamin as soon as you find out you are pregnant or, ideally, before pregnancy. These multivitamin supplements are available without a prescription. They contain the recommended daily allowances for the vitamins and minerals you will need during your pregnancy, such as vitamins A, C, and D; folic acid; and minerals such as iron. During pregnancy, taking prenatal vitamins can ensure that you're getting all of the important nutrients you need, especially if you're battling nausea and finding it hard to eat all of the foods you should.

At your first **prenatal care** visit, tell your health care provider if you have been taking prenatal vitamins; you may want to bring the bottle with you. It's important to tell your health care provider that you're taking vitamins because excess amounts of some vitamins can be harmful.

If the smell of your vitamins makes you queasy or if you find it difficult to keep them down, you can take two children's chewable vitamins. Be sure to tell your health care provider that you're taking children's vitamins.

## Weight Gain

A certain amount of weight gain is normal during pregnancy. However, too much or too little weight gain can be a problem (see box "Where Does the Weight Come From?").

How much weight you should gain while you're pregnant depends on your weight before you became pregnant. Your **body mass index (BMI)** is an indication of whether you are at a healthy weight for your height. If your BMI falls between 18.5 and 24.9, you are at a normal, healthy weight. A BMI below 18.5 is considered underweight, and a BMI of 25 or greater is considered overweight. Table 2-1 shows the amount of weight that you should gain during pregnancy based on your prepregnancy BMI.

Now that you know the total weight you should gain, how does this translate into how much to eat each day? An easy guideline to follow is that if you were a normal weight before pregnancy and are carrying only one baby, you need only about 300 extra **calories** per day to provide all of the necessary nutrients to keep your body running efficiently and to fuel the extra growth and development of your baby. If you are carrying twins or multiple babies, you need about 300 extra calories per baby. It may sound like a lot, but 300 extra calories adds up fast; it's the amount in a bowl of cereal with fruit

## Where Does the Weight Come From?

The average newborn weighs approximately 7.5 pounds, yet most mothers-to-be are advised to gain 25–35 pounds when they are pregnant. Where do the other pounds come from? Here's a breakdown of the weight gain for a normal-weight woman who gains 30 pounds during pregnancy:

- Baby—7.5 pounds
- Amniotic fluid—2 pounds
- Placenta—1.5 pound
- Uterus—2 pounds
- Breasts—2 pounds
- Body fluids—4 pounds
- Blood—4 pounds
- Maternal stores of fat, protein, and other nutrients—7 pounds

and low-fat milk, a whole-wheat bagel with cream cheese, or a hard-boiled egg and half a dozen crackers. If you are overweight to begin with, you may need less than 300 extra calories a day.

Keep in mind that you will gain weight differently throughout the different months of your pregnancy. During the first 3 months, you may see little gain. In fact, some women lose a few pounds because of morning sickness. You will gain most of your weight during the second and third trimesters, when your baby is growing at a faster pace. However, your rate of weight gain should stay within a certain range.

Do not worry about how much weight other pregnant women gain. Also, if you are pregnant for the second time, you may gain weight differently. Your health care provider will check your weight gain at each of your prenatal care visits and will let you know whether you are on a healthy track.

## ⤳ Exercise

You're tired. You're gaining weight. For many pregnant women, exercise is the last thing they want to do. But exercise actually can boost your energy

## Table 2-1 Amount of Weight You Should Gain During Pregnancy

| Prepregnancy Body Mass Index | Recommended Total Weight Gain During Pregnancy | Recommended Rate of Weight Gain per Week in the Second and Third Trimesters* |
|---|---|---|
| Underweight (BMI less than 18.5) | 28–40 lb | 1.0–1.3 lb |
| Normal weight (BMI 18.5–24.9) | 25–35 lb | 0.8–1 lb |
| Overweight (BMI 25–29.9) | 15–25 lb | 0.5–0.7 lb |
| Obese (BMI more than 30) | 11–20 lb | 0.4–0.6 lb |

*Assumes a first-trimester weight gain between 1.1 lb and 4.4 lb.
Abbreviation: BMI, body mass index.
Data from Institutes of Medicine (US). Weight gain during pregnancy: reexamining the guidelines.
Washington, DC: National Academies Press; 2009.

levels. Being active and exercising—even just walking—at least 30 minutes on most days of the week can benefit your pregnancy in many ways:

- Reduces backaches, constipation, bloating, and swelling
- Boosts your mood
- Promotes muscle tone, strength, and endurance
- Helps you sleep better

The ideal exercise routine during pregnancy gets your heart pumping, keeps you limber, and controls your weight gain without causing too much physical stress for you or the baby. Exercising now also will make it easier for you to get back in shape after the baby is born. Some exercise routines can help you relieve pregnancy-related aches and pains. For instance, the extra weight you are carrying affects your posture and can be hard on your back. Exercise may help ease back pain by toning muscles and making them stronger.

Before you start your exercise program, talk with your health care provider to make sure you do not have any health conditions that may limit your activity. If you have heart disease, are at risk of preterm labor, or have vaginal bleeding, your health care provider may advise you not to exercise. Women with any of the following conditions are advised not to exercise during pregnancy:

- Some forms of heart and lung disease
- Cervical problems
- *Multiple pregnancy* that is at risk of preterm labor
- Vaginal bleeding
- Preterm labor during the current pregnancy
- *Premature rupture of membranes*
- *Preeclampsia* or *high blood pressure* that occurs for the first time during pregnancy

Unless your health care provider tells you not to, you should do moderate exercise for 30 minutes or more on most days, if not every day. The 30 minutes do not have to be all at one time; it can be a total of different exercise periods. If you have not been active, start with a few minutes each day and build up to 30 minutes or more.

Pay attention to your body while you exercise. If you have any of the signs or symptoms listed in the box "Warning Signs to Stop Exercise," stop exercising and call your health care provider immediately.

### Pregnancy Changes That Can Affect Your Exercise Routine

Some of the changes in your body during pregnancy affect the kinds of activities you can do safely. Consider the following things when choosing an exercise program that will be safe for you during pregnancy:

- Joints—Some pregnancy hormones cause the ligaments that support your joints to stretch. This makes them more prone to injury.

- Balance—The weight you gain in the front of your body shifts your center of gravity. This puts stress on your joints and muscles—mostly those in the lower back and pelvis. It also can make you less stable and more likely to fall.

## Warning Signs to Stop Exercise

Whether you're a seasoned athlete or a beginner, watch for the following warning signs during exercise. If you have any of them, stop exercising and call your health care provider.

- Dizziness or faintness
- Increased shortness of breath
- Uneven or rapid heartbeat
- Chest pain
- Trouble walking
- Calf pain or swelling
- Headache
- Vaginal bleeding
- Uterine contractions that continue after rest
- Fluid gushing or leaking from your vagina
- Decreased fetal movement

- Heart rate—Extra weight also makes your body work harder than it did before you were pregnant. This is true even if you are working out at a slower pace. Intense exercise boosts oxygen and blood flow to the muscles and away from other parts of your body, such as your uterus. If you can't talk normally during exercise, then you are working too hard.

### Starting an Exercise Program During Pregnancy

If you've never exercised, pregnancy is a great time to start. Discuss your plan to start exercising with your health care provider. Also, remember to start slowly. Begin with as little as 5 minutes of exercise a day and add 5 minutes each week until you can stay active for 30 minutes per day.

Many sports are safe during pregnancy, even for beginners:

- Walking is a good exercise for anyone. Brisk walking gives a total body workout and is easy on the joints and muscles. If you were not active before getting pregnant, walking is a great way to start an exercise program.

- Swimming is great for your body because it works so many muscles. The water supports your weight so you avoid injury and muscle strain. It also helps you stay cool and may prevent your legs from swelling.

- Cycling provides a good aerobic workout. However, your growing belly can affect your balance and make you more prone to falls. You may want to stick with stationary or recumbent biking later in pregnancy.

### Activities to Avoid

Although there are many sports that you can do while you're pregnant, such as walking and swimming, there are some activities that you should avoid because they can be too risky for you and the baby:

- Downhill snow skiing—Downhill skiing poses a risk of severe injuries and hard falls. In addition, exercising at heights of more than 6,000 feet carries various risks. If you do engage in physical activities at high altitude, know the signs of altitude sickness (throbbing headache, nausea, vomiting, dizziness, weakness, and difficulty sleeping). Be prepared to descend to a lower altitude and seek medical help if you have any of the signs.

- In-line skating, gymnastics, horseback riding—Your balance is affected, and there is a risk of crashes and falls.

## Exercise of the Month: Kegel Exercises

As your uterus grows in the coming months, it will put more pressure on your bladder. Even if your bladder is almost empty, it still may feel like it's full. The weight of your uterus on your bladder even may cause you to leak a little urine when you sneeze or cough. Doing Kegel exercises may help improve your bladder control. Kegel exercises strengthen the muscles that surround the opening of the vagina. Here's how they're done:

• Squeeze the muscles that you use to stop the flow of urine.

• Hold this position for 10 seconds, then release.

Do this 10–20 times in a row at least three times per day. You can do Kegel exercises anywhere—while working, driving in your car, or watching television.

• Water skiing, surfing, diving—Hitting the water with great force can be harmful. Taking a fall at such fast speeds could harm you or your baby.

• Contact sports—Avoid playing fast-paced team sports, such as ice hockey, soccer, basketball, and volleyball. Collisions or falls could result in harm to you and your baby.

• Scuba diving—Scuba diving puts your baby at risk of decompression sickness.

Some sports should be avoided if you haven't done them before. In racquet sports, such as badminton, tennis, and racquetball, your changing body may affect your balance and put you at an increased risk of falls. If you're an experienced player, however, you may be more adept at compensating for these changes. If you're not sure about your ability to maintain your balance, you may want to avoid these sports.

### Healthy Decisions

In the first 2 months of pregnancy, you may have a lot of questions to ask and decisions to make. The decisions facing you now may include making important lifestyle changes, picking a practitioner who will care for you during pregnancy, and deciding when to tell others your news.

## Things to Avoid During Pregnancy

It's perfectly normal to be anxious about what you can and cannot do while you are pregnant. The list of "don'ts" may seem long, but most are easy to remember.

**Smoking.** If you smoke, it's best to quit before pregnancy or as soon as you know that you are pregnant. Cigarette smoke contains thousands of harmful chemicals, including lead, tar, nicotine, and carbon dioxide. When you smoke, these *toxins* go directly to your baby and increase the risk of the following complications:

- Vaginal bleeding
- Preterm birth
- A low birth weight baby (weighing less than 5 ½ pounds)
- *Stillbirth*
- *Sudden infant death syndrome*

It is best to stop smoking before pregnancy or as soon as you find out you are pregnant. Stopping smoking during pregnancy is better than not stopping at all. It is unclear whether cutting down on the amount that you smoke has any benefits. Quitting completely is best for you and your baby. You even may be able to quit for a lifetime. You and your family will be healthier as a result.

If you are pregnant and you smoke, tell your health care provider. He or she can help you find support and quitting programs in your area. You also can call the national "quit line" at 1-800-QUIT-NOW. One of the best things to do when quitting smoking is to join a stop-smoking group or to get individual counseling on the phone, in person, or online. Sharing your experiences with others trying to quit assures you that you're not alone and that you have people to turn to if you run into problems. Knowing that others have experienced the same things as you can make you feel less alone. The American Cancer Society states that there is a strong link between how often and how long counseling lasts (its intensity) and the success rate of the counseling: The more intense the program, the greater the chance of success. To find out more about quitting programs in your area, to get information about quitting, or to find support, see the "Resources" section in this chapter.

Although many smokers quit with the help of nicotine replacement products (such as nicotine gum or the patch) or prescription medications, these aids need to be used with caution during pregnancy. Not enough tests have been done to determine their safety during pregnancy. Over-the-counter nicotine replacement products should be used only if other attempts to quit have not worked and you and your health care provider have weighed the known risks of continued smoking against the possible risks of these products. Smokeless tobacco, electronic cigarettes, and nicotine gel strips are not safe substitutes for cigarettes. They should not be used to quit smoking.

Secondhand smoke—smoke from cigarettes smoked by other people nearby—can be harmful as well. Breathing secondhand smoke during pregnancy increases the risk of having a low-birth-weight baby by as much as 20%. Infants who are exposed to secondhand smoke have an increased risk of sudden infant death syndrome and are more likely to have respiratory illnesses than those not exposed to secondhand smoke. If you live or work around smokers, take steps to avoid secondhand smoke. You may want to ask family members who smoke to smoke outside or quit altogether.

Once the baby is born, it can be tempting to start smoking again. Be prepared. Before the baby is born, think about how you will handle wanting to smoke and have a plan in place to avoid smoking. Talk with your health care provider about your plan to remain smoke-free.

**Drinking Alcohol.** Alcohol can harm your baby's health. It's best to stop drinking before you become pregnant. If you did have some alcohol before you knew you were pregnant, it most likely will not harm your baby. The important thing is to avoid alcohol once you learn you're pregnant.

When a pregnant woman drinks alcohol, it quickly reaches the baby. Alcohol is much more harmful to a baby than it is to an adult. In an adult, the liver breaks down the alcohol. A baby's liver is not fully developed and is not able to break down alcohol.

"Fetal alcohol spectrum disorders" is a term that describes different effects that can occur in the baby when a woman drinks during pregnancy. These effects may include physical, mental, behavioral, and learning disabilities that can last a lifetime. The most severe disorder is *fetal alcohol syndrome (FAS)*. Fetal alcohol syndrome can cause growth problems, mental or behavioral problems, and abnormal facial features. It is most likely to occur in infants whose mothers drank heavily (three or more drinks per occasion or more than seven drinks per week) and continued to drink heavily throughout pregnancy, but it also can occur with lesser amounts of alcohol use. Even moderate alcohol use during pregnancy (defined as one alcoholic drink per day) can cause lifelong learning and behavioral problems in the child.

It is not known how much alcohol it takes to harm the baby. The best course is not to drink at all during pregnancy. Also, there are no types of drinks that are safe. One beer, one shot of liquor, one mixed drink, or one glass of wine all contain approximately the same amount of alcohol.

It may be hard to stop drinking. Some questions to ask yourself about your dependence on alcohol are listed in the box "Do You Have a Drinking Problem?" Talk honestly to your health care provider about your drinking habits. If you are dependent on alcohol, you may need specialized counseling and medical care. Your health care provider can help you connect with these resources.

**Substance Abuse.** Substance abuse is the use of illegal drugs such as heroin, cocaine, methamphetamines, marijuana, and prescription drugs used for a nonmedical reason. Drug abuse is a widespread problem in the United States. A survey conducted in 2011 found that about 5% of pregnant women admitted to using an illegal substance in the past 30 days. Often, more than one

## Do You Have a Drinking Problem?

Do you use alcohol or abuse it? Sometimes it's hard to tell. If you're not sure, ask yourself these questions:

1. On average, how many standard-sized drinks containing alcohol do you have in a week? If your answer is more than 7 drinks per week, that is at-risk alcohol use.
   *Note:* If you are pregnant, any amount of alcohol use is at-risk use.

2. When you drink, what is the maximum number of standard-sized drinks you have at one time? If your answer is 3 drinks or more, that is at-risk alcohol use.
   *Note:* If you are pregnant, any amount of alcohol use is at-risk use.

If you do drink alcohol, answer the following questions:

**T** How many drinks does it take to make you feel high? (TOLERANCE)

**A** Have people ANNOYED you by criticizing your drinking?

**C** Have you felt you ought to CUT DOWN on your drinking?

**E** Have you ever had a drink first thing in the morning to steady your nerves or get rid of a hangover? (EYE OPENER)

Scoring:

• 2 points if your answer to the first question is more than two drinks.
• 1 point for every "yes" response to the other questions.

If your total score is 2 or more, you may have an alcohol problem.

*Modified from Sokol RJ, Martier SS, Ager JW. The T-ACE questions: practical prenatal detection of risk drinking. Am J Obstet Gynecol 1989;160:865.*

substance has been used. Use of these substances during pregnancy may cause preterm birth, interfere with the baby's growth, or cause birth defects or learning and behavioral problems.

It has been difficult for researchers to link a particular problem to the use of a specific drug because women who use illegal drugs often use alcohol and tobacco as well, which also place pregnant women and their babies at risk. In addition, women who use illegal drugs may have other unhealthy behaviors, such as poor nutrition, that are known to adversely affect pregnancy.

The bottom line is that you should make all illegal drugs and prescription drugs used for nonmedical reasons off limits while you are pregnant. If you are addicted to any of these drugs, tell your health care provider that you need help. Trying to break an addiction on your own while you are pregnant may result in more harm for you and your baby. This is especially true if you are addicted to an opioid, such as heroin or the prescription drug oxycodone. Suddenly stopping use of these drugs can cause serious complications, including preterm labor and fetal death. For this reason, many pregnant women who are addicted to opioids are placed on maintenance therapy with another drug to avoid the complications of withdrawal. Substance abuse treatment programs specifically tailored for pregnant women are available that include prenatal care, counseling and family therapy, nutritional education, and other services. Your health care provider can help you enroll in one of these programs. To find one of these programs in your area, you can go to the Substance Abuse and Mental Health Services Administration's web site (http://dpt2.samhsa.gov/treatment/directory.aspx) or call them at 1-800-662-HELP (4357).

It is very important to be open and honest with your health care provider about substance abuse issues. Help is available in the form of treatment programs, addiction medicine specialists, and other types of assistance.

### What Do I Do About Medications?

Most medications are not known to cause harm during pregnancy. However, it is a good idea to tell your health care provider about all of the medications that you are taking, including prescription medications, over-the-counter drugs, and herbal remedies. Don't stop taking a medication prescribed for you until you have consulted your health care provider. The risks of taking some medicines during pregnancy may be outweighed by the effects of not taking them. For instance, certain diseases are more harmful to a developing baby than the drugs used to treat them. If a medication you are taking poses a risk, your health care provider may recommend switching to a safer drug while you are pregnant.

Over-the-counter medicines, including herbal medications and vitamin supplements, can cause problems during pregnancy too. Check with your health care provider before taking any over-the-counter drug. This includes pain relievers, *laxatives*, cold or allergy remedies, and skin treatments. However, you don't have to go through the discomfort of headaches or colds without relief. Your health care provider can give you advice about medicines that are safe for pregnant women to use. For more information about medication use during pregnancy, see Chapter 21, "Reducing Risks of Birth Defects."

## Choosing a Health Care Provider for Your Pregnancy

If you don't already have one, finding a health care provider for your pregnancy is probably one of the most important choices you'll make early on. Talk to your regular health care provider for recommendations, or ask women you know to share their opinions about the health care providers who delivered their babies.

You also can find a pregnancy care provider through your health insurance provider list. All health plans offer a "find a doctor" service on their web sites, or you can call the insurance provider directly. The American College of Obstetricians and Gynecologists' web site also provides a "Find a Physician" resource tool. To access this tool, go to www.acog.org/About-ACOG/Find-an-Ob-Gyn.

**Types of Health Care Providers.** Four types of practitioners offer medical care for pregnancy, childbirth, and the postpartum period: *obstetrician–gynecologists* (ob-gyns), *maternal–fetal medicine subspecialists* (high-risk obstetricians), family physicians, and certified nurse–midwives (CNMs) and certified midwives (CMs).

1. Obstetrician–gynecologists—Obstetrician–gynecologists are doctors who specialize in the health care of women. After completing medical school, obstetrician–gynecologists complete 4 years of specialized training in obstetrics and gynecology. To be certified, an obstetrician–gynecologist must pass written and oral tests to show that he or she has obtained the knowledge and skills required for the medical and surgical care of women. A certified obstetrician–gynecologist then can become a Fellow of the American College of Obstetricians and Gynecologists. This group helps doctors stay up to date on the latest medical advances.

2. Maternal–fetal medicine subspecialists—These doctors, who also are called perinatologists, have completed 4 years of training in obstetrics and gynecology and then received further training in high-risk obstetrics for 2–3 years. Maternal–fetal medicine subspecialists must pass written and

oral exams to become certified. Women who have high-risk pregnancies may be referred to maternal–fetal medicine subspecialists for care.

3.  Family physicians—Doctors in family practices provide general care for most conditions, including pregnancy. After completing medical school, family physicians complete 3 years of advanced training in family medicine (including obstetrics) and become certified by passing an exam. They are able to care for women with normal pregnancies and deliveries.

4.  Certified nurse–midwives and certified midwives—Certified nurse–midwives (CNMs) and certified midwives (CMs) are specially trained practitioners who provide care for women with low-risk pregnancies and their babies from early pregnancy through labor, delivery, and the weeks after birth. Certified nurse–midwives are registered nurses who have completed an accredited nursing program and have a graduate degree in midwifery. To be certified, they must pass a national written exam administered by the American Midwifery Certification Board and must maintain an active nursing license. Certified midwives have graduated from a midwifery education program accredited by the American College of Nurse-Midwives Division of Accreditation. They have successfully completed the same requirements, have passed the same American Midwifery Certification Board national certification exam, and adhere to the same professional standards as CNMs. Both CNMs and CMs generally work with a qualified doctor who will provide backup support.

Certified professional midwives (CPMs) also may be called "licensed direct-entry midwives," "registered midwives," or "licensed midwives" and are recognized legal medical practitioners in some U.S. states but not in others. There is no standard education program for CPMs. Certified professional midwives can learn by following a training program, through an apprenticeship, or through self-study, and they receive certification through the Midwife Education Accreditation Council.

**Types of Practices.** Another factor to think about is whether a health care provider is in a solo practice, group practice, or collaborative practice. In a solo practice, one health care provider works alone but may have help from other health care providers to cover deliveries. In a group practice, two or more health care providers share duties for constant coverage of their patients' health care. A collaborative practice brings together a team of health care professionals—such as nurses, CNMs or CMs, *laborists*, nurse practitioners, physician assistants, and childbirth educators—with different knowledge and skills. The contributions of each member are key to the health care of the patient.

Another type of prenatal care you might consider is called Centering Pregnancy, a form of group prenatal care. Instead of individual medical appointments, a group of 8–12 women with similar due dates meets regularly with a health care provider for health assessments, education, and support. Physical exams are performed in a private room. If this model of group prenatal care appeals to you, ask your health care provider for more information.

**Questions to Ask.** Once you find a health care provider who seems promising, it's a good idea to ask him or her questions that are important for you and your partner. Don't hesitate to write down a list of your concerns to take with you on your first prenatal care visit. Use this list as a guide for some questions you may want to ask:

- How does the office work? Are you in practice alone, or is there a group of doctors or health care providers?

- If it is a group, how often will I see the same health care provider when I come for my prenatal care visits?

- If you are in solo practice, who covers you when you are not available?

- Which hospital will I go to when I give birth?

- Do you have an after-hours office number I can call in case of an emergency or if I have questions?

- Who takes the after-hours calls?

- Who will deliver my baby?

- What are your views on **anesthesia** during labor, **episiotomy**, alternative birthing positions, **cesarean delivery**, and operative delivery?

- Who can be with me during delivery?

## When to Spread the News

When to tell family and friends that you're pregnant is your personal choice. Many women choose to wait until after the first 12 weeks have passed. Others may decide to tell as soon as they get the positive pregnancy test result. Deciding when to deliver the news is a personal decision, but you may want to keep a few things in mind:

- The risk of **miscarriage** is highest in the first 3 months of pregnancy. You may want to wait until your second trimester to tell friends, coworkers, and extended family members that you're pregnant.

- Discrimination against pregnant women is illegal. However, you may want to wait to spread the news at work until you've worked out the logistics of your maternity leave with your supervisor.

- Women who have had problems with past pregnancies, especially early problems, may feel more secure waiting until the second trimester to tell others. Your friends' and family members' concern about you may be heartfelt, but it may make your own anxiety about your pregnancy worse.

## Other Considerations

Many pregnant women have jobs outside the home. Pregnant women often work right up until delivery and return to their jobs within weeks or months of the baby's birth. Women often can keep doing their normal jobs while they are pregnant. However, some jobs may not be safe for a pregnant woman. Also, fatigue, nausea, and other discomforts can make working during early pregnancy a challenge.

### A Safe Workplace

Most women can continue working throughout their pregnancies. However, small changes may be needed depending on the work that you do. Jobs that require heavy lifting, climbing, carrying, or standing may not be safe during pregnancy. That's because the dizziness, nausea, and fatigue common in early pregnancy can increase the chance of injury. Later on, the change in body shape can throw off your balance and lead to falls.

Some substances found in the workplace pose a risk during pregnancy. Although being exposed to harmful substances on the job is fairly rare, it makes sense to think about the things you come into contact with during the course of your workday. You also may come into contact with these agents through a hobby. Agents that pose a pregnancy risk are discussed in detail in Chapter 21, "Reducing Risks of Birth Defects."

If you think your job may bring you into contact with something harmful, find out for sure by asking your personnel office, employee clinic, or union. Let your health care provider know right away if you think you and your baby are at risk. Workplace safety hazards and tips can be found at the web sites of the Occupational Safety and Health Administration and the National Institute for Occupational Safety and Health. Also see the "Your Workplace Rights" section in Chapter 4, "Month 4 (Weeks 13–16)."

## *Tips for Working During Early Pregnancy*

Working when you are experiencing the nausea and fatigue of early pregnancy can be difficult. To cope, you may want to try the following:

- Take advantage of flex time—If your workplace has flex time, use this benefit to your advantage. What is the time of day when you feel the most energized? Consider coming in later if the early morning is bad for you. If afternoons are a problem, arrive earlier so that you can leave earlier.

- Bring snacks with you—Healthy snacks throughout the day may help keep nausea at bay and supply a source of energy. Crackers; fresh, raw vegetables; or fruit and cheese are good choices.

- Cat nap, if you can—If you have an office, you can shut the door and rest during your lunch hour.

- Stay hydrated—Being dehydrated can make you feel worse. Make sure you are drinking enough fluids throughout the day.

## Prenatal Care Visits

As soon as you know you're pregnant, call your health care provider to schedule an appointment so you can start prenatal care right away. You'll have regular appointments throughout your pregnancy. At each visit, the health care provider will monitor your health as well as that of your growing baby.

Your first or second prenatal care visit will probably be one of your longest visits. Your health care provider will need to ask a lot of questions about your health and perform several tests. It's important to answer all the questions honestly and with as much detail as you can. A health history form is provided in Appendix B. You can fill out this form before your visit, or you can just read it through to see what questions will be asked. It may be helpful to bring a support person with you on your prenatal care visits. During these early visits, your health care provider may do the following:

- Ask about your health history, including your previous pregnancies, surgeries, or medical problems.

- Ask about any prescription and over-the-counter medications you're taking (bring them with you, if possible).

- Ask about the health history of your family and the baby's father.

- Do a complete physical exam with blood and urine tests.

- Do a **pelvic exam**.
- Measure your blood pressure, height, and weight.
- Calculate the baby's expected due date.

Some health care providers perform an **ultrasound exam**, which uses sound waves to show features inside the body, to confirm pregnancy. This exam may be done transvaginally, in which a special **transducer** (the instrument that transmits the sound waves) is placed in the vagina. If you are less than 5 weeks pregnant, the embryo may not be visible. If you are more than 5 weeks pregnant, don't expect to see much more than a small, circular shape that represents the amniotic sac in which the baby is growing. You will not be able to see arms or legs or any other distinct features until later in pregnancy.

A first-trimester ultrasound exam is considered to be the most accurate way of estimating the due date. The gestational age can be estimated using a measurement called "crown–rump length." This is the length of the embryo or fetus measured from the top of the head ("crown") to the bottom of the area that will become the buttocks ("rump"). If you are less than 7 weeks pregnant, it is not possible to see the embryo's crown or rump, so the greatest length of the embryo is measured. A formula then is used to estimate the gestational age based on this measurement. The heart rate also can be detected at about 6 weeks of pregnancy during an ultrasound exam.

## ✒ Special Concerns

Although it's normal for pregnant women to worry about complications, most women have perfectly healthy pregnancies and give birth to healthy babies. However, it's best to be alert to signs and symptoms that may signal a problem. Often, the earlier you see your health care provider, the more likely that the complication can be managed successfully.

### Miscarriage

The loss of a pregnancy in the first trimester is called a miscarriage. About 15–20% of pregnancies end this way. Some miscarriages take place before a woman misses her menstrual period or even knows that she is pregnant.

The most common sign of a miscarriage is bleeding. Call your health care provider if you experience any of the following warning signs:

- Spotting or bleeding without pain

- Heavy or persistent bleeding with abdominal pain or cramping
- A gush of fluid from your vagina but no pain or bleeding
- Passed fetal tissue

Most miscarriages are caused by a problem with the **chromosomes** of the fertilized egg that occurs by chance and is not likely to occur again in a later pregnancy. In most cases, there is nothing wrong with the woman's or man's health. Most women who have a miscarriage go on to have healthy, successful pregnancies. Miscarriage is discussed in detail in Chapter 33, "Early Pregnancy Loss: Miscarriage, Ectopic Pregnancy, and Molar Pregnancy."

### Ectopic Pregnancy

An **ectopic pregnancy** is one in which the fertilized egg implants outside of the uterus. The egg usually implants in one of the fallopian tubes, but it also can implant in other locations, such as the **cervix** or abdomen. An ectopic pregnancy in a fallopian tube can cause serious health problems. The fallopian tube can burst (rupture), resulting in internal bleeding that can be life threatening. Approximately 2% of all pregnancies are ectopic.

An ectopic pregnancy may feel like a normal pregnancy with some of the same symptoms, such as a missed menstrual period and nausea. If you have any vaginal bleeding, have pain in your pelvis, or feel dizzy or light-headed (caused by internal bleeding)—especially if you haven't yet had an ultrasound exam to confirm that your pregnancy is in your uterus—call your health care provider. Ectopic pregnancy is discussed in detail in Chapter 33, "Early Pregnancy Loss: Miscarriage, Ectopic Pregnancy, and Gestational Trophoblastic Disease."

## ASK THE EXPERTS

**I'm a coffee drinker, but I'm worried about the caffeine. How much caffeine can I safely consume per day?**

Many women have been told to limit their caffeine consumption during pregnancy because of a possible association with an increased risk of miscarriage, preterm birth, and **low birth weight**. However, recent research regarding caffeine consumption and miscarriage risk is conflicting. Some research suggests that women who consume 200 mg of caffeine (equal to one 12-ounce cup of coffee) or more a day are more than twice as likely as women who consume no caffeine to have a miscarriage. Yet other research found no relationship between caffeine consumption and the risk of miscarriage, regardless of the amount consumed. There also is no clear evidence that caffeine intake increases the risk of having a low-birth-weight baby. Because of these conflicting research results, it is not possible to give a recommendation about how much caffeine is safe to consume during pregnancy. As for the links between moderate caffeine intake and preterm birth, results from much of the research show that caffeine consumption does not appear to affect this complication.

Still, it may be a good idea to limit your caffeine intake for other reasons. Excess caffeine can interfere with much-needed sleep and can contribute to nausea and light-headedness. The diuretic effect of caffeine can increase urination and lead to dehydration. If you do cut down on caffeine, don't just focus on coffee. Remember that caffeine also is found in tea, chocolate, energy drinks, and soft drinks.

### Is it safe to douche during pregnancy?

No. It is best to avoid douching at all times, whether you're pregnant or not. Women do not need to douche to wash away blood, semen, or vaginal discharge. Most experts say that it's better to let your vagina clean itself naturally. Douching can even increase your chances of getting a vaginal infection. Keep in mind that even healthy, clean vaginas may have a mild odor.

---

# RESOURCES

The following resources offer more information about some of the topics discussed in this chapter:

**How to Survive Morning Sickness Successfully**
Motherisk
www.motherisk.org/women/morningSickness.jsp
*Booklet that addresses how to prepare for and manage nausea and vomiting of pregnancy.*

**SAMHSA's National Helpline**
Substance Abuse and Mental Health Services Administration
www.samhsa.gov/find-help/national-helpline
1-800-662-HELP (4357)
*Provides a locator service for substance abuse programs in your area.*

**Smokefree Women: Pregnancy and Motherhood**
Smokefree Women
http://women.smokefree.gov/pregnancy-motherhood.aspx
*Developed by numerous health organizations dedicated to helping pregnant women quit smoking, this web site offers information about smoking during pregnancy and how to quit, maintains current information about quit lines and online programs, and even offers an instant messaging service.*

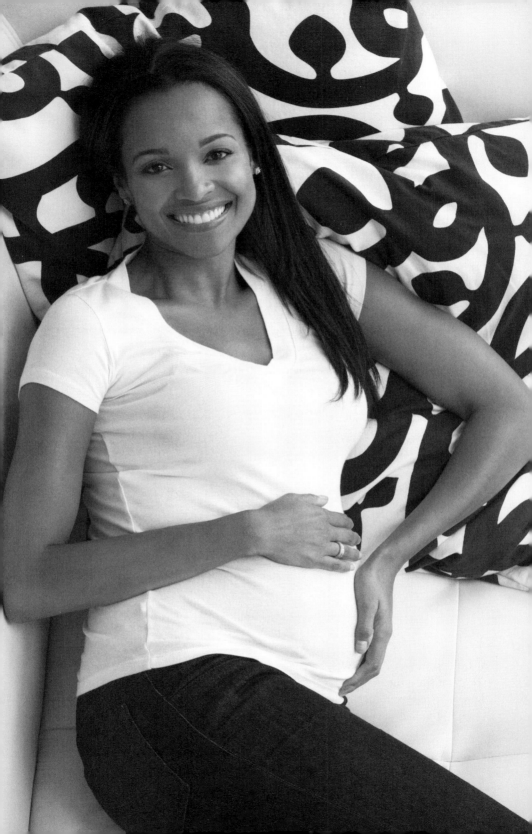

Chapter 3

# Month 3

(Weeks 9–12)

---

## YOUR GROWING BABY

### Week 9

The baby is close to ½ inch long now. Buds for future teeth appear, and the intestines begin to form.

### Week 10

Fingers and toes continue to grow, and soft nails begin to form. During this week, it may be possible to hear your baby's heart beat with a Doppler auscultation device (although it's more likely to be heard by week 12 of pregnancy).

### Week 11

Bones are starting to harden, and muscles begin to develop. The backbone is soft and can flex. The skin is still thin and transparent but will start to thicken soon.

### Week 12

At this point, your baby weighs about ½ ounce and is about 2 inches long. The hands are more fully developed than the feet, and the arms are longer than the legs. Your baby moves on his or her own now, but it is still too early to feel these movements.

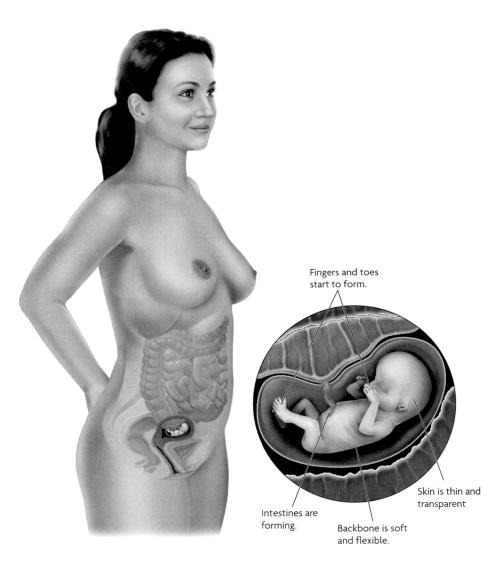

Fingers and toes start to form.

Skin is thin and transparent

Intestines are forming.

Backbone is soft and flexible.

**Mother and baby: Weeks 9–12.** At this point, the baby weighs about ½ ounce and is about 2 inches long.

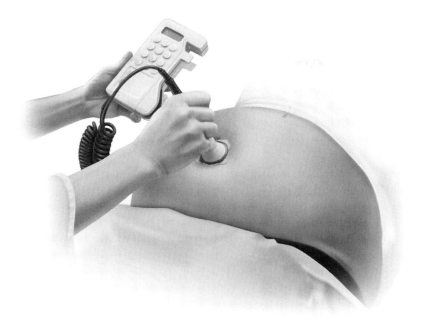

**Listening to the fetal heartbeat.** A small, handheld Doppler device is pressed against your abdomen to detect your baby's heartbeat.

# YOUR PREGNANCY

## ◢ Your Changing Body

You still may not look pregnant to others even though you may be able to tell your waist is getting a little thicker. When you are not pregnant, the uterus is about the size of a small pear. By around week 10, it is as big as a large orange.

## ◢ Discomforts and How to Manage Them

As you begin your third month of pregnancy, you may notice that your morning sickness is decreasing. At the same time, you may notice changes in your breasts, skin, and digestion. All of these changes are normal during pregnancy.

## Nausea

Most women start to feel relief from nausea this month. While you wait for your symptoms to pass, remember to keep handy the remedies that help ease your queasiness and to drink as much fluid as you can during the day.

## Fatigue and Sleep Problems

You probably still are feeling exhausted during the day from all the changes happening in your body. But, as these first few months pass, it may become more difficult to get a good night's sleep. As your abdomen grows larger, it will be harder to find a comfortable position. To help you get the rest you need, you may find the following suggestions useful:

• Try sleeping on your side with a pillow under your abdomen and another pillow between your legs.

• Take a shower or warm bath at bedtime to help you relax.

• Exercise can promote good sleep. Try a relaxing exercise, like yoga, before bedtime to help initiate a restful sleep.

• Make sure your bedroom area is pleasant and relaxing. The bed should be comfortable, and the room should not be too hot or cold or too bright.

## Acne

Acne is common during pregnancy. If you are prone to acne, you may notice that it gets worse during pregnancy. If you've never had it, you may find yourself dealing with acne breakouts during these months. If you get acne during pregnancy, you can take the following steps to treat your skin:

• Wash your face twice a day with a mild cleanser and lukewarm water.

• If you have oily hair, shampoo every day and try to keep your hair off your face.

• Avoid picking or squeezing acne sores to lessen possible scarring.

• Choose oil-free cosmetics.

Many medications can be used to treat acne. Some are available as the active ingredients in over-the-counter products. Others are available only by prescription. As with any medication you take during pregnancy, ask your health care provider before trying any over-the-counter product to treat your acne. Tell any health care provider who is treating you for acne that you are pregnant.

Most over-the-counter acne products are applied directly on the skin (topical). Because the amount of medication absorbed through the skin is very low, they are considered safe to use during pregnancy, even if they have not been tested in pregnant women. Over-the-counter products containing the following ingredients can be used during pregnancy:

- Topical benzoyl peroxide
- Azelaic acid
- Topical salicylic acid
- Glycolic acid

If you want to use an over-the-counter product that contains an ingredient not on this list, contact your health care provider.

Some acne medications can seriously harm your unborn baby. The following medications should not be used while you are pregnant:

- Hormonal therapy
- **Isotretinoin**
- Oral tetracyclines
- Topical retinoids

Some topical retinoids are available by prescription (tretinoin). However, retinols can be found in some over-the-counter products. Read labels carefully. If you are concerned about which products to use to treat your acne, talk with your dermatologist or health care provider. Together you can decide which option is best for you. For more information about medication use in pregnancy, see Chapter 21, "Reducing Risks of Birth Defects."

## Breast Changes

Early in pregnancy, your breasts begin changing to get ready for feeding the baby. By now, your breasts may even have grown a whole bra-cup size. They may be very sore. Many changes are taking place:

- Fat builds up in the breasts, making your normal bra too tight.

- The number of milk glands increases as your body prepares for making milk.

- The nipples and areolas (the pink or brownish skin around your nipples) get darker.

- Your nipples may begin to stick out more, and the areolas will grow larger.

Your breasts may keep growing in size and weight during these first 3 months. If they are making you uncomfortable, now is the time to switch to a good maternity bra. These bras have wide straps, more coverage in the cups, and extra rows of hooks so you can adjust the band size. You also might want to buy a special sleep bra for nighttime support. If you exercise regularly, you may want to consider an athletic bra with good support.

By the end of your third trimester, your breasts may start leaking a thick, yellow fluid called **colostrum**. Colostrum contains proteins and **antibodies** that nourish your newborn until your breasts start making milk a few days after birth. Don't worry, however, if your breasts don't leak, because it doesn't happen to all women.

## Constipation

Increased levels of hormones cause your digestive system to work more slowly. This slower functioning of your gut may lead to constipation. The iron in prenatal vitamin supplements also can contribute to constipation. To help ease this problem, drink plenty of liquids and increase your intake of fiber, which is found in fruits, vegetables, and whole grains. A side effect of increased fiber consumption, however, is gas formation. To combat this problem, try eating your meals more slowly, and avoid anything that causes you to swallow air, such as gum chewing and carbonated drinks. Your body eventually will adjust to the dietary changes. Talk to your health care provider if these measures don't ease constipation.

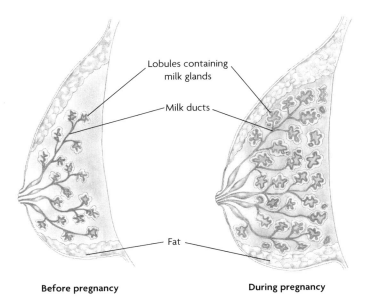

Lobules containing milk glands

Milk ducts

Fat

Before pregnancy

During pregnancy

**Breast changes during pregnancy.** During pregnancy, the fat layer of your breasts thickens, and the number of milk glands increases. Because of these changes, your breasts enlarge.

## 〰 Nutrition

This month, you may have started to put on a few extra pounds. Your health care provider will track your weight each month. As you plan your meals, make sure that you are getting enough iron—a key mineral that most women need more of during pregnancy.

### Weight Gain

You may be noticing that your clothes are starting to fit a little snugly around the waist. By the end of week 12, most women have gained between 1 ½ pounds and 4 ½ pounds, although some women will have lost weight due to morning sickness. Don't worry if you have lost a pound or two; you will gain it back in the coming months. The chart on the next page gives you a general picture of the weight gain that is recommended during pregnancy.

### Sugar and Sugar Substitutes

Limit the amount of simple sugars you eat daily. Simple sugars are found in foods such as table sugar, honey, syrup, fruit juices, soft drinks, and many processed foods. Although they may give you a quick energy boost, they have more **calories** than other **nutrients**, and the energy they give is used up quickly. They also contribute to excess weight gain.

### Focus on Iron

Iron is used by your body to make the extra blood that you and your baby need during pregnancy. Pregnant women need 27 mg of iron a day (nonpregnant women need 18 mg a day). This increased amount is found in most prenatal vitamin supplements. Vitamin supplements with higher iron levels may cause digestion problems, such as constipation.

You also can eat foods rich in a certain type of iron called heme iron. Heme iron is absorbed more easily by the body. It is found in animal foods, such as red meat, poultry, and fish. Nonheme iron is found in vegetables and legumes, such as soybeans, spinach, and lentils. Although it is not as easily absorbed as heme iron, nonheme iron is a good way to get extra iron if you do not eat animal foods. Iron also can be absorbed more easily if iron-rich foods are eaten with vitamin C-rich foods, such as citrus fruits and tomatoes.

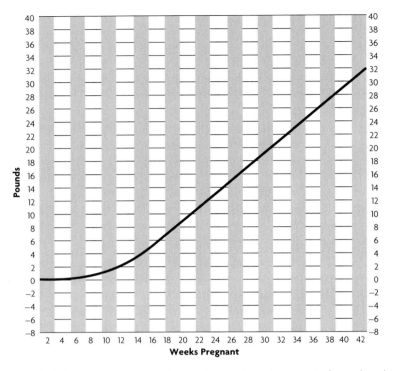

**Weight gain during pregnancy.** This graph shows how much weight a woman of normal weight should gain throughout pregnancy. Copyright 2009 March of Dimes.

If you normally use some of the following artificial sweeteners, which are 200–600 times sweeter than sugar, they are still safe to use while you're pregnant as long as you use them in moderation:

- Saccharin (Sweet'n Low)
- Aspartame (Equal and NutraSweet)
- Sucralose (Splenda)
- Acesulfame-K (Sunett)
- Stevia (Truvia and SweetLeaf)

## Exercise

If you haven't been exercising regularly, try simple things—like taking the stairs instead of the elevator—to get more exercise into your life. If you have been exercising, this month's exercise can help you start toning strategic muscles in your hips and abdomen.

## Exercise of the Month: 4-Point Kneeling

This exercise strengthens and tones the abdominal muscles.

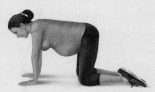

1. Kneel on all fours. Make sure that your hips are positioned directly over your knees and your shoulders are positioned directly over your hands. Your back should be straight, not curved upward or downward.

2. Inhale deeply. Then, exhale. As you exhale, pull your abdominal muscles in. Imagine that you are pulling your belly button inward up to your spine. Breathe normally; do not hold your breath. Make sure your back stays straight. This is called "engaging" your abdominal muscles.

3. Return to the starting position and repeat five times.

### Get Moving

Ideally, pregnant women should get at least 30 minutes per day of exercise that increases the heart rate and some strength exercises on most days of the week. However, it may be tough to get started if you're not used to exercising regularly. There are simple ways of adding additional movement into your daily life. Try going to your local shopping mall and walking to the farthest end and back. Or, while you're at the grocery store, do a couple of laps around the perimeter of the store—where the most healthy and least processed foods are found. Take the stairs instead of the elevator. The important thing is to get moving a little more each day while you're pregnant to get the best benefits.

### Healthy Decisions

If you have had a previous *cesarean delivery*, you will need to think about how you will have your baby this time around and discuss your options with your health care provider. Another important decision to consider is genetic screening for *birth defects*.

### Vaginal Birth After Cesarean Delivery

If you have had a baby by cesarean delivery in the past, it is important to talk about your delivery plans with your health care provider early in your *prenatal care*. Many women who have had a past cesarean delivery can try to have a *vaginal birth after cesarean delivery (VBAC)*. Vaginal birth after cesarean provides many benefits for women. Women who have a VBAC avoid major surgery and the risks that go along with it. Recovery is shorter after a vaginal delivery compared with a cesarean delivery. If you want more children, having a VBAC can help you avoid some of the potential future complications of multiple cesarean deliveries, such as infection, bowel or *bladder* injury, or *hysterectomy*.

However, there are some risks involved with a VBAC that may not make it the right choice for every woman. The decision of whether to try a vaginal delivery or to have a repeat cesarean delivery can be complex. Let your health care provider know if you're interested in trying to have a VBAC with this pregnancy. Together, you and your health care provider can consider the risks and benefits that apply to your individual situation. For detailed information about VBAC, see Chapter 15, "Cesarean Delivery and Vaginal Birth After Cesarean Delivery."

### Prenatal Genetic Screening and Diagnosis

There are now many ways to screen for certain birth defects and *genetic disorders* during pregnancy and to provide diagnostic testing for those who desire it. Prenatal *screening tests* are available for certain chromosomal defects such as *Down syndrome* and for *neural tube defects* such as *spina bifida*. Prenatal *diagnostic tests* are available for chromosomal defects as well as many specific inherited disorders, such as *cystic fibrosis*, *sickle cell disease*, *Tay–Sachs disease*, and *thalassemias.*

*Screening tests* for birth defects are offered to all pregnant women. *Diagnostic tests* also are available as a first choice for all pregnant women, even for those who do not have risk factors. Screening tests can tell you whether you are at increased risk of having a child with a certain birth defect, but they cannot tell you for sure whether your baby has the disorder or not. Diagnostic tests can tell you whether the *fetus* has a certain birth defect. Results are either "positive" (a defect is present) or "negative" (no defect is present).

Deciding if you want to be tested, and if so, what types of tests to have, involves considering a lot of different factors. Here are some important things to consider when making a decision:

- Screening tests for neural tube defects and chromosomal disorders carry no risks for the fetus. They are done using a specialized *ultrasound exam* called a **nuchal translucency screening** and a sample of your blood. Diagnostic tests are invasive, meaning that a sample of **amniotic fluid** or tissue from the **placenta** needs to be obtained through **amniocentesis** or **chorionic villus sampling (CVS)**. There is a small risk of pregnancy loss with these diagnostic procedures (about 1 pregnancy loss for every 300–500 procedures performed).

• First-trimester screening tests are able to detect approximately 85% of cases of Down syndrome, and second-trimester screening tests can detect approximately 80% of cases of Down syndrome. Combining results of first-trimester and second-trimester screening tests provides a Down syndrome detection rate of 94–96%. Diagnostic testing has a detection rate of more than 99% for many disorders.

• Screening tests for neural tube defects and chromosomal disorders can be performed in the first trimester or in the second trimester. Diagnostic tests also are performed in the first trimester (between 10 weeks and 12 weeks of pregnancy for CVS) and in the second trimester (between 15 weeks and 20 weeks of pregnancy for amniocentesis). Getting results in the first trimester from a diagnostic procedure is appealing to many parents-to-be because it gives more time to make decisions.

Your health care provider can explain all of the options to you and help you decide which tests are best for your particular situation. Your personal beliefs and values are important factors in this decision. The choice that's right for one woman may not be right for another. Some parents want to know beforehand if their child will have a birth defect so that they can be prepared. Knowing beforehand also gives you the opportunity to learn about the disorder and to organize the care that the child will need. Some parents may decide to end the pregnancy in certain situations. Pregnancy termination carries less risk of complications if it is performed before 13 weeks of pregnancy. This timing may affect which tests a woman chooses to have.

**Genetic counselors** or other health care provider with expertise in genetics can help you understand whether you are at risk of having a child with certain genetic disorders. In genetic counseling, a genetic counselor or someone with special training in genetics asks you and the baby's father for a detailed family history. If a family member has a problem, the counselor may ask to see that person's medical records. You also may be referred for physical exams or tests. Using all the information gathered, the counselor will assess the baby's risk of having a problem. The counselor then will discuss the options for prenatal testing. A detailed discussion of all of the available screening and diagnostic tests that are offered can be found in Chapter 25, "Screening and Diagnostic Testing for Genetic Disorders."

## ≋ Other Considerations

This month, you may notice other changes that may concern you. Your mood may be up one minute and down the next. These sudden mood shifts can be disconcerting if you were not expecting them. You also may be noticing changes in your skin, such as dark pigmentation on your face or abdomen. Another common concern is what to do if you become sick with the flu, a cold, or diarrhea. There are steps you can take to deal with these illnesses safely during pregnancy.

### Emotional Changes

Your body is going through big changes now, and so are your emotions. Don't blame yourself if you are sad or moody. The emotions you are feeling—happy or sad—are normal. Ask loved ones to support you and be patient. If your emotions are affecting your work or personal relationships and you're concerned about these issues, talk to your health care provider.

### Skin Changes

During pregnancy, your body produces more *melanin*—the pigment that gives color to skin. This increase in melanin is the reason your nipples become darker, for example. It also causes the skin condition known as *melasma* during pregnancy. Melasma causes brown patches to appear on the face around the cheeks, nose, and forehead. When it appears in pregnant women, it is called *chloasma* or the "mask of pregnancy." Spending time in the sun can make chloasma worse, so protect yourself by wearing sun block and a hat and limiting your exposure to direct sunlight. Melasma usually fades on its own after you have the baby. Some women, however, may have dark patches that last for years.

Some women also notice a faint, dark line that runs from their belly button to their pubic hair. This is called the *linea nigra*. This line is always there, but before you become pregnant it is the same color as the skin around it.

Stretch marks may appear later in pregnancy. The skin on your belly and breasts may become streaked with reddish brown, purple, or dark brown marks, depending on your skin color. Some women also get them on their buttocks, thighs, and hips. Stretch marks are caused by changes in the elastic supportive tissue that lies just beneath the skin. There are no proven remedies that keep them from appearing or make them go away. Keeping your belly well moisturized as it grows may reduce itching, though. Once your baby is born, some of these streaks will slowly fade in color.

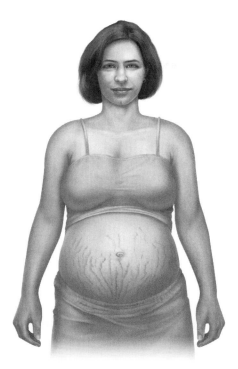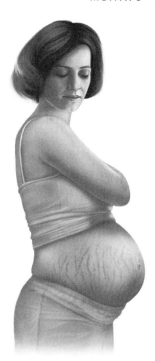

**Stretch marks**

## Getting Sick

Pregnant women can get a cold or come down with the flu just like anyone else. Here are some tips to follow if you become sick:

- Colds—Catching a cold can make you feel miserable whenever it happens, but getting sick while you're pregnant may make you more miserable than ever. Ask your health care provider about the safety of taking any over-the-counter medication while you are pregnant. Also, get plenty of rest and drink plenty of fluids.

- Flu—Flu symptoms are more severe than those of colds. Pregnancy can increase the risk of complications from the flu, such as pneumonia. Depending on your general health and other factors, your health care provider may prescribe an antiviral drug that can help shorten the flu's duration. For antiviral medication to be effective, it must be taken within 48 hours of the onset of symptoms. If you think you are getting the flu, call your health care provider right away. Don't wait for your symptoms to get worse (see box "Common Symptoms of the Flu").

## Common Symptoms of the Flu

- Fever over 101°F
- Muscle aches and pains
- Extreme fatigue and weakness
- Headache
- Dry cough
- Sore throat
- Loss of appetite

All pregnant women should get the flu vaccine as soon as it becomes available (usually a month or two before "flu season"—from October to May—starts). Protection from the vaccine usually begins 1–2 weeks after getting the shot. The protection lasts 6 months or longer. A flu shot is considered safe at any stage of pregnancy. However, the nasal flu mist is not approved for use in pregnant women.

- Diarrhea—If you come down with a bout of diarrhea, drink plenty of liquids to avoid getting dehydrated. If it continues, call your health care provider to report your symptoms and find out whether there are any over-the-counter antidiarrhea medications that you should take.

## ➣ Prenatal Care Visits

Prenatal care involves tests, physical exams, and imaging exams (such as ultrasound exams) that are performed to assess the health and well-being of you and your baby. It gives you the opportunity to learn about your pregnancy and to ask your health care provider questions. Prenatal visits also allow your health care provider to detect any medical or psychological problems and provide care. Some of the tests that are performed during pregnancy may be mandated by state law. Most commonly, state-regulated tests are those that screen for certain *sexually transmitted infections (STIs)*.

How often you will see your health care provider for prenatal care depends on your health history, obstetric history, and other factors. Typically, if this is your first pregnancy and you do not have any complications, you will see your health care provider every 4 weeks for the first 28 weeks of pregnancy, every 2 weeks until 36 weeks of pregnancy, and weekly thereafter. If you have had a successful prior pregnancy and you're healthy, you may be able to have less frequent scheduled visits as long as you are able to see your health care provider on an as-needed basis.

## Ultrasound Exam

An ultrasound exam makes an image of your baby from sound waves. These sound waves are produced by a device called a *transducer*. The transducer is either moved across your abdomen, which is called a *transabdominal ultrasound* scan, or placed in your vagina, which is called a *transvaginal ultrasound* scan. The method chosen depends on the purpose of the exam and the *gestational age* of the fetus.

Some women have an ultrasound exam performed early in pregnancy. This exam often is done to confirm the pregnancy and to help estimate the gestational age. Other reasons for performing a first-trimester ultrasound exam include the following:

- Determine whether the baby's heart is beating
- Check whether there is more than one baby
- Screen for birth defects (in combination with a maternal blood test)
- Examine the uterus and *ovaries*

## Pelvic Exam

Your health care provider may do a *pelvic exam* to assess the size of the pelvis and uterus. Cervical cancer screening may be done to check for changes in the *cervix* that could lead to cancer depending on whether you are due for this screening .

## Lab Tests

The following tests are performed early in pregnancy and may not be done at the same prenatal care visit:

- *Complete blood count (CBC)*—The CBC counts the numbers of different types of *cells* that make up your blood. The number of red blood cells can show whether you have a certain type of *anemia*. The number of white blood cells shows how many disease-fighting cells are in your blood, and the number of platelets can reveal whether you have a problem with blood clotting.

- Blood type—During the first trimester of pregnancy, you will have a blood test to find out your blood type and whether you are Rh positive or

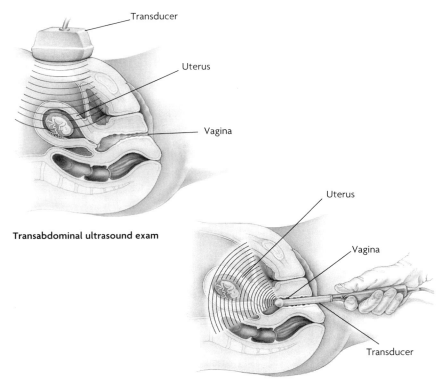

**Transabdominal ultrasound exam**

**Transvaginal ultrasound exam**

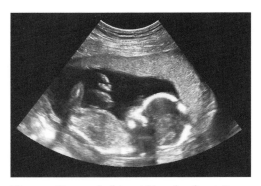

**Ultrasound image of a fetus at 17 weeks of gestation**

**Ultrasound exam.** During an ultrasound exam, sound waves are produced by a transducer. These sound waves are reflected off the fetus. The reflected sound waves are changed into pictures that you and your health care provider can view on a screen.

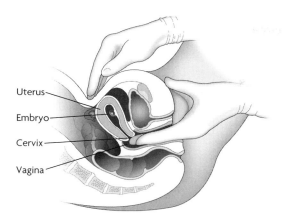

Uterus
Embryo
Cervix
Vagina

**Pelvic exam.** During a pelvic exam, your health care provider checks your internal organs by inserting one or two fingers into the vagina while pressing on your abdomen with the other hand.

Rh negative. Just as there are different major blood groups, such as type A and type B, there also is an ***Rh factor***. The Rh factor is a protein that can be present on the surface of red blood cells. Most people have the Rh factor—they are Rh positive. Others do not have the Rh factor—they are Rh negative. If the fetus is Rh positive and the woman is Rh negative, the woman's body can make antibodies against the Rh factor that can damage the fetus's red blood cells. Problems usually do not occur in a first pregnancy when only a small number of antibodies are made, but they can occur in a later pregnancy. These problems can be prevented by giving ***Rh immunoglobulin*** during pregnancy. More information about Rh incompatibility can be found in Chapter 28, "Blood Type Incompatibility."

• Urinalysis—Your urine may be tested for red blood cells (to see if you have urinary tract disease), white blood cells (to see if you have a urinary tract infection), and ***glucose*** (high levels may be a sign of ***diabetes***). The amount of protein also is measured. The protein level early in pregnancy can be compared with levels later in pregnancy. High protein levels may be a sign of ***preeclampsia***, a serious complication that usually occurs later in pregnancy or after the baby is born.

• Urine culture—This test looks for ***bacteria*** in your urine, which can be a sign of a urinary tract infection. Sometimes these infections do not cause symptoms. Your urine will be tested early in pregnancy and again later in pregnancy. If your test result shows that you have bacteria in your urine, you will be treated with ***antibiotics***. After you finish treatment, you may have a repeat test to see if the bacteria are gone.

- *Rubella*—Your blood is tested to check whether you have had a past infection with rubella (sometimes called German measles) or if you have been vaccinated against this disease. Rubella can cause birth defects if a woman is infected during pregnancy. If you had this infection before or you have been vaccinated, you are not likely to get it again—you are *immune* to the disease. If your blood test shows you are not immune, you should avoid anyone who has the disease while you are pregnant because it is highly contagious. The vaccine contains a live *virus* and is not recommended for pregnant women. If you have not had the vaccine, you should get it after the baby is born, even if you are breastfeeding.

- *Hepatitis*—Hepatitis B and hepatitis C are viruses that infect the liver. Pregnant women who are infected with hepatitis B or hepatitis C can pass the virus to their babies. All pregnant women are tested for *hepatitis B virus* infection. If you have risk factors, you also may be tested for the *hepatitis C virus.* If you are infected with either virus, you may need special care during pregnancy. Your baby also may need special care after birth. You still can breastfeed if you have either infection. A vaccine that protects against hepatitis B is available. It is given in a series of three shots, with the first dose given to the baby within a few hours of birth.

- Sexually transmitted infections—All pregnant women are tested for *syphilis* and *chlamydia* early in pregnancy. Tests for these STIs may be repeated later in pregnancy if you have certain risk factors. If you have risk factors for *gonorrhea* (you are aged 25 years or younger or you live in an area where gonorrhea is common), you also will be tested for this STI.

- *Human immunodeficiency virus (HIV)*—This virus attacks cells of the body's immune system and causes *acquired immunodeficiency syndrome (AIDS)*. If you are infected with HIV, there is a chance you could pass it to your baby. While you are pregnant, you can be given medication that can greatly reduce this risk and get specialized care to ensure that you stay as healthy as possible throughout your pregnancy. Your baby also can get specialized care after birth.

- *Tuberculosis (TB)*—Women at high risk of TB (for example, women who are infected with HIV or who live in close contact with someone who has TB) should be tested for this infection.

### Genetic Testing

First-trimester screening tests for chromosomal defects and other birth defects may be performed this month. If you have chosen to have CVS, a technique used for diagnostic testing for certain birth defects, it is performed between 10 weeks and 12 weeks of pregnancy. Amniocentesis is performed later, usually between 15 weeks and 20 weeks of pregnancy.

 ## Special Concerns

It's important to be alert to things that may be harmful during pregnancy, including sexually transmitted infections and domestic violence. Recognizing these risks early will allow you to get the treatment or help you need sooner and prevent harm to yourself and your unborn baby.

### Sexually Transmitted Infections

Sexually transmitted infections are passed from one person to another through sexual contact. There are many different STIs (see Chapter 30, "Protecting Yourself From Infections"). Some STIs can be harmful during pregnancy. For instance, if you have an STI, you are more likely to have **preterm** labor. You are tested for certain STIs early in your pregnancy. Some tests are repeated later in pregnancy, depending on your risk factors. That's why it is important to be honest with your health care provider about your risks. But by far the best strategy to prevent complications associated with STIs is to be tested and treated before pregnancy.

For some STIs, such as chlamydia, gonorrhea, and syphilis, treatment is available. For other STIs, such as **genital herpes** and HIV, there is no treatment, although signs and symptoms often can be managed. If you are diagnosed with a treatable STI during pregnancy, you will receive treatment. You may be tested again to see if the treatment has worked. Your sex partner or partners also should be treated.

### Intimate Partner Violence

An abusive relationship is one in which one partner subjects the other to emotional, physical, or sexual abuse. Emotional abuse can take the form of constant name-calling, criticism, and extreme jealousy. In physical abuse, a partner may push, slap, or kick you. Sexual abuse involves sexual activity without your consent. But whether the abuse is emotional, physical, or sexual, it is all considered intimate partner violence.

Intimate partner violence (also called domestic violence) is a common and tragic problem in the United States. Intimate partner violence is the leading cause of injury to women in the United States between the ages of 15 years and 44 years and is estimated to be responsible for 20–25% of hospital emergency room visits by women.

Intimate partner violence can happen to people of any race, age, sexual orientation, religion, or gender. It can happen to couples who are married, living together, of the same sex, or dating. It happens to people of all socioeconomic and educational backgrounds. Abuse doesn't have to happen every day or every week for it to be classified as intimate partner violence.

Pregnancy often offers no break from the abuse. In fact, one in six abused women is first abused during pregnancy. More than 320,000 women each year are abused by their partners while they are pregnant. Abuse puts both the pregnant woman and her baby at risk. The dangers of physical abuse include *miscarriage*, vaginal bleeding, *low birth weight*, and fetal injury.

It isn't easy to realize or admit that the person whom you love or once loved, or who is the parent of your child, is an abuser. But if you are in a violent relationship, it's vital to take steps to protect yourself and your baby. Abusers often blame others for their own actions. No matter what your partner says, it is not your fault. You do not make it happen. The abuser is the one to blame for the abusive actions.

The first step to breaking the pattern of violence is to tell someone about it. Tell someone you trust—a close friend, a family member, your health care provider, a nurse, a counselor, or a clergy member. Talking about a problem can be a huge relief. You also can seek out resources in your area, such as crisis hotlines, intimate partner violence programs, legal aid services, and shelters for abused women.

Getting ready to leave an abusive relationship can be difficult, but knowing these tips can help:

- Contact your local shelter for domestic violence victims and find out about laws and other resources available to you. For example, some shelters and programs offer donated cell phones that can allow you to make arrangements to leave or contact the police. Your abuser can't track your phone calls on a donated phone.

- Keep any evidence of physical abuse, such as pictures, and write down dates of when the abuse happens.

- If you are injured, go to the emergency room and report what happened to you.

- Try to set money aside or ask friends or family members to hold money for you.

Once you decide to leave, be prepared for a safe, quick escape:

- You may request a police stand-by or escort while you leave.

- Make a plan for how you will escape and where you will go.

- Hide an extra set of car keys.

- Pack an extra set of clothes for yourself and your children and store them at a trusted friend or neighbor's house. Don't forget toys for the children.

- Take with you important phone numbers of friends, relatives, doctors, and schools, as well as other important items, including the following:
  —Your driver's license
  —Regularly needed medication
  —Credit cards or a list of credit cards you hold yourself or jointly
  —Pay stubs
  —Checkbooks and information about bank accounts and other assets
  —Birth certificates for you and your children

It's hard to break the cycle of violence. If you do nothing though, chances are the abuse will happen more often and will become more severe. Leaving your partner or having him or her arrested during your pregnancy takes great courage. But you owe your baby a safe and loving home, and you owe yourself an end to the violence. For more information or to get help, call the National Domestic Violence Hotline (see Resources).

## ASK THE EXPERTS

### Are saunas and hot tubs safe?

Some studies have suggested that prolonged time in a sauna or hot tub use may cause an increase in a woman's core body temperature and may lead to birth defects in a developing baby. The American College of Obstetricians and Gynecologists advises pregnant women to remain in saunas for no more than 15 minutes and hot tubs for no more than 10 minutes at a time. It's also suggested that a pregnant woman avoid submerging her head, arms, and shoulders in the hot tub to decrease the areas exposed to heat.

### Do I have to get rid of my cat?

No. You may have heard that cat feces are a source of the infection **toxoplasmosis**, but there's no need to give away your pet. The infection is only present in cats that have access to the outdoors and hunt prey. If your cat never goes outside, only eats cat food, and does not hunt any prey (for example, mice and other rodents), your risk of toxoplasmosis is extremely low. The infection can be very serious for pregnant women. If you have a cat that goes outdoors or may eat prey, have someone else take over cleaning the litter box. (Note that clean cat litter is not dangerous; the feces and the litter that has come in contact with it are what you should avoid.) The litter should be changed daily. If you do it yourself, wear disposable gloves and wash your hands thoroughly afterwards. Keep in mind that toxoplasmosis also can be acquired when working with soil or eating raw or undercooked meat. It's essential to wear gloves when gardening and to avoid raw or rare meat.

### Is hair dye safe to use during pregnancy?

There are different types of hair dyes, including permanent, semipermanent, and temporary hair dyes. All contain different types and levels of chemicals. Studies on animals indicate that high doses of these chemicals (100 times the amount that humans would use) do not cause serious birth defects. In addition, only a very small amount of the chemicals in hair dye are absorbed through the scalp into the bloodstream. Most experts conclude that using hair dye during pregnancy is not a cause for concern.

---

# RESOURCES

The following resources offer more information about some of the topics discussed in this chapter:

**Making Sense of Your Genes: A Guide to Genetic Counseling**
Genetic Alliance
www.geneticalliance.org/publications/guidetogeneticcounseling
*Web site that discusses genetic counseling and how it's used in various situations, including prenatally.*

**National Domestic Violence Hotline**
1-800-799-SAFE (7233)
www.thehotline.org

*Hotline to call for help and resources to deal with intimate partner violence and abuse. Caution: Internet use can be tracked. If you think that your abuser is monitoring the sites you visit, use the phone hotline instead, preferably from a phone only you have access to.*

**Skin and Hair Changes During Pregnancy**
Medline Plus
www.nlm.nih.gov/medlineplus/ency/patientinstructions/000611.htm

*Describes the normal changes that can happen to skin and hair during pregnancy and provides guidance about when to call your health care provider.*

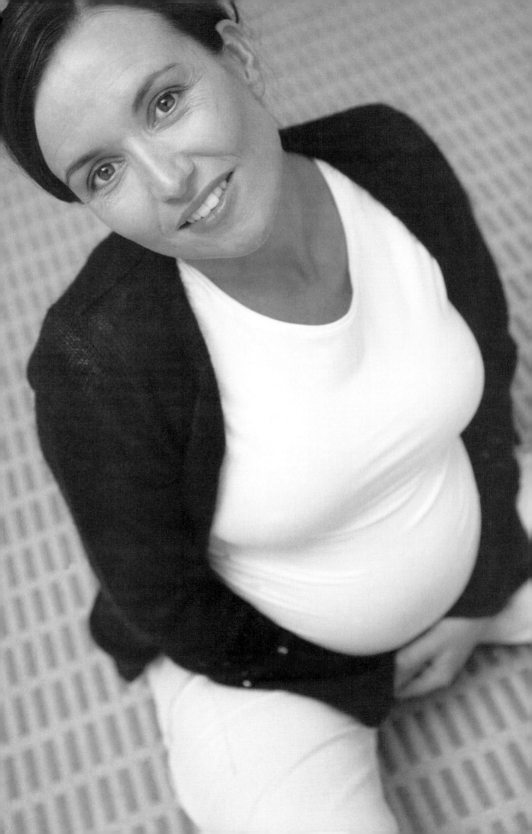

# Chapter 4

# Month 4

### (Weeks 13–16)

## YOUR GROWING BABY

### Week 13

Your baby is beginning to grow at a quicker pace. The organs are fully formed and will grow even more this trimester. For instance, the spleen is working to produce red blood **cells**. Your baby's sex hormones (**testosterone** and **estrogen**) also are being made. On an ultrasound exam, you may see your baby making breathing-like movements and swallowing **amniotic fluid**.

### Week 14

The eyes are beginning to move, and the arms and legs now can flex. The hands will soon open and close into fists, and movements such as putting the hands to the mouth are happening more frequently. The organs of taste and smell are developing. Also, the baby's skin is starting to become thicker, and hair follicles are appearing just below the skin surface.

### Week 15

The baby is becoming more active now in the **amniotic sac**, rolling around and doing flips. The heart is pumping about 100 pints of blood each day, and the **kidneys** are now producing urine.

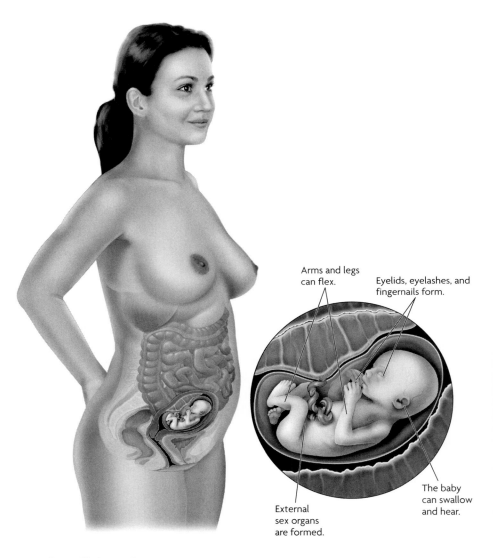

Arms and legs can flex.

Eyelids, eyelashes, and fingernails form.

External sex organs are formed.

The baby can swallow and hear.

**Mother and baby: Weeks 13–16.** Your baby weighs about 5 ounces and is about 5 inches long now.

## Week 16

Your baby weighs about 5 ounces and is about 5 inches long now. Facial features, such as eyelids, ears, and an upper lip, can be seen. He or she can hear sounds now. The digestive system is working, even the stomach. The baby's external genitals also are defined, and you may be able to see them if you have an ultrasound exam.

# YOUR PREGNANCY

## 〜 Your Changing Body

Welcome to the second trimester! Most women feel their best during these next couple of months—so much so that the second trimester is called the "honeymoon period" of pregnancy. Your morning sickness has probably subsided, your energy level may be back to normal, and your pregnancy may be starting to show. The second trimester also marks the time when many women worry a little less because the risk of *miscarriage* is lower. And beginning this month, your uterus is large enough that it is no longer completely within the pelvis.

## 〜 Discomforts and How to Manage Them

This month's discomforts may include spider veins and changes in your gums, teeth, and mouth—even strange dreams. You also may experience aches and pains in your abdomen, which can be worrying. It helps to know what pain is normal and what isn't—and when you should call your health care provider.

### Lower Abdominal Pain

As the uterus grows, the round ligaments (bands of tissue that support the uterus on both sides) are pulled and stretched. You may feel this stretching as either a dull ache or a sharp pain on one side of your belly. The pain may be most noticeable when you cough or sneeze. Not moving for a short time or changing position may help relieve the pain.

If abdominal pain doesn't go away or gets worse, call your health care provider. It could be a sign of a problem.

### Mouth and Dental Changes

Another surprising change that you may not have expected during pregnancy are changes in your mouth, teeth, and gums. Pregnancy can cause a variety of changes that include the following:

• Your gums may be more sensitive to flossing and brushing and may swell or bleed. This is called *gingivitis*. Untreated gingivitis can progress to *periodontal disease*, in which inflammation leads to the buildup of plaque below the gum line, which in turn can create pockets of infection. This infection can destroy the teeth, gums, and bone. Periodontal disease has been linked to an increased risk of *preterm* birth. Rinsing with saltwater (1 teaspoon of salt in 1 cup of warm water) and switching to a softer toothbrush may help lessen irritation.

- You may develop sores in your mouth known as granuloma gravidarum. These sores are a caused by the *immune system* working overtime to get rid of any disease-causing germs in your mouth. They usually go away after pregnancy.

- Your teeth may feel looser. This happens because during pregnancy, a hormone is produced that relaxes ligaments in the pelvis, which makes giving birth easier. This same hormone, however, also may relax the tiny ligaments that hold the teeth in place. It's usually not enough to cause you to lose a tooth, but it can be annoying.

- You may have tooth erosion. If you've had morning sickness, frequent vomiting may expose your teeth to higher-than-normal levels of acid, which can erode the enamel on the teeth. This acid also may make you more susceptible to dental caries (or "cavities").

It's important to continue your usual dental care during pregnancy, which means continuing to brush and floss and seeing your dentist for routine checkups every 6 months. A dental checkup early in pregnancy helps make sure that your mouth stays healthy. The American Dental Association recommends timing any elective dental procedures to occur during the second trimester or first half of the third trimester and to postpone any major dental work until after you've had your baby. If an emergency dental issue arises— you need a root canal, for instance— it's usually recommended that you have the procedure in order to prevent the problem from getting worse. If you will need *general anesthesia* or sedation, your dentist should consult with your pregnancy health care provider.

## Strange Dreams

It's normal to have unusual dreams—especially in the last trimester—that may be vivid and scary. Experts believe these types of dreams may provide a way for your subconscious to cope with any fears and doubts you have about pregnancy and becoming a mother.

### Excessive Salivation

Some women notice that they have excessive salivation during pregnancy, especially when they're nauseated. This condition is more common among women who have severe morning sickness.

The exact cause of excessive salivation is not known, but hormonal changes may be a reason. Also, nausea might make some women try to swallow less, causing saliva to build up in the mouth. If this is a problem for you, tell your health care provider.

### Spider Veins

You may have tiny red veins that show up under the skin of your face or legs. Spider veins are a normal part of the changes in your circulation and usually fade once you give birth.

## ✐ Nutrition

This month may bring food cravings that you didn't expect, which can be a challenge when you are trying to eat a healthy diet. One thing you can do to eat more healthfully is to learn about high- and low- glycemic foods.

### Weight Gain

Eating a healthy diet and gaining a healthy amount of weight during pregnancy is important for your well-being and that of your growing baby. Different stages of pregnancy can present certain challenges to healthy eating. In the first trimester, morning sickness can affect your eating habits. You may crave certain foods or not feel like eating. Usually, though, your appetite increases in the second trimester. Some women again lose their appetites in the third trimester because nausea sometimes returns. Throughout your pregnancy, it is important to stick to a healthy diet to ensure that you and your baby are getting all of the **nutrients** you need. It's a balancing act that may often prove challenging. See Chapter 17, "Nutrition During Pregnancy," for more detailed information about how to keep eating a healthy diet throughout your pregnancy. Also see the weight gain chart in Chapter 3, "Month 3 (Weeks 9–12)," to check that your weight gain is on track.

## Food Cravings

Pregnant women often have food cravings. Occasionally giving in to these cravings is okay. Cravings can cause problems, however, if you eat only a few types of food for long periods. They also can be less than healthy if you indulge your cravings for one type of food and neglect the rest of your diet. Eating lots of sugary foods, for instance, can lead to excessive weight gain and tooth problems.

Some women may feel a strong urge to eat nonfood items, such as laundry starch, clay, or chalk. This condition is called *pica*. If you feel these urges, don't indulge in them. Eating nonfood items can be harmful and can prevent you from getting the nutrients you need. Call your health care provider if you think you have pica.

### Focus on High- and Low-Glycemic Foods

As you learn to eat a healthier diet, it may be a good idea to be familiar with which foods have a high and low glycemic index. Foods with a low glycemic index are part of an overall healthier eating plan.

The glycemic index is a ranking of how quickly foods that contain the complex sugars called carbohydrates increase your blood **glucose** (sugar) level. A food with a high glycemic index increases blood glucose levels more rapidly than a food with a medium or low glycemic index. Foods with a high glycemic index provide a quick burst of energy, whereas foods with a low glycemic index provide a slower, more even burning of energy. You may feel less hungry when you eat foods with a low glycemic index, and you may be able to sustain higher energy levels for a longer period of time.

Foods with a high glycemic index tend to be white: white breads, potatoes, white rice, and popcorn; however, not all foods with a high glycemic index are white—pretzels also fall into this category. The following foods have a low glycemic index:

- 100% whole-wheat, multigrain, or pumpernickel bread
- Oatmeal (rolled or steel cut), oat bran, and muesli
- Whole-wheat pasta, brown rice, and barley
- Sweet potatoes, corn, yams, lima or butter beans, peas, and legumes and lentils
- Apples, oranges, and peaches
- Nonstarchy vegetables and carrots

## 〰 Exercise

You may be feeling much more energized this month, so now is a good time to rev up your exercise routine. This month's exercise will help tone your back muscles, which may be getting a workout in the coming months as your uterus grows larger.

### Walking: A Great Way to Stay Motivated

With your energy returning, you may have more motivation to exercise. Walking is a great form of exercise—and one of the easiest. All you need is a good pair of shoes and comfortable clothing. Wear walking shoes or tennis shoes that fit well and give good support, flexibility, and cushioning.

If you need motivation, ask a friend to join you on your walks. If you have other small children, try walking them in their stroller. Make it a family activity. Another way to stay motivated is to keep track of your progress. If you're a beginner, gradually increasing the time and distance that you walk can be a great incentive to keep at it. Various apps and web sites are available that track your distance, speed, *calories* burned, and other factors. Some use a tracking device or bracelet that you can wear all day to monitor your daily activity. You may be surprised by how active you are during the course of a normal day.

### Exercise of the Month: Seated Ball Balance

This exercise strengthens abdominal muscles and helps with balance and stability.

1. Sit on the center of an exercise ball, keeping your spine in a neutral position. Your feet should be flat on the floor, about hips-width apart. Start near a wall for additional balance if needed.

2. Engage you abdominal muscles by imagining that you are pulling your belly button inward to your spine. Your tailbone should relax. Do not hold your breath. Your arms should be relaxed.

3. Raise the left foot off the ground by extending your knee. At the same time, raise your right arm. Hold for a few seconds.

4. Return to the starting position. Alternate four to six times.

## ⤳ Healthy Decisions

Some women with medical conditions may have to take time off before the baby is born. And what about after the baby born? If you work outside the home, it's not too early to start thinking about how much time you or your partner will take off to care for your new arrival. You also may want to give some thought about where you would like to have your baby.

### Your Workplace Rights

Three federal laws protect the health, safety, and employment rights of many pregnant working women. If you think you are being denied your rights, contact the agencies discussed in the following sections. Many states also have laws that protect pregnant workers.

### Pregnancy Discrimination Act

The Pregnancy Discrimination Act prohibits employers from discriminating against a woman because she is pregnant. It states that women affected by pregnancy, childbirth, or related medical conditions are to be treated the same for all employment-related purposes—such as hiring, firing, promotions, and fringe benefits—as other employees or applicants similar in their ability or inability to work. If you think you are the being discriminated against because of pregnancy, contact the U.S. Equal Employment Opportunity Commission (see the "Resources" section in this chapter). The commission's web site also gives details about how to file a claim.

### Occupational Safety and Health Act

The Occupational Safety and Health Act requires employers to provide a workplace free from known hazards that cause or are likely to cause death or serious physical harm. It also requires employers to give workers facts about harmful agents. If you think your employer may be breaking these rules, call the Occupational Safety and Health Administration (OSHA), or go to the OSHA web site (see the "Resources" section in this chapter).

The National Institute for Occupational Safety and Health (NIOSH) is the agency that researches workplace hazards and makes recommendations for preventing workers' injury and illness. Established by OSHA, NIOSH finds workplace hazards, decides how to control them, and suggests ways to limit the dangers. You or your union can request that NIOSH conduct a Health Hazard Evaluation. Call NIOSH or visit the web site where you can ask an occupational safety and health question (see the "Resources" section in this chapter).

Certain state and city laws also give workers and unions the right to ask for the names of chemicals and other substances used in the workplace. If you have questions or concerns, ask your employer or consult OSHA or NIOSH.

## Family and Medical Leave Act

The Family and Medical Leave Act (FMLA) provides eligible employees with up to 12 work weeks of leave without pay in any 12-month period. Under FMLA, you have a right to return to your same job or to an equivalent job at the end of your leave. To qualify for FMLA, you must meet the following conditions:

- Work for a company where there are at least 50 employees of the same employer within a 75-mile area (at a branch office, for instance)
- Have worked there for at least 12 months (these months do not need to be consecutive but need to have occurred within the last 7 years)
- Have worked at least 1,250 hours during the past 12 months

During pregnancy and after your baby is born, FMLA can be taken for the following reasons:

- Prenatal appointments
- Any period of incapacity due to pregnancy (such as severe morning sickness)
- Recovery from childbirth
- To care for a newborn (until the baby is aged 12 months)

Dads also can use FMLA during pregnancy to care for spouses who have an illness caused by pregnancy and after childbirth to care for their newborns.

The 12 weeks do not have to be taken all at once. They can be taken intermittently, but your FMLA cannot exceed a total of 12 weeks per 12-month period. This means that if you use some of the 12 weeks for a difficult pregnancy, you will have less than 12 weeks to take after the baby is born.

You may have to use vacation time or personal or sick leave for some or all of your FMLA leave. If your employer provides health care benefits, this coverage must be kept at the same level during the leave period. If you believe that your FMLA rights are being violated or to file a complaint, contact the Wage and Hour Division (WHD) of the Department of Labor at 1-866-487-9243 to locate the WHD office nearest you or go to www.dol.gov/whd/america2.htm.

Many states have laws that are similar to FMLA. In some cases, a state's FMLA gives more weeks of job-protected leave than the federal FMLA. To find out if your state has a law similar to FMLA, go to www.dol.gov/whd/state/fmla/.

## Birth Places

The setting in which you give birth can have a major effect on your experience. Many hospitals offer a range of settings; in others, the choice may be limited. There also are freestanding birthing centers that are not in a hospital. The safest places to give birth are thought to be a hospital, a birthing center within the hospital complex that meets the standards jointly outlined by the American Academy of Pediatrics and the American College of Obstetricians and Gynecologists, or an accredited freestanding birth center that meets the standards of the Accreditation Association for Ambulatory Health Care, the Joint Commission, or the American Association of Birth Centers. Depending on where you live, the following options may be available at the hospital:

• Labor and delivery—You go through labor in one room and give birth in another room. You will be transferred to a recovery room and then to a hospital room for the rest of your stay.

• Labor–delivery–recovery—You will be in the same room throughout labor, delivery, and recovery and then transferred to a hospital room for the rest of your stay.

• Labor–delivery–recovery–postpartum—You will be in the same room throughout your stay at the hospital.

Your choice will depend on what your area offers, where your health care provider performs deliveries, and what your health insurance will cover. Your health care provider will let you know about the choices available. You can tour the hospitals in your area to see which settings appeal to you.

What about giving birth at home? Although some women choose this option, you should be aware that even the healthiest pregnancies could have complications that arise with little or no warning during labor and delivery. If problems occur, a hospital setting offers the expert staff and equipment to give you and the baby the best care in a hurry. For this reason, the American College of Obstetricians and Gynecologists believes that a hospital, hospital-based birthing center, or accredited freestanding birthing center is the safest place for you and your baby during labor, delivery, and the day or two afterward.

## 〰️ Other Considerations

Many parents have lots of questions about how their new arrival will affect their finances. This month is a good time to think about financial issues, including health insurance. Many options now are available for health insurance (see the "Health Insurance" section in this chapter).

### Financial Issues

It's no secret that a new baby can drastically alter your family's finances (see box "How Much Does Raising a Child Cost?"). If you stay home on an extended maternity leave, you and your family will have to adjust to a lower income, and you will have more expenses related to the baby's care:

• Child care expenses—Child care can be very expensive. Do some research and compare the costs of different types of care, such as day care centers, home providers, and nannies.

• Income taxes—You can claim your baby as a new dependent on your income tax form, so it is a good idea to apply for his or her Social Security number soon after birth. The federal government offers a Child Tax Credit for each child under age 17 years if you meet certain criteria. You also may be able to get a tax credit for the money you spend on child care. If you have questions, talk to a tax preparer or check the Internal Revenue Service's web site.

• Being a stay-at-home parent—Can you or your partner afford to stop working and stay home with the baby full time? Although there are other things to consider when making the decision to stay at home, finances are a major issue. Take a good look at your family's income and expenses and weigh them against the average cost of child care in your area. Also factor in the money you'll save by staying at home, such as decreased spending on work clothes, carryout lunches, commuting costs, or dry cleaning.

### Health Insurance

Today, there are many options for health insurance. If you are employed, you may have health insurance through your employer. Employers with 50 or more full-time employees must provide insurance to their full-time employees or pay a tax penalty. If you are not employed, or if your employer does not offer health insurance, you can purchase a health insurance plan through the health insurance "Marketplace." Marketplace plans are offered through "State Health Insurance Exchanges." You can go to www.healthcare.gov

## How Much Does Raising a Child Cost?

Many parents-to-be wonder how much it costs to raise a child. The U.S. Department of Agriculture offers a handy online calculator that allows you to estimate these annual costs. The calculator is based on a report called Expenditures on Children by Families, a comprehensive study of families across the country. It takes into account how many children you already have, their ages, your marital status, where you live, and your annual income.

After you enter this information and click on "calculate," you will receive a report that breaks down your expenses into several categories: housing, food, transportation, clothing, health care, child care and education, and other expenses. You also can enter specific amounts in each category.

Note that the calculator applies only to children younger than 18 years—it does not, for example, include the costs of a college education. If you are interested in trying this calculator, go to www.cnpp.usda.gov/calculatorintro.htm.

to access the main web site for getting health insurance. You must sign up for this coverage during an open enrollment period. Insurance plans cannot deny you coverage because you are pregnant or have a preexisting medical condition.

With some exceptions, all health insurance plans—whether sold through the Marketplace or offered by employers—must provide certain essential benefits, including maternity care, preventive care, and pediatric care services. All health insurance plans must provide breastfeeding support, counseling, and equipment (such as breast pumps) for as long as you breastfeed your baby. The type of pump provided, whether you need to return the pump after you are finished with it, and when you will receive the pump differ among insurance plans. Usually, a health insurance plan follows your health care provider's recommendations. Talk to your health care provider about how to access these benefits and services. Also, see Chapter 18, "Breastfeeding and Formula-Feeding Your Baby," for more information about breastfeeding and how to acquire a breast pump through your insurance plan.

Tax credits are available to help qualified individuals and families purchase insurance through the Marketplace. People at certain income levels may qualify for government-funded health care, such as Medicaid. When you sign up for health insurance coverage at healthcare.gov, you will answer questions about your annual income to see if you qualify. The government-funded health care offered in the United States includes the following programs:

- Medicaid—Medicaid is a state-run program that is funded by the federal government. Medicaid provides medical assistance for low-income families and individuals.

- State Children's Health Insurance Program—The State Children's Health Insurance Program (SCHIP) provides health coverage to children, up to age 19 years, whose families have incomes too high to qualify for Medicaid but can't afford private coverage. Signed into law in 1997, SCHIP provides federal matching funds to states to provide this coverage. States can use these funds to expand their Medicaid programs or they can fund a separate SCHIP program. Some states do both. To find out more about SCHIP in your state, go to www.insurekidsnow.gov.

## Prenatal Care Visits

Your **prenatal care** visit in your fourth month will be much shorter than your first visit. Still, you will have to have some tests and procedures to check your health and your baby's health.

### Tests

Your health care provider will do a routine check of your weight and blood pressure and may do a urine test to check for glucose and protein. You may have additional **screening tests** for **birth defects**. For example, if you are having second-trimester screening for birth defects, it will be performed this month. If you have chosen to have diagnostic testing with **amniocentesis**, this technique usually can be performed after 15 weeks of pregnancy.

### Exams

Your health care provider also will monitor how the baby is developing. Your health care provider may perform an ultrasound exam to check the baby's growth.

## Special Concerns

Because infections of the urinary tract and vagina are more common during pregnancy, it is important to know the signs and symptoms of each. Left untreated, some of these infections can result in pregnancy complications. The earlier you receive treatment, the better. Another special concern for pregnant women is stress. Being aware of your stress and taking steps to alleviate it are essential to your health and well-being.

## Urinary Tract Infections

Urinary tract infections are common in pregnancy. They are caused by different kinds of *bacteria*. Bacteria from the bowel live on the skin near the *anus* or in the vagina. These bacteria can enter the urinary tract through the *urethra*. If they move up the urethra, they may cause infections in the *bladder*. If untreated, the infection can become severe and lead to a more serious kidney infection. Be alert to the signs and symptoms of a urinary tract infection and call your health care provider if you have any of them:

- Pain when you urinate
- Urge to urinate right away
- Urine that is cloudy or that has blood in it
- Urine that has a strong smell
- Fever
- Back pain

If a urinary tract infection is diagnosed, *antibiotics* will be prescribed for treatment. These medications are safe to take during pregnancy.

Another type of bladder infection is caused by a bacterium called *Group B streptococci (GBS)*. A GBS bladder infection may not cause any symptoms. If it is not diagnosed and treated, it can lead to serious problems for you and for the baby. Women are routinely screened for GBS in the third trimester of pregnancy.

## Vaginal Discharge

Vaginal discharge often increases during pregnancy. A sticky, clear, or white discharge is normal, and it's usually nothing to worry about. The increased discharge is caused by the normal pregnancy-related changes in the vagina and *cervix*. A discharge, however, that has changed from its normal color, that has a bad odor or that is accompanied by pain, soreness, or itching in the vaginal area can be a sign of a vaginal infection:

- *Bacterial vaginosis* is an infection caused by an imbalance of the bacteria growing in the vagina. The main symptom is increased discharge with a strong fishy odor. The odor may be stronger after sex. There have been some studies linking symptomatic bacterial vaginosis to *low birth weight*, preterm birth, and **premature rupture of membranes**. For this reason, symptomatic infections during pregnancy should be treated. Two antibiotics that are used to treat bacterial vaginosis are metronidazole and clindamycin. They can be taken by mouth or inserted into the vagina as a cream or gel. They both are considered safe to use during pregnancy.

* A **yeast infection** usually causes symptoms such as a vaginal discharge that is thick, white, and curd-like; itching around the vagina; and painful urination. It is caused by the overgrowth of yeast in the vagina. Yeast infections are treated with a single dose of an oral antifungal medication called fluconazole or with an antifungal vaginal cream that is applied for 7 days. A single dose of fluconazole at the dosage usually prescribed to treat yeast infections (150 mg) has not been shown to cause birth defects or other problems during pregnancy. Higher doses over many weeks, which sometimes are used to treat chronic (long-lasting) yeast infections, may be linked to some types of birth defects and should probably be avoided during pregnancy.

If you have had a yeast infection before and recognize the symptoms, you should talk to your health care provider before using an over-the-counter medication. If this is the first time you have had vaginal symptoms, you should see your health care provider.

## Pregnancy-Related Stress

It is perfectly normal to worry about your pregnancy and whether you are doing all the right things for the baby—what you eat, drink, and feel. The changes happening in your life and thoughts about how your life will change once the baby comes can be stressful. However, it's important to make sure this type of normal stress doesn't become too much, to the point that it makes you anxious or upset every day.

If you think your stress is becoming too much to handle, talk to your family, friends, and especially your health care provider. You will need help to ease your feelings. One good way to start is by realizing that you can't do everything and may need to ask for help sometimes—from your partner, family, and friends. Here are a few more tips that can help reduce your stress:

* Let the household chores go undone sometimes, and use that time to do something relaxing.

* Take advantage of sick days or vacation whenever possible. Spending a day, or even an afternoon, resting at home will help you get through a tough week.

* Get regular exercise. Yoga especially helps to reduce stress.

- Go to bed early. Your body is working overtime to nourish your growing baby, and you need all the sleep you can get.

# ASK THE EXPERTS

### What if I need surgery while I'm pregnant?

Whether having surgery during pregnancy is OK depends on what type of procedure is needed and what types of medications will be necessary. Talk to your health care provider about your particular situation. The decision is based on whether the risks of having the surgery outweigh the benefits.

### Can I have my regularly scheduled dental X-ray during my pregnancy?

Yes. The amount of radiation in a dental X-ray is extremely low. A dental X-ray doesn't pose any risk as long as it is done with your baby's safety in mind. Be sure to let your dentist know that you are pregnant. Your abdomen, pelvis, and neck area (where the thyroid gland is located) will be covered by a lead apron that will protect you and the baby.

### I have terrible allergies. Can I take a prescription medication? What about over-the-counter remedies?

Many people with allergies depend on drugs called antihistamines for relief. Some are available over the counter, and others are available only by prescription. Two antihistamines that have been extensively studied and found to be safe during pregnancy are chlorpheniramine and tripelennamine. However, both of these drugs can cause drowsiness, and they may not be as effective as some of the newer antihistamines. Newer antihistamines that do not cause drowsiness, such as loratadine, cetirizine, fexofenadine, and desloratadine, also may be considered for pregnant women. Studies performed thus far have found that these medications are safe to use in pregnancy.

Oral decongestants help decrease nasal congestion and can be useful in treating allergies. Use of one of the most common decongestants, pseudoephedrine, during pregnancy has been linked to a slightly increased risk of abdominal wall birth defects. For this reason, it has been suggested that women avoid taking this decongestant during the first 3 months of pregnancy. There have been few studies on the safety of two other decongestants, phenylephrine and phenylpropanolamine, during pregnancy, so it is difficult to say whether they can cause harm to an unborn baby.

Another allergy medication available by prescription is **corticosteroid** nasal spray, such as fluticasone propionate (Flonase) and beclomethasone dipropionate (Beconase). Most experts agree that these medications are safe to use during pregnancy. However, the bottom line on allergy (and all other) medications is to check with your health care provider before taking any over-the-counter drug.

---

# RESOURCES

The following resources offer more information about some of the topics discussed in this chapter:

**Family Medical Leave Act (FMLA)**
www.dol.gov/whd/fmla/
*Web site that provides detailed information about FMLA for workers and employers.*

**Healthcare.gov**
www.healthcare.gov
*Portal for the Health Insurance Marketplace that provides information about coverage under the Affordable Care Act and information about how to sign up during open enrollment.*

**Insure Kids Now**
www.insurekidsnow.gov
*Provides information about finding free or low-cost health insurance coverage for your child.*

**National Institute for Occupational Safety and Health (NIOSH)**
www.cdc.gov/niosh/
*Part of the Centers for Disease Control and Prevention that conducts research into and makes recommendations for prevention of work-related hazards and injuries.*

**Occupational Safety and Health Administration (OSHA)**
www.osha.gov
*Federal agency that prevents work-related injuries, illnesses, and deaths by enforcing laws designed to protect workers' health and safety.*

**U.S. Equal Employment Opportunity Commission (EEOC)**
www.eeoc.gov/laws/types/pregnancy.cfm
*Enforces federal laws that make it illegal to discriminate against applicants or employees because of race, color, religion, sex, national origin, age, or disability. Investigates charges of discrimination and may take action against employers to protect employees and the public.*

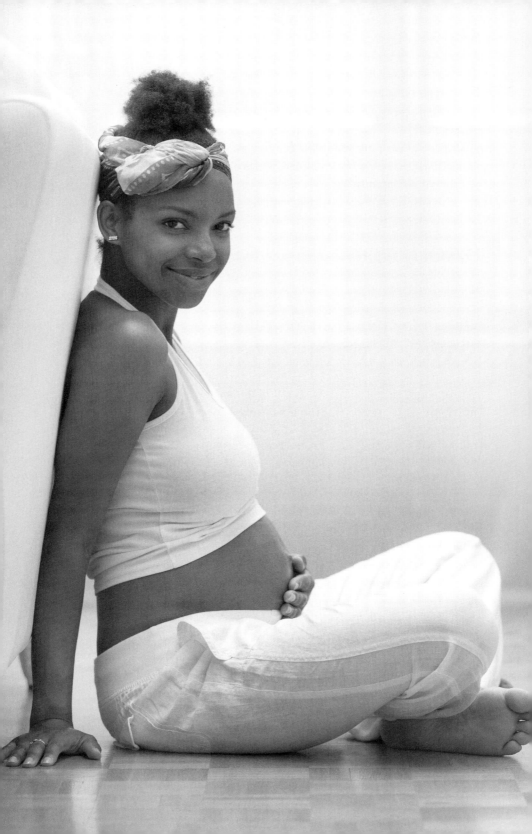

# Chapter 5

# Month 5
### (Weeks 17–20)

---

## YOUR GROWING BABY

### Week 17

The baby is a little over 5 inches long and weighs about 5 ounces, but in the next few weeks he or she will double in weight. Glands in the skin begin to produce a greasy material called **vernix**. This material acts as a waterproof barrier that protects the baby's skin. The skin will be completely covered with this material by the time the baby is born.

### Week 18

Your baby sleeps and wakes regularly and now can be awakened from sleep by noises and your movements. Soft, downy hair called **lanugo** is starting to form and will cover your baby's body. In girls, **ovaries** containing **eggs** have formed, and in boys, the **testes** have begun to descend.

### Week 19

Your baby's kicks and turns are stronger now. If you have already felt your baby move, the movements are more noticeable now. The sucking reflex is developing. If the hand floats to the mouth, the baby may suck his or her thumb.

### Week 20

Your baby may weigh as much as 1 pound now and is about 10 inches long. The digestive system is producing **meconium**, a greenish-black, sticky

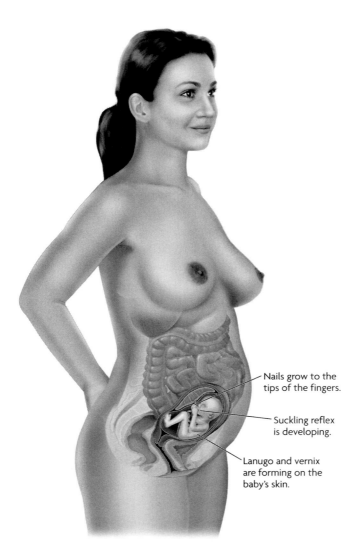

Nails grow to the
tips of the fingers.

Suckling reflex
is developing.

Lanugo and vernix
are forming on the
baby's skin.

**Mother and baby: Weeks 17–20.** The baby may weigh as much as 1 pound and is about 10 inches long. You may be able to feel your baby move this month.

by-product of digestion. This substance will accumulate in the baby's bowels, and you'll see it in your baby's first soiled diaper (some babies pass meconium in the womb or during delivery). Your baby's nails grow to the ends of the fingers and may get so long that they will need to be trimmed once he or she is born.

# YOUR PREGNANCY

## Your Changing Body

Soon you will feel your baby move for the first time. This is known as **quick-ening**. Some women, especially those who have had another child, experience quickening as early as 16 weeks of pregnancy. If this is your first baby, however, you may not be aware of your baby's movements until about 18 weeks of pregnancy, and sometimes even later.

Another thing you may be noticing now is that your feet are getting bigger. They may continue to increase in size until late in pregnancy. The growth in your feet is partly caused by your weight gain and the swelling from the extra fluid your body retains while you're pregnant, called **edema**. Another reason for this is a hormone called relaxin, which loosens the joints around your pelvis so your baby can make his or her way down the birth canal. Relaxin also loosens the ligaments in your feet, causing the foot bones to spread. To help with the swelling, soak your feet in cool water and prop them on a pillow as much as you can. You may have to buy new shoes in a bigger size too.

## Discomforts and How to Manage Them

If you were not expecting it, nasal congestion may seem like a strange pregnancy symptom. But there is actually a reasonable explanation for that stuffy feeling. You also may feel dizzy at times, and you may find yourself forgetting the simplest things. Another uncomfortable symptom—one that may stay with you throughout the rest of your pregnancy—is low back pain.

### Congestion and Nosebleeds

During pregnancy, your hormone levels increase, and your body makes extra blood. Both of these changes cause the mucous membranes inside your nose to swell up, dry out, and bleed easily. This may cause you to have a stuffy or runny nose. You also may get nosebleeds from time to time. Here are some remedies:

- Try saline drops or a saline rinse to relieve congestion. (Never use other types of nose drops, nasal sprays, or decongestants without your doctor's approval.)

- Drink plenty of liquids.

- Use a humidifier to moisten the air in your home.

- Dab petroleum jelly around the edges of your nostrils to keep the skin moist.

### Lower Back Pain

Backache is one of the most common pregnancy problems, especially in the later months. You can probably blame your growing uterus and hormonal changes for your aching back. Your expanding uterus shifts your center of gravity and stretches out and weakens your abdominal muscles, changing your posture and putting a strain on your back. The extra weight you're carrying means more work for your muscles and increased stress on your joints, which is why your back may feel worse at the end of the day. Here are some tips to help lessen back pain:

- Wear low-heeled (but not flat) shoes with good arch support, such as walking shoes or athletic shoes. High heels tilt your body forward and strain your lower back muscles.

- Do exercises to stretch and strengthen your back muscles. Many of the exercises in this book are designed to do just that.

- Don't bend at the waist to pick something up. If you must lift something, squat down, bend your knees, and keep your back straight.

- Get off your feet. If you have to stand for a long time, rest one foot on a stool or a box to take the strain off your back.

- Sit in chairs with good back support, or tuck a small pillow behind your lower back.

- Use an abdominal support garment (for sale in maternity stores and catalogs). It looks like a girdle and helps take the weight of your belly off your back muscles. Also, some maternity pants come with a wide elastic band that fits under the curve of your belly to help support its weight.

- Apply a heating pad using the lowest temperature setting, warm-water bottle, or cold compress to ease the pain. Be sure to use a towel for wrapping to avoid burns.

### Dizziness

Early in your second trimester, it's normal if you feel dizzy or light-headed at times. Your body is going through a lot of changes in circulation, such as less blood flow to your head and upper body. To prevent feelings of dizziness, move slowly when you stand up or change positions. Drinking lots of fluids may help. Also, avoid standing for long periods of time or getting too hot. If you feel dizzy, lie down on your side.

### Forgetfulness

You may find it harder to concentrate at work these days or may forget ordinary things that you never did before, such as appointments or tasks. Don't be too alarmed because forgetfulness is common during pregnancy. In the meantime, if it helps, start keeping lists of things to do at work or home to help jog your memory.

## Nutrition

You may have heard that fish is a good source of omega-3 fatty acids. But you also may have heard that eating some types of fish is not recommended for pregnant women. This month's nutrition focus is aimed at sorting out the latest information on fish. As your appetite increases in the second trimester, you also may be wondering about healthy snacking—which snack foods pack the most nutritional punch and which snack foods you should avoid.

### Fish Precautions During Pregnancy

Fish and shellfish are important parts of a healthy and balanced diet at any time in your life and especially during pregnancy. They are good sources of protein, omega-3 fatty acids, and other **nutrients** that are crucial to your health and to the development of your baby. However, certain kinds of fish contain high levels of a form of mercury that can be harmful to young children and to women who are or who may become pregnant or who are breast-feeding. The following four types of fish contain the highest levels of mercury and should not be fed to young children nor eaten while you are pregnant, may become pregnant, or are breastfeeding:

1. Shark
2. Swordfish
3. King mackerel
4. Tilefish

You should eat at least 8 ounces and up to 12 ounces (about 2–3 servings) a week of fish that are low in mercury, such as are shrimp, salmon, pollock,

## Focus on Omega-3 Fatty Acids

Although you should limit your intake of many high-fat foods in your diet, omega-3 fatty acids are "good" fats that should be part of a healthy diet. Research shows that omega-3 fatty acids, especially docosahexaenoic acid and eicosapentaenoic acid, may help reduce the risk of heart disease and can slightly lower blood pressure. Results of some research suggest additional benefits, including boosting the *immune system* and decreasing the symptoms of *depression*. Omega-3s also play an important role in the development of the nervous system during fetal development and early childhood.

To get these benefits, pregnant women should eat at least two to three servings of a variety of fish every week. A good source of omega-3 fatty acids is fatty fish, such as salmon, bluefin tuna, and sardines. About 1 ½ ounces of fish contains 1 gram of omega-3 fatty acids.

Even if you don't like fish, you can still get what you need from other foods. Flaxseed (either as whole seeds or oil) is a good source, and so are canola oil, broccoli, cantaloupe, kidney beans, spinach, cauliflower, and walnuts. One handful of walnuts, for instance, has about 2½ grams of omega-3s. Supplements also can be taken, but tell your health care provider before taking any over-the-counter supplement. High doses may have harmful effects.

tilapia, catfish, and canned light tuna (not albacore, which has a higher mercury content) while you're pregnant. If you want to eat albacore tuna, limit the amount of this type of fish to 6 ounces a week. Check local advisories about any mercury or other pollution warnings if you eat fish caught locally. If no information is available, limit your intake to no more than 6 ounces of such fish a week (and limit young children's intake to 1–3 ounces a week), and don't eat any other fish that week. If you follow these guidelines, you and your baby will get all of the health benefits of fish while reducing your and your baby's exposure to mercury. For more information about fish advisories, see the "Resources" section in this chapter.

### Healthy Snacking

Snacking is a good way to get the extra *calories* you need during pregnancy, as long as you choose some healthy snacks that are low in fat and good for you:

- Whole-grain crackers, pretzels, and crisp breads

- Fruits and vegetables

- Nuts and seeds

- Low-fat cheese and yogurt

- Fruit shakes (for example, whip together frozen yogurt, a banana, a splash of fruit juice, and a handful of berries in a blender)

Remember to count any snacks in your total calorie count for the day.

## Weight Gain

Steady weight gain is more important in the second and third trimesters, especially if you start out at a healthy weight or you're underweight. In general, you should gain about one third of your total pregnancy weight by your 20th week of pregnancy. If you are gaining weight too quickly, you may have to adjust how much food you're eating and get more exercise.

## Exercise

If traditional exercise, such as walking or swimming, does not appeal to you, you may want to try alternative exercise, such as yoga or Pilates. No matter which type of exercise you choose, it's very important to learn a few safety tips. This month's exercise of the month is a safe exercise that stretches and strengthens your back muscles.

## Alternative Exercises

Exercise is beneficial for you and your baby. Walking and swimming are generally safe, but what if neither appeals to you? There are other options that can get you moving, build muscle strength, and help lower your stress:

- Yoga—Yoga exercises or postures can stretch and strengthen muscles and help develop good breathing techniques. This age-old practice keeps you limber, tones your muscles, and improves your balance and circulation, with little, if any, impact on your joints. Yoga also is beneficial because it helps you learn to breathe deeply and relax, which may be helpful during labor and birth. Yoga is safe for pregnant women, with the exception of Bikram and other forms of yoga that are performed in a hot environment. Also, some poses aren't recommended for pregnant women, such as those in which you lie flat on your back (after the first trimester) and those that require a lot of abdominal stretching. Tell your yoga instructor that you are pregnant. You may want to consider joining a yoga class that is designed especially for pregnancy.

## Exercise of the Month: Ball Wall Squat

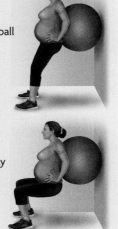

This exercise stretches the muscles of the legs and buttocks.

1.  Place exercise ball against wall. Stand and firmly press the ball into the wall using your low back.

2.  Distribute the weight between both feet. With a slow, controlled movement, squat down while firmly pressing against the ball. Do not let your knees collapse inward. Keep your feet flat and avoid lifting the heels. Maintain an open chest and avoid rounding your shoulders.

3.  Start with squatting halfway if you cannot squat all the way down. Caution: If you have any knee pain, do not do this exercise.

4.  Repeat four to six times, working up to 10–12 times.

- Pilates—With its focus on healthy breathing and improving flexibility, a Pilates exercise program is a good way to improve posture and build muscle strength. As with yoga, some Pilates moves shouldn't be done during pregnancy. Make sure that your instructor knows that you are pregnant, or join a special class for pregnant women.

- Tai chi—Tai chi involves performing a series of postures or movements in a slow, graceful manner. Each posture flows into the next without pausing. Anyone can do tai chi, and it's known to reduce stress, increase flexibility and energy, and improve muscle strength and balance.

### Tips for Safe and Healthy Exercise

Although getting regular exercise is important, it's just as important to be sure that you protect yourself from injury. For starters, make sure you have all the equipment you need for a safe workout. Wear shoes that have plenty of padding and that give your feet good support. Wear a sports bra that fits well and gives plenty of support. Here are a few more tips on keeping exercise safe:

- Drink enough fluids. Take a bottle of water with you for a drink before, during, and after your workout. If you're getting hot or feeling thirsty, take a break and drink more water or a sports drink.

- Begin your workout with stretching and warming up for 5 minutes to prevent muscle strain. Slow walking or riding a stationary bike are good warm-ups.

- Work out on a wooden floor or a tightly carpeted surface. This gives you better footing.

- Don't do jerky, bouncy, or high-impact motions. Jumping, jarring motions, or quick direction changes can strain your joints and cause pain.

- Get up slowly after lying or sitting on the floor. This will help keep you from feeling dizzy or faint. Once you're standing, walk in place briefly.

- Don't do deep knee bends, full sit-ups, double leg lifts (raising and lowering both legs at once), or straight-leg toe touches. After the first trimester, you also should avoid exercises in which you lie flat on your back. This can cut down the blood flow to your baby.

- Follow intense exercise with cooling down for 5–10 minutes. Slow your pace little by little and end your workout by gently stretching. Don't stretch too far, though. Intense stretching can injure the tissue that connects your joints.

## Healthy Decisions

Do you want to know the baby's sex? You may be able to find out during this month's **ultrasound exam**. Now is also a good time to start thinking about choosing your baby's health care provider.

### Knowing the Baby's Sex

If you'd like to find out whether your baby is a male or a female, you usually can do so at the ultrasound exam often done around 18–20 weeks. In some cases, it's important for your practitioner to know your baby's sex—for example, if the baby is believed to be at risk of certain conditions. Sometimes it's not possible to determine the sex because the baby is not facing the right way.

The American College of Obstetricians and Gynecologists recommends that ultrasound exams be performed only for medical reasons. Although ultrasound exams generally are considered safe, it's not possible to rule out all potential risks. Having an ultrasound exam only to determine the baby's sex is not recommended.

### Choosing Your Baby's Physician

Now is a good time to start thinking about choosing a health care provider for your baby. Newborns usually have their first physical examination on the day of birth, so make your selection early. Most parents choose a pediatrician—a physician who specializes in the medical care of children from birth until young adulthood. Or you may wish to use a family practitioner who treats the entire family.

If you need suggestions on a physician, ask other parents you know, the team who cared for you during pregnancy, or search your health insurance's network of physicians. Make sure your choices are accepting new patients and your current health insurance.

Most pediatricians will meet with parents and parents-to-be for brief interviews to answer questions. During the interview, ask yourself whether you feel comfortable with the physician. Do you like his or her manner and communication style? Here are some other questions you might ask:

- When will the physician see your baby for the first time? How often will your baby be seen for checkups?

- Is the physician available by phone or email for questions? If not, is there a nurse who can answer your concerns without an office visit?

- Does the physician take calls afterhours (nighttime or weekends) or must you go to an emergency room or urgent care center?

- What are the fees for sick visits, routine examinations, and immunizations?

For links to more information about pediatricians and how to choose one, see the "Resources" section in this chapter.

### ◢ Other Considerations

The second trimester is a good time to travel. If you're planning a trip, you may want to learn about how to take care of yourself away from home. Paying attention to the way you feel is the best guide for your activities, whether you are on the road or at home. The second trimester also is the time when women may begin having problems finding a good position to sleep in.

### Travel During Pregnancy

In most cases, travel during pregnancy is safe. If you are planning a trip, it's a good idea to check with your health care provider about safety measures to take during travel. Most women can travel safely until close to their due dates. Travel may not be recommended for women who have pregnancy complications, however.

The best time to travel is midpregnancy (14–28 weeks of pregnancy). During midpregnancy, your energy has returned, morning sickness is over, and you are still mobile. After 28 weeks, often it's harder to move around or sit for a long time.

When choosing your mode of travel, think about how long it will take to get where you are going. The fastest way often is the best. Whether you go by train, plane, car, or boat, take steps to ensure your comfort and safety. Here are some tips for healthy travel:

- Have a prenatal checkup before you leave.

- If you'll be far from home, take a copy of your health record with you.

- Know how to locate a health care provider in case you need one. If you need a doctor while traveling in the United States, visit the American Medical Association's web site (see "Resources") and search for "Doctor Finder." The American College of Obstetricians and Gynecologists' web site (www.acog.org) can help you locate an obstetrician; click on "Find an Ob-Gyn." (For international travel, see box "International Travel".)

- Keep your travel plans flexible. Pregnancy problems can come up at any time and prevent you from leaving. Buy travel insurance to cover tickets and deposits that can't be refunded.

- Wear comfortable shoes and clothing that doesn't bind. Wear a few layers of light clothing.

- Take time to eat regular meals to boost your energy. Be sure to get plenty of fiber to ease constipation, a common travel problem.

- Drink extra fluids. Take some juice or a bottle of water with you. In an airplane, the cabin is very dry. Choose water instead of a soft drink.

A concern for all travelers—not just pregnant women—is **deep vein thrombosis (DVT)**. Learn all that you can about this condition before you embark on your trip (see box "Deep Vein Thrombosis and Travel").

## By Car

During a car trip, make each day's drive brief. Spending hours on the road is tiring, even when you're not pregnant. Try to limit driving to no more than 5 or 6 hours each day. Stop every few hours to stretch, get a drink, and

## International Travel

If you are planning a trip out of the country, your health care provider can help you decide if foreign travel is safe for you and figure out what steps to take before your trip. Visit your health care provider at least 4–6 weeks before your trip. During this visit, you can go over your travel plans, get advice about specific health issues (such as food and water precautions), and get any vaccines that are recommended for the area you are traveling to. The Travelers' Health web site at the Centers for Disease Control and Prevention (see the "Resources" section in this chapter) provides a wealth of useful information, such as safety tips, vaccination facts, and special concerns for pregnant travelers.

While you are pregnant, you shouldn't travel to areas where there is a risk of getting malaria, including Africa, Central and South America, and Asia. Malaria is a major risk to your pregnancy. If travel to these areas can't be avoided, have your health care provider prescribe an antimalarial drug (a drug to prevent malaria), such as chloroquine or mefloquine. Pregnant women should not take the antimalarial drugs atovaquone and proguanil, doxycycline, or primaquine.

Even if you are in perfect health before going on a trip, you never know when an emergency will come up. Be sure to get a copy of your health record to take with you. Also, before leaving home, locate the nearest hospital or medical clinic in the place you are visiting. The International Association for Medical Assistance to Travelers has a worldwide directory of doctors who provide quality health care for travelers. Call this agency to obtain a free directory of doctors or visit their web site (see the "Resources" section in this chapter). You must become a member to view their directory of doctors, but membership is free.

If you need to see a doctor who doesn't speak English, it's a good idea to have a dictionary with you of the language spoken. After you arrive, register with an American embassy or consulate. This will help if you need to leave the country because of an emergency.

empty your bladder. Be sure to wear your seat belt every time you ride in a car or truck, even if your car has an air bag (see box "Buckling Up During Pregnancy"). If you get in a crash—even a minor one—notify your health care provider. You may need to have tests to check the health of the baby.

### By Plane

For healthy pregnant women, air travel is almost always safe during pregnancy. Most airlines allow pregnant women to fly until about 36 weeks of

## Deep Vein Thrombosis and Travel

Deep vein thrombosis (DVT) is a condition in which a blood clot forms in the veins in the leg or other areas of the body. It can lead to a dangerous condition called pulmonary embolism, in which a blood clot travels to the lungs. Research shows that any type of travel lasting 4 hours or more—whether by car, train, bus, or plane—doubles the risk of DVT. This finding suggests that it is not the mode of travel that increases the DVT risk, but the length of time a person remains seated and not moving. Being pregnant is an additional risk factor for DVT.

If you are planning a long trip, you should take the following steps to reduce your risk of DVT:

- Drink lots of noncaffeinated fluids.

- Wear loose-fitting clothing.

- Walk and stretch at regular intervals (for example, when traveling by car, make frequent stops to allow you to get out and stretch your legs).

Special stockings that compress the legs below the knee also can be worn to help prevent blood clots from forming. However, talk to your health care provider before you try these stockings because some people should not wear them (for example, those with diabetes and other circulation problems).

pregnancy, but check with your airline to be sure about their rules. (If you are planning an international flight, however, the cut-off point for traveling on international airlines is often earlier.)

If you have a medical or pregnancy condition that may be made worse by flying or could require emergency medical care, you should avoid flying during your pregnancy. Keep in mind that most common pregnancy emergencies usually happen in the first and third trimesters.

If you're worried about air pressure and cosmic radiation at high altitudes, these issues don't normally cause any problems for the occasional traveler. Although decreased air pressure during a flight may slightly reduce the amount of **oxygen** in your blood, your body will naturally adjust. Radiation exposure also increases at higher altitudes, but the level of exposure for the occasional traveler usually isn't a concern. There are concerns, however, for pregnant women whose jobs require them to fly often (such as pilots, flight attendants, or air marshals). Frequent fliers may exceed the cosmic radiation exposure limits set by the federal government. Most airlines, in fact, restrict

## Buckling Up During Pregnancy

For the best protection in a vehicle, wear a lap–shoulder belt every time you travel. The safety belt will not hurt your baby. You and your baby are far more likely to survive a car crash if you are buckled in. Follow these rules when wearing a safety belt:

- Always wear both the lap and shoulder belt.
- Buckle the lap belt low on your hip bones, below your belly.
- Never put the lap belt across your belly.
- Place the shoulder belt across the center of the chest (between your breasts)— never under your arm.
- Make sure the belts fit snugly.

The upper part of the belt should cross your shoulder without chafing your neck. Never slip the upper part of the belt off your shoulder. Safety belts worn too loosely or too high on the belly can cause broken ribs or injuries to your belly if you are in an accident.

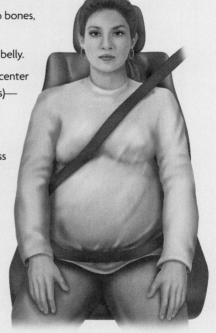

their flight attendants from flying after 20 weeks of pregnancy. Some even prohibit pilots from flying once pregnancy is diagnosed. If you are a frequent flyer, be sure to check with your health care provider about how long it is safe to fly during your pregnancy. When traveling by air, you can follow these tips to help make your trip as comfortable as possible:

- If you can, book an aisle seat so that it's easy to get up and stretch your legs during a long flight.

- Avoid gas-producing foods and carbonated drinks before your flight. Gas expands at high altitude and can cause discomfort.

- Wear your seat belt at all times. Turbulence can occur without warning during air travel.

- Move your feet, toes, and legs often. If you can, get up and walk around a few times during your flight.

## By Ship

If you are thinking about taking a cruise, check with the cruise line to see if they accept pregnant passengers. Most cruise ships restrict pregnant passengers after 28 weeks of pregnancy, and some won't accept pregnant passengers past week 24 of pregnancy. Before you book your trip, make sure a doctor or nurse is on board the ship. Also, check that your scheduled stops are places with modern medical facilities in case there is an emergency.

If you have never taken a cruise, planning your first one while you are pregnant may not be a good idea. Many travelers on cruise ships have the unpleasant symptoms of seasickness, also called motion sickness. Seasickness occurs when conflicting signals about your position from the body, eyes, and inner ear (which controls your sense of balance) are sent to the brain. Seasickness causes nausea and dizziness, and sometimes weakness, headache, and vomiting. If seasickness usually is not a problem for you, traveling by sea during pregnancy may not upset your stomach. To be on the safe side, ask your health care provider about which medications are safe for you to carry along to calm seasickness. Seasickness bands are useful for some people, although there is little scientific evidence that they work. The bands use acupressure to help ward off an upset stomach. For many people, seasickness goes away on its own after a few days as the body adjusts to the boat's motion.

Another concern for cruise ship passengers is norovirus infection, which can cause severe nausea and vomiting for 1 or 2 days. This infection is caused by a **virus**. It is very contagious and can spread rapidly throughout cruise ships. People can become infected by eating food, drinking liquids, or touching surfaces that are contaminated with the virus.

There is no vaccine or drug that prevents this infection, but you can help protect yourself from it by frequently washing your hands and by washing any fruits and vegetables before you eat them. If you are pregnant and get this infection (or any other illness that causes diarrhea and vomiting), see a health care provider. Dehydration can lead to certain pregnancy problems. You may need to receive **intravenous (IV)** fluids.

## Sleeping Positions

You may be finding it difficult to get into a comfortable position for sleep. Your belly has grown, and sleeping face down is uncomfortable. Sleeping on your back may not be good for you either because it puts the weight of your uterus on your spine and back muscles. In the second and third trimesters, lying on your back may compress a major blood vessel, making you feel dizzy.

The best position is to sleep on your side. Keep one or both knees bent. It may also help to place one pillow between your knees and another under your abdomen, or use a full-length body pillow.

Don't worry if you wake up and find yourself on your back. You won't harm the baby. Also, trust your body. Some pregnant women find that their bodies automatically find the best positions for sleep.

## Prenatal Care Visits

The timing of your **prenatal care** visits during your second trimester depends on your health and any special needs you may have during your pregnancy. Healthy moms-to-be with no known risk factors often need fewer visits than women with medical or obstetric problems.

As long as you and the baby are well, from your first prenatal care visit until 28 weeks of pregnancy, you most likely will have a checkup every 4–6 weeks. During your second-trimester visits, you may have the following procedures:

- Ultrasound exam—This standard ultrasound scan is done after approximately 18 weeks of gestation and provides information about your baby's basic anatomy. Your health care provider may be able to tell the baby's sex if the baby is in a good position for the genitals to be seen. The amount of **amniotic fluid** is checked, and the baby's heart activity is assessed. Despite all of the benefits, a normal ultrasound exam does not preclude the possibility of some fetal abnormalities.

- Fundal height—As your baby grows, the top of the uterus (the fundus) grows up and out of the pelvic cavity. At about 12 weeks of pregnancy, it can be felt just above the pubic bone. At 20 weeks, it reaches the navel. Starting at this prenatal care visit, your health care provider will measure the fundal height—the distance from your pubic bone to the top of your uterus. This measurement allows your health care provider to assess your baby's size and growth rate. As a rule of thumb, the fundal height (in centimeters) should roughly equal the number of weeks you're pregnant. For example, at 20 weeks, the fundal height should be about 18–22 centimeters.

- **Amniocentesis**—If you have decided to have amniocentesis but didn't have the test last month, you will have it this month (see Chapter 25, "Screening and Diagnostic Testing for Genetic Disorders").

## Special Concerns

Exposure to lead may be a concern for some pregnant women, such as those who work in certain industries or who live with someone who does. A *screening test* for lead is recommended for women with at least one risk factor for lead exposure. Another question that many pregnant women have is whether the amount of movement that they feel the baby making is normal.

### Prenatal Lead Exposure

Lead is a heavy metal that is used in certain industries (battery manufacturing, construction, and printing,) and, until the late 1970s, was a component in paint. In the United States, the use of lead in industry is strictly regulated and standards and protocols are in place to help reduce workers' exposure. In other areas of the world, however, lead use and exposure is not as strictly enforced, and items such as pottery, jewelry, and even candy that contain lead are readily available. Certain folk remedies and medicines used in different cultures also may contain high levels of lead.

Lead can be inhaled in dust, absorbed through the skin, or ingested. It readily crosses the *placenta* in pregnant women. Studies show that children whose mothers were exposed to high levels of lead during pregnancy have an increased risk of learning and behavioral problems. Lead exposure also can increase the risk of certain pregnancy problems, including **miscarriage**, **low birth weight**, and **preterm** birth.

A blood test that measures the level of lead in your body is available and can be used to evaluate how much lead you have been exposed to. Pregnant women who have at least one risk factor for lead exposure should have this blood test. If any of the following apply to you, let your health care provider know:

- You have recently emigrated from a country or area where there are high concentrations of lead, such as countries where leaded gasoline is still being used (or was recently phased out) or where pollution is not well controlled.

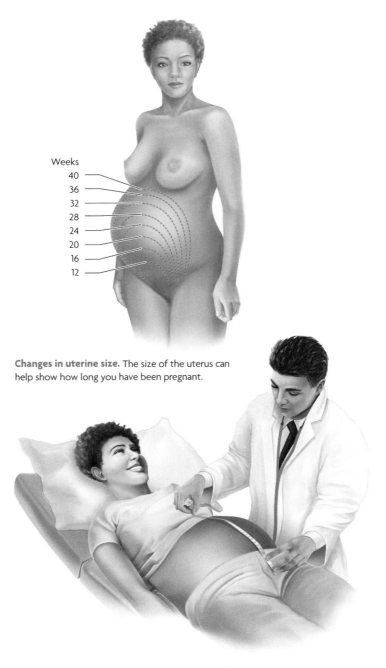

Weeks
40
36
32
28
24
20
16
12

**Changes in uterine size.** The size of the uterus can help show how long you have been pregnant.

**Measuring fundal height.** Starting at around the fifth month of pregnancy, your health care provider will measure the height of your uterus to check your baby's growth during each prenatal care visit.

MONTH 5 • 125

- You live near a source of lead, such as a lead mine, smelter, or battery recycling plant (even if the establishment is closed).

- You work in an industry that uses lead (eg, lead production, battery manufacturing, paint manufacturing, ship building, ammunition production, or plastic manufacturing), have a hobby that may expose you to lead (stained glass production or pottery making with certain leaded glazes and paint), or live with someone who works with lead or who has a hobby with potential lead exposure.

- You cook, store, or serve food in lead-glazed ceramic pottery made in a traditional process.

- You have *pica* (a condition in which a pregnant woman eats nonfood substances, such as soil).

- You use traditional East Indian, Indian, Middle Eastern, West Asian, and Hispanic alternative or complementary substances, herbs, or therapies; imported cosmetics such as kohl or surma; or certain imported foods or spices.

- You are renovating an older home without lead hazard controls in place.

- Your home has lead pipes or water sources that are lined with lead.

- You have a history of previous lead exposure or evidence of elevated lead levels, or you live with someone identified with an elevated lead level.

If your lead level is elevated, steps may need to be taken to identify the source of lead exposure and to avoid future exposure. Depending on how much lead is found in your body, you may need ongoing follow-up testing of your lead levels for the rest of your pregnancy or treatment to prevent problems for you and your baby.

## Assessment of Your Baby's Movement

For many women, feeling their babies move is reassuring, and not feeling their babies move for a while is a cause for concern. A decrease in fetal movement does not always signal that something is wrong. However, research studies show that women who report a decrease in their babies' movement are more likely to have certain problems. Nevertheless, obsessively worrying about how often your baby moves is not good for either you or the baby. It can be helpful to know that as the baby's brain and nervous system grows, the part that regulates sleeping and waking is also developing. Fetuses begin to have definite sleeping and waking cycles at about 17–20 weeks of pregnancy.

If you have not felt your baby move in a while, he or she could just be asleep. It's important to note that your perception of a decrease in your baby's activity relative to a previous level is more important than any single guideline about how much movement is normal.

A simple way of keeping track of your baby's movements is to use the "10 movements in 2 hours" rule of assessing how often your baby moves. If you can feel 10 distinct movements in a period of up to 2 hours, it most likely means that everything is normal. Once you have felt this amount of movement, you can stop counting for that day. If you don't feel 10 movements in 2 hours, let your health care provider know.

# ASK THE EXPERTS

### Can I eat sushi?

It's a good idea to eat only cooked sushi or vegetable sushi during your pregnancy. Although many fish are safe to eat when fully cooked, you should avoid all raw or seared fish when you're pregnant. Raw fish, including sushi and sashimi, is more likely to contain parasites or *bacteria* than cooked fish.

### Can I get a massage?

Sure. Massage is a good way to help relax your muscles, improve circulation, and get some well-deserved pampering. The best position for a massage while you're pregnant is lying on your side, rather than face-down. However, some massage tables have a cutout for the abdomen, allowing a pregnant woman to lie face down comfortably. Be sure to let your massage therapist know that you are pregnant if you're not showing yet. Many health spas now offer special prenatal massages done by therapists who are trained to treat pregnant women.

# RESOURCES

The following resources offer more information about some of the topics discussed in this chapter:

**American College of Obstetricians and Gynecologists: Find an Ob-Gyn**
www.acog.org/About_ACOG/Find_an_Ob-Gyn

**American Medical Association DoctorFinder**
https://apps.ama-assn.org/doctorfinder/home.jsp
*Online, searchable directories of physicians that can help you locate doctors in the United States.*

**Choosing Fish and Shellfish Wisely**
Environmental Protection Agency
http://epa.gov/choose-fish-and-shellfish-wisely
*Provides information about safe fish consumption.*

**The International Association for Medical Assistance to Travelers**
www.iamat.org
*Nonprofit organization that provides medical information for international travelers. Membership is free and allows you to access detailed information for your destination, such as doctors and hospitals.*

**Travelers' Health**
Centers for Disease Control and Prevention
www.cdc.gov/travel
*Trusted medical advice for travelers for national and international destinations, including food and water precautions, disease outbreak information, and vaccine recommendations.*

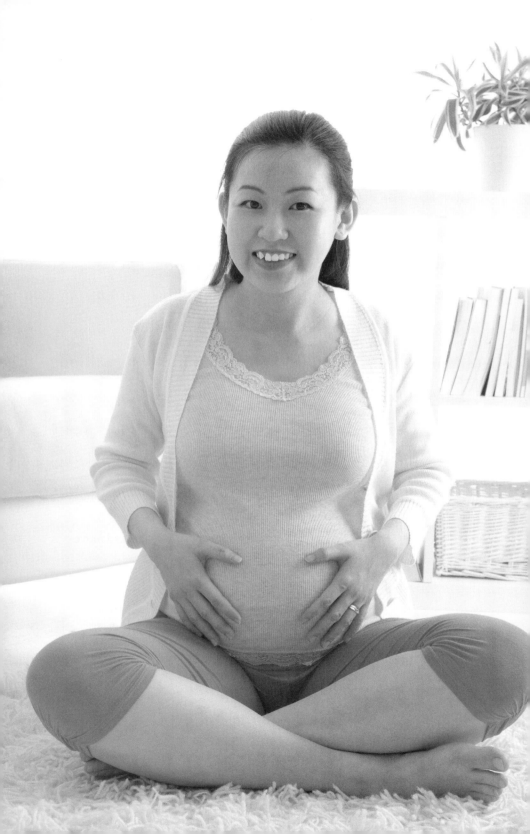

Chapter 6
# Month 6
## (Weeks 21–24)

---

## YOUR GROWING BABY

### Week 21

Your baby's fingers and toes are completely formed now, even down to finger prints and toe prints. You may notice jerking movements—it's the baby hiccuping.

### Week 22

Although the eyelids are still shut, your baby's eyes are moving behind the lids. Tear ducts also are developing. You may notice that the baby responds to sounds now. Loud sounds may make your baby respond with a startled movement and contract his or her arms and legs.

### Week 23

Your baby can respond with movement to familiar sounds, such as the sound of your voice. About 80% of the baby's sleep time is now spent in rapid eye movement (REM) sleep. During this stage of sleep, the eyes move and the brain is very active.

### Week 24

The baby has added more weight by the last week of month 6. He or she now weighs just over 1 pound and is almost 12 inches long. There also is much more muscle tone than in earlier weeks. The lungs are now fully formed but are not yet ready to function outside the womb.

MONTH 6

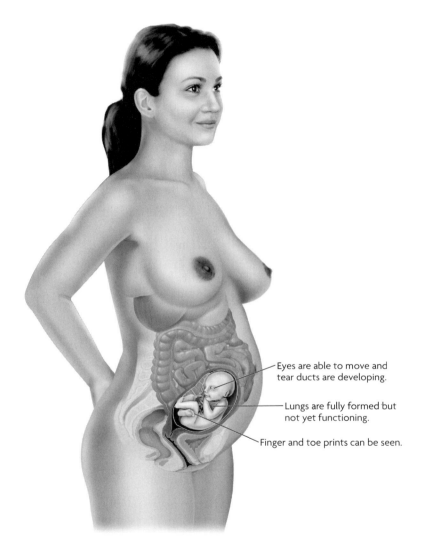

Eyes are able to move and tear ducts are developing.

Lungs are fully formed but not yet functioning.

Finger and toe prints can be seen.

**Mother and baby: Weeks 21–24.** This month, your baby has fingerprints, and you may feel the baby hiccup.

# YOUR PREGNANCY

## ﹌ Your Changing Body

Week 21 marks the start of the second half of your pregnancy. You'll begin to feel the baby's kicks and to feel stronger movements a lot more now.

## ﹌ Discomforts and How to Manage Them

You may already have experienced acid reflux—otherwise known as heartburn—earlier in your pregnancy. But now, as your uterus grows larger and pushes up against your stomach, heartburn may become more frequent. Other discomforts include hot flashes (caused by pregnancy hormones) and aches and pains (caused by the increased weight of your uterus).

### Heartburn

Heartburn is a burning feeling or pain in the throat and chest and is common among pregnant women. Heartburn doesn't mean that something is wrong with your heart. Pregnancy hormones, which relax the valve between your stomach and esophagus (the tube leading from the mouth to the stomach), are a main cause of heartburn. When the valve between your esophagus and stomach doesn't close, stomach acids leak into the esophagus. As your uterus grows, it adds to the problem by pressing up against your stomach.

If you are bothered by heartburn, try these remedies:

- Eat six small meals per day instead of three big ones (a "grazing" eating pattern).

- Eat slowly and chew your food well.

- Don't drink a lot of liquid with your meals. Drink fluids between meals instead.

- Don't eat or drink within a few hours of bedtime. Don't lie down right after meals, either.

- Try raising the head of your bed. Place a few extra pillows under your shoulders, or put a couple of books or wood blocks under the legs at the head of the bed.

- Avoid foods that are known to make acid reflux worse, such as citrus fruits, chocolate, and spicy or fried foods.

Over-the-counter antacids are safe to use during pregnancy, as long as they do not contain aluminum or a salicylate such as aspirin (avoid Alka Seltzer and Pepto Bismol). Antacids that contain magnesium or calcium are fine, such as Tums, Rolaids, or Mylanta. Read labels carefully, and if you have any doubts, contact your health care provider. If you have tried these remedies and your acid reflux persists or gets worse, see your health care provider.

## Hot Flashes

If you're feeling hot and sweaty when everyone else says they feel fine, blame your pregnancy hormones and your increased **metabolism**. You are burning more **calories** and generating more heat. Try to stay cool just as you would on the hottest summer days: Wear loose clothing, drink plenty of water, and stay close to a fan or air conditioner for a blast of cool air.

## Aches and Pains

It is normal for the extra weight of your growing belly to cause aches and pains as you move around during the day or even when you're trying to rest. Although you may not be able to take the medications you normally would to get rid of the pain, you can find some relief from over-the-counter acetaminophen medications that are safe to use during pregnancy. Check with your health care provider first, however, to make sure that you are not taking any other medications containing acetaminophen. Aspirin or nonsteroidal anti-inflammatory drugs (sometimes referred to as NSAIDs), such as ibuprofen, are not the pain relievers of choice during pregnancy. There are concerns about a possible association with certain **birth defects** when they are taken in the third trimester.

You also might consider alternative ways to relieve the pain. If your muscles are sore and aching, try a warm bath or massage. A heating pad on its lowest setting or a heat wrap may help. For mild headaches, try lying down with a cool pack on your head. (Note: If you have a severe headache or if it doesn't go away, call your health care provider.)

## ⟿ Nutrition

Vitamin B and choline are important to your baby's development. Although vitamin B is found in most prenatal vitamin supplements, choline is not. You

## Focus on B Vitamins and Choline

B vitamins, including B$_1$, B$_2$, and B$_6$, are key **nutrients** your growing baby needs. These vitamins supply energy for your baby's development, promote good vision, and help build the **placenta** and other tissues in your body. Your prenatal supplement should provide the right amount of B vitamins that you need each day, but eating foods rich in these nutrients is a good idea too. Foods such as liver, pork, milk, poultry, bananas, whole-grain cereals and breads, and beans are packed with B vitamins.

Choline is another nutrient that's thought to be needed in higher amounts during pregnancy. Choline plays a role in your baby's brain development and may help prevent some common birth defects. Experts recommend that pregnant women get 450 mg of choline each day. Although the body produces some choline on its own, it doesn't make enough to fulfill all your needs while you are pregnant. It's important to get choline from your diet because the nutrient is not found in most of the prenatal vitamin supplements and multivitamin supplements taken by pregnant women. Make sure your diet contains a healthy amount of foods rich in choline, such as chicken, beef, eggs, milk, and peanuts.

may want to learn which foods are high in choline and to make sure that your diet includes them. This month, you also will learn about salt and monosodium glutamate as well as the different kinds of food poisoning and how to prevent food-borne illnesses.

### Salt and Monosodium Glutamate

You may be wondering if it is okay to keep eating salty foods while you're pregnant. The answer is yes, but do so in moderation. Current dietary guidelines recommend consuming no more than 2,300 mg of sodium per day, which is the equivalent of about 1 teaspoon of table salt. Foods that are extremely high in sodium are frozen processed foods, canned soups and broths, and other processed products.

Another seasoning used in many foods is monosodium glutamate (MSG). It is used to enhance the flavor of many foods, especially Asian food. However, the U.S. Food and Drug Administration (FDA) requires that all foods that contain MSG list this ingredient on the label because some people develop an adverse reaction to it, pregnant or not. However, the FDA hasn't found any evidence that MSG is harmful to a developing baby.

## Avoiding Food Poisoning

Pregnant women can get food poisoning like anyone else. However, food poisoning in a pregnant woman can have serious consequences for the baby. It's important to know the signs and symptoms of the most common forms of food poisoning so that you can get treatment as soon as possible:

* Salmonellosis—*Salmonella* is a common cause of food poisoning. These **bacteria** often are found in raw poultry, fish, eggs, and milk. Salmonellosis (infection with *Salmonella* bacteria) causes vomiting, diarrhea, fever, and abdominal cramps that can last for a couple of days. People with salmonellosis can become dehydrated because of the loss of body fluids. When you are pregnant, you may become dehydrated more quickly than someone who is not pregnant. Dehydration can disrupt the body's chemical balance and has been linked to **preterm** labor and **miscarriage**. In addition, one type of *Salmonella* bacteria, called *Salmonella typhi,* can be passed to the baby if you are infected during pregnancy. If you have signs and symptoms of salmonellosis, see your health care provider as soon as possible. You may receive fluids through an **intravenous (IV) line** to prevent dehydration. Drug treatment also may be needed in some cases.

* **Listeriosis**—Listeriosis is a serious infection caused by *Listeria* bacteria found in unpasteurized (raw) milk; soft cheeses made with unpasteurized milk, such as queso, feta, and Brie; hot dogs; luncheon meats; and smoked seafood. Listeriosis can cause fever and other flu-like symptoms, such as chills and aches. Even if the infection doesn't make you seriously ill, it can have serious effects on your developing baby. If it's not treated right away, listeriosis can cause miscarriage and **stillbirth**. Babies can become infected during passage through the birth canal during delivery. Pregnant women with listeriosis should be treated with **antibiotics**.

* Campylobacteriosis—This infection is caused by bacteria known as *Campylobacter*. Most people who become ill with campylobacteriosis get diarrhea, cramping, abdominal pain, and fever within 2–5 days after being exposed to the bacteria. The illness usually lasts about 1 week. Most cases of the infection are from eating raw or undercooked poultry or from contamination of other foods by raw poultry. Animals also can be infected, and some people have gotten campylobacteriosis from contact with the stool of a sick dog or cat.

* *Escherichia coli*—*E. coli* are a large and diverse group of bacteria. Although most strains of *E. coli* are harmless, others can make you sick. Some kinds of *E. coli* can cause diarrhea, whereas others cause urinary tract infections,

respiratory illness and pneumonia, and other illnesses. Most often, people are exposed to *E. coli* by eating or drinking contaminated food, unpasteurized milk, and water that has not been disinfected.

To avoid getting these types of food poisoning, follow these tips:

- Wash your hands and kitchen surfaces with hot, soapy water after you prepare a meal.

- Avoid all raw and undercooked seafood.

- Avoid raw eggs, which can be found in homemade mayonnaise and caesar salad (if you haven't made it yourself, ask whether the dressing has been made with raw egg). Avoid undercooked eggs as well.

- Wash raw fruits and vegetables thoroughly before eating them.

- To prevent listeriosis, don't eat cold cuts, deli meat, or smoked or pickled fish unless they are cooked until they are steaming hot.

## Weight Gain

You may have gained between 10 pounds and 15 pounds by this time. If your health care provider thinks you are gaining weight too quickly, you may have to adjust how much food you're eating and get more exercise. If you gain too much weight during pregnancy, it often is very difficult to lose after pregnancy, and the extra weight can have negative consequences for your future health.

## ⟫ Exercise

For your aching back and pelvis, try this month's exercise, the rocking back arch. You also should be aware of how your growing belly affects your balance.

## Loss of Balance

As you continue to exercise in your second and third trimesters, be aware that your growing belly changes how your weight is balanced when you move around. The weight you gain in the front of your body shifts your center of gravity. This puts stress on your joints and muscles—mostly those in the lower back and pelvis. It also can make you less stable and more likely to fall. If you do fall, contact your health care provider if you have bleeding or are experiencing contractions.

## Exercise of the Month: Ball Shoulder Stretch

This exercise stretches the upper back, arms, and shoulders.

1. Kneel on the floor with the stability ball in front of you. Put your hands on either side of the ball.

2. Move your buttocks back toward your hips while rolling the ball in front of you. Keep your eyes on the floor; do not arch your neck. Go only as far as is comfortable for you to feel a gentle stretch. Hold the stretch for a few seconds.

3. Return to starting position. Repeat four to six times.

## Healthy Decisions

With about 3 months to go, now is a good time to give some thought to labor and delivery as well as your baby's care after birth. You have quite a few decisions to make, including how you will feed your baby, whether you want your baby circumcised (if it's a boy), and other important choices. You also may have heard about *cesarean delivery* on request and are wondering whether it is right for you.

### Labor and Delivery: Things to Start Thinking About

It is best to think about your childbirth options and resolve as much as you can well before you give birth. You also should make choices about your baby's birth and care after delivery. Some options you may want to think about ahead of time include the following:

• What kind of childbirth preparation do you want, and what classes are offered nearby?

• Do you want pain relief during labor, or will you try natural childbirth?

• If you have a boy, do you want him circumcised?

- Will you breastfeed your baby? Are there lactation classes in your area that you can attend?

Another issue to think about is whom you'd like at your side during labor and delivery. It's a good idea to choose someone who will help you stay relaxed and calm. A childbirth partner can be a spouse, partner, relative, or close friend. A growing trend is the use of a **doula**, a layperson who has received special training in labor support and childbirth (doulas are discussed in more detail in the "Doulas" section in Chapter 7, "Month 7 [Weeks 25–28]").

If possible, your childbirth partner should come with you to **prenatal care** visits and tests. Your partner also needs to attend childbirth classes with you because this person has almost as much to learn as you do. Your childbirth partner will help you practice breathing or relaxation exercises. When you're in labor, your partner will coach you through contractions and help you carry out what you learned in class.

## Labor and Delivery in Water

A growing trend is to undergo labor and sometimes give birth while immersed in a tub of water. Although there are lots of videos online and on television showing women giving birth underwater, not much is known about the benefits and risks of water birth, especially about how being born underwater affects newborns. Laboring in water may have some benefits for the woman, including a shorter labor and less pain. Pushing and delivering the baby underwater, however, has not been shown to have any benefits for the baby and has been associated with several complications, including infection (in the woman and baby) and injury. One of the most serious concerns is that the baby will breathe water into its lungs and develop severe breathing problems. Until more studies are performed, the American College of Obstetricians and Gynecologists recommends that immersion in water be limited to the first stage of labor.

## Cesarean Delivery on Request

Some pregnant women ask to undergo a cesarean delivery even though there is no medical reason it must be done. This type of delivery is known as cesarean delivery on request. It is estimated that 2.5% of all births in the United States are by cesarean delivery on request. Some women ask for a cesarean delivery because they are anxious about labor and childbirth. Other women are concerned about developing **incontinence** after a vaginal delivery.

If you are thinking about requesting a cesarean delivery, you and your health care provider will discuss whether it is right for you. This discussion will focus on the potential risks and benefits of requesting a cesarean delivery compared with the risks and benefits of a vaginal delivery. Some of the risks and benefits depend on your age, your **body mass index**, and whether you want to have more children.

The benefits of having a planned cesarean delivery compared with a planned vaginal delivery include a decreased risk of **postpartum hemorrhage** for the mother and a decrease in urinary incontinence during the first year after delivery. However, at 2 years and 5 years after delivery, there is no difference in incontinence rates between women who had a vaginal delivery and those who had a cesarean delivery.

A cesarean delivery is major surgery. Like all surgical procedures, it has risks, including infection, **hemorrhage**, and problems related to the **anesthesia** used. Multiple cesarean deliveries are associated with bowel or **bladder** injury and certain problems with the placenta. With each cesarean delivery, the chance that you will have a serious complication—including **uterine rupture** and needing a **hysterectomy** at the time of delivery—increases. For these reasons, cesarean delivery on request is not recommended for women who desire more children.

Having a cesarean delivery "early" (before 39 weeks of pregnancy) increases health risks for newborns. Babies who are born even a few weeks early may not be as developed as those who are born after 39 weeks of pregnancy. Because they may be less developed, they may have an increased risk of short-term and long-term health problems, including breathing problems, feeding difficulties, hearing and vision problems, and learning and behavioral issues. When there is no medical reason to do so, having a planned cesarean delivery before 39 weeks of pregnancy is not recommended and may not even be offered at certain hospitals.

If you are considering cesarean delivery on request because you are afraid of the pain of childbirth, talk to your health care provider about the pain relief options that are available and learn all you can about the birth process. If you have had a prior bad experience giving birth, talk with your health care provider about your concerns. Make sure that you have adequate emotional support during your delivery, such as a doula.

## Other Considerations

A common concern that many moms-to-be have is whether their baby would survive if they were to give birth prematurely. The answer to this question is complex and depends on many factors.

As your baby grows larger, you may experience a change in how you view your body. How you feel about sex may change too. Also, if you already have children, you may be wondering about the best way to involve them in your pregnancy.

### Early Preterm Birth

A baby is considered preterm or premature when he or she is born before 37 weeks of pregnancy. When babies are born before 32 weeks of pregnancy, they are considered to be early preterm. Early preterm babies are at risk of many short-term and long-term problems:

* **Respiratory distress syndrome**
* Bleeding in the brain
* **Cerebral palsy** and other neurologic problems
* Vision problems
* Developmental delays, such as learning disabilities

Babies born before the 23rd week of pregnancy are not likely to survive. By the 26th week, the chances that your baby will survive are higher—75%—but serious lifelong health problems are likely. The chances that a baby born this early will survive depends on several factors, including the type of hospital the baby is born in, the baby's sex and weight, whether medications have been given to the mother to promote the baby's development, and whether there is more than one baby.

Some measures can be taken if you are at risk of preterm labor or have symptoms of preterm labor. Being aware of the symptoms of preterm labor is important; these symptoms are listed in the "Preterm Labor" section in this chapter.

### Body Image

Some women love the way they look during pregnancy. Others don't. Mixed feelings about your pregnant body also are normal. Some days, you may love your growing body. Other days, however, you may feel fat and wonder if your body will ever be the same.

Eating a healthy diet and exercising will help you feel better about how you look. If you're in good shape and don't gain more than the suggested weight during pregnancy, you'll have an easier time losing weight after delivery.

### Sex

If you're having a normal pregnancy, you and your partner can keep having sex right up until you go into labor. Don't worry; you won't hurt the baby by having intercourse. The *amniotic sac* and the strong muscles of the uterus keep the baby protected.

It is normal to have cramps or spotting after sex. *Orgasm* can cause cramps, and semen contains chemicals called *prostaglandins* that stimulate uterine contractions. If you have severe, persistent cramping, or if your bleeding is heavy (like normal menstrual bleeding), call your health care provider.

As your belly grows, you'll have to find a position that is most comfortable for you. Let your partner know if anything feels uncomfortable, even if it's something you're used to doing all the time. You may want to try these positions:

- Side-by-side—You and your partner can face each other or your partner can enter you from behind.

- Woman-on-top—This position takes the pressure off your belly.

- Man-behind—Support yourself on your knees and elbows so your partner can enter from behind.

It's up to you whether you feel up to having sex. Some women do, and some don't. Some women find that their desire for sex changes throughout pregnancy. During the first trimester of your pregnancy, you may have felt too nauseated and tired to have sex. But you may find that your sex drive comes back during the second trimester after morning sickness goes away and you have your energy again. It's also normal for your desire for sex to wane again during the third trimester, particularly in the last month or two. Whatever your mood is, talk with your partner.

If you are having any complications with your pregnancy or you have a history of preterm labor, you may be advised to restrict sexual activity or to monitor yourself for contractions after sex. If you cannot have intercourse, there are other ways to be intimate, such as cuddling, kissing, fondling, oral sex, and mutual masturbation. In some (rare) cases, you may be advised to avoid orgasm. It's important that you ask your health care provider specifically what sexual activity is and is not off-limits.

## Involving Your Other Children in Your Pregnancy

If you already have children, they may have many different feelings about your pregnancy and the new baby soon to join the family. Small children may have lots of questions about where babies come from, or they may not want to talk about the baby at all. Some children are eager to be a big brother or sister. Others resent losing center stage to the new baby. A busy teenager with his or her own hobbies and friends may show little interest in your pregnancy and the new baby.

When is the best time to share the news about your pregnancy and talk about the changes soon to come? It really depends on your child. You may want to tell your school-aged children before you tell people outside your family. This way, you can be sure that they hear the news from you, and not others. With young children, it may be a good idea to wait until they ask about your changing body. The idea of a baby growing inside you may be too hard for small children to grasp before they can see your expanded belly.

## Prenatal Care Visits

Your prenatal care visit this month will focus on checking your baby's growth and making sure you are not having any complications. Your weight and blood pressure will be checked, and the fundal height also will be measured. It should now be around 21–24 centimeters.

Be sure to tell your health care provider if you are experiencing any symptoms that are causing discomfort. Don't hesitate to ask any questions that may be of concern.

## Special Concerns

Preterm birth can occur if labor starts before the end of the 37th week. It's important to recognize the signs and symptoms of preterm labor. If preterm labor is diagnosed early, your health care provider may try to postpone birth to give your baby extra time to grow and mature. Even a few more days in the womb may mean a healthier baby. *Preeclampsia* is another concern that you should be aware of. It is most common in the third trimester, but it can occur any time after 20 weeks of pregnancy and during the postpartum period.

Have you ever wondered about those keepsake ultrasound facilities you have seen in shopping malls? You may want to think twice about using one. And if you are concerned about a racing heartbeat, rest assured that it is a normal effect of pregnancy (although you should contact your health care provider in certain situations).

### Preterm Labor

Call your health care provider right away if you notice any of these signs of preterm labor:

- Change in vaginal discharge (becomes watery, mucus-like, or bloody)

- Increase in amount of vaginal discharge

- Pelvic or lower-abdominal pressure

- Constant, low, dull backache

- Mild abdominal cramps, with or without diarrhea

- Regular or frequent contractions or uterine tightening, often painless (four times every 20 minutes or eight times an hour for more than 1 hour)

- Ruptured membranes (your water breaks—either a gush or a trickle)

Diagnosis and treatment of preterm labor are discussed in more detail in Chapter 27, "Preterm Labor, Premature Rupture of Membranes, and Preterm Birth."

### Preeclampsia

Preeclampsia is a medical condition of pregnancy that can occur after 20 weeks of pregnancy or after childbirth. This condition can affect all organs of the mother's body, including the **kidneys**, liver, brain, and eyes. It also affects the placenta. It is a serious condition that requires prompt diagnosis and treatment.

Preeclampsia is diagnosed by your health care provider when your blood pressure is elevated above a certain point and you have signs of organ injury, such as an abnormal amount of protein in your urine, a low number of platelets, abnormal kidney or liver function, pain over the upper abdomen, fluid in the lungs, or a severe headache or changes in vision. Preeclampsia may cause the following signs and symptoms:

- Swelling of face or hands
- A headache that will not go away
- Seeing spots or changes in eyesight
- Pain in the upper abdomen or shoulder
- Nausea and vomiting (in the second half of pregnancy)
- Sudden weight gain
- Difficulty breathing

If you notice any of these symptoms, call your health care provider right away. Chapter 22, "Hypertension and Preeclampsia," gives more details about how preeclampsia is diagnosed and treated.

## Fast or Racing Heartbeat

You may notice throughout your pregnancy that your heart is beating faster. This is normal. It occurs because your heart is pumping more blood faster than normal. You also may be surprised to know that as your pregnancy progresses, your heart pumps up to 30–50% more blood than when you aren't pregnant. These increases in heart rate and blood volume allow the efficient delivery of **oxygen** and nutrients to the baby through the placenta. Another reason for the faster heartbeat may be caffeine. Pregnant women may be more sensitive to its effects. If you notice that your heart rate stays elevated or if you also have shortness of breath, contact your health care provider right away.

## Keepsake Ultrasound Photos

Some centers offer **ultrasound exams** to create keepsake photos or videos. However, the American College of Obstetricians and Gynecologists and other experts recommend that, although there is no reliable evidence of physical harm to a human **fetus**, casual use of ultrasound exams without a valid medical reason, especially during pregnancy, should be avoided. Having an ultrasound exam only to obtain a keepsake picture or find out the sex of the baby without a physician's order may even violate state or local laws or regulations. An ultrasound exam is a medical technology that should be used only for a medical reason.

Many parents are excited about the three-dimensional ultrasound exams that use special equipment to show a view of your baby that's almost as detailed as a photograph. However, at the present time, there is no evidence that a three-dimensional ultrasound exam is any better at diagnosing problems than a conventional ultrasound exam. Until a clear advantage is established, three-dimensional ultrasound exams remain optional.

# ASK THE EXPERTS

**I've been exposed to chickenpox. What should I do now?**

If you've been around someone who has **chickenpox**, you've never had the illness, and you did not get the **varicella** vaccination before becoming pregnant, tell your health care provider immediately. Sometimes steps can be taken to avoid problems and decrease any risk to your baby.

**My friend says she had "back labor." What does that mean?**

Back labor refers to the intense lower back pain that many women feel during contractions when they're giving birth. Some women even feel it between contractions. It's caused by the pressure your baby's head puts on your lower back. During your prenatal classes, you and your pregnancy partner may learn ways to deal with back labor, such as massage or changes in position.

# RESOURCES

The following resources offer more information about some of the topics discussed in this chapter:

**Food Safety for Pregnant Women**
U. S. Food and Drug Administration
www.fda.gov/downloads/Food/FoodborneIllnessContaminants/UCM312787.pdf
*Comprehensive guide that provides practical information for avoiding food-borne illness during pregnancy (and at any time).*

**Preeclampsia Foundation**
www.preeclampsia.org
*Provides in-depth information about signs and symptoms, diagnosis, and treatment of preeclampsia and offers a supportive community for women and their families who have had this condition.*

**Preparing Your Child for a New Sibling**
KidsHealth
http://kidshealth.org/parent/emotions/feelings/sibling_prep.html
*Tips and advice for getting your kids ready for the new arrival.*

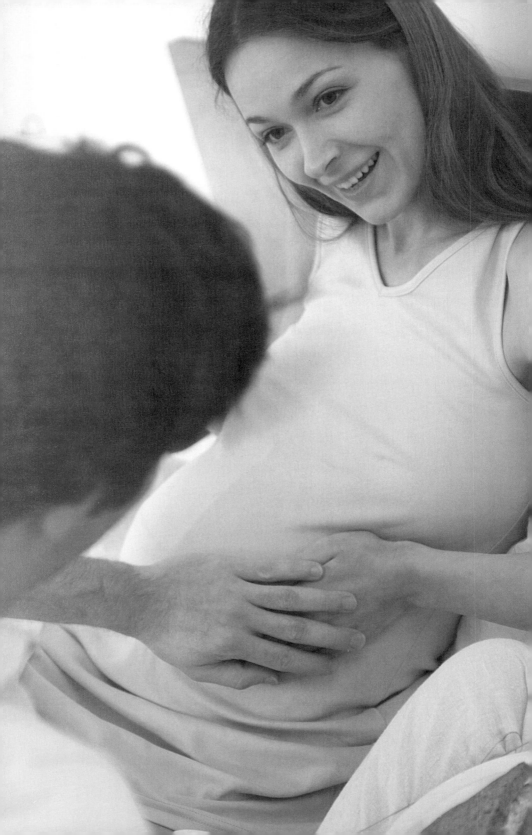

Chapter 7
# Month 7
### (Weeks 25–28)

---

# YOUR GROWING BABY

### Week 25

Your baby is entering a time of rapid growth and further development, particularly of the nervous system. More fat is being added too, which will make the baby's skin look smoother and less wrinkled.

### Week 26

Your baby's skin has taken on color because of the *melanin* that is now being produced. The lungs are starting to produce *surfactant*, a substance that's necessary for the baby's lungs to function after he or she is born. The highest levels of surfactant production occur during the third trimester.

### Week 27

The baby kicks and stretches and can make grasping motions. A smile, especially during rapid eye movement (REM) sleep, may be seen in a baby at this age. At the sound of familiar voices, your baby's heart rate may decrease, which may mean that your baby is calmed by these sounds.

### Week 28

The eyes can open and close and sense changes in light. Your baby now weighs about 2 ½ pounds and is about 14 inches long.

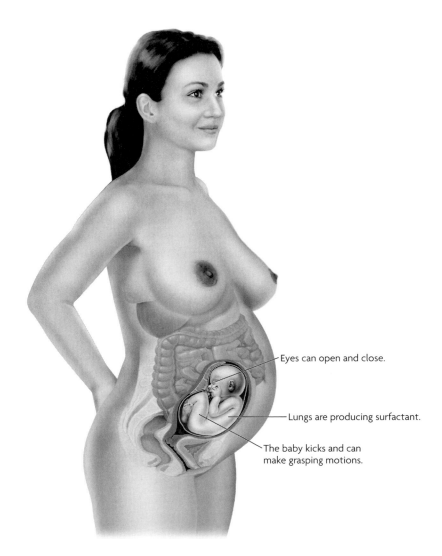

Eyes can open and close.

Lungs are producing surfactant.

The baby kicks and can make grasping motions.

**Mother and baby: Weeks 25–28.** By the end of this month, your baby will weigh about 2 pounds and will be about 14 inches long.

# YOUR PREGNANCY

## ⬳ Your Changing Body

At 28 weeks of pregnancy, you will start the third—and last—trimester. The end is finally in sight. Now's the time to start making plans for the baby's birth and giving some thought to what your life will be like after the baby is born.

## ⬳ Discomforts and How to Manage Them

The third trimester is a time of rapid fetal growth, and you will probably start seeing—and feeling—the extra weight of your baby. The increasing size and weight of your uterus may trigger lower back pain and other pains as your body adjusts. Constipation may become a problem. You also may experience "practice contractions" called *Braxton Hicks contractions*.

### Lower Back Pain

Many pregnant women experience lower back pain, especially during the later stages of pregnancy. There are several causes that may be responsible for pain in the lower back. One of the most common is the loosening of the ligaments in the sacroiliac joints, the strong, weight-bearing joints in the pelvis, which occurs during pregnancy. To make your baby's passage through your pelvis easier, a hormone called relaxin relaxes the sacroiliac ligaments, making the joints more mobile and flexible. Although this loosening is normal, pain may occur, especially during activities such as getting up from a chair, walking up a flight of stairs, or getting out of a car. If you have these symptoms, see your health care provider. He or she may suggest exercises that strengthen the muscles surrounding the joints. Usually, the problem goes away on its own after the baby is born. However, the more pregnancies a woman has, the greater her risk of sacroiliac joint problems.

Another cause of lower back pain is *sciatica*, a condition caused by the pressure of the growing uterus on the sciatic nerve. Sciatica causes pain in the lower back and hip that radiates down the back of the leg. Sciatica often resolves on its own after the baby is born. But if you have numbness in your feet or leg weakness with this pain, or if you have severe calf pain or tenderness, you should let your health care provider know.

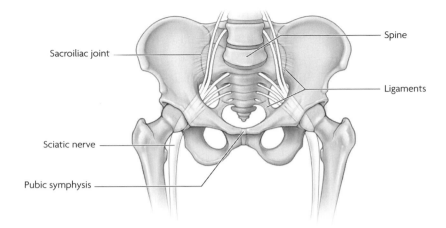

Spine

Sacroiliac joint

Ligaments

Sciatic nerve

Pubic symphysis

**Causes of pain during pregnancy.** Pregnancy-related changes in the sacroiliac joint, the sciatic nerve, and the pubic symphysis all may cause pain during pregnancy.

## Pelvic Bone Pain

The two halves of your pelvis are connected at the front by a joint called the pubic symphysis, which is normally stiff and hardly moves. The hormone that loosens the sacroiliac joints also affects the pubic symphysis, making it more flexible during and just after pregnancy. Sometimes, the increased movement in the joint can cause pain in the pelvic area. To get some relief, try to avoid prolonged standing and heavy lifting. Exercises for the abdomen and pelvic muscles also can help.

## Constipation

If you didn't have constipation earlier in your pregnancy, you most likely will have it now, in the later stages. Constipation occurs when you have infrequent bowel movements with stools that are firm or hard to pass. It can occur for many reasons. High levels of **progesterone** may slow digestion. Constipation can be aggravated by iron supplements. Toward the end of pregnancy, the weight of the uterus puts pressure on your **rectum**, adding to the problem.

Although there is no miracle cure for constipation, the following tips may help:

• Drink plenty of liquids, especially water and prune juice or other fruit juices.

- Eat high-fiber foods, such as fruits, vegetables, beans, whole-grain bread, and bran cereal.

- Walk or do another safe exercise every day to help your digestive system.

- Eat frequent, smaller meals instead of larger, less frequent meals. Smaller amounts of food eaten more frequently may be easier to digest.

You also can ask your health care provider about over-the-counter medications. Bulk-forming agents absorb water and add moisture to the stool to make it easier to pass. If you do take these agents, you need to drink plenty of liquids. Stool softeners add liquid content to the stool to soften it. Stimulants use a chemical to increase bowel activity, which moves the stool through the intestines. Before taking any over-the-counter remedy, talk to your health care provider to get his or her approval.

### Braxton Hicks Contractions

As early as the second trimester, many women experience Braxton Hicks contractions. Sometimes Braxton Hicks contractions are very mild. They can barely be felt or feel like a slight tightness in your abdomen. Other times, they can be painful. These contractions help your body gear up for birth but do not open the *cervix*. Braxton Hicks contractions often occur in the afternoon or evening, after physical activity, or after *sexual intercourse*. They are more likely to occur when you are tired or dehydrated, so be sure to drink plenty of fluids to stay hydrated. Braxton Hicks contractions tend to occur more often and become stronger as your due date draws near.

## Nutrition

If constipation is a problem for you, you may want to increase your intake of water and fiber. If you are concerned or just curious about whether you are on track for a healthy weight gain, see the weight gain chart in Chapter 3, "Month 3 (Weeks 9–12)," which shows the average weight gain by week of pregnancy. Some advice also is provided for how to handle those well-meaning comments about your weight.

### Weight Gain

It is not uncommon for other people to comment on how much weight you have (or haven't) gained. These comments may make you feel that you aren't gaining weight the way you should, and you may become worried or upset. To cope with the comments, first understand that your pregnancy and your weight are your private concerns. A well-timed reply, such as "Thank you for your concern" or "I don't feel comfortable discussing my weight with you," can let your questioner know that his or her comments are off-limits. If you're concerned about your weight, talk to your health care provider. By this stage in your pregnancy, if you have been gaining weight too quickly or too slowly, your health care provider probably has addressed the issue with you already. If not, bring up the issue yourself.

## Focus on Water and Fiber

Getting enough water and fiber in your diet are the keys to avoiding or relieving constipation. But water and fiber are useful in other ways. Water performs the following functions:

- Allows **nutrients** and waste products to circulate within and out of the body
- Aids digestion
- Helps form **amniotic fluid** around the baby

While you're pregnant, it's important to drink water throughout the day—not just when you're thirsty. A good goal is to aim for drinking six to eight 8-ounce cups a day.

Fiber also is known as roughage and is found mostly in fruits, vegetables, whole grains, beans, and nuts and seeds. In addition to its well-known benefit of helping with constipation, fiber also can lower your risk of **diabetes mellitus** and heart disease. You should get about 25 grams of fiber in your diet each day. Good sources of fiber are raspberries, apples, bananas, whole-wheat pasta, split peas, and lentils.

A word of caution: if you have not been eating a high-fiber diet and you suddenly introduce lots of high-fiber foods, you may experience gas and bloating as your body adjusts to the increased fiber intake. It's best to introduce high-fiber foods gradually. If you have not been getting your 25 grams a day, increase the amount of grams you take in slightly each day. Remember to drink lots of water as you increase your fiber intake.

## ➤ Exercise

Exercise can help ease some of the aches and pains that you may be feeling this month. Good exercises to try are swimming and the back press.

### Swimming

Swimming is a good exercise because it uses your arms and your legs. Although it is a low-impact activity, swimming has good cardiovascular benefits and lets you feel weightless in the water, despite the extra pounds you're carrying. Another benefit of swimming is that it keeps you cool. It also poses a very low risk of injury. Many pregnant women use swimming as a way to exercise right up until their last month.

## Exercise of the Month: Seated Side Stretch

This exercise eases tension on the side of your body; stretches your hip muscles.

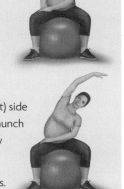

1. Sit up tall on the center of an exercise ball, keeping your spine in a neutral position and your abdominals engaged. Your feet should be flat on the floor, about hips-width apart. Start near a wall for additional balance if needed. Put your left hand on the opposite knee.

2. Raise your right arm and bend it toward the opposite (left) side until you feel a gentle stretch. Breathe normally. Do not hunch down or round your shoulders. Hold the stretch for a few seconds.

3. Return to the starting position. Alternate four to six times.

## ➤ Healthy Decisions

As your due date nears, you will need to make decisions about many different issues. This month, you may want to concentrate on your birth experience, including whether you would like to use a **doula**. Another issue to think about this month is whether you will want to save the baby's cord blood.

## Doulas

As you and your pregnancy partner discuss the role he or she will have during your labor, you may want to consider hiring a professional labor assistant, or doula. The main role of these trained labor coaches is to help you during childbirth and the postpartum period. They also provide you and your partner with emotional support. Doulas don't have medical training, and they don't replace the doctors and nurses caring for you in the hospital.

If you're interested in hiring a doula, ask your health care provider or the instructor of your childbirth class whether they can recommend a few for you to choose from. Ask friends and family members as well. You also can try the association of doulas, DONA International, which has an online locator service (see the "Resources" section in this chapter). Most health insurance plans do not cover doula expenses. Doulas charge different rates for their services, so be sure to ask about their fees.

## Birth Plan

Some childbirth education classes will help you draft a birth plan, a written outline of what you would like to happen during labor and delivery. A birth plan might include the setting you want to deliver in, the people you want to have with you, and whether you plan to use pain medications. A birth plan is useful to help your health care provider and labor nurses be aware of your wishes for your labor and delivery.

Keep in mind, though, that having a birth plan does not guarantee that your labor and delivery will go according to that plan. Changes may need to be made based on unexpected events that arise or how your labor is progressing. Remember that you and your health care provider have a common goal: the safest possible delivery for you and your baby. A birth plan is a great starting point, but you should be prepared for alterations as the circumstances dictate.

It's a good idea to go over your plan with your health care provider well before your due date. Your health care provider can advise you about how your plan fits with his or her policies and practice as well as the hospital's resources and policies. Not every hospital or birthing center can accommodate every request. Nevertheless, a plan can help you make your wishes clear, and discussion about your expectations up front can help reduce surprises and disappointments later.

When writing your birth plan, think about how you would like labor and delivery to proceed. What things do you want during labor and delivery? What would enhance the experience for you? What would make you more comfortable? A sample form that you can use to create your own birth plan is provided in the box "Birth Plan." A separate section is provided for your baby's care that you can give to the baby care staff members. Here are some additional pointers:

- Keep it short.

- Bring two or three copies to the hospital or birth center.

- Don't be surprised if your own wishes change once you are in labor. Give yourself permission to change your plan.

Don't think that you need to have a birth plan before you have your baby. It's not a requirement. If the idea of drawing up a plan doesn't appeal to you, that's perfectly OK.

## Cord Blood Banking

Cord blood is blood from the baby that is left in the **umbilical cord** and **placenta** after birth. It contains **cells** called hematopoietic (blood-forming) **stem cells** that can be used to treat some diseases, such as disorders of the blood, **immune system**, and **metabolism**. For some of these diseases, stem cells are the only treatment. For others, treatment with stem cells is considered when other treatments have not worked. Other uses are being studied. It's now possible to collect some of this cord blood after birth and store it.

Some states have laws that require physicians to inform their patients about umbilical cord blood banking options. But before you make a decision about banking your baby's cord blood, it's important to get all of the facts.

There are two ways in which stem cells can be used to treat disease. Rarely, a child's stem cells can be used to treat a disease in that child or in a family member. This type of use is called an autologous transplant. Stem cells are more likely to be used to treat people who are unrelated to the stem cell donor. This type of use is called an allogenic transplant.

Cord blood is kept in one of two types of banks: public or private. Public cord blood banks operate like blood banks. Cord blood is collected for later use by anyone who needs it. The stem cells in the donated cord blood can be used by any person who "matches." There is no fee for storing cord blood in a public bank. Donors must be screened before birth. This screening entails a detailed medical history of the mother and father and their families. Listed are some factors that rule out donating to public banks:

- Travel to certain countries
- Exposure to some vaccines
- Use of illegal drugs

# Birth Plan

Name: _____

Health care provider's name: _____

Your baby's health care provider's name: _____

Type of childbirth education: _____

**Labor** *(choose as many you wish)*
- ❏ I would like to be able to move around as I wish during labor.
- ❏ I would like to be able to drink fluids during labor.

I prefer:
- ❏ An intravenous (IV) line for fluids and medications
- ❏ A heparin or saline lock (this device provides access to a vein but is not hooked up to a fluid bag)
- ❏ I don't have a preference

I would like the following people present with me during labor (check your hospital's policy on the number of people who can be in the room):

_____

It's OK_____ not OK_____ for people in training (eg, medical students or residents) to be present during labor and delivery.

I would like to try the following options if they are available (choose as many as you wish):
- ❏ A birthing ball
- ❏ A birthing stool
- ❏ A birthing chair
- ❏ A squat bar
- ❏ A warm shower or bath during labor (not during delivery)

**Anesthesia Options** *(choose one):*
- ❏ I do not want anesthesia offered to me during labor unless I specifically request it.
- ❏ I would like anesthesia. Please discuss the options with me.
- ❏ I do not know whether I want anesthesia. Please discuss the options with me.

**Delivery**

I would like the following people present with me during delivery (check hospital policy):

_____

**Birth plan.** Feel free to make a copy of this plan and to check off your preferences. Remember that it's a good idea to discuss your birth plan with your health care provider well before your due date.

❏ Unless it needs to be done to ensure the safety of the baby, I would prefer not to have an episiotomy.

❏ I have made prior arrangements for storing umbilical cord blood.

For a vaginal birth, I would like (choose as many as you wish):

❏ To use a mirror to see the baby's birth

❏ For my labor coach to help support me during the pushing stage

❏ For the room to be as quiet as possible

❏ For one of my support persons to cut the umbilical cord

❏ For the lights to be dimmed

❏ To be able to have one of my support persons take a video or pictures of the birth. (Note: Some hospitals have policies that prohibit videotaping or taking pictures; also, if it is allowed, the photographer needs to be positioned in a way that does not interfere with performing medical care.)

❏ For my baby to be put directly onto my abdomen immediately after delivery

❏ To begin breastfeeding my baby as soon as possible after birth

In the event of a cesarean delivery, I would like the following person to be present with me: _____

❏ I would like to see my baby before he or she is given eye drops.

❏ I would like one of my support persons to hold the baby after delivery if I am not able to.

❏ I would like one of my support persons to accompany my baby to the nursery.

## Baby Care Plan

### Feeding the Baby

*I would like to (check one):*

❏ Breastfeed exclusively

❏ Bottle-feed

❏ Combine breastfeeding and bottle-feeding

*It's OK to offer my baby (check as many as you wish):*

❏ A pacifier

❏ Formula

❏ Sugar water

❏ None of the above

### Nursery and Rooming In

*I would like my baby to stay (check one):*

❏ In my room with me at all times

❏ In my room with me except when I am asleep

❏ In the nursery but be brought to me for feedings

❏ I don't know yet; I will decide after the birth

### Circumcision

❏ If my baby is a boy, I would like my baby circumcised at the hospital or birthing center.

- High-risk sexual behavior
- History of cancer in the mother, father, or siblings

Many people do not pass the screening required for a public bank. A limited number of hospitals participate in the public cord blood banking option. To find out more about public banks, visit the National Marrow Donor Program web site (see the "Resources" section in this chapter).

The other storage choice is a private bank, which charges a yearly fee. Private banks store cord blood for use in treating only your baby and for directed donation for an immediate family member. One thing to keep in mind is that the chances that your child will need to use his or her own cord blood is very low. One estimate is approximately 1 in 2,700, and some estimates are even lower. Also, if your baby is born with a genetic disease, the stem cells from the baby's cord blood cannot be used for treatment because they will have the same **genes** that cause the disorder. The same is true if your child has leukemia. However, stem cells from a healthy child can be used like any other donated organ to treat another child's leukemia.

Whether to donate or store cord blood is up to you. You have three choices:

1. Donate the cord blood to a public bank.
2. Store the cord blood in a private bank.
3. Do not donate or store cord blood.

If you decide to donate or store cord blood, you will need to choose a cord blood bank. Here are some questions to ask yourself when deciding on a bank:

- What will happen to the cord blood if a private bank goes out of business?

- Can you afford the yearly fee for a private bank?

- What are your options if results of the screening tests show you cannot donate to a public bank?

You must let your health care provider know far in advance of your due date (preferably 2 months) if you want to collect and store your baby's cord blood. If you have chosen a private bank, you will need to arrange for the collection equipment to be sent to your health care provider. Also, there usually is a fee charged by your health care provider for collecting cord blood. Often, this fee is not covered by insurance.

Keep in mind that even if you have planned to donate or store cord blood, it may not be possible to collect the blood after delivery. For example, if the baby is born prematurely, there may not be enough cord blood for this purpose. Delayed cord clamping also reduces the amount of blood in the cord. If you have an infection, the cord blood may not be usable.

## 〰 Other Considerations

*Depression* and anxiety are serious conditions that can affect a woman's pregnancy. It's important to know the signs and symptoms and to talk to your health care provider if you think you may be experiencing any of them.

Do you know the best sleep positions for your baby after he or she is born? Now is a good time to learn about the latest recommendations.

### Depression, Anxiety, and Stress

Depression and anxiety are common during pregnancy. Some women experience depression and anxiety for the first time in their lives during pregnancy or after delivery. If you have had depression in the past, or if you are currently taking medication for depression, talk with your health care provider about your management options during pregnancy. Management of preexisting depression during pregnancy is covered in more detail in Chapter 24, "Other Chronic Conditions."

The signs of depression can seem like the normal ups and downs of pregnancy. A blue mood now and then is normal. However, you may have depression if you are sad most of the time or have any of these symptoms for at least 2 weeks:

• Depressed mood most of the day, nearly every day

• Loss of interest in work or other activities

• Feeling guilty, hopeless, or worthless

• Sleeping more than normal or lying awake at night

• Loss of appetite or losing weight (or eating much more than normal and gaining weight)

• Feeling very tired or without energy

• Having trouble paying attention and making decisions

Depression that is untreated during pregnancy may cause problems for you and your baby after delivery. For example, a woman who is depressed may have trouble eating or getting enough rest. She may be more likely to use drugs or alcohol or to smoke. For these reasons, it's important to tell your health care provider if you have any signs or symptoms of depression. Your health care provider also may ask you questions like those in the box "Depression Screening Test" during your *prenatal care* visits to check whether you are at risk of this condition.

## Depression Screening Test

The following questionnaire is called the Edinburgh Postnatal Depression Scale. This questionnaire can help you find out if you have signs and symptoms that are common in women who have **postpartum depression** or depression during pregnancy. It is not intended to diagnose postpartum depression; only a health care provider can do that. It is strongly recommended that you answer these questions with a health care professional.

### In the past 7 days (not just today)

I have been able to laugh and see the funny side of things.
- ❏　0　As much as I always could
- ❏　1　Not quite so much now
- ❏　2　Definitely not so much now
- ❏　3　Not at all

I have looked forward with enjoyment to things.
- ❏　0　As much as I always could
- ❏　1　Not quite so much now
- ❏　2　Definitely not so much now
- ❏　3　Not at all

I have blamed myself unnecessarily when things went wrong.
- ❏　3　Yes, most of the time
- ❏　2　Yes, some of the time
- ❏　1　Not very often
- ❏　0　No, never

I have been anxious or worried for no good reason.
- ❏　0　No, not at all
- ❏　1　Hardly ever
- ❏　2　Yes, sometimes
- ❏　3　Yes, very often

I have felt scared or panicky for no very good reason.
- ❏　3　Yes, quite a lot
- ❏　2　Yes, sometimes
- ❏　1　No, not much
- ❏　0　No, not at all

Things have been getting the best of me.
- ❏ 3 Yes, most of the time I haven't been able to cope at all
- ❏ 2 Yes, sometimes I haven't been coping as well as usual
- ❏ 1 No, most of the time I have coped quite well
- ❏ 0 No, I have been coping as well as ever

I have been so unhappy that I have had difficulty sleeping.
- ❏ 3 Yes, most of the time
- ❏ 2 Yes, sometimes
- ❏ 1 Not very often
- ❏ 0 No, not at all

I have felt sad or miserable.
- ❏ 3 Yes, most of the time
- ❏ 2 Yes, quite often
- ❏ 1 Not very often
- ❏ 0 No, not at all

I have been so unhappy that I have been crying.
- ❏ 3 Yes, most of the time
- ❏ 2 Yes, quite often
- ❏ 1 Only occasionally
- ❏ 0 No, never

The thought of harming myself has occurred to me.
- ❏ 3 Yes, quite often
- ❏ 2 Sometimes
- ❏ 1 Hardly ever
- ❏ 0 Never

**NOTE:** If you have thoughts of harming yourself, it is important to get help right away. Contact your health care provider or emergency medical services.

**Scoring:** Add the numbers next to the items you have selected. A score of 10 or higher means that you should consult your health care provider to discuss your signs and symptoms.

Cox J, Holden J, Sagovsky R. (1987) Detection of postnatal depression: development of the 10-item Edinburgh postnatal depression scale. Brit J Psychiatry 1987;150:782–86. Developed as the Edinburgh Postnatal Depression Scale and validated for use in both pregnancy and in the postnatal period to assess for possible depression and anxiety.

Treatment of depression may include medication and counseling. Support from your partner, family members, and friends also can be helpful. In addition to providing support, they can help you determine if your symptoms are worsening because you may not be the first to notice.

If an *antidepressant* is prescribed, your health care provider and you can determine which drug is best for your individual situation. As with any medication, the benefits of taking an antidepressant drug during pregnancy need to be weighed against the risks. Studies of pregnant women who took antidepressants called selective serotonin reuptake inhibitors do not show an increase in the risk of **birth defects** above that found in the general population. However, there is conflicting evidence about some antidepressants and their potential to cause certain birth defects. If your health care provider prescribes antidepressant medication for you, the type and the dosage should be individualized. Keep in mind that not treating depression also can have negative effects on your developing baby.

Another problem that can affect pregnant women is anxiety and stress. Anxiety disorders are the most common psychiatric disorders in the United States—about 18% of all adults have an anxiety disorder. Pregnancy also can trigger a specific anxiety disorder called obsessive–compulsive disorder, or can make existing obsessive–compulsive disorder worse. Anxiety and stress have been associated with some pregnancy problems and a more difficult delivery. If you are experiencing anxiety and stress, tell your health care provider so that you can get the help you need. Treatment may include behavioral therapy to learn coping strategies and relaxation techniques, and sometimes medication.

## Safe Sleep Position

Before you bring your newborn home, you and anyone who will care for your baby should learn about how to safely put your infant to sleep. Studies have shown that the risk of **sudden infant death syndrome (SIDS)** can be reduced by following certain guidelines:

- Always place the baby on his or her back to sleep or nap or whenever the baby is left alone in a room.

- Place the baby on a firm sleep surface, such as a mattress covered with a fitted sheet.

- Don't use blankets, quilts, or bumper pads in the baby's sleeping area.

- Remove soft toys and loose bedding from your baby's sleeping area.

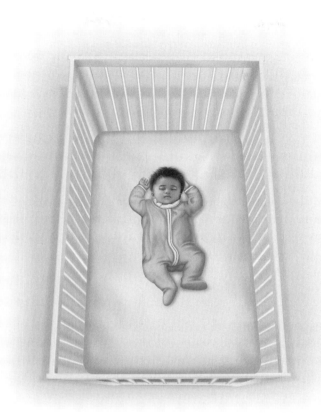

**Safe sleep position for infants.** Always place the baby on his or her back on a firm sleep surface for nap time, sleep time, and whenever the baby is left alone in a room. Do not use bumper pads, stuffed animals, blankets, or other soft objects in the crib.

- Dress your baby in light clothing for sleeping. Do not cover your baby with a blanket, and make sure nothing is covering the baby's head.

- Do not smoke or let anyone else smoke around the baby.

- Do not let your baby sleep in an adult bed, couch, or chair, alone or with you or another adult.

Use of a pacifier also may reduce the risk of SIDS. It's recommended, though, that breastfeeding infants not use a pacifier until they are about 1 month of age to ensure that breastfeeding gets off to a good start.

## ᐳ Prenatal Care Visits

During this month's prenatal care visit, your health care provider likely will track the baby's growth by measuring the fundal height. It probably will measure between 25 centimeters and 28 centimeters, about equal to the number of weeks of your pregnancy.

Your health care provider will check your weight and blood pressure and may give you a blood test to check for *anemia*, a condition in which there are too few red blood cells, which can cause fatigue. In addition to checking you for anemia, you are likely to have the following tests:

- *Glucose* challenge test—This test measures your body's response to glucose (sugar) and is usually done between 24 weeks and 28 weeks of pregnancy to see whether you have *gestational diabetes mellitus*—a type of *diabetes mellitus* that develops only during pregnancy. The test is done in two steps: 1) you drink a sugary solution, and 2) 1 hour later, a blood sample is taken to measure your sugar level. If the test result is positive, more testing is needed to confirm the diagnosis. Some women who are at high risk of gestational diabetes are given this test earlier in pregnancy. If the earlier test result was negative, you may have a repeat test at 24–28 weeks.

- Rh *antibody* screening—In earlier prenatal care visits, your health care provider tested your blood to see if you are Rh negative or Rh positive. If you tested Rh negative then, you'll probably be tested for Rh antibodies this month. If the test result shows you are not producing antibodies, your health care provider will prescribe an **Rh immunoglobulin** shot to prevent antibodies from forming during the remainder of your pregnancy (see Chapter 28, "Blood Type Incompatibility").

- Tdap vaccination—The *tetanus toxoid, reduced diphtheria toxoid, and acellular pertussis (Tdap) vaccine* helps prevent **pertussis** (whooping cough) as well as *tetanus* and *diphtheria*. Pertussis can be very serious in newborns. You should have a Tdap shot during each pregnancy, even if you have had this immunization in the past. The best time to get the vaccine during pregnancy is between 27 weeks and 36 weeks. Getting the shot at this time ensures that you will make enough antibodies against pertussis to protect the baby after he or she is born. However, it can be given at any time during pregnancy. If you don't get the vaccine during pregnancy, it should be given after you have your baby and before you leave the hospital. The Tdap vaccine is safe for pregnant women and their unborn children as well as breastfeeding women.

## ➤ Special Concerns

Because **preterm** labor is such a serious issue, each of the remaining month-to-month chapters addresses its signs and symptoms. Other complications that can occur during this time are vaginal bleeding and amniotic fluid problems. Remember, though, that most women do not have any complications during pregnancy. If you do have unusual signs and symptoms, it's best to see your health care provider right away so that any potential complication can be diagnosed and treated as soon as possible.

### Preterm Labor

Preterm birth can happen if labor starts before the 37th week of pregnancy. If you notice any signs and symptoms of preterm labor, call your health care provider right away:

- Mild abdominal cramps, with or without diarrhea
- Change in type (watery, mucus, or bloody) of vaginal discharge
- Increase in amount of discharge
- Pelvic or lower abdominal pressure
- Constant, low, dull backache
- Regular or frequent contractions or uterine tightening, often painless
- Ruptured membranes (your water breaks with a gush or a trickle of fluid)

Keep in mind that Braxton Hicks contractions may get stronger as your uterus grows. But if they come at regular intervals—four times every 20 minutes or eight times an hour for more than 1 hour—you should contact your health care provider.

### Vaginal Bleeding

Vaginal bleeding in pregnancy can have many causes in the third trimester. Sometimes bleeding can become serious and require prompt treatment. You should report any bleeding to your health care provider so that the proper course of action can be taken.

Bleeding may be caused by something minor. Bleeding might occur if the cervix becomes inflamed, for instance. However, some bleeding can be severe and may pose a threat to you or the baby. Heavy vaginal bleeding can suggest a problem with the placenta. The most common problems are **placenta previa** and **placental abruption**. In placenta previa, the placenta lies low in the uterus and covers all or part of the cervix, blocking the baby's exit from the uterus. This condition often causes painless vaginal bleeding. In placental abruption, the placenta starts to separate from the wall of the uterus before the baby is delivered. This condition often causes a constant severe pain in the abdomen; contractions, which may be mild or severe; and heavy bleeding. This condition is very serious and requires prompt attention.

With both placental abruption and placenta previa, the baby may need to be delivered early. If bleeding is severe, you may need a blood **transfusion**. **Cesarean delivery** may be necessary for either of these conditions. In some cases, the bleeding may stop. If it does, the pregnancy may continue normally, although you will need to be monitored closely.

### Amniotic Fluid Problems

The amount of amniotic fluid in your uterus should increase until the beginning of your third trimester. After that, it gradually decreases until you give birth. Sometimes, though, a pregnant woman may have too much amniotic fluid, which can cause discomfort or pain, or too little amniotic fluid. Abnormal amounts of amniotic fluid could be a sign of potential problems with the baby or the placenta.

During your regular prenatal care visits, your health care provider will be monitoring the growth of your uterus. If he or she suspects a problem, you likely will need an additional **ultrasound exam** to assess the fetal size and amount of amniotic fluid.

# ASK THE EXPERTS

**What kind of birth control should I use after I have the baby? What if I want my tubes tied?**

You have many birth control options. What you were using before pregnancy might not be a good choice now. For example, birth control pills that contain **estrogen** may affect your milk supply while you are starting to breastfeed. Birth control is discussed in detail in Chapter 16, "The Postpartum Period."

If you're considering **sterilization**, talk to your health care provider about your wishes ahead of time. **Tubal sterilization,** in which the **fallopian tubes** are closed off or removed, can be performed after delivery, often while you are still in the hospital. This procedure requires a small abdominal incision. The operation is easy to do after birth because the fallopian tubes are easy to access at this time. *Laparoscopic sterilization*, which uses instruments inserted through small incisions in the abdomen, or *hysteroscopic sterilization*, which does not require any incision, also can be performed as separate procedures later on. If you want to have hysteroscopic sterilization, it can be performed 3 months after childbirth. This method involves inserting an instrument called a hysteroscope into the uterus though the vagina and placing a small device into each fallopian tube. The devices cause scar tissue to form, which blocks the fallopian tubes and prevents the *egg* from being fertilized. Because it takes up to 3 months for the scar tissue to completely block the fallopian tubes, you are not immediately sterile after this procedure, and you must use another form of birth control during this time. A procedure called a *hysterosalpingogram* is performed usually at the 3-month mark to confirm that the tubes are blocked.

You should not have sterilization if you have any doubts about having another child. Sterilization is permanent. If you are sure, you may want to talk with your partner about *vasectomy*, which is not as invasive as tubal sterilization. If you are not sure, there are many forms of birth control that you can use that provide long-term, but reversible, protection against pregnancy that are just as effective as sterilization. These forms include the *intrauterine device* and the birth control implant. Make sure you explore all of the options so that you know what's available and what would best suit your needs.

### Is breastfeeding really the best way to feed my baby?

Yes. Although there are a few exceptions (for example, if you are infected with *human immunodeficiency virus [HIV]*), breastfeeding is by far the best way to feed your baby. Breast milk contains all of the nutrients to nourish your baby fully. It contains antibodies that help your baby's immune system fight off illnesses. The protein and fat in breast milk are better used by the baby's body than the protein and fat in formula. Babies who are breastfed have less gas, fewer feeding problems, and often less constipation than those given formula. They also are at lower risk of sudden infant death syndrome. But breastfeeding isn't just good for babies; it's good for mothers too. It's convenient, cheaper than formula, and always available. Breastfeeding burns *calories*, helping you lose those extra pounds you gained during pregnancy. By releasing the hormone *oxytocin*, breastfeeding helps your uterus contract and return to its normal size more quickly. The American College of Obstetricians and Gynecologists recommends exclusive breastfeeding for the first 6 months of the baby's life and continuing as new foods are introduced up to the baby's first birthday or beyond if both mother and baby are willing.

### What is vitamin D deficiency? Am I at risk of it?

Vitamin D deficiency happens when a person does not get enough of the vitamin in her daily diet. Although vitamin D can be made in the body through exposure to sunlight, most people do not get enough vitamin D through sunlight exposure alone. Food sources of vitamin D include fortified milk; fatty fish, such as salmon and mackerel (avoid king mackerel, however, due to concerns about high levels of mercury); and fish liver oils. Most prenatal vitamins contain 400 international units of vitamin D, although the Institute of Medicine recommends 600 international units of vitamin D each day for pregnant and breastfeeding women. However, at this time, there isn't enough evidence to recommend vitamin D supplementation during pregnancy beyond the amount contained in prenatal vitamins.

Severe vitamin D deficiency during pregnancy can interfere with the development of the fetal skeleton and cause skeletal disorders after birth. Some women are at greater risk of vitamin D deficiency than others, including women who get only limited sun exposure (those who live in cold climates or live in northern areas) and some ethnic groups, especially those with darker skin. If your health care provider suspects that you may be vitamin D deficient, a test can be done to measure the levels in your body. Vitamin D supplements may be recommended if your levels are too low.

---

# RESOURCES

The following resources offer more information about some of the topics discussed in this chapter:

### Cord Blood Collection and Donation
National Bone Marrow Donor Program
www.bethematch.org
*Offers information, maintains a donor registry, and facilitates donor–recipient matching of donated bone marrow and cord blood.*

### National Cord Blood Program
www.nationalcordbloodprogram.org
*Site for the largest public cord blood bank in the United States; provides information for patients, families, caregivers, health care professionals, expectant parents and the general public about cord blood collection, storage, banking, and retrieval.*

**Safe Sleeping**
Safe to Sleep Public Education Campaign
*Eunice Kennedy Shriver* National Institute of Child Health and Human
    Development
P.O. Box 3006
Rockville, MD 20847
Phone: 1-800-505-CRIB (2742)
TTY: 1-888-320-6942
Fax: 1-866-760-5947
Email: NICHDInformationResourceCenter@mail.nih.gov

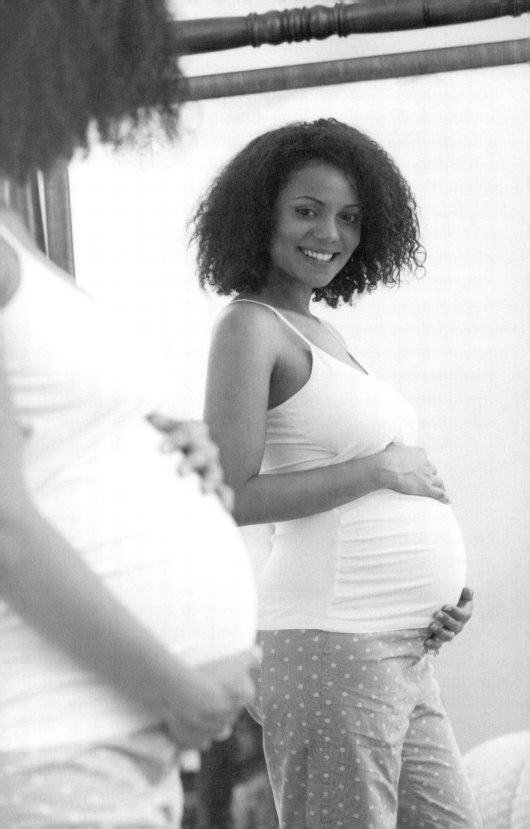

# Chapter 8

# Month 8

## (Weeks 29–32)

## YOUR GROWING BABY

### Week 29

With major development finished, the baby gains weight very quickly. During the last 2½ months of pregnancy, one half of the baby's weight at birth will be added. Your baby is going to need plenty of ***nutrients*** to finish growing.

### Week 30

This week, the fine hair that covered the baby's body (***lanugo***) begins to disappear. Some babies, however, never fully rid themselves of lanugo and are born with patches of it on their shoulders, back, and ears. Meanwhile, the hair on the baby's head starts to grow and thicken. Some babies are born with a full head of hair, although it normally is lost within the first 6 months of life.

### Week 31

The baby's brain is growing and developing rapidly. Parts of the brain can now control the body's temperature too, so the baby is not just relying on the temperature of the ***amniotic fluid***. The bones harden, but the skull remains soft and flexible.

### Week 32

More fat is accumulating under the skin, which changes the skin from being "see-through" to opaque. The baby is about 18 inches long and may weigh about 5 pounds.

MONTH 8

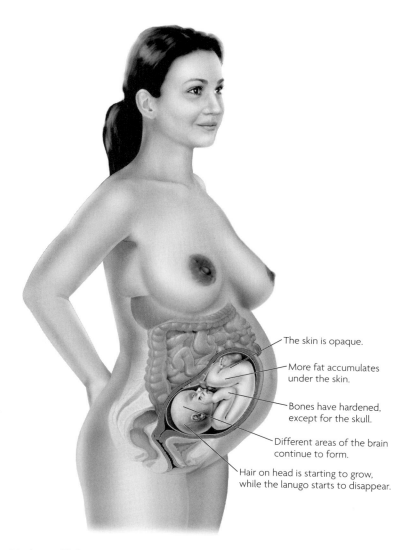

The skin is opaque.

More fat accumulates under the skin.

Bones have hardened, except for the skull.

Different areas of the brain continue to form.

Hair on head is starting to grow, while the lanugo starts to disappear.

**Mother and baby: Weeks 29–32.** With major development now complete, your baby will put on weight rapidly in the last 2 months of pregnancy.

# YOUR PREGNANCY

## ◢ Your Changing Body

You're reaching the homestretch of your pregnancy now. You are probably excited but anxious as well. In these last weeks, your body is working hard to help your baby fully develop. As a result, you may find that you tire more easily, just as you did during the first trimester.

## ◢ Discomforts and How to Manage Them

By this month, your uterus has expanded to midway between your navel and breasts. The size of your uterus may now be causing some unpleasant side effects.

### Shortness of Breath

In these later weeks of pregnancy, you may start to experience shortness of breath from time to time. Your uterus is now starting to take up more room in your abdomen, pressing the stomach and the diaphragm (a flat, strong muscle that aids in breathing) up towards the lungs. Although you may feel short of breath, your baby is still getting enough **oxygen**. To help make breathing easier, move more slowly and sit or stand up straight to give your lungs more room to expand. If there is a major change in your breathing or if you have a cough or chest pain, call your health care provider right away.

### Hemorrhoids

Pregnant women often have hemorrhoids—painful, itchy varicose veins in the rectal area. The main causes of hemorrhoids are the extra blood flow in the pelvic area and the pressure that the growing uterus puts on veins in the lower body. Constipation can make hemorrhoids worse because straining during bowel movements traps more blood in the veins.

Hemorrhoids often improve after the baby is born. Talk to your health care provider about using over-the-counter creams and suppositories. You also can try these tips for relief (or to avoid the problem in the first place):

• Eat a high-fiber diet and drink plenty of liquids.

• Keep your weight gain within the limits your health care provider suggests.

- Sitting for a long time puts pressure on the veins in your pelvic area. Get up and move around to shift the weight of your uterus off these veins.

- If you do get hemorrhoids, apply an ice pack or witch hazel pads to the area to relieve pain and reduce swelling.

- Try soaking in a warm (not hot) tub a few times a day.

### Varicose Veins and Leg Swelling

The weight of your uterus pressing down on a major vein called the inferior vena cava can slow blood flow moving from your lower body to your heart. The result may be sore, itchy, blue bulges on your legs called varicose veins. These veins also can appear near your vagina, **vulva**, and **rectum** (see the previous section, "Hemorrhoids"). In most cases, varicose veins do not cause significant problems and are more of a cosmetic issue.

Varicose veins are more likely to occur if this isn't your first pregnancy. They also tend to run in families. Although there is nothing you can do to prevent varicose veins, there are ways to relieve the swelling and soreness and perhaps help stop them from getting worse:

- If you must sit or stand for long periods, be sure to move around often.

- Don't sit with one leg crossed over the other.

- Prop up your legs—on a couch, chair, or footstool—as often as you can.

- Wear support hose that do not constrict at the thigh or knee.

- Don't wear stockings or socks that have a tight band of elastic around the legs.

### Leg Cramps

Cramps in the lower legs are another common symptom in the second and third trimesters. During late pregnancy, you may experience sharp, painful cramps in your calves that can awaken you from a sound sleep. No one is sure what actually causes leg cramps. It once was thought that these cramps were caused by not getting enough calcium or potassium in your diet, but experts no longer think these deficiencies are the reason. The following tips may help:

- Stretch your legs before going to bed.

- If you experience a cramp, flex your foot upward and then back down, which often brings immediate relief.

- Massage the calf in long downward strokes.

## Fatigue

Most women find that they are more tired during the third trimester than they were during the second trimester. Feeling tired is normal at this time. Your body is working hard to support a developing new life, and your increasing size may make it difficult for you to find a comfortable sleeping position. Try to get as much rest as you can, even if it's a short 15–30-minute nap during the day. Continue to exercise and eat healthily because both will help boost your energy.

## Itchy Skin

Some women find that their skin is very itchy during pregnancy, especially the skin over the expanding abdomen and breasts. If you're bothered by itchy skin, keep well hydrated. Applying a moisturizer to your skin in the morning and at night also can help. Adding cornstarch to your bath water may help as well. If your itching is severe or you have a rash, let your health care provider know. Some skin conditions that can occur during pregnancy should be treated.

## Nutrition

It's important to stick to a healthy diet in these last weeks of pregnancy. Eating well will give you more energy and will ensure that your baby is getting the nutrients he or she needs.

### Focus on Calcium

Calcium is a mineral that is used to build your baby's bones and teeth. The recommended dietary allowance for calcium is 1,000 mg each day (teenagers younger than 19 years need 1,300 mg a day). Dairy products are great sources of calcium, as are dark, leafy greens; fortified cereals, breads, and juices; almonds; and sesame seeds. Your health care provider also may recommend calcium supplements if your diet does not contain enough calcium.

## ～ Exercise

Even if you are feeling more tired, you should still try to keep up with your exercise routine. Monitor how you feel, and stop if you are out of breath or feeling winded. You may find that learning some relaxation techniques will be helpful as you count down these final weeks.

### Relaxation Techniques

Relaxation techniques are a great way to help reduce the stress of pregnancy and any anxiety you have about your upcoming childbirth. It's important to do your best to stay calm and stress-free so that you can conserve energy in these coming weeks. Learning some basic relaxation techniques can improve your health in many ways:

- Slows your heart rate
- Lowers your blood pressure
- Slows your breathing rate
- Reduces your need for oxygen
- Increases blood flow to major muscles
- Reduces muscle tension

## Exercise of the Month: Kneeling Heel Touch

This exercise tones muscles of the upper and lower back; tones abdominals; and stretches arm muscles.

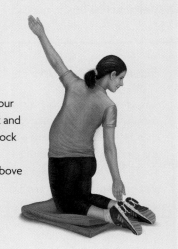

1. Kneel on an exercise mat.

2. Using a slow, controlled movement, rotate your torso to the right. Bring your right hand back and touch your left heel. You can place a yoga block next to each ankle, and aim to touch them instead of your heels. Extend your left arm above your head for balance.

3. Return to starting position. Alternate four to six times.

Listening to music or getting a massage are two easy ways to relax. Try burning a scented candle that has a calming aroma, such as lavender, and just closing your eyes and resting. You may want to find a class in your neighborhood or buy or rent a DVD that teaches the relaxation techniques of yoga, tai chi, or meditation. Whatever you do, just make sure it calms you for some part of your day, whenever you're feeling most stressed.

## Healthy Decisions

Planning and making decisions may seem like all you and your partner are doing these days, but rest assured, planning can help make your life less stressful. If you have a boy, you and your partner will have to decide whether to circumcise him. You also need to decide what kind of child care you will use if you and your partner are going to work outside the home after the baby is born. Just as you're thinking about your child's care arrangements, it's important to start getting ready for your labor and delivery too.

### Circumcision for Boys

Circumcision means removing the foreskin—a layer of skin that covers the tip of the penis. An **anesthetic** will be used for pain relief. Circumcision usually is done before the baby leaves the hospital.

For some parents, circumcision is performed for cultural or religious reasons, or it can be a matter of family tradition. There also can be medical benefits to circumcision, including a decreased risk of urinary tract infections during the first year of life and a lower risk of getting some **sexually transmitted infections**, including **human immunodeficiency virus (HIV)**, the **virus** that causes **acquired immunodeficiency syndrome (AIDS)**. The most common complications that occur from circumcision are bleeding and infection, but these are not likely to occur. If you want your son circumcised, tell your health care provider ahead of time. Also, check with your insurance provider to find out if the procedure is covered.

### Child Care

If you and your partner are planning to work outside the home after having the baby, finding good child care will be a top priority. Give yourself some time to figure out which option is best for your family. You may want to arrange child care during these final weeks before the baby arrives. Ask around for recommendations for child care; your friends, neighbors, and

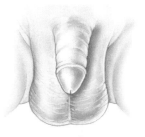
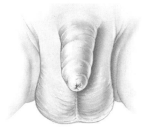

**Circumcised penis**                    **Uncircumcised penis**

**Circumcision.** In this procedure, the baby's foreskin is removed.

coworkers are all good sources of information. The box "Finding Good Child Care" can help direct your search.

There are three basic child care options: 1) care in your home, 2) care in a caregiver's home, or 3) care in a child care center. If you want to hire someone to care for your baby in your home (such as a nanny or au pair), contact agencies that focus on child care placements. Keep in mind that this type of care can be very costly. To cut costs, some parents share a caregiver with another family. The caregiver in these "share-care" setups is paid to watch two babies in one family's home.

A less costly option is having a relative or a licensed provider care for your baby in their home. In most cases, these caregivers watch more than one child.

Child care centers are yet another option. This type of setting may take care of many groups of children of all different ages. Some accept babies as young as 6 weeks, whereas some do not take infants until they are out of diapers, so be sure to ask questions while you're doing your research.

## Getting Ready for Delivery

There is a lot you can do to help delivery go as smoothly as possible. You can start by practicing with your partner all the exercises you learned in childbirth classes, such as breathing, relaxation, stretching, or meditation. You also can have the answers to the following questions well before your delivery day:

- Have I filled out all the paperwork needed to begin my maternity leave and collect disability pay?

- Do I need to register at the hospital before I check in for delivery? If so, have I done this?

- At what point in my labor should I leave for the hospital?

# Finding Good Child Care

Getting answers to the following questions can help you find a child care provider who is right for you and your baby:

1. **Gather the facts.** Make a list of child care providers, family child care homes, and child care centers in your area. Then find out the following about each of them:

   Where are they located? _____

   Do they care for newborns or infants up to 1 year of age?_____

   What hours are they available? _____

   Do they provide year-round care (do they work during holidays)? _____

   What's the cost for care (are there extra charges for some circumstances)?_____

   _____

2. **Check them out.** If you are thinking about family home or center care, visit more than once. Make an appointment the first time. If you like what you see during this visit, drop in the next time. (If drop-in visits aren't allowed, keep looking.) During your tour, find out the following:

   Is the facility clean, safe, and well equipped?_____

   Are there enough care providers (one adult per three to four infants, four to five toddlers, or six to nine preschoolers)?_____

   Are the caregivers attentive and loving? _____

   Do the children seem happy and well cared for? _____

   What's a normal day like?_____

   What's served at meal and snack times? _____

3. **Set up an interview.** Schedule a chat with a family child care provider, nanny, or center director. Have your baby with you and note how the caregiver responds to him or her. Ask the following:

   What experience and training do the care providers have? _____

   _____

   For an individual caregiver, why did she leave her last job? _____

   For a center, what's the staff turnover rate?_____

   Do the child care providers have training in first aid and CPR?_____

   Are they willing to give your child prescribed medications? _____

   What plans are in place in case of a medical emergency? _____

   Is the home or center licensed, or is the caregiver certified?_____

   Can you visit during the day to breastfeed? _____

4. **Check credentials.** Never leave your baby with someone until you have checked out his or her background. Ask for the following:

   ❏ The document showing that the home or center is licensed or registered, or that the caregiver is certified; call the licensing agency to ask about any complaints.

**Finding Good Child Care,** *continued*

❑ Written policies on philosophy, procedures, and/or discipline

❑ At least three references from other parents who have used the caregiver, home, or center

5. **Try them out.** Once you have chosen a caregiver, do a few "practice" runs before you go back to work. This way, if anything strikes you as being "off," you still have time to keep looking. It also will help you and your baby get used to the setup before your maternity leave ends.

- Should I go straight to the hospital or call the health care provider's office first?
- What number do I call if I have questions?
- Have I made arrangements for the care of my other children and pets while I'm in the hospital?
- When can family and guests visit me after I have the baby?
- What friends and family do we need to spread the news to once the baby arrives?
- Do we have their phone numbers or e-mail addresses?
- Have I purchased an infant car seat, and do I know how to install it?

## ⤳ Other Considerations

Women now have many choices about childbirth preparation methods. There is something out there for everyone. This month also is a good time to familiarize yourself with your *anesthesia* options, and a hospital tour may make you feel more secure as your due date approaches.

### Childbirth Preparation Methods

Childbirth preparation is a means of coping with pain and reducing the discomfort associated with labor and delivery. Childbirth preparation classes are available that teach these various techniques. The most common methods of preparation—Lamaze, Bradley, and Read—are based on the theory that much of the pain of childbirth is caused by fear and tension. Although specific techniques vary, these childbirth preparation methods seek to relieve discomfort through the general principles of education, support, relaxation, paced breathing, and touch. For a complete description of childbirth preparation methods, see Chapter 11, "Pain Relief During Childbirth."

With all of the choices available, you are likely to find something that will appeal to you and your individual beliefs. As you consider your options, keep the following tips in mind:

- Contact the instructor, if possible. The instructor's approach and knowledge are important factors in determining whether the class is right for you. Call or e-mail the instructor to ask questions and get a sense of how the class is taught.

- Find out the location and schedule. Is the class offered nearby? What is the schedule? How many weeks does it meet? You want to find a class that fits your lifestyle and schedule.

- How many people are in the class? Some classes are small and offer individual attention. Others are larger. Talk with your childbirth partner about whether a small or large class is more suitable for you and your needs.

- Find out how much the class costs and what's included in the fee. Also, check whether your insurance policy covers all or part of the cost.

Don't think, though, that you have to select a particular childbirth method. It's not a requirement for giving birth. Your nurses and health care provider will give you the instructions and information you need while you're at the hospital or birthing center.

## Hospital Tour

Most hospitals offer tours of where you'll give birth, and it's a good idea to take advantage of this opportunity if it's available. In fact, if you're taking childbirth education classes at the hospital where you'll be giving birth, you'll probably get a tour at some point during the course. If it will be your first time at the hospital, going for a tour also will give you a chance to learn the quickest route there and where to park the car when it's time for the birth. During the tour is a good time to ask about the hospital's policies on when your partner can be in the room during labor and delivery (even cesarean deliveries), whether your partner can stay overnight in the room with you and the baby, and whether your partner can take pictures or videos of the birth itself.

## Pain Relief During Labor

You may want to start thinking about whether you would like medications for pain relief during labor and delivery. You don't have to decide now, but it's a good idea to know your options. Even if you do make a decision now, you may change your mind once you're in labor.

Each woman's labor is unique. The amount of pain a woman feels during labor may differ from that felt by another woman. Pain depends on many factors, such as the size and position of the baby, the strength of contractions, and how you handle pain.

Some women take classes to learn breathing and relaxation techniques to help cope with pain during childbirth. Others may find it helpful to use these techniques along with pain medications.

There are two types of pain-relieving drugs. An **analgesic** lessens the pain, whereas an **anesthetic** can block all pain or sensation. Some forms of anesthesia, such as **general anesthesia**, cause you to lose consciousness. Other forms, such as **regional anesthesia** (eg, **epidural block** or **spinal block**), remove pain or sensation from certain regions of the body while you stay conscious. General anesthesia usually is not used for vaginal births.

Not all hospitals are able to offer all types of pain relief medications. However, at most hospitals, an **anesthesiologist** will work with your health care team to help you choose the best method. See Chapter 11, "Pain Relief During Childbirth," for more discussion about pain relief during labor.

### Bed Rest

Your health care provider may recommend that you restrict certain activities during the late stages of your pregnancy and may even advise bed rest or avoidance of **sexual intercourse** in some circumstances. Bed rest or activity restriction sometimes is recommended if you show signs of **preterm** labor, if you are having a **multiple pregnancy**, or if you have **high blood pressure.** However, there is no scientific evidence that bed rest helps alter the course of pregnancy. If bed rest is recommended, talk to your health care provider about whether you need to stay in bed or whether you can do some forms of activity.

### ᗞ  Prenatal Care Visits

During the third trimester, your health care provider will ask you to come in for more frequent checkups, usually every other week beginning at week 32 and every week beginning at week 36 of pregnancy. As in your earlier visits, your health care provider will check your weight and blood pressure and ask about any symptoms you may be experiencing.

Your health care provider also will check your baby's size and heart rate. A vaginal exam may be done to check whether your **cervix** has started preparing for birth.

## Special Concerns

As in previous months, you should know the signs and symptoms of preterm labor. You also should be alert to the signs and symptoms of *premature rupture of membranes (PROM)*, a condition that occurs in almost 1 out of 10 pregnancies.

### Preterm Labor

Preterm labor is still a problem to watch out for during this month of pregnancy, but babies born now have a better outcome than those who are born earlier. If you notice any of the signs and symptoms of preterm labor (see Chapter 27, "Preterm Labor, Premature Rupture of Membranes, and Preterm Birth"), call your health care provider or go to the hospital right away. *Braxton Hicks contractions* may start to intensify as you approach your due date. It's normal to have these contractions during the later stages of pregnancy. However, if they become regular, persist, or are associated with vaginal bleeding, pelvic pressure, or a change in vaginal discharge, these are signs to contact your health care provider.

### Premature Rupture of Membranes

In most cases, when your water breaks, it's followed by other signs of labor. When doctors refer to your water breaking, they are referring to the rupture of the *amniotic sac* that holds the amniotic fluid. When the membranes rupture at term but before labor begins, it is called premature rupture of membranes. When the membranes rupture before 37 weeks of pregnancy, it's called *preterm PROM*.

If you have any leakage of fluid from your vagina, you should go to the hospital. The health care provider will want to examine you to confirm whether your membranes have ruptured. Other reasons for fluid leakage are urine leakage, cervical mucus, vaginal bleeding, or a vaginal infection. PROM is diagnosed on the basis of your medical history, physical exam results, and lab test results. It is confirmed when there is amniotic fluid in the vagina. Labor frequently starts after the membranes rupture. If it does not and the pregnancy is at term, labor often is induced. If the pregnancy is not at term, a decision needs to be made about whether to deliver the baby. More information about PROM can be found in Chapter 27, "Preterm Labor, Premature Rupture of Membranes, and Preterm Birth."

# ASK THE EXPERTS

### Are there any particular signs or symptoms that should alert me to call my health care provider?

In your eighth month of pregnancy, you should be aware of the signs of preterm labor and PROM and call your health care provider or go to the hospital if you experience any of them. Also go to the hospital or call your health care provider if you have any vaginal bleeding, a fever, severe abdominal pain, or a severe headache. It's always a good idea to be cautious, so if you have any symptoms that cause you concern, don't hesitate to call your health care provider.

### What is delayed cord clamping?

Delayed cord clamping is the practice of waiting for a short period of time (usually at least 1 minute) before cutting the **umbilical cord.** This allows blood from the umbilical cord, along with extra iron, **stem cells**, and **antibodies**, to flow back into the baby. A potential benefit of delayed cord clamping is a decreased risk of **anemia** during the first year of life. However, there are risks involved, including an increased risk of newborn **jaundice** requiring treatment. Because anemia in healthy, term infants is rare in the United States, there is no compelling reason to recommend delayed cord blood clamping in most situations. There may be more benefits with this practice for preterm infants (those born between 24 weeks and 36 weeks of pregnancy), including a decreased need for blood **transfusion.** If you are planning to store your baby's cord blood in a cord blood bank, delayed cord clamping may interfere with this process, and there may not be enough cord blood left for storage.

### I am *lactose intolerant*. How can I get all the calcium I need if I can't eat dairy products?

Lactose intolerance is also known as lactase deficiency and means you cannot fully digest the milk sugar (lactose) in dairy products. Pregnant women with this condition still need to get the daily amount of calcium in their diet to nourish their baby's growing muscles and organs. The following tips can help lessen the symptoms of lactose intolerance without limiting your calcium intake:

- Try different kinds of dairy products. Not all dairy products have the same amount of lactose. For example, hard cheeses such as Swiss or cheddar have small amounts of lactose and generally cause no symptoms.

- Buy lactose-free products, such as Lactaid. They contain all of the nutrients found in regular milk and dairy products.

- Get calcium from other foods. Good sources are canned pink salmon; almonds; dark, leafy greens like spinach, kale, and collard greens; molasses; and calcium-fortified breads and juices.

# RESOURCES

The following resources offer more information about some of the topics discussed in this chapter:

**Childbirth Education**
International Childbirth Education Association
www.icea.org
*Search for childbirth classes or find educators or doulas in your area.*

**Circumcision**
HealthyChildren.Org
American Academy of Pediatrics
www.healthychildren.org/English/ages-stages/prenatal/decisions-to-make/
Pages/Circumcision.aspx
*Describes the risks and benefits of male circumcision, how the procedure is performed, and what to expect after the procedure.*

**Lactose Intolerance**
National Institute of Diabetes and Digestive and Kidney Diseases, National Institutes of Health
www.niddk.nih.gov/health-information/health-topics/digestive-diseases/
lactose-intolerance/Pages/facts.aspx
*Gives detailed information about the causes, signs and symptoms, diagnosis, and management of lactose intolerance.*

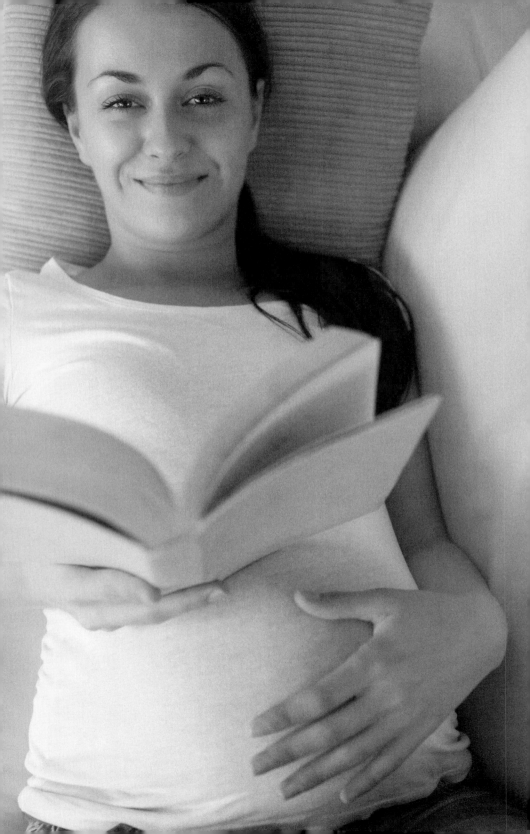

Chapter 9
# Month 9
### (Weeks 33–36)

## YOUR GROWING BABY

### Week 33

The baby is gaining weight more quickly—about ½ pound a week—and is getting ready for birth in a few weeks. He or she now weighs about 5 ½ pounds and is about 20 inches long. Babies at this stage won't get too much longer than 20 inches but will continue to put on weight.

### Week 34

The skin is less wrinkled because of the fat that's been added underneath. During these weeks, most babies turn into a head-down position for birth.

### Week 35

The lungs continue to develop, as do the brain and nervous system. The circulatory system is complete, and so is the musculoskeletal system.

### Week 36

The baby probably weighs about 6–7 pounds and is taking up a lot of space in the *amniotic sac.* There's not much room for rolling around and turning somersaults. You will continue to feel kicks and fetal movement.

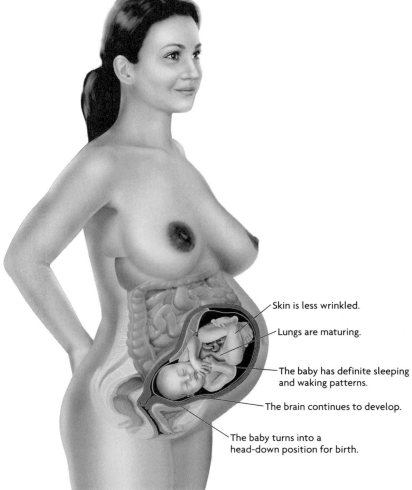

Skin is less wrinkled.

Lungs are maturing.

The baby has definite sleeping and waking patterns.

The brain continues to develop.

The baby turns into a head-down position for birth.

**Mother and baby: Weeks 33–36.** This month, your baby will most likely gain about 2 pounds of weight but won't get much longer than 20 inches.

# YOUR PREGNANCY

## ～ Your Changing Body

Today starts the ninth month of pregnancy. It's probably a busy time for you as you prepare your life, your home, and your family to welcome the new baby.

## ～ Discomforts and How to Manage Them

This month, the discomforts of pregnancy are probably at their peak. Remember to take good care of yourself and get plenty of rest during these last weeks.

### Frequent Urination

In the final weeks of your pregnancy, you'll feel more pressure on your **bladder** as the baby moves deeper into your pelvis. You will urinate much more often during the day and may have to go several times during the night. Some women also leak urine during these later weeks, especially when laughing, coughing, sneezing, or even just with simple bending and lifting. This, too, is caused by the baby pressing on your bladder.

### Prelabor (Braxton Hicks) Contractions

As you near your due date, **Braxton Hicks contractions** may get stronger. You even may mistake them for labor contractions. It's easy to be fooled by these prelabor contractions. If you have contractions, time them. Note how long it is from the start of one contraction to the start of the next. Keep a record for an hour and also jot down how your contractions feel. The time between contractions will help tell you if you are truly in labor. When it's true labor, your contractions will come at regular intervals, get closer together, and can last 30–90 seconds. The intensity of the contractions is also important. It's more likely to be true labor if you have trouble walking and talking during a contraction.

No matter what your watch says about the timing of contractions, it's better to be safe than sorry. If you think you may be in labor, call your health care provider. Even a doctor, midwife, or nurse can have a hard time telling prelabor from the real thing. You may need to go to the office or hospital for a few hours for observation. A *pelvic exam* also may need to be done to see if your *cervix* is opening.

## Trouble Sleeping

It's normal for insomnia to return in these last few weeks of pregnancy. It's also normal for it to be almost impossible to find a comfortable position for sleep. Try not to worry about losing sleep. Make your bedroom as comfortable as possible, use as many pillows as you need to prop yourself up to get support, and get a few hours of rest whenever you can.

## Leg Swelling and Pain

Most pregnant women have some swelling in their legs and feet. To relieve the swelling, try to limit prolonged standing. When sitting, prop your legs up on a pillow or use a footrest. Comfortable, supportive shoes may help relieve some of the discomfort.

## Pelvic Pressure

The baby will soon settle into a deeper position in your pelvis to get ready for birth. You may feel this settling as the baby "dropping" in your pelvis. When your baby drops, it can cause some increased pressure in the pelvis, bladder, and hips, but you may feel less pressure against your diaphragm and lungs. There is not much you can do about the pressure other than try to stay off your feet when you are most uncomfortable. Soaking in a warm bath (make sure that the water is no more than 100°F) may give some relief.

## Numbness of Legs and Feet

If you have numbness or tingling in your hands or feet, it is a normal reaction caused by your body's swelling tissues pressing on the nerves. Some women may develop *carpal tunnel syndrome*. Carpal tunnel syndrome is discomfort in the hand caused by the compression of a nerve within the carpal tunnel, a passageway of bones and ligaments in the wrist. These symptoms usually go away after you give birth and the tissues return to normal. However, if you have these symptoms, don't hesitate to mention them to your health care provider at the next *prenatal care* visit. Wrist splints and resting the affected hand are typically used to treat these symptoms during pregnancy.

## Nutrition

Continue your healthy eating, and make sure you are drinking plenty of water. Your baby needs lots of **nutrients** these last few weeks to fully mature and be ready for birth. You'll need the energy a healthy diet provides too.

---

### Focus on Vitamin C

Getting the right daily amount of vitamin C is important for a healthy **immune system** as well as for building strong bones and muscles. During your pregnancy, you should get at least 85 mg of vitamin C each day (80 mg if you are younger than age 19 years). You can get the right amount in your daily prenatal vitamin supplement, but you also can find vitamin C in foods such as citrus fruits and juices, strawberries, broccoli, and tomatoes.

---

## Exercise

Keep up with your exercise this month. Go for walks and continue the strengthening and stretching exercises you learned early in your pregnancy.

---

### Exercise of the Month: Standing Back Bend

This exercise helps counteract the increased forward bending that happens during pregnancy as your uterus grows.

1. Stand upright with your palms on the back of each hip.

2. Slowly bend backward about 15–20 degrees. Hold for 20 seconds. Repeat five times.

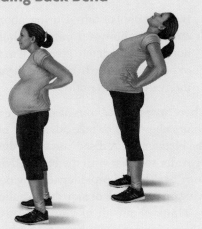

Don't forget, you can still do your yoga poses too. Yoga will help with your breathing exercises once labor begins. You can speak with a yoga instructor about which poses are appropriate for late pregnancy.

## Healthy Decisions

There are many important decisions for you and your partner to make this month, from how you want to give birth to how to feed your baby.

### Positions for Labor and Childbirth

You and your partner may want to start thinking about positions you may want to use during labor and delivery. It is a good idea to discuss your thoughts with your health care provider, who can help you learn what options are available at your hospital or birthing center. Some options to consider include the following:

- Birthing bed—A bed that can be adjusted to numerous positions for you, such as squatting, sitting on the end of the bed with your feet supported, or lying on your side.

- Birthing chair—A chair that has been especially designed to allow you to give birth in a seated position.

- Birthing stool—A frame that stabilizes and supports you while you squat.

- Birthing ball—A large rubber ball that you can sit on during labor and that allows you to rock back and forth on a soft surface.

- Birthing pool or tub—During labor, you get into a tub of water that is large enough for both you and your childbirth partner, if desired. However, it is not recommended to give birth in water. Many hospitals do not have a tub or pool, so be sure to check with your hospital or birthing center if you are interested in this option.

There are pros and cons of each type of birthing position. Birthing stools and chairs allow you to take advantage of gravity as the baby descends through the birth canal. A disadvantage is that it may be difficult for the health care provider to assist with the birth. Giving birth in a bed may make it easier for your health care provider to provide assistance to you during delivery, but lying on your back or side doesn't allow gravity to do its work.

Think about all of your options and ask lots of questions. Find out which options your hospital or birthing center offers. You also should remember that you won't know which positions feel best to you until you are in labor. Don't get too attached to a specific method or position before-hand, and be open to alternatives once you get to the hospital or birthing center.

## Your Baby's Hospital Stay

The hospital where you give birth may offer several options for your baby's stay. Some hospitals now encourage the option of "rooming in," in which the baby stays with you at all times in your room. Others have a nursery that the baby can stay in for all or part of your hospital stay.

Rooming in is a good way to get to know your new baby. It's also the best way to get started with breastfeeding. However, having the baby stay in the hospital nursery may be a good choice as well, especially if you are exhausted or have had a difficult labor. The baby will be brought to your room for feedings.

Be sure you know the options offered by your hospital. If rooming in is encouraged, you may want to have someone stay with you at the hospital to help take care of the baby.

## Packing for the Hospital

The last thing you want to be doing once labor starts is tossing items into a suitcase in a panic. To avoid this, pack your bag a few weeks before your due date. Leave it in a handy place, such as a hall closet or the trunk of your car. You can't pack everything ahead of time—you will need some things in the meantime, such as your glasses and slippers (see box "Things You May Want to Pack"). Make a list of these last-minute items that need to be packed before you leave for the hospital, and put the list in a place that will trigger your memory, such as on the refrigerator door.

Don't worry if you forget something. A friend or family member can bring you whatever you need. The hospital also may have some items, but you may be charged for them.

## Feeding Your Baby

Deciding whether to breastfeed or bottle-feed your new baby is a personal decision that each new mother should make on her own. There are a few important facts that you need to know when making this decision. Most experts agree that breastfeeding is the best way to feed your baby.

## Things You May Want to Pack

*For labor:*

___ Your health insurance card, photo ID, and hospital registration forms

___ Lotion or oil for massage

___ Lip balm

___ A nightgown or nightshirt (if you don't want to wear a hospital gown)

___ A bathrobe, slippers, and socks

___ Glasses, if you wear them (you may not be allowed to wear contact lenses)

___ Camera

___ Music to play during labor

___ Back-up charger for your cell phone and any other electronic devices

*For your hospital stay:*

___ Two or three nightgowns (be sure the gowns open at the front if you plan to nurse)

___ Two or three nursing bras

___ A few pairs of socks and panties

___ Toiletries, such as toothbrush, toothpaste, and deodorant

___ Contact lenses, if you wear them

___ Phone numbers of people you want to call after the birth

___ Reading material

*For discharge from the hospital:*

___ A receiving blanket and clothes for your newborn to wear home

___ Loose-fitting clothes for you to wear home

___ Infant car seat

## What not to bring:

*Many hospitals do not allow the following things:*

___ Portable TVs, DVD players, or CD players

___ Cell phones—you may be asked to turn off your cell phone in certain areas because they can interfere with medical equipment.

___ Valuables, such as jewelry—leave your jewelry at home; if it is stolen, the hospital is not responsible for replacing it.

___ Cigarettes, alcohol, and illegal drugs

Breastfeeding gives newborns the perfect food, with numerous advantages over baby formula. It also can help you lose weight quicker after giving birth. Breast milk is good for several reasons:

- It is always available.

- It is free.

- It contains active infection-fighting white blood **cells** and **antibodies** that give increased protection against respiratory and digestive tract infections in the first months of a baby's life, when these infections can be the most serious.

- It lowers the risk of **sudden infant death syndrome**.

- It contains the perfect proportion of nutrients that your baby needs, including protein, carbohydrates, fats, and calcium.

- It is easily digestible.

There are numerous advantages for women who breastfeed as well:

- Women who breastfeed tend to lose weight more quickly after the birth.

- Breastfeeding helps the uterus contract and return to its normal size more rapidly, which decreases postpartum bleeding.

- Breastfeeding may reduce the risk of certain types of cancer, such as breast cancer and ovarian cancer. However, more research needs to be done to clarify these associations.

Of course, not everyone is able to breastfeed, and some women prefer not to. Here are some facts about bottle-feeding:

- Infant formulas have gotten better at matching the ingredients and their proportions to those of human milk. However, some babies need to try several formulas before the right one is found.

- It gives the mom some flexibility because using formula allows more than one person to feed the baby (although this option is also possible with breast milk if you pump it into a bottle).

- It can be expensive. You will need to buy infant formula, nipples, and bottles.

- It's time consuming. You will need to keep the bottles clean and sterilized so you always have a bottle ready at feeding time.

If you need more questions answered to help make a decision between breast-feeding or bottle-feeding, ask your health care provider. You also can go online to the La Leche League International web site. This organization aims to help mothers breastfeed worldwide (see the "Resources" section in this chapter). The American Academy of Pediatrics also has extensive informa-tion about breastfeeding (see the "Resources" section in this chapter).

Many mothers-to-be wonder if there's anything they should do to get ready to breastfeed. The truth is, there is very little you need to do to prepare your breasts for breastfeeding other than purchasing a good nursing bra.

There usually is no need to put lotion on your breasts. Your nipples are already producing what they need for their protection. Also, do not use soap on your breasts because soap can dry them out. When you bathe or shower, rinsing with plain water is fine.

If you have any questions about breastfeeding before the baby arrives, contact the lactation specialist at your hospital or your local La Leche League chapter. Keep in mind, though, that the nurses at the hospital will show you how to breastfeed the baby once you give birth, so you won't be left on your own to learn the proper technique. Chapter 18, "Breastfeeding and Formula-Feeding Your Baby," provides more detailed information about feeding your baby.

## Other Considerations

The last few weeks are always a busy time for new parents as they make sure they are prepared to bring the baby home from the hospital. Now is the time to shop for a car seat if you haven't done so already and to make sure that you have all the clothes and supplies you'll need once the baby comes home.

### Preparing Your Home for the Baby

A trip to any baby supply retailer or a look at the many online baby supply web sites will give you plenty of ideas about what you'll need at home to get ready. Talk to other new moms as well to get an idea of what products they used and liked best.

This also is a great time to start lining up family and friends who can help once the baby arrives. Don't be afraid to ask for help. You'll welcome the extra pair of hands once you're at home and spending some sleepless nights with the new baby. Make a list of some things you can use help with, such as the following tasks, and ask family and friends to take their pick:

- Cook a few meals and place them in the freezer for later.

- Go grocery shopping.
- Help with the laundry.
- Help out with your other children.
- Take care of family pets.

Remember that you may need help for a few weeks, not just for a few days after the baby comes home. Make sure that you have help lined up for the weeks ahead and not just the first couple of days after the baby comes home.

### Buying a Car Seat

You will not be able to take the baby home from the hospital unless you have a car seat already secured in your car. All 50 states have laws requiring child safety seats for infants and children at different ages.

All infants should ride in rear-facing car seats in the back seat starting with their first ride home from the hospital. In a rear-facing car seat, the baby is turned to face the back windshield of the car. Infants and toddlers should ride in a rear-facing car seat until they are 2 years of age or until they reach the highest weight or height allowed by the car seat's manufacturer. They then can sit facing the front but still must ride in the back seat of a car until they are age 13 years to avoid risk of injury associated with the passenger air bag inflating.

There are different types of rear-facing car safety seats: 1) infant-only seats, 2) convertible seats, and 3) 3-in-1 seats. An infant-only seat is for babies weighing up to 35 pounds. Most infant-only seats are made to pop out of a base; that way you can carry the seat by its handle or place it in a special stroller. An infant-only seat must be replaced when your baby reaches 35 pounds or the specific weight listed by the car seat maker. A convertible seat isn't as portable as an infant-only seat, but it can be converted to a forward-facing seat when your child turns 2 years old or reaches the height and weight limit for riding in a rear-facing seat. A 3-in-1 seat can be used as a rear-facing seat and a forward-facing seat as well as a booster seat when your child outgrows the forward-facing seat.

Many moms pass on baby supplies to new mothers once their own children no longer use them. Be careful, however, with used car seats. If you do borrow or reuse a car seat, you need to make sure that you know its history, such as whether it's been in an accident. Check the seat carefully for missing parts and defects. If you find any problems, do not use the car seat. The label with the car seat's model number should still be attached, and the instructions should be included with the car seat. Keep in mind that car seats have expiration dates. Check the expiration date for any car seat on

## Tips for Buying and Installing a Car Seat

Some safety seats will fit in your car better than others. A well-designed seat that is easy to use is the best for you and your child. When buying a seat, keep these tips in mind:

• Know whether your car has the LATCH system. LATCH stands for Lower Anchors and Tethers for Children. Special anchors, instead of safety belts, hold the seat in place. Newer cars and trucks will have the LATCH system. If either your car or your safety seat is not fitted with LATCH, you will need to use safety belts to install the car safety seat.

• Try locking and unlocking the buckle while you are in the store. Try changing the lengths of the straps.

• Try the seat in your car to make sure it fits.

• Read the labels to check weight limits.

• Do not decide just based on price. Seats that cost more are not always better.

When installing the seat, follow these tips:

• Decide whether to place the seat in the middle of the rear seat or in one of the side seats. Some experts think that placing the car seat in the middle is best. However, some cars do not have a middle seat or have a middle seat that is too narrow or uneven. Some LATCH systems do not work in the middle seat. The safest option is to place the car seat in the rear seat location where it can be tightly anchored with the seatbelt or LATCH system.

• Lock the seat into its base, if it has one. The base should not move more than 1 inch when pushed front to back or side to side. If you are using the safety belts, make sure the lap part of the belt is tightly fastened to the car seat frame.

If you have questions about installing a car seat, contact your local fire department or other local agency, which may be able to check your seat's placement and make sure it's properly installed.

the manufacturer's web site. If you can't afford to buy a seat, some communities and hospitals have programs for new parents to borrow an approved safety seat at no charge.

Once you have the car seat, it's important to install it correctly (see box "Tips for Buying and Installing a Car Seat." Even the best car seat won't protect your baby if it's not installed properly. Some fire departments and other

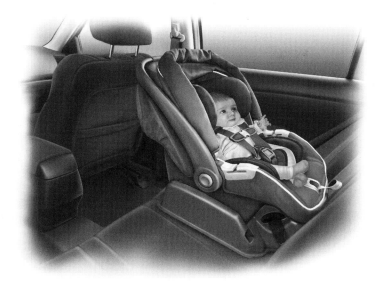

**Car safety for infants.** A baby should ride in a rear-facing car seat until he or she is 2 years old or reaches the top height and weight limit set by the rear-facing car seat manufacturer.

local agencies will check the placement of your car seat. If your infant seat has a base, practice putting it in and out of the base properly to make sure you know how it is done before leaving the hospital.

## Prenatal Care Visits

During this month of pregnancy, you'll have health care appointments every other week. At these visits, your health care provider will check your weight, blood pressure, and urine as usual. Fundal height will be measured again and the heartbeat will be monitored. You may have a vaginal exam to check whether your cervix is preparing for labor. Your health care provider also may estimate the baby's weight and determine his or her position in the uterus.

### Group B Streptococci Screening

At one of your prenatal care visits during weeks 35–37, you will be screened for **group B streptococci (GBS)**. Group B streptococci are common **bacteria** that are usually harmless in adults. Some pregnant women may develop a urinary tract infection or infection of the uterus caused by GBS. A baby can become infected with GBS as he or she moves through the birth canal of a woman who has the bacteria. A small number of babies who develop these early-onset infections can become critically ill. Babies also can become infected a few days or weeks after birth, but these late-onset infections usually are not related to the baby's delivery.

To help prevent early-onset infections, women are tested for GBS between week 35 and week 37 of pregnancy. In this test, your health care provider uses a swab to take a sample from your vagina and rectum. This procedure is quick and painless. The sample is sent to a lab where it is processed. It may take a few days to get the results.

If you test positive for GBS, you may receive *antibiotics* during labor to decrease the chances of passing the bacteria to your baby during birth. The antibiotics work only if they are given during labor. If treatment is given earlier in pregnancy, the bacteria may regrow and be present during labor.

Some women do not need to be tested for GBS. If you had a previous baby with a group B streptococcal infection or if your urine has had group B streptococcal bacteria during this pregnancy, you are at high risk of passing group B streptococci on to your baby during labor and delivery. You will receive treatment during labor to protect your baby from infection, and you don't need to be tested between 35 weeks and 37 weeks of pregnancy.

It's important for you to know what your GBS status is after you are tested. If you go into labor far from home or if your health care provider is not available, it will be helpful for your caregivers to know whether you need to receive antibiotics during labor. If your GBS status is not known when you go into labor, you may be given antibiotics if you go into labor early, if your membranes have ruptured early, if you have a fever, or if GBS is found in your urine.

## Other Screening Tests

Depending on your risk factors and state laws, you may have the following *screening tests* repeated during the last month of pregnancy:

- *Human immunodeficiency virus (HIV)*
- *Syphilis*
- *Chlamydia*
- *Gonorrhea*

## ⤳ Special Concerns

Be aware of the signs and symptoms of **preterm** labor (see Chapter 7, "Month 7 [Weeks 25–28]"). If you have any doubts about whether you are experiencing signs and symptoms of preterm labor, contact your health care provider.

### Preeclampsia

As discussed in Chapter 5, "Month 5 (Weeks 17–20)," **preeclampsia** is a serious medical condition of pregnancy that can occur after 20 weeks of pregnancy, typically in the third trimester, or after childbirth. It is important to be aware of the following signs and symptoms:

- Swelling of face or hands
- A headache that will not go away
- Seeing spots or changes in eyesight
- Pain in the upper abdomen or shoulder
- Nausea and vomiting (in the second half of pregnancy)
- Sudden weight gain
- Difficulty breathing

If you notice any of these symptoms, call your health care provider right away. Chapter 22, "Hypertension and Preeclampsia," gives more details about how preeclampsia is diagnosed and treated.

### Breech Presentation

Most babies move into a head-down position a few weeks before birth. This is called a **vertex presentation**. If the baby's buttocks, or buttocks and feet, are positioned to come out first, this is called a **breech presentation**. Sometimes, the baby can be turned into a head-down position using a technique called **external cephalic version (ECV)**. External cephalic version can be done after 36 completed weeks of pregnancy. In ECV, your health care provider will apply firm external manual pressure on your abdomen to try to turn the baby inside the uterus. There is some risk of complications with this procedure (see more information in Chapter 14, "Operative Delivery and Breech Presentation"). If there is only one baby and he or she is still breech by the due date, a planned **cesarean delivery** is the most common and safest option, but a vaginal delivery may be possible in certain situations.

# ASK THE EXPERTS

**I'd like to get a pedicure, since I can't see, let alone reach, my feet. I've heard you can get infections from pedicures. Is this true?**

While it is true that you can get fungal nail infections if the instruments used for your pedicure are not sanitized, this happens very rarely. Pedicures are a great way to pamper yourself during pregnancy, so indulge yourself and enjoy! To reduce the small risk of a fungal infection, bring along your own pedicure tools. Also, make sure that the soaking tub is disinfected before you put your feet in it.

**How soon after I have my baby can I start breastfeeding?**

If you feel up to it, you can start breastfeeding as soon as the baby is delivered. A healthy baby is perfectly capable of breastfeeding in the first hour after birth. Keeping your baby directly next to your skin also is the best way to maintain his or her body temperature. Your labor nurses can help you and your baby get into the right position.

**I have inverted nipples. Can I still breastfeed?**

Yes, breastfeeding is still possible. You first should determine whether your nipples are truly flat or inverted—there are degrees of inversion, and your nipples may not be completely flat. The way to find out is to pinch your nipple. If it does not become erect, then it is flat. If it does not protrude, it is truly inverted. However, many babies can exert enough suction to draw the nipple out on their own. Before the baby is born, you can wear breast shells, which provide gentle traction on the nipples. You also can use breast shells when you first start breastfeeding your baby. Keep in mind that a nurse or lactation specialist will be on hand at the hospital to provide assistance.

# RESOURCES

The following resources offer more information about some of the topics discussed in this chapter:

**Breastfeeding**
La Leche League International
www.llli.org
*Provides information and support for breastfeeding moms and offers referrals to local support groups.*

**Car Seats: Information for Families**
HealthyChildren.Org/American Academy of Pediatrics
www.healthychildren.org/English/safety-prevention/on-the-go/Pages/
Car-Safety-Seats-Information-for-Families.aspx
*Provides the latest recommendations for car seat safety and gives tips about shopping for and installing car seats.*

**Group B Streptococci**
Group B Strep International
www.groupbstrepinternational.org
*Promotes awareness and prevention of group B streptococcal infection in babies before birth through early infancy.*

**Parents Central**
National Highway Traffic Safety Administration
www.safercar.gov/parents/index.htm
*Gateway to information about all aspects of child safety and transportation, including choosing the right car seat and a car seat installation inspection station locator.*

**Safe Roads/Safe Kids**
Safe Kids Worldwide
www.safekids.org
*Maintains a list of child safety seat inspection events and keeps track of car seat safety recalls.*

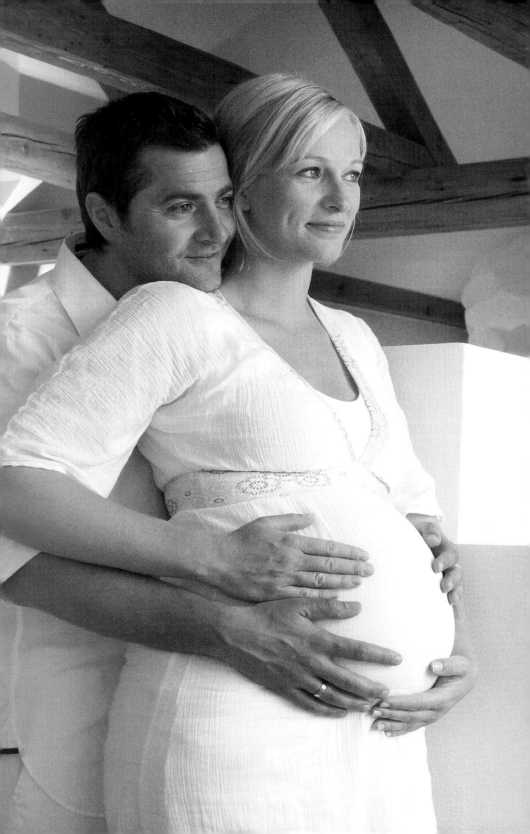

# Chapter 10

# Month 10
## (Weeks 37–40)

---

## YOUR GROWING BABY

### Week 37

The *lanugo* (body hair) that covered the baby has mostly been shed. Fat is being added all over—the elbows, knees, and shoulders—to keep your baby warm after birth. Your baby also grows in length by about 10%. At this stage, your pregnancy is considered to be *early term*. Babies who are born between this week and week 38 have not yet finished growing, but they are very close to doing so.

### Week 38

The baby's brain continues to develop—it grows by one third between week 35 and week 39 of pregnancy. The liver and lungs also are completing their growth during these last few weeks.

### Week 39

At 39 weeks of pregnancy, your baby is considered to be *full term*. Once he or she is born, the lungs and brain continue to develop—the brain completes its growth when your child is about 2 years of age.

### Week 40

The baby is ready to be born. By now, the baby's head may have dropped lower into position in your lower pelvis. At 40 weeks of pregnancy, he or she weighs about 6–9 pounds and is probably between 18 inches and 20 inches long.

MONTH 10

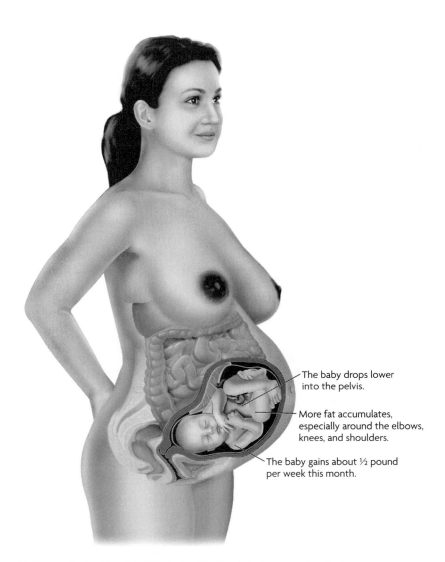

The baby drops lower into the pelvis.

More fat accumulates, especially around the elbows, knees, and shoulders.

The baby gains about ½ pound per week this month.

**Mother and baby: Month 10 (Weeks 37–40).** Your baby is now ready to be born.

# YOUR PREGNANCY

## ➣ Your Changing Body

You've reached the end of your pregnancy! In these final weeks before your due date, you probably can't wait until the pregnancy is over. This month, your uterus will finish expanding; it has grown from only about 2 ounces before you were pregnant to about 2 ½ pounds now.

## ➣ Discomforts and How to Manage Them

You're probably very uncomfortable now. Walking is an effort, and lying down is not much better. Many women report sleepless nights during the last few weeks. It may be difficult to get in and out of the car. You may be getting bored with just waiting for the baby to come, or you may be keyed up and anxious.

Try to keep your mind off the waiting. Spend some quality time with your partner, read a good book, or go see a movie. Staying active will help the days pass more quickly. Now is the time to complete some last-minute items that can help prepare you, your family, and your home for the new arrival (see box "Things to Do This Month to Get Ready").

### Frequent Urination

The uterus is bigger than it has ever been now and it is pressing much more on your bladder, causing many trips to the bathroom throughout the day. But don't cut back on drinking plenty of liquids during this time because your body needs the fluids more than ever.

### Snoring

If your partner says you've been snoring a lot more than usual, blame it on normal changes in breathing during pregnancy. If your snoring is a real problem, try sleeping with nasal strips across the bridge of your nose or using a humidifier in your bedroom.

MONTH 10

## Things to Do This Month to Get Ready

- Put a waterproof sheet or mattress cover on your bed to protect it in case your water breaks during the night.

- Wash and organize the baby's clothes. Some advise leaving the tags on and only washing them if you're sure your baby is going to need them. You may want to wait if you think you will be returning baby clothes to the store. However, you can always donate any clothes that you don't end up using.

- Line up your helpers. Make sure everyone knows what they should do and when they should do it. You may want to make a schedule to see on what days you may be shorthanded and to avoid an overload of people on any one day. Also, keep in mind that you still may need helpers a few weeks after the birth, not just in the first few days.

- Prepare meals that can be frozen and defrosted easily. Soups, stews, and casseroles are great to have on hand and easy to microwave when needed.

- Write in a journal. You may want to write down your thoughts and feelings as you get ready for the birth. Your child may enjoy reading your journal later on, and you'll have a record of how you felt during this special time.

## Nutrition

It's not unusual for symptoms of mild nausea to return in the final weeks of pregnancy. In fact, some women even lose a few pounds. Nausea may be a sign that labor is starting. If nausea is severe or persistent, call your health care provider.

In these last weeks, you may feel better eating four or five small meals during the day instead of three big ones. If mild nausea is a problem for you, try to eat bland foods, such as the BRATT (banana, rice, applesauce, tea, and toast) diet. Just remember that you must keep eating regularly throughout the day. You and the baby will need the energy to cope with the strain of labor and birth.

## Focus on Docosahexaenoic Acid

Docosahexaenoic acid (DHA) is an omega-3 fatty acid (see Chapter 5, "Month 5 [Weeks 17–20]") found in fish, such as salmon and tuna, as well as flaxseeds and their oil. Although research still is being conducted to learn more about its effects, some studies suggest that DHA plays a role in the development of the brain before and after the baby is born. The U.S. Food and Drug Administration states that DHA also may be useful in helping to protect against heart disease in adults. Fish and shellfish are great sources of DHA, and pregnant women are advised to eat at least 8 ounces and up to 12 ounces of fish a week. Choose fish that contain low amounts of mercury, such as shrimp, salmon, and halibut, and avoid tilefish, shark, swordfish, and king mackerel, which contain the highest levels of mercury.

## What to Eat if You Think You Are Going Into Labor

If you think you're in the early stages of labor, you may be wondering whether you can eat and if so, what. Here are the latest guidelines from the American College of Obstetricians and Gynecologists about eating and drinking during labor:

- If you are having a planned *cesarean delivery*, you should not eat any solid food for 6–8 hours before your surgery is scheduled. Depending on your hospital's or health care provider's policies, you may have small amounts of clear liquids up to 2 hours before surgery. Clear liquids include water, fruit juices without pulp, carbonated beverages, tea, and sports drinks.

- Women who are having an uncomplicated labor can have small amounts of clear liquids during labor. However, because it's not possible to predict whether you will need a cesarean delivery, you won't be allowed to eat solid foods during labor at the hospital.

- Women with certain conditions that may increase their risk of problems with *anesthesia*, such as *obesity* or *diabetes mellitus*, may be told to further restrict their intake of food and liquids beyond these guidelines.

  Your health care provider or the hospital or birth center may have their own policies regarding eating and drinking during labor. You need to know these policies before your labor starts, so be sure to ask at one of your prenatal visits.

## ~~ Exercise

Exercise this month will be a challenge. Now is a good time for you and your partner to practice the breathing exercises you learned in childbirth class. Practice now while you are relaxed so you both remember exactly what to do once labor starts.

## Exercise of the Month: Paced Breathing

Different childbirth methods teach different breathing techniques. Paced breathing is one type of breathing technique that many women use in the early stages of labor. Using paced breathing has many benefits. It ensures that you and the baby are getting enough **oxygen**. It promotes both physical and mental relaxation. Controlling your breathing gives you a sense of control over your body, which can be helpful during childbirth. It also allows you to focus on pacing your inhalation and exhalation instead of focusing on the pain from contractions.

Paced breathing is slow, deep breathing. The idea is to slow your respirations to about one half the number of breaths that you usually take in 1 minute. If you usually take 15 breaths per minute, try to breathe eight full, deep breaths per minute during paced breathing. Don't try to do less than half though, or you may not be breathing enough. Taking six to nine breaths per minute is the goal—each inhalation and exhalation should last about 5 seconds each. Try counting to five with each inhalation and counting to five on each exhalation.

As you breathe in, breathe all the way down into your chest. Your rib cage should expand a bit. As you breathe out, relax the muscles of your chest, arms, and neck. It doesn't matter if you breathe in or out through your mouth or your nose—do whatever is most relaxing and comfortable for you. If you do breathe in or out through your mouth, your mouth can become dry. You may need to have clear liquids or ice chips on hand to counteract this. Also, use both your abdomen and your chest—just as you do in "normal" breathing—during paced breathing. You can practice paced breathing for 10 minutes a day. Paced breathing may help you relax during pregnancy before the delivery of your baby as well, so practicing during these last few weeks can both relax you now and help you remember this breathing technique to use during labor.

## 〰 Healthy Decisions

When do you go to the hospital? Can your children be in the delivery room? These are common decisions that you may be asking during these final weeks.

### Delivery Before 39 Weeks

It was once thought that babies born a few weeks early—between 37 weeks and 39 weeks—were just as healthy as babies born after 39 weeks. Experts now know that babies grow throughout the entire 40 weeks of pregnancy. This is important if you are thinking about scheduling your baby's birth—by having your labor induced or requesting a cesarean delivery—for a non-medical reason, which is called an *elective delivery*. Some nonmedical reasons include wanting to schedule the birth of the baby on a specific date or living far away from the hospital. Some women request delivery because they are uncomfortable in the last weeks of pregnancy. Some women request a cesarean delivery because they fear vaginal birth.

Babies who are born before 39 weeks may not be as developed as those who are born after 39 weeks. As a result, they may have an increased risk of short-term and long-term health problems, including breathing problems, difficulty eating and sleeping, hearing and visual problems, and learning problems later in life.

If you or the baby develop complications, early delivery may be necessary to save your or your baby's life. But if you are having a healthy pregnancy and there are no complications, early delivery is not recommended. If you're considering elective delivery because of discomfort, it may help to know that it is normal to feel uncomfortable at the end of pregnancy. If you live far away from the hospital, you might want to stay with someone who lives closer. You also may be able to travel to the hospital when you are in very early labor. Talk to your health care provider to get other suggestions and advice.

### When to Go to the Hospital

During the final weeks, you and your partner will no doubt spend anxious moments wondering when is the right time to go to the hospital. It will depend mostly on the timing and intensity of your contractions or whether your water breaks. Your health care provider will give you clear instructions as you approach your due date, so follow them exactly. You may be able to call and talk with your health care provider or the staff to discuss the signs and symptoms of labor that you are experiencing.

### Children in the Delivery Room

Some families invite their older children into the delivery room to witness their sibling's birth. Only you can know if this is right for your child or for you. If you would like to make your baby's birth a family affair, talk with your health care provider first. Find out what the hospital policy is about children in the delivery room. Many won't allow young children to be present. If your other children are going to be in the room, each needs to have their own adult support person. Even if your child isn't with you during delivery, he or she can meet the new brother or sister shortly after birth.

## Other Considerations

Sometimes it's hard to tell if labor is starting or if it is simply a false alarm. There may be times when you wonder, "Is this it?" Telling real labor from false labor often is difficult, even for health care providers. While you are waiting for labor to begin, some women wonder whether it is still OK to have sex. Some women also may experience a burst of energy, commonly called the "nesting instinct," during these weeks.

### Knowing When You're in Labor

It sometimes can be difficult to tell when you're in labor. **Braxton Hicks contractions** can occur for many weeks before labor actually begins. These "practice" contractions can be very painful and can make you think you are in labor when you really are not. But painless contractions don't always mean that you're not in labor, either. Each woman feels pain differently, and it can differ from one pregnancy to another. Nevertheless, there are certain changes in your body that signal labor is near:

- Lightening—You feel as if the baby has dropped lower. Because the baby isn't pressing on your diaphragm, you may feel "lighter." The baby's head has settled deep into your pelvis. Lightening can occur anywhere from a few weeks to a few hours before labor begins.

- Loss of the mucus plug—A thick mucus plug has accumulated at the **cervix** during pregnancy. When the cervix begins to dilate (several days before labor begins or at the onset of labor), the plug is pushed into the vagina. You may notice an increase in vaginal discharge that's clear, pink, or slightly bloody. Some women expel the entire mucus plug.

- Rupture of membranes—The fluid-filled sac that surrounded the baby during pregnancy breaks (your "water breaks"). You may experience this as a discharge of watery fluid from your vagina in a trickle or gush. Your membranes can rupture from several hours before labor to any time during labor.

• Contractions—As your uterus contracts, you may feel pain in your back or pelvis that's similar to menstrual cramps. Contractions occur in a regular pattern and get closer together over time.

How can you tell the difference between "real" labor contractions and Braxton Hicks contractions? One good way to tell the difference is to time the contractions) and to note whether the contractions go away with movement. Table 10-1 shows other differences between true labor and false labor contractions that may be helpful.

If you have doubts about whether you are in labor, call your health care provider. There also are other signs that should prompt you to call your health care provider or go to the hospital:

• Your membranes have ruptured and you are not having contractions.
• You are bleeding from the vagina (other than bloody mucus).
• You have constant, severe pain with no relief between contractions.
• You notice the baby is moving less often.

## Having Sex

If you and your partner feel the desire, it is perfectly OK to have sex right up to the time you give birth unless your health care provider has told you otherwise. Some women find *sexual intercourse* uncomfortable in the final

**Table 10-1 Differences Between False Labor and True Labor**

| Type Of Change | False Labor | True Labor |
| --- | --- | --- |
| Timing of contractions | Often are irregular and do not get closer together (called Braxton Hicks contractions) | Come at regular intervals and, as time goes on, get closer together. Each lasts about 30–70 seconds. |
| Change with movement | Contractions may stop when you walk or rest or may even stop with a change of position. | Contractions continue, despite movement. |
| Strength of contractions | Usually weak and do not get much stronger (may be strong and then weak) | Increase in strength steadily |
| Pain of contractions | Usually felt only in the front | Usually starts in the back and moves to the front |

weeks of pregnancy. You and your partner can give each other pleasure in ways that do not involve intercourse, including oral sex and mutual masturbation.

### Nesting

Many moms-to-be approaching their due dates feel a strong urge to complete work projects and organize the house for the baby. This urge is known as the "nesting instinct." While there is no scientific evidence to prove that there is such a thing, many women attest that it indeed exists.

If the nesting urge strikes, go ahead and do what you need to do in order to satisfy your feelings. However, remember not to overdo it, and don't exhaust yourself. Ask for help. You need to conserve your energy for labor and delivery as well as for caring for the new baby.

## Prenatal Care Visits

You usually will see your health care provider once a week this month until you go into labor. Your weight, blood pressure, and uterus size will be measured just as they were last month. The baby's position will be checked, and you will be asked about the baby's movements. Your cervix may be checked to see if it has started preparing for labor.

## Special Concerns

Although **preeclampsia** can occur earlier in pregnancy (any time after 20 weeks), it most commonly occurs in the last weeks of pregnancy. For some women, rupture of the membranes signals the start of labor, as does vaginal spotting. Heavy bleeding, however, may be a sign of a problem that needs to be checked by your health care provider.

### Signs of Preeclampsia

Preeclampsia may cause the following signs and symptoms:

- Swelling of the face or hands
- A headache that will not go away
- Seeing spots or changes in eyesight
- Pain in the upper abdomen or shoulder

- Nausea and vomiting (in the second half of pregnancy)
- Sudden weight gain
- Difficulty breathing

If you notice any of these symptoms, call your health care provider right away. Chapter 22, "Hypertension and Preeclampsia," gives more details about how preeclampsia is diagnosed and treated.

## Rupture of Membranes

You may feel a trickle or a gush of fluid at the beginning of labor or during labor. When your membranes rupture, also known as your water breaking, the fluid-filled *amniotic sac* that surrounds the baby has broken. Call your health care provider if your membranes rupture, and follow his or her instructions. Once your membranes rupture, your health care provider will want to make sure labor begins soon if it hasn't already.

## Changes in the Baby's Movement

You may notice that the baby's movement is different now from the movements you felt in previous weeks. It's normal for movements to feel different because there is less room in the uterus. The rate of movement is actually the same; it just doesn't feel the same to you.

Your health care provider may have you monitor the baby's movements by keeping track of how long it takes for you to feel 10 movements. To do this test (which sometimes is called a "kick count"), choose a time when the baby usually is active. Often, a good time is after you've eaten a meal. Each baby has its own level of activity, and most have a sleep cycle of 20–40 minutes. Call your health care provider if it takes longer than 2 hours for the baby to make 10 movements.

## Vaginal Spotting

If you have light spotting in weeks 37–40, it could be a sign that labor is beginning. Vaginal discharge that is pink or slightly bloody may be an indication of early labor as the cervix starts to dilate and the thick mucus plug that seals off the cervix during pregnancy is beginning to loosen. However, if vaginal bleeding is heavy—as heavy as a normal menstrual period—it could be a sign of a problem. In this situation, contact your health care provider right away.

## Late-Term and Postterm Pregnancy

A *late-term pregnancy* is defined as one that is 41 weeks and 0/7 days through 41 weeks and 6/7 days. A *postterm pregnancy* is one that is 42 weeks and 0/7 days or longer. Women who are having a baby for the first time or who have had postterm pregnancies before may give birth later than expected. One reason for postterm pregnancy is an inaccurate due date. However, sometimes postterm pregnancy occurs because the pregnancy is actually lasting longer than normal. Postterm pregnancy is not all that rare—in the United States, 6% of pregnancies last 42 weeks or longer.

If your due date has come and gone, your health care provider most likely will do some type of fetal evaluation to check your baby's health. If you don't start labor on your own by 41–42 weeks, your health care provider will discuss the option of inducing labor with you.

**Risks.** When a pregnancy goes longer than 40 weeks, it can increase the risks to the baby's and mother's health. After 42 weeks, the *placenta* may not work as well as it did earlier in pregnancy. Also, as the baby grows, the amount of *amniotic fluid* may begin to decrease. Less fluid may cause the *umbilical cord* to become pinched as the baby moves or as the uterus contracts. The baby can grow larger than normal, which can complicate a vaginal delivery. Postterm pregnancy doubles the mother's risk of needing a cesarean delivery.

Despite these risks, most women who give birth after their due dates have healthy newborns. When a baby is not born by the due date, certain tests can help monitor the baby's health. Some tests, such as a kick count, can be done on your own at home. Others are done in the health care provider's office or in the hospital. These include the *nonstress test, biophysical profile*, assessment of amniotic fluid levels, and *contraction stress test* (see Chapter 26, "Testing to Monitor Fetal Well-Being," for a detailed description of these tests).

**Deciding to Induce Labor.** Labor induction is the use of medication or other methods to start labor. Whether your labor will be induced depends on the following factors:

- Your condition and your baby's condition

- How far along you are in your pregnancy

- If your cervix has begun to soften (called "*cervical ripening*") and open in preparation for delivery

- Results of tests for fetal well-being

In preparation for labor and delivery, the cervix begins to soften, thin out (a process called **effacement**), and open (called **dilation**). Your health care provider will perform a vaginal exam in the last few weeks of pregnancy to see if your cervix has started these processes.

If you've gone past your due date and your cervix has not begun these changes, your health care provider may recommend techniques to help ripen the cervix. Cervical ripening techniques include devices that open the cervix or medications containing **prostaglandins**, chemicals that are made by the body that ripen the cervix and cause uterine contractions.

**Laminaria** is a natural or artificial substance inserted into the cervix that expands when it absorbs water. A **catheter**, or small tube, also can be used to dilate the cervix, as well as special dilators. Medications that dilate the cervix can be given by mouth or placed in the vagina.

The decision to use cervical ripening techniques is based on several factors, including whether the risks outweigh the benefits. There is an increased risk of infection with the use of dilators. Risks of cervical ripening medication include an increase in the rate and strength of uterine contractions and changes in fetal heart rate. Monitoring of the baby's heart rate and the strength of uterine contractions is done for at least a short period after medications for cervical ripening are given.

In cases in which continuing the pregnancy is more risky than delivering the baby, your health care provider might induce labor. More than one method of labor induction may be used. Some of the methods used to induce labor also can speed up a labor that's not progressing as it should. Details about labor induction can be found in Chapter 12, "Labor Induction."

## Old Wives' Tales

You may have heard other women talk about ways you can make labor start on your own. Many women believe doing such things as taking long walks, having sex, or eating spicy foods can bring on labor. There is, however, no evidence that any of these methods work.

One nonmedical method of labor induction that is somewhat more effective is nipple stimulation. Research on this method found that it did bring on labor in some women, but only when the cervix was ready for labor. However, you should not attempt to bring on labor with nipple stimulation without your health care provider's supervision.

# ASK THE EXPERTS

### What is an episiotomy and why might I need one?

An *episiotomy* is a procedure in which a small cut is made to widen the opening of your vagina when you're giving birth. It may be done to assist delivery of the baby or to avoid tearing the skin at the opening of the vagina. Episiotomies used to be performed routinely, but current guidelines from the American College of Obstetricians and Gynecologists suggest restricting their use. It is helpful to discuss this issue with your health care provider before labor. Ask about his or her rate of episiotomy and the situations in which it could be performed.

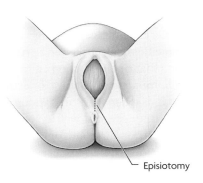

Episiotomy

### I've heard about *operative vaginal delivery*. What is it and when is it done?

In an operative vaginal delivery, the baby is delivered using *forceps* or *vacuum extraction* (a special suction cup). Operative vaginal delivery may be done if you have pushed for a long time without progress or you are not able to push the baby out because of a medical condition. It also can be done if there are suspected problems with the baby, such as a slow or erratic heartbeat. See Chapter 14, "Operative Delivery and Breech Presentation" for more details about operative vaginal delivery.

# RESOURCES

The following resources offer more information about some of the topics discussed in this chapter:

**40 Reasons to Go to the Full 40**
Healthy Mom & Baby
www.health4mom.org/zones/go-the-full-40
*40 reasons to go the full 40 weeks of pregnancy.*

**Thinking About Inducing Your Labor: A Guide for Pregnant Women**
Agency for Healthcare Research and Quality
http://effectivehealthcare.ahrq.gov/index.cfm/search-for-guides-reviews-and-repo
rts/?productid=353&pageaction=displayproduct
*Discusses why it's best to wait until after 39 weeks of pregnancy if you are thinking about elective labor induction.*

**Why at Least 39 Weeks Is Best for Your Baby**
March of Dimes
www.marchofdimes.com/pregnancy/why-at-least-39-weeks-is-best-for-your-baby.
aspx
*Explains why healthy babies need 39 weeks of development.*

# Part II
# Labor, Delivery, and Postpartum Care

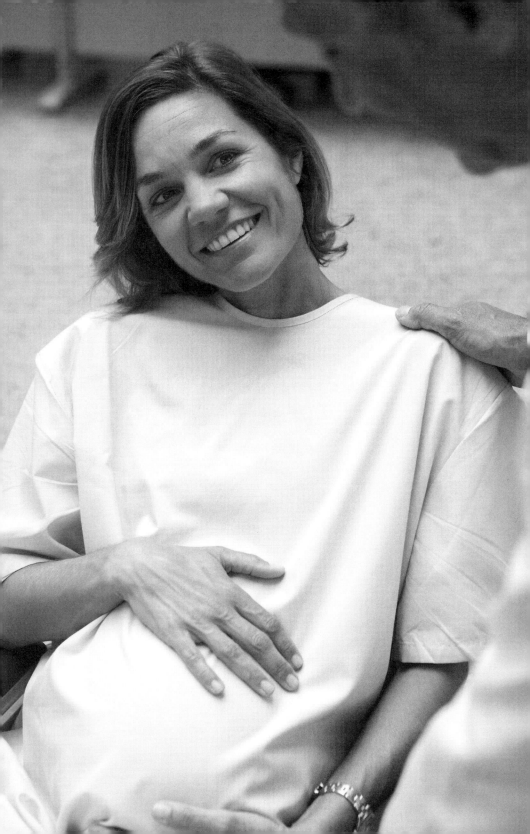

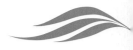

Chapter 11

# Pain Relief During Childbirth

The pain felt during childbirth is different for every woman. It also can be different from your past deliveries if you have had other children. How you experience the pain depends on many factors, such as the size and position of the baby, the strength of your contractions, and how well you handle pain.

To cope with the pain of childbirth, many women take classes that teach breathing and relaxation techniques. Others find it helps to use these techniques along with pain medication. Despite the expected pain of labor, some women worry that getting pain relief medication during labor and delivery will make the childbirth experience less natural. But many women find that receiving pain relief medications allows them to participate more fully in childbirth and gives them better control.

Start thinking about the type of pain relief you would like to use during labor and delivery while you are pregnant. Talk to your health care provider about your options. Not all types of pain relief are available at every hospital or birthing center.

## Medications for Pain Relief

There are two main types of pain relief drugs. An ***analgesic*** drug relieves pain without total loss of feeling or muscle movement. These drugs lessen pain but usually do not stop pain completely. An ***anesthetic*** drug relieves pain by blocking all feeling, including pain.

### Systemic Analgesics

Systemic analgesics act on the body's entire nervous system, rather than a specific area, to lessen pain. They will not cause you to lose consciousness (put you to sleep). Types of drugs used for this purpose include *narcotics*, which block the feeling of pain, and *sedatives*, which make you drowsy. These medications often are used during early labor to allow you to rest.

Systemic analgesics usually are given as a shot. Depending on the type of medication, the shot is given into either a muscle or a vein. With patient-controlled analgesics, you can control the amount of medication you receive through an *intravenous (IV) line*.

Systemic pain medications can have side effects. Most are minor, such as nausea, feeling drowsy, or having trouble concentrating. Sometimes another drug is given along with a systemic analgesic to relieve nausea. Another side effect is that these medications can make it more difficult to detect problems with the fetal heart rate. High doses of systemic pain medications can cause you to have breathing problems and can slow down the baby's *respiratory system*, especially right after delivery. You and the baby will be monitored closely during and after this medication is given.

### Local Anesthesia

*Local anesthesia* provides complete relief from pain in a small area of the body. You already may have had local anesthesia if you've had a cavity filled at the dentist's office. During childbirth, a local anesthetic can be used to block pain in the *perineum*. It's also used when an *episiotomy* is needed or if any vaginal tears that happen during birth need to be repaired. It does not lessen the pain of contractions.

Local anesthesia is injected into the area around the nerves that carry feeling to the vagina, *vulva*, and perineum. When used to relieve pain during childbirth, the drug is given just before the baby is delivered. The drug rarely affects the baby and there usually are no side effects once the local anesthesia wears off.

### Regional Analgesia and Regional Anesthesia

*Regional analgesia* and *regional anesthesia* act on a specific region of the body. For labor and delivery, these types of medication lessen or block pain below the waist. There are several types available.

**Epidural Analgesia or Anesthesia.** An *epidural block* (or "an epidural") is the most common type of pain relief used during childbirth in the United States. In this type of pain relief, medication is given through a **catheter** (a small tube) that is inserted with a needle into the lower back.

An epidural may be started soon after your contractions start or later as your labor progresses. An *anesthesiologist* or other specialized health care provider typically gives an epidural.

Before an epidural is given, your skin will be cleaned and local anesthesia will be used to numb an area of your lower back. As you sit or lie very still on your side, a needle is inserted into the small area in your lower back called the epidural space. After the epidural needle is inserted, a catheter usually is inserted and the needle is removed. The catheter remains in place. Medication then can be given as needed through the catheter to reduce the discomfort of labor. Patient-controlled epidural analgesia also is an option. With this option, you can give yourself a dose of medication by pushing a button. The device is programmed so that you can't give yourself too much medication. Medications also can be given continuously without another injection.

Because the medication needs to be absorbed into several nerves, it may take about 10–20 minutes for you to feel pain relief. The medication that is given is usually a combination of an anesthetic and an analgesic. Depending on your level of pain, your anesthesiologist can adjust the amount of medication as needed throughout labor and delivery. With an epidural, you usually will be able to move, but you may not be able to walk around once the medication starts to work. You still may feel your contractions, but you will be more comfortable.

The risk of side effects from an epidural is low, but there is a chance that you may have a drop in blood pressure, a fever, or back soreness in the injection area. About 1% of women will have a severe headache that can occur within 1 day to 1 week after receiving an epidural. This headache happens if the needle used to place the epidural punctures the covering of the spinal cord, causing leakage of spinal fluid. Standard headache medications are tried first to relieve the headache. If they don't work, you may need to have a simple procedure called a blood patch. In this procedure, some of your own blood is injected into the epidural space near the site where the needle went in. As this blood clots, it stops the spinal fluid from leaking out.

In a very small number of women, the anesthesia medication might be injected into one of the veins in the epidural space. This can cause dizziness, rapid heartbeat, or a funny taste. To reduce the chance of these problems, you will be monitored closely while you are receiving epidural medication. Tell your labor and delivery team if you have any of these symptoms.

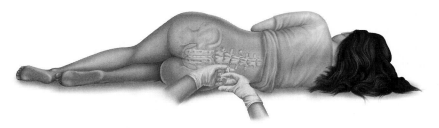

**Regional anesthesia and analgesia.** Regional pain relief is given through a needle that delivers pain medication to the nerves that carry pain signals.

**Spinal Block.** With a *spinal block*, a small amount of medication is injected with a thin needle into the sac of spinal fluid below the level of the spinal cord. The medication starts to relieve pain right away but only lasts for an hour or two. A spinal block usually is given only once.

Depending on the medications used, a spinal block can be used for analgesia or anesthesia. A combination of analgesics and anesthetics can be injected to provide short-term pain relief during labor. Higher doses of anesthetics can give a complete loss of feeling for *cesarean delivery*. A spinal block can cause the same side effects as an epidural.

**Combined Spinal–Epidural Block.** A *combined spinal–epidural (CSE) block* has the benefits of both a spinal block and an epidural block. A spinal block is given first to give pain relief right away. An epidural catheter then is placed to provide pain medication throughout labor. The CSE block sometimes is called a "walking epidural." Depending on your hospital's policy, you may be able to walk for a short distance after the CSE is in place, such as to the bathroom. However, you most likely will not be allowed to walk the hallways or to use gravity-assisting labor positions. In most hospitals, women who receive any type of pain relief need to stay in bed.

## General Anesthesia

With *general anesthesia*, you are not awake and you feel no pain. It can be started quickly and causes a rapid loss of consciousness. This type of anesthesia is used most commonly in emergency situations and may not be offered as an option you can choose.

The drugs that put you to sleep are given through an IV line or through a mask. After you are asleep, your anesthesiologist will place a breathing tube into your mouth and windpipe.

A rare but major risk during general anesthesia is aspiration of food or liquids from the stomach into the lungs. Labor usually causes undigested food to stay in the stomach longer than usual. While you are unconscious, the contents of your stomach can come back into the mouth and go into the lungs. This can cause a lung infection (pneumonia) that can be serious.

General anesthesia usually requires the placement of a breathing tube into the lungs to help you breathe while you are unconscious. Difficulty placing this tube is another risk of general anesthesia.

General anesthesia can cause the newborn baby's breathing rate to decrease. It also can make the baby less alert. In rare cases, the baby may need help breathing after birth. The effects of general anesthesia usually wear off quickly. There are no permanent effects from general anesthesia on the baby's brain or development.

## Childbirth Preparation Methods

Childbirth preparation methods are ways of coping with pain and reducing the discomfort of labor and delivery. Childbirth preparation classes are available that teach mothers-to-be the various techniques. Although specific techniques are different, all childbirth preparation methods seek to relieve discomfort through the general principles of education, support, relaxation, paced breathing, and touch. Here is a brief description of some of these methods:

• Lamaze—The Lamaze method of childbirth preparation was developed in the 1950s by French obstetrician Dr. Fernand Lamaze. This method is based on the idea that a woman's inner wisdom guides her through childbirth. Lamaze childbirth education helps women gain confidence in their bodies and learn to make informed decisions about pregnancy, birth, breastfeeding, and parenting. To learn more about this method, go to the Lamaze International web site (see the "Resources" section in this chapter).

• Bradley—The Bradley method views childbirth as a natural process and is based on the belief that a healthy pregnancy and birth can be achieved through education, preparation, and support from a childbirth coach. This method involves the active participation of the mother and her coach during the labor process and teaches a variety of relaxation techniques. Information about the Bradley method is available online (see the "Resources" section in this chapter).

• Read—One of the first methods to introduce the concept of prepared childbirth, the Read method seeks to eliminate fear and anxiety by educating mothers and coaches about labor and delivery. The Read method is explained in the book *Childbirth Without Fear,* written by its founder, Dr. Grantly Dick-Read.

- Hypnosis—"Hypnobirthing" consists of using relaxation and self-hypnosis techniques to teach women how to harness the body's natural painkilling chemicals—endorphins—to achieve a natural and fear-free childbirth. Information about this method is available online (see the "Resources" section in this chapter).

- Yoga and Sophrology—Both of these methods derive from Indian culture and teach control of the body and mind. Through relaxation, concentration, and meditation, these techniques can lessen the pain of labor. Ask your health care provider about prenatal yoga classes offered in your area.

- Music therapy—Listening to soft, relaxing music during early labor and music that has a steady beat during the later stages has been shown to reduce pain for some women.

- Massage therapy—A gentle, firm massage on the lower back and shoulders with a partner's knuckles or a tennis ball can relieve some of the pressure from uterine contractions.

With all of the choices available, you're likely to find something that appeals to you and your own beliefs. As you consider your options, keep the following tips in mind:

- Contact the class instructor—The instructor's approach and knowledge are important factors in determining whether the class is right for you. Ask questions to get a sense of how the class is taught.

- Find out the location and schedule—Is the class offered nearby? How many weeks does it meet? You want to find a class that is convenient for your lifestyle.

- Figure in price—Find out how much the class costs and what's included in the fee. Also, check whether your insurance policy will cover any of the cost.

- How many people are in the class?—Some classes are small and offer individual attention. Others are larger. Talk with your childbirth partner about whether a small or large class is more suitable for you and your needs.

Don't think, though, that you have to select a particular childbirth method. It's not a requirement for giving birth. Your health care providers will give you the instructions and information you need while you're at the hospital or birthing center.

## Pain Relief Techniques

Starting centuries before epidurals were invented, women have used different methods to ease the pain of labor. If you are interested in using some of these techniques, you may want to make sure they are available at the hospital where you will give birth.

### Positions

There has long been a healthy debate about the best position in which to labor and give birth. Many women in the United States give birth while lying on their backs with their feet supported in stirrups. This is called the lithotomy position. Giving birth in this position may make it easier for your health care provider to give assistance and provides support for your back and legs.

Other positions besides lying on your back or side also can be tried, as long as your health care provider gives approval. Squatting, standing, kneeling, or sitting allow gravity to help move the baby downward in the birth canal. Being upright instead of lying down alleviates the pressure of the baby pressing on your spine, which can feel more comfortable for some women. Squatting positions stretch the birth canal to its widest diameter, making it easier for the baby to slide out.

Many hospitals and birth centers offer beds, chairs, and other equipment to accommodate various positions. Some of the options that may be available are as follows:

- Birthing bed—A birthing bed can be adjusted to numerous positions for you, such as squatting, sitting on the end of the bed with your feet supported, or lying on your side. A squatting bar that you can hang on to can be attached over the bed.

- Birthing chair—Birthing chairs are specially designed to allow you to give birth in a seated position.

- Birthing stool—Birthing stools stabilize and support you while you squat.

- Birthing ball—Although you cannot give birth on one, a birthing ball can be used during labor. Sitting on the ball opens up your pelvis and birth canal, giving gentle support and stability. You also can rock back and forth on the ball to help ease the pain of contractions or lean your upper body on the birthing ball if it is placed on the bed. You can bring a birthing ball from home if the hospital does not have one.

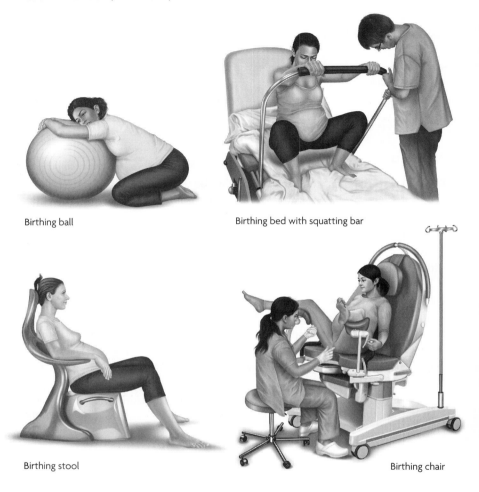

Birthing ball

Birthing bed with squatting bar

Birthing stool

Birthing chair

**Positions for labor.** Many hospitals offer special chairs and other equipment to help you get into comfortable positions for labor and delivery.

Consider all your options and ask plenty of questions. You may want to make a plan before labor begins, but be aware that not all birthing positions or equipment may be available at your facility.

## Warm Baths and Showers

Undergoing labor in water has become more popular in recent years as more hospitals and birthing centers have started offering this service. The use of water for pain relief, also known as "hydrotherapy," is a method that has been used in medicine for centuries. Some studies have shown that sitting in water during the first stage of labor can lessen pain and shorten labor, but results are not consistent. There appears to be no benefit to immersion in water during actual delivery of the baby, and there also is no indication that laboring in water has any benefits for the baby.

Although it may be acceptable from a safety standpoint to go through the first stage of labor in a pool of water, giving birth underwater is not recommended. Even if you do not plan to give birth underwater, the baby may be born accidentally while you are in the birthing pool or tub. There have been reports of serious harm to babies born underwater, including breathing problems, seizures, and near drowning. For these reasons, it's recommended that underwater birth not be performed routinely, but only in the setting of a research trial for which you have given informed consent.

There are a few precautions that you should keep in mind if you want to try laboring in water. It should not prevent your health care provider from being able to monitor your condition and the condition of your baby. There should be a process in place to quickly and safely move you from the tub if concerns or problems arise. Finally, to avoid the possibility of the baby being born underwater accidentally, you should move out of the tub when the second stage of labor begins (ie, when you start to push the baby out).

Many women report that taking a warm shower is helpful during labor. Having warm water flow on your back and abdomen can ease tense muscles, promote relaxation, and help diffuse pain sensations. As a safety precaution, you should have someone standing nearby to support you in case you need it.

## Walking

During the early stages of labor, walking may help you stay relaxed and ease some of the pain. If your health care provider says it's OK, take short walks down the hall with your birthing coach. You will not be able to walk if you have an epidural or spinal analgesia. If you are connected to the electronic fetal monitor, you still can walk or pace close to your bed. You also can ask your health care provider if it is OK to monitor the baby intermittently, for example, for 15 minutes every hour. Some hospitals have wireless electronic fetal monitor devices that monitor the baby continuously and allow you to move around more freely.

## Continuous Labor Support

"Continuous labor support" is a term that experts use to describe when a woman has someone with her throughout labor and delivery. Studies that involved thousands of women from across the world have proven that women who have a support person from the time labor begins until the baby is born have a better birthing experience. The women studied had shorter labor times, needed less pain medication, and were less likely to need a cesarean delivery or help from the use of *forceps* or a vacuum device.

Your support person can be someone familiar to you, including your partner, family member, or friend. This person can be a big help, emotionally and physically. He or she can assist in many ways, such as offering comfort and encouragement, timing your contractions, massaging your back and shoulders, allowing you to lean on them while walking or swaying, and acting as a focal point during contractions. Even hearing that you're doing a good job and being reassured that everything is going well can be beneficial.

Continuous labor support also can come from a trained professional such as a nurse, midwife, or *doula*. Doulas are professional labor coaches who don't have any medical training but can be hired to help during childbirth. Many doulas have training in relaxation techniques, such as breathing techniques and massage. If you'd like to find a doula in your area, see the "Resources" section in this chapter.

---

# RESOURCES

The following resources offer more information about pain relief during labor:

**DONA International**
www.dona.org
*International organization for doulas.*

**International Childbirth Education Association**
www.icea.org
*Search for childbirth classes or find educators or doulas in your area.*

**Lamaze International (www.lamaze.org)**
**The Bradley Method of Natural Childbirth (www.bradleybirth.com)**
**HypnoBirthing (www.hypnobirthing.com)**
*These web sites offer three popular options for childbirth preparation; there are many more out there. Ask your health care provider for his or her recommendations as well.*

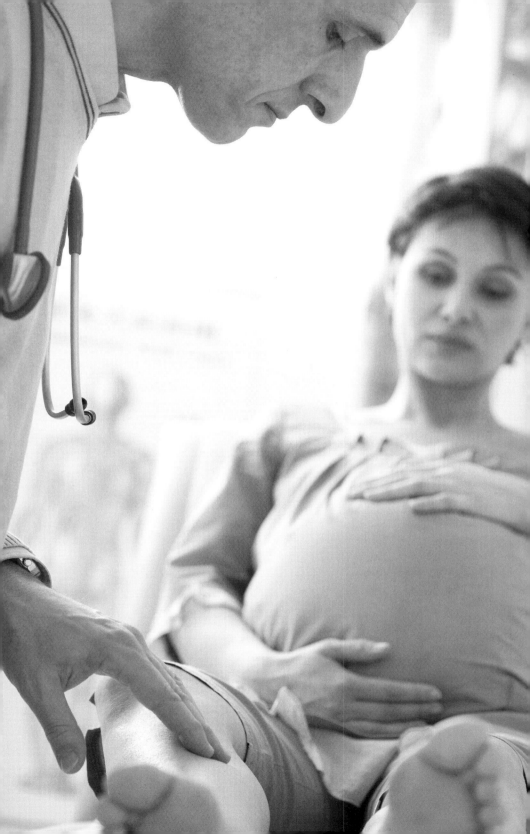

Chapter 12

# Labor Induction

Sometimes situations occur that make continuing your pregnancy too risky for your health and the health of your baby. When this happens, your health care provider may decide to bring on (induce) labor. Labor is induced to stimulate contractions of the uterus so that you can try to have a vaginal birth.

More than 20% of pregnant women in the United States undergo labor induction each year. The procedure is done more often now than in years past. In fact, the number of induced labors has doubled since 1990. In general, labor is induced when the benefits of having the baby soon outweigh the risks of continuing the pregnancy. Labor induction itself can increase the risk of certain complications for you and your baby. If your health care provider is thinking about inducing your labor, these risks also must be taken into consideration.

## Reasons for Labor Induction

There are many reasons why your health care provider may decide to induce your labor. Labor may be induced in the following situations:

- If you have health problems, such as *diabetes mellitus*, *high blood pressure*, or conditions of the heart, lungs, or *kidneys*

- *Placental abruption* (the *placenta* begins to separate from the inner wall of the uterus before the baby is born)

- Problems with the baby, such as poor growth or lack of *amniotic fluid*

- Your pregnancy has lasted more than 41–42 weeks

- Uterine infection

- *Gestational hypertension*

- *Preeclampsia* or *eclampsia*

- *Premature rupture of membranes*

Before labor is induced, your health care provider will assess your and the baby's condition to determine the possible risks that labor induction may have for either of you. In some situations, labor induction may be needed even if it means the baby will be born early. Babies born before reaching *full term*—before 39 weeks and 0 days (often written as "39 and 0/7 weeks")— have an increased risk of health problems. Some of these problems can be serious and lifelong. The risks of these problems occurring and their severity increase the earlier a baby is born. If labor induction is recommended even though your baby will be born early, it usually means that the risks of continuing the pregnancy are greater than the risks of an early birth.

Sometimes, labor is induced at a woman's request for nonmedical reasons, such as her physical discomfort or living far away from the hospital. This is called an elective induction. Elective induction should not be done before 39 and 0/7 weeks of pregnancy. Researchers now know that babies grow and develop throughout the entire 40 weeks of pregnancy. For example, the brain, liver, and lungs are among the last organs to mature and aren't fully developed before 39 weeks of pregnancy. Babies who are born even a little before 39 weeks may not be as developed as those who are born after 39 weeks of pregnancy, and they may have an increased risk of short-term and long-term health problems. If you are considering elective induction, your health care provider will review your obstetric records to be reasonably sure that you have reached 39 and 0/7 weeks of pregnancy. This is done by confirming one of the following:

- You had an *ultrasound exam* at less than 20 weeks of pregnancy that supports a *gestational age* of 39 weeks or greater.

- The baby's heartbeat has been documented as present for 30 weeks.

- It has been 36 weeks since a positive pregnancy test result.

## When Is Labor Not Induced?

There are some conditions that make labor induction or vaginal delivery unsafe for you and the baby. These conditions include the following:

- **Placenta previa**—The placenta is covering part or all of the opening of the uterus.
- Transverse lie—The baby is lying sideways in the uterus instead of head down.
- **Umbilical cord prolapse**—The **umbilical cord** has dropped down into the vagina ahead of the baby.
- Active **genital herpes** infection
- Some types of previous uterine surgery

## How Induction Is Done

There are several ways to start labor if it hasn't started naturally. The method used depends on several factors, including your health and the experience and preferences of your health care provider. Sometimes, several of these methods are used together.

If you are undergoing labor induction, electronic monitoring of the fetal heart rate and your contractions may be done initially. If you have additional risk factors, such as a preexisting medical condition or a complication with your pregnancy, electronic monitoring is recommended throughout labor.

### Ripening the Cervix

Ripening the **cervix** is a procedure that helps the cervix soften and thin out so that it will dilate (open) during labor. If labor is going to be induced but the cervix is not yet "ripe" (or soft), labor may not be able to progress. Before inducing labor, your health care provider will check to see if your cervix has started this change. Health care providers use the Bishop score to rate the readiness of the cervix for labor. With this scoring system, a number ranging from 0 to 13 is given. A score of 6 or less means that your cervix is not yet ready for labor. In this case, your health care provider may choose to start your induction by ripening the cervix.

Medications called **prostaglandins** commonly are used to ripen the cervix. Prostaglandins are forms of chemicals produced naturally by the body. These drugs can be inserted into the vagina or taken by mouth. Some of these drugs are not used in women with a previous **cesarean delivery** or other uterine surgery because of the possible risk of **uterine rupture**.

The cervix also can be widened with special dilators. For example, inserting **laminaria** (a natural or artificial substance that absorbs water) expands the cervix. A thin tube with an inflatable balloon on the end also can be inserted to widen the cervix. This device is called a Foley bulb.

### Stripping the Amniotic Membranes

"Stripping the **amniotic membranes**" is another common way to start labor. This can be done in your health care provider's office or in the hospital. The health care provider uses a gloved finger to separate the **amniotic sac** from the wall of your uterus. This action may cause your body to release prostaglandins, which soften the cervix and may cause contractions.

### Amniotomy

The amniotic sac also is called "the bag of waters." If the sac hasn't broken already, rupturing the sac can start contractions. It also can make them

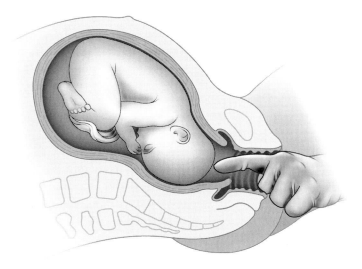

**Stripping the amniotic membranes.** Your health care provider may strip the amniotic membranes to help start your labor.

stronger if they have already begun. The health care provider makes a small hole in the amniotic sac with a special tool. This procedure, called an **amniotomy**, may cause some discomfort.

Amniotomy is done to start labor when the cervix is dilated and thinned and the baby's head has moved down into the pelvis. Most women go into labor within hours after their water breaks.

## Oxytocin

**Oxytocin** is a hormone that causes the uterus to contract and is produced naturally in your body. Synthetic oxytocin is used to induce labor or to speed up labor that began on its own. Oxytocin is given through an **intravenous (IV) line** in the arm. A pump hooked up to the IV line controls the amount given. Contractions usually start within about 10 minutes.

## Risks

Problems sometimes can happen with both cervical ripening and labor induction. When oxytocin or prostaglandins are used, the uterus can be overstimulated, causing it to contract too frequently. This is called uterine tachysystole. Tachysystole is defined as more than five contractions in a 10-minute period, averaged over 30 minutes. It can be concerning because it can lead to changes in the baby's heart rate. If tachysystole occurs while you are receiving oxytocin and there are problems with the fetal heart rate, the oxytocin dosage may be decreased or the oxytocin may be stopped. Other treatment also may be needed to stabilize the fetal heart rate.

In addition to tachysystole, additional risks of cervical ripening and labor induction include

* infections in you or the baby
* uterine rupture (rarely)
* increased risk of **cesarean birth**
* death of the baby

Another risk of labor induction is that sometimes it doesn't work. This is called a "failed induction." A failed induction is diagnosed when the first stage of labor lasts for a certain length of time, usually 24 hours and sometimes longer.

When an induction fails, a cesarean delivery is done. The chance of having a cesarean delivery is greatly increased for women giving birth for the first time who have induction, especially if the cervix is not ready for labor. Cesarean deliveries pose additional risks for you, including infection, **hemorrhage**, and problems with the *anesthesia* used. The recovery time for a cesarean delivery usually is longer than that for a vaginal delivery. There also are considerations for future pregnancies. With each cesarean birth, the risk of serious problems occurring with the placenta in future pregnancies increases. In addition, the number of cesarean deliveries you have had is a major factor in how you will give birth to any future babies.

## If Your Labor Is Going to Be Induced

If your health care provider recommends labor induction, make sure that you understand why the induction is being done, the method or methods that will be used, and what you can reasonably expect to happen during your induction. The first stage of labor typically lasts longer when labor is induced than when it starts on its own. The contractions may be stronger and more painful. Pain relief during labor, such as an *epidural block* or *spinal block*, can be given if you are undergoing induction. Discuss your options with your health care provider before labor.

# RESOURCES

The following resources offer more information about labor induction:

**Inducing Labor**
Medline Plus
www.nlm.nih.gov/medlineplus/ency/patientinstructions/000625.htm
*Provides a basic overview of the different ways labor can be induced.*

**Labor Induction: Resource Overview**
The American College of Obstetricians and Gynecologists (ACOG)
http://www.acog.org/Womens-Health/Labor-Induction
*Lists ACOG's articles and patient education resources about labor induction.*

**Thinking About Inducing Your Labor: A Guide for Pregnant Women**
Agency for Healthcare Research and Quality
http://effectivehealthcare.ahrq.gov/index.cfm/search-for-guides-reviews-and-reports/?productid=353&pageaction=displayproduct
*Discusses why it's best to wait until after 39 weeks if you are thinking about elective labor induction.*

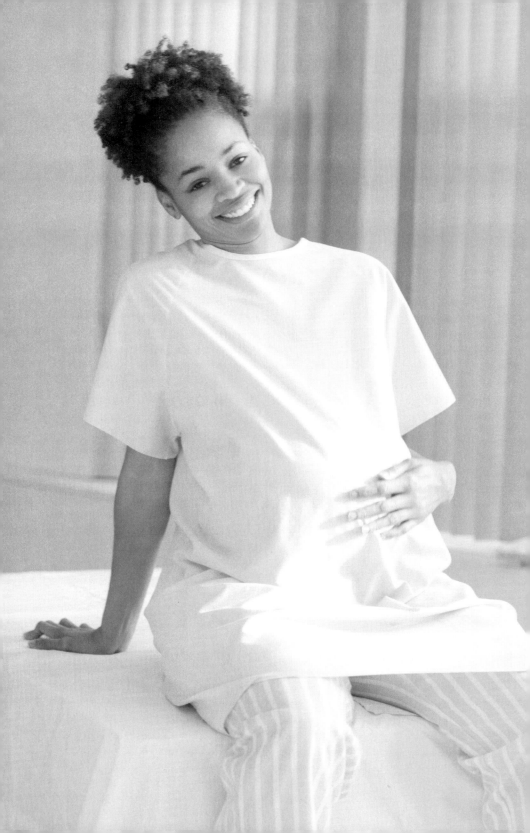

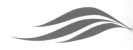

# Chapter 13
# Labor and Delivery

*Labor* occurs when a woman has regular contractions that result in a change in her *cervix*. For a woman having her first baby, labor typically lasts 12–18 hours. For women who have given birth before, it typically lasts 8–10 hours. However, every woman is different. Your labor may not be like your sister's or your friend's. It may even differ with each child you have. Despite these differences, labor and delivery usually follow a pattern. The more you know about what to expect during labor, the better prepared you will be once it begins.

## Common Terms

You may hear your health care provider and nurses use specific terms to describe how your labor is progressing:

- *Effacement*—Shortening and thinning of the cervix. Normally, your cervix looks like a tube that connects the top of the vagina to the bottom of the uterus. Prior to labor, the average length of the cervix is 3.5–4 cm. As your labor progresses, the cervix will start to draw up and thin out until it is right up against the uterine wall. Effacement is estimated in percentages, from 0% (no effacement) to 100% (complete effacement). Effacement makes it possible for your cervix to open and for the baby to pass through the opening.

- *Dilation*—The amount that the cervix has opened. It is measured in centimeters, from 0 cm (no dilation) to 10 cm (fully dilated).

- *Cervical ripening*—The process of softening, thinning, and dilation of the cervix in preparation for birth.

- *Presentation*—The part of the baby's head that is lowest in the vagina. Normally, the fetal head is the presenting part. This is called a **vertex presentation.**

- *Station*—The location of the presenting part in the vagina. The ischial spines, the bony parts of the pelvis that stick out into the birth canal, are used as a reference point. Station is measured in numbers, describing the position of the presenting part of the baby relative to the ischial spines. A negative station (from –1 to –5) means that the presenting part is above the spines. At –5, the baby is 5 cm above the spines. A positive station (from +1 to +5) describes a presenting part that has progressed down the birth canal. At +5, the baby is **crowning** and is visible during a **pelvic exam** just at the opening of a woman's vagina.

## Stages of Childbirth

Childbirth is divided into three different stages—Stages 1, 2, and 3. Stage 1 is labor; Stage 2 is the "pushing and delivery phase," in which you actively participate in pushing the baby out; and Stage 3 is the delivery of the **placenta**.

When reading the following sections, it is important to remember that every woman's labor is unique to her. The descriptions of the typical labor below may not describe exactly what you ultimately experience.

### Stage 1: Early Labor

Stage 1 is divided into two separate phases: early labor and active labor. The beginning of early labor can be difficult to define, but it usually means that you are having regular contractions until the cervix dilates to 6 cm. You may hear this stage described as "latent labor."

**What Happens During Early Labor.** During early labor, you may feel mild contractions that occur 5–15 minutes apart and last about 60–90 seconds. The contractions gradually will get closer together, and toward the end of early labor, they will be less than 5 minutes apart. During these contractions, you may feel pain or pressure that starts in your back and moves around to your lower abdomen. When this happens, your belly will tighten and feel hard. Between contractions, the uterus relaxes and your belly

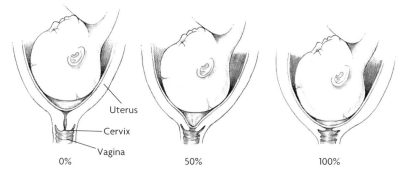

0%  50%  100%

**Effacement.** During effacement, your cervix draws upward and becomes part of the lower uterus. It is measured in percentages, from 0% (no effacement) to 100% (full effacement).

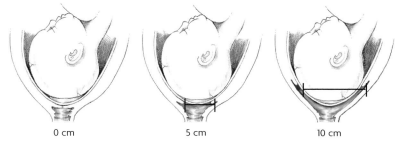

0 cm  5 cm  10 cm

**Dilation.** During dilation, the opening of the cervix enlarges. It is measured in centimeters, usually from 0 cm (no dilation) to 10 cm (fully dilated).

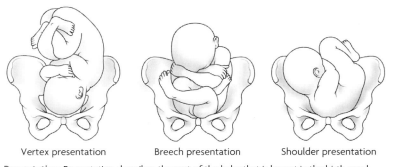

Vertex presentation  Breech presentation  Shoulder presentation

**Presentation.** Presentation describes the part of the baby that is lowest in the birth canal.

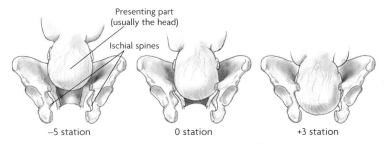

−5 station  0 station  +3 station

**Station.** Station describes the location of the presenting part of the baby in the birth canal.

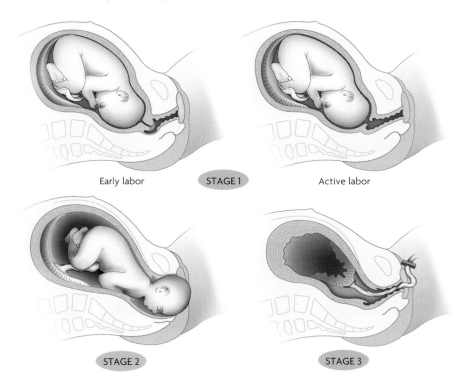

Early labor    STAGE 1    Active labor

STAGE 2    STAGE 3

**The three stages of childbirth.** In Stage 1, the cervix dilates. In Stage 2, the cervix completely dilates, and the mother pushes the baby out of the vagina. In Stage 3, the placenta detaches from the uterus and is delivered.

softens. These contractions are doing vital work. They help dilate the cervix and push the baby lower into the pelvis.

The first stage of labor is almost always the longest. How long it lasts is different for every woman. For some, it's a few hours. For others, it's longer. For first-time moms, the average is from 6 hours to 12 hours, but it can last as long as 20 hours for first-time moms and 14 hours for women who have had children. The intensity of early labor also varies. Some women do not feel any contractions in very early labor. For others, contractions are more intense but usually are still manageable.

You probably will spend most of early labor at home, waiting for the contractions to get closer together. Your health care provider most likely will have given you instructions on when to leave for the hospital, so follow them exactly. If you are not sure about what to do, call your health care provider. If your water breaks or if you have significant bleeding, contact your health care provider right away and be prepared to go to the hospital immediately for an evaluation.

**What You Can Do.** During early labor, try to stay as relaxed as possible. Staying relaxed will help your cervix thin out and dilate. You may want to alternate active movements with rest. Here are some things you can do during early labor:

- Go for a walk.
- Take a nap.
- Take a shower or bath.
- Play some relaxing music.
- Do the relaxation and breathing techniques taught in childbirth class.
- Change positions often.
- Make sure you have everything you need for the hospital.

Slow, relaxing breathing may be helpful during this stage:

- Take a deep, cleansing breath at the beginning of the contraction.
- Breathe slowly, focusing on the in-and-out movement of your breath.
- Try counting during the contraction.
- At the end of the contraction, take a deep, cleansing breath.

**How Your Labor Coach Can Help.** Your labor partner can be a big help to you during the early stage of labor, both emotionally and physically. Now is the time for him or her to help you with the strategies you both learned in childbirth class about how to relax and cope with the pain. Other ways your labor partner can help include the following:

- Keeping you distracted by playing cards or other games
- Massaging your back and shoulders
- Timing your contractions
- Placing a heating pad or ice pack on your lower back
- Making phone calls with you

### Stage 1: Active Labor

As active labor begins, your contractions will have progressed and are coming closer together. It is during this stage that the cervix dilates most rapidly. Active labor is typically considered to have started when a woman is having regular contractions and her cervix has dilated to 6 cm. It's hard to know precisely when that occurs, so when your contractions are stronger, closer together, and regular, it's time to go to the hospital.

**What Happens When You Go to the Hospital.** Before you are admitted to the hospital, the hospital staff will determine whether you are in labor. You may be taken to a special triage room, or this may be done in the hospital's emergency department. The following signs usually are assessed:

- Your vital signs (temperature, blood pressure, pulse)
- Fetal heart rate
- Frequency and duration of your contractions
- Vaginal exam to check cervical dilation and effacement
- Whether your water has broken
- Position of the baby
- Estimated weight of the baby

The only way to diagnose labor is for your health care provider to see changes taking place in the cervix. You may need two or more cervical exams over a period of time to tell if you are really in labor. If you are found to be in labor, you will be admitted to the hospital. If you're not in labor, you'll be told to return home. If you are in very early labor, and you and the baby are doing well, you also may be told to return home until your labor contractions are more regular.

If you are admitted to the hospital, the following events usually occur:

- Room assignment—You'll be taken to a hospital room. In some hospitals you will stay in the same room for both labor and delivery. Other hospitals have a separate delivery room.

- Changing clothes—You'll be asked to put on a hospital gown. You can ask the nurse if you can wear your own gown, but keep in mind that it may get stained or ruined.

- *Intravenous (IV) line*—An IV line may be placed so that medications and fluids can be administered if you need them.

- Fetal heart rate monitor—Depending on your hospital's policy, you may be connected to an electronic fetal monitor. *Electronic fetal monitoring* allows your health care provider and the hospital staff to monitor the fetal heart rate and the strength of your contractions.

After you have been examined and your condition is assessed, you may be asked to sign consent forms. These forms vary, but most spell out who will be taking care of you, why a procedure is being done, and the risks that are involved. Read this form and be sure to ask about anything that's not clear. Signing the consent form means that you understand your medical condition and agree to the care described. You may need to sign separate consent forms for **anesthesia** and for **cesarean delivery**.

Once you're in your hospital room, a labor-and-delivery nurse will be checking on you from the time you check in until after your baby is born. These nurses are trained to help women through the physical and emotional demands of labor. In teaching hospitals, a resident doctor, student nurse, or medical student also may be a part of your birth team.

Your own health care provider may be there from start to finish, or he or she may arrive shortly before you give birth. During this stage, the following things will be monitored closely:

- Your heart rate and blood pressure (these will be checked at least every 4 hours)

- The time between and length of your contractions

- How much your cervix has dilated

- Fetal heartbeat, either continuously with an electronic fetal monitor or periodically with a Doppler device or a special stethoscope.

**What Happens During Active Labor.** Active labor generally is when the cervix dilates from 6 cm to 10 cm. Contractions get stronger and come as often as 3 minutes apart, and each one lasts about 45 seconds. Active labor can last about 4–8 hours. During this time, you may experience the following:

- Your water may break if it hasn't already.

- You'll have back pain if the fetal head presses down on your backbone during contractions.

- Your legs may cramp.

- You may feel the urge to push.

- You may feel nauseated.

**What You Can Do.** Your contractions will become more intense, so focus on your breathing and take each contraction one at a time. Let your childbirth partner and nurse help you through all the breathing and relaxation exercises. When each contraction passes, try to relax and don't think about the next one. It may help to move around to find a position that is most comfortable for you. Medications for pain relief also can be given at this time (techniques for pain relief are discussed in Chapter 11, "Pain Relief

During Childbirth"). There are some other things you can do now to cope with the contractions:

- If you feel like it and your health care provider says it's OK, walk the halls.

- Urinate often because an empty **bladder** gives the baby's head more room to move down.

- If you feel the urge to push, tell your health care provider. Don't give in to the urge just yet—pant or blow to keep yourself from bearing down.

Eating solid food during active labor is not recommended. If you need to have a cesarean delivery, having food in your stomach can lead to serious complications. You can have modest amounts of clear liquids, such as water, ice chips, popsicles, fruit juices without pulp, carbonated beverages, clear tea, black coffee, sports drinks, and ices. Your hospital may have some of these things on hand, or you can bring your own liquids from home.

**How Your Labor Coach Can Help.** You'll depend on your labor partner more and more as the labor pains intensify. Let him or her help you through the pain-management methods you learned in childbirth class. Your partner also can help in the following ways:

- Apply counterpressure to your back: press firmly on the lower back or massage with knuckles or tennis balls.

- Flex your feet to help relieve your leg cramps.

- Act as a focal point during contractions.

- Offer comfort and support.

- Give you small amounts of clear liquids (see above) if you want them.

Sometimes if your labor isn't progressing as quickly as it should, your health care provider may decide to augment your labor by rupturing your membranes (if they haven't already ruptured) or giving you a synthetic form of **oxytocin**, the hormone that causes the uterus to contract. This drug increases the frequency and duration of your contractions. Labor is augmented if contractions are thought to be infrequent or mild enough that they won't cause the cervix to dilate and the woman is in active labor.

## Transition to Stage 2

Towards the end of the active phase of labor, it is common for labor to intensify. For many, this will be the toughest stage and the most painful. If you've been given an epidural or other pain medication, however, the pain may not be as intense. The contractions come closer together and can last 60–90 seconds. With each contraction, you may start to feel an urge to bear down. You'll feel a lot of pressure in your lower back and **rectum**. This can feel like the urge to move your bowels but much stronger. Tell your health care provider or nurse as soon as you feel like pushing. He or she will check your cervix to see how much it has dilated. Until your cervix is fully dilated and your health care provider or nurse gives you the go-ahead, you should try not to push. Pushing before your cervix is fully dilated can exhaust you as well as cause some swelling of the cervix, which may prevent it from fully dilating. Controlling your breathing or blowing air out in short puffs can help you resist the urge to bear down. The transition phase does not last too long, usually 15–60 minutes. You should be ready to start Stage 2 soon.

### Stage 2: Pushing and Delivery

This is the stage in which you actively participate in pushing your baby out. It is different for every woman and for every pregnancy. The second stage of labor typically is shorter than the first stage but usually involves the most work for the mother. Once your cervix is fully dilated, you can begin to push your baby out. During Stage 2, you'll notice a change in the way your contractions feel. They may be slower, come 2–5 minutes apart, and last about 60–90 seconds.

The second stage of labor can last anywhere from 20 minutes to 2–3 hours. If you have had an **epidural block** or if the baby is in an abnormal position, it may take longer to push the baby out. In general, if no anesthesia has been given and the second stage lasts longer than 3 hours for a first-time mom or 2 hours for a woman who has given birth before, it may be necessary to intervene to help get the baby out. This may mean an **operative vaginal delivery** (see Chapter 14, "Operative Delivery and Breech Presentation"), turning the baby so that it is in a more favorable presentation for birth, or a cesarean delivery (see Chapter 15, "Cesarean Delivery and Vaginal Birth After Cesarean Delivery"). If you have had an epidural, a longer time may be given for the second stage, especially if you are making progress.

**What You Can Do.** If you have been in a standard labor room, you'll be moved to a room for delivery. If you are in a labor–delivery–recovery room, your health care provider and nurse will help you get into a good delivery position. Many women give birth to their babies while propped up in bed, with their legs braced against foot rests. There are other birth positions you can try as long as your health care provider approves (for more on birth positions, see Chapter 11, "Pain Relief During Childbirth").

Once your health care provider gives you the go-ahead, bear down with each contraction or when you are told to push. Your attendants will tell you how to help the baby move down the birth canal. When the baby's head appears at the opening of your vagina, you'll feel a burning or stinging feeling as the *perineum* stretches and bulges. This is normal.

After the head emerges from the birth canal, the baby's body turns. First one shoulder slips out and then the other. After the shoulders are delivered, the rest of the baby's body follows quickly. Your health care provider or your labor coach then will cut the **umbilical cord**. The blood in the umbilical cord (called cord blood) routinely is obtained for newborn blood tests, such as blood typing.

**How Your Labor Coach Can Help.** Your coach can make a real difference during this stage of labor. For some birth positions, your coach is needed to give you physical support. For squatting positions, you may need to lean on or hold onto your partner for balance. If you are lying on your back, your partner can support one of your legs. Offering words of support also can be a big help. Tell your coach what kind of support you need. If you need your coach to be hands off, that's OK at this stage as well.

### Stage 3: Delivery of the Placenta

After your baby is delivered, one more part of childbirth remains: delivery of the placenta. This last stage is the shortest of all. It likely will last from just a few minutes to about 20 minutes. During this stage, you still will have contractions. They will be closer together and less painful. These contractions help the placenta separate from the wall of the uterus. Then the contractions move the placenta down into the birth canal. Once there, a push or two by you will help expel the placenta from the vagina. Some health care providers help deliver the placenta by reaching inside the vagina to the uterus and grasping the placenta. If you had an *episiotomy* or tear, it will be repaired. If you have elected to store cord blood, it's collected either before or after delivery of the placenta.

After the placenta is delivered, your uterus will continue to contract. These contractions help your uterus return to its smaller size. Medication is given (either before or after the placenta is delivered) to help the uterus contract and prevent excessive bleeding. A nurse will palpate (squeeze and press on) your abdomen to make sure that the uterus feels normal. As the uterus shrinks, the blood vessels that brought **nutrients** and **oxygen** to the placenta and removed wastes are sealed, which helps control blood loss.

## After the Baby Is Born

If you had a normal labor and delivery, immediately after your baby is born, he or she will be placed on your abdomen next to your skin and covered with a blanket. A newborn baby has to adjust from the warmth inside your body to a new place that's much cooler. Your newborn also is wet with **amniotic fluid**. The baby can lose a lot of heat as the moisture on his or her skin evaporates. Skin-to-skin contact helps regulate the baby's body temperature and is the best way to keep the baby warm. If you had any problems during labor or delivery or if the baby is **preterm**, your baby may need to be evaluated by medical staff first or placed under a warming light.

If all is well, you most likely will be able to spend as much time as you want with your baby after he or she is born. A physical exam and tests of your newborn can be done when you and the baby are ready (see Chapter 16, "The Postpartum Period").

Your vital signs will be measured frequently for the next few hours. This is done to monitor you for signs of infection or **hemorrhage**. If you have had regional anesthesia, you will be observed for a few hours by hospital staff for complications. If you were moved to a delivery room for the birth, you will be returned to a regular room once it is determined that your condition is stable.

Welcome to motherhood! The next stage in your journey is described in Chapter 16, "The Postpartum Period." This will be a time of adjustment and change, but being prepared for both will make the transition easier.

# RESOURCES

The following resources offer more information about childbirth:

**Childbirth**
National Library of Medicine
www.nlm.nih.gov/medlineplus/childbirth.html
*A great starting point with links to detailed resources on many childbirth topics.*

**Labor and Delivery: Resource Overview**
The American College of Obstetricians and Gynecologists (ACOG)
http://www.acog.org/Womens-Health/Labor-and-Delivery
*Lists ACOG's articles and patient education resources about labor and delivery.*

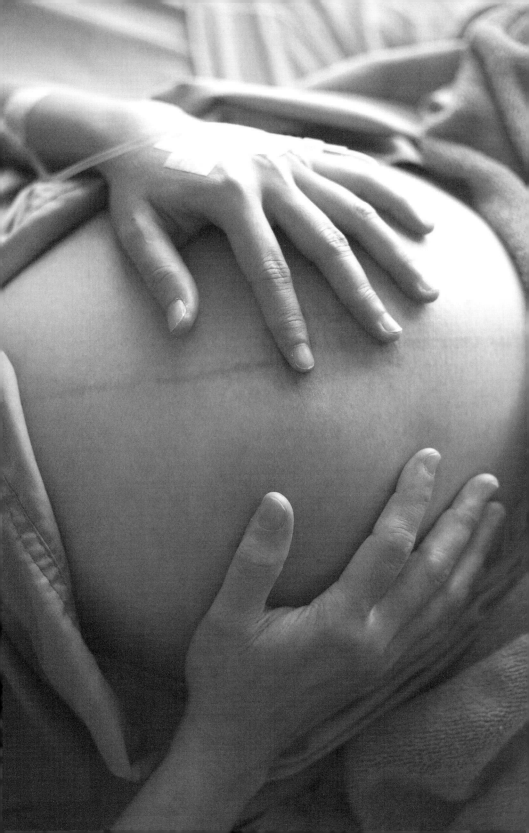

## Chapter 14

# Operative Delivery and Breech Presentation

Labor sometimes does not go as planned. Labor can slow down or stop. Problems with the baby or with your condition may arise. If your health care provider thinks that continuing labor or a vaginal delivery would be unsafe for you or your baby, he or she may decide that the best option is to deliver the baby another way—either by *operative vaginal delivery* or *cesarean delivery*. This chapter covers operative vaginal delivery. A separate chapter (Chapter 15, "Cesarean Delivery and Vaginal Birth After Cesarean Delivery") addresses cesarean delivery.

A *breech presentation*—in which the baby is positioned to come out feet or buttocks first—often is detected a few weeks before labor starts. If your baby is in a breech presentation, it may be possible to turn the baby before delivery, a procedure called *external cephalic version (ECV)*. If the baby does not turn, you will need to discuss a plan for delivery with your health care provider.

## Operative Vaginal Delivery

Once labor starts, it usually progresses steadily. No one can predict just how the birth of a baby will proceed. Sometimes birth happens fairly quickly and there are no problems. With some births, however, the mother may push for hours and not make much progress, or problems may occur during labor. In some cases, your health care provider may need to assist delivery by using *forceps* or a vacuum device. This type of delivery is called operative vaginal delivery. Operative vaginal delivery is done in about 4% of vaginal deliveries in the United States. Some of the reasons why an operative vaginal delivery may be done include the following:

- Suspected problem with the baby (for example, your baby's heartbeat becomes slow or erratic)

- You have pushed for a long time without any progress

- You aren't able to push effectively because of a medical condition

### Types of Operative Vaginal Delivery

There are two types of operative vaginal delivery: 1) forceps delivery and 2) **vacuum extraction**. Both types of deliveries are safe. The choice of which type of delivery is done depends on several factors, including the experience of your health care provider and your individual situation.

- Forceps delivery—Forceps look like two large spoons. They are inserted into the vagina and placed around the baby's cheekbones and jaw. The forceps then are used to gently guide the baby's head out of the birth canal while you continue to push.

- Vacuum extraction—A **vacuum extractor** is a device that has a suction cup with a handle attached. The suction cup is inserted into the vagina and is pressed to the baby's head. Suction holds the cup in place. Your health care provider uses the handle to guide the baby's head out through the birth canal while you continue to push.

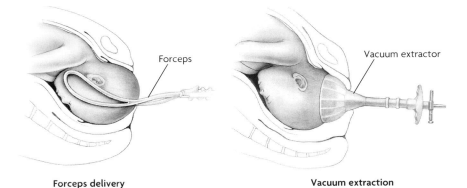

| Forceps |
| Vacuum extractor |

**Forceps delivery** · **Vacuum extraction**

**Types of operative vaginal delivery.** Operative vaginal delivery involves the use of forceps or a vacuum extractor.

## Risks

In most cases, using these tools to help with delivery causes no major problems. There are, however, some risks associated with operative delivery:

- Risks for the baby—With forceps delivery, the baby's face may be injured, but these injuries usually are minor. In rare situations, more serious complications, such as seizures or bleeding in the brain, have been known to occur. Vacuum extraction can cause injury to the fetal head and bleeding of the blood vessels in the eye. *Jaundice* occurs more frequently in newborns delivered by vacuum extraction. Most of the injuries caused by vacuum extraction have no lasting consequences for the baby.

- Risks for you—Both forceps delivery and vacuum extraction may cause injury to the tissues of the vagina, *perineum*, and *anus*. These problems can lead to *pelvic organ prolapse* and *incontinence* of urine, stool, or gas after delivery. In some cases, surgical repair may be necessary. It should be noted, though, that any vaginal delivery may potentially cause these injuries.

It is important to discuss all of these risks with your obstetrician before operative delivery is performed. If you do have an operative vaginal delivery, your baby's health care provider should be notified so that he or she can watch for any problems that might arise.

## Breech Presentation

By 3 or 4 weeks before the due date, most babies change position in the uterus so their heads are down near the birth canal. This is called a

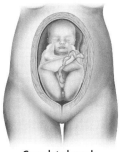 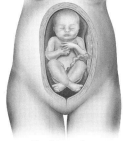 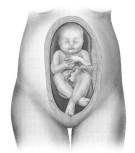

| Complete breech | Frank breech | Footling breech |

**Breech presentations.** In a breech birth, the baby's buttocks, feet, or foot may be in place to come out first during birth.

*vertex presentation*. If the baby does not change position, he or she may be in a breech presentation. This happens in 3–4% of babies who are born *full term*. It occurs more frequently in *preterm* babies.

Although the reasons why a baby is in a breech position are not always known, it is more common if one or more of the following conditions apply to you:

- You have had more than one pregnancy.

- You are having twins.

- The uterus has too much or too little *amniotic fluid*.

- The uterus is abnormal in shape or has abnormal growths (*fibroids*, for example).

- The *placenta* covers all or part of the opening of the uterus (*placenta previa*).

Occasionally, babies with certain *birth defects* also will stay in a breech presentation at term, but most babies in a breech presentation at term are otherwise normal.

### The Baby's Position

During the last weeks of your pregnancy, your health care provider will perform a physical exam to find out the baby's position. Your health care provider will place his or her hands on your abdomen and try to feel the outline of the baby. By locating the baby's head, back, and buttocks, your health care provider can tell what position the baby is in. If a breech presentation is suspected, an *ultrasound exam* may be done to confirm the position.

The baby's position can change until the end of pregnancy. As the time of delivery nears, some babies turn on their own. Your health care provider may not know for sure if your baby has settled in a breech presentation until labor starts. Sometimes a breech presentation is first found during a *pelvic exam* of a woman in labor.

### Turning the Baby

If the baby is in a breech presentation—and depending on your and the baby's condition—your health care provider may try to turn the baby head down so that you can deliver the baby vaginally without complications. This procedure is known as external cephalic version, or ECV. The chances that ECV will be successful are about 50-50.

External cephalic version won't be tried if you are carrying more than one baby, there are possible fetal heart rate problems, you have certain abnormalities of the reproductive system, or the placenta is in the wrong place (placenta previa) or has detached from the wall of the uterus (*placental abruption*). External cephalic version may be considered if you have had a previous cesarean delivery, depending on the reason why the previous cesarean delivery was done and the type of uterine scar that you have (see Chapter 15, "Cesarean Delivery and Vaginal Birth After Cesarean Delivery"). Your health care provider will discuss with you the risks and benefits of ECV in this situation so that you can make an informed decision.

Usually, ECV is not done until you are at least 37 weeks pregnant. If it is done before this time, the baby may go back to a breech presentation. If that happens, the procedure may be tried again. However, it tends to be harder because the baby is bigger and there is less room for him or her to move.

External cephalic version is performed as follows:

• It usually is done near a delivery room because if a problem occurs, the baby then can be delivered quickly by cesarean if necessary.

• The baby's heart rate is checked before and after ECV.

• Sometimes a medicine is given to relax the uterus, which may make turning the baby easier. You also may receive pain medicine, such as an *epidural block* or medicine given through an *intravenous (IV) line*.

• To turn the baby, the health care provider places his or her hands on your abdomen.

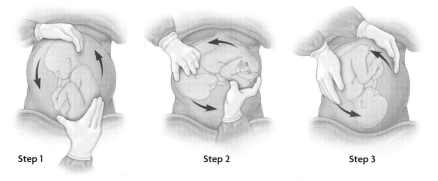

Step 1           Step 2           Step 3

**External cephalic version.** In this procedure, the health care provider attempts to lift and turn the baby from a breech presentation to a vertex (head-down) presentation. Reprinted from Beckmann CRB, Ling FW, Barzansky BM, Herbert WNP, Laube PW, Smith RP. Obstetrics and gynecology. 6th ed. Baltimore: Lippincott Williams & Wilkins; 2010.

- Firm pressure is applied to your abdomen to try to turn your baby.

- In some cases, a second health care provider may be asked to help turn the baby or perform an ultrasound exam to monitor the baby.

Complications can occur with ECV, although the chance that these complications will occur is low. They include the following:

- ***Premature rupture of membranes***
- Problems with the baby's heart rate
- Placental abruption

After the procedure, you will be monitored for a period of time to make sure your and the baby's condition are stable.

## Options for Delivery

If your baby is in a breech presentation, your health care provider will talk with you about the best type of birth for you and your baby. If the baby can be turned with ECV, vaginal birth may be an option. If the baby is breech as the time of delivery nears, ***cesarean birth*** may be best. Your health care provider will review the risks and benefits of both types of birth in detail. Together you will decide on the best plan for you and your baby.

**Cesarean Birth.** Most breech babies are born by planned cesarean delivery. However, it is not always possible to plan for cesarean birth. The baby may move into the breech position just before labor begins. Although very rare, some babies even move from head down to breech during labor.

**Vaginal Birth.** Vaginal birth can be more difficult when a baby is breech. At birth, the head is the largest and firmest part of the baby's body. In the head-down position, the head comes out first, and the rest of the body follows. In a breech presentation, the body comes out first, leaving the largest part of the body to be delivered last. The baby's body may not stretch the ***cervix*** enough to allow room for the baby's head to come out easily, and the head or shoulders may become stuck. You and the baby can be injured if this occurs. There also is an increased risk that the ***umbilical cord*** will slip through the cervix into the birth canal before the baby does. This is called a prolapsed cord. If the cord becomes pinched, it can stop the flow of blood through the cord to the baby.

Vaginal birth may be possible in certain situations. Before making a decision, you should be informed of all the possible risks of a vaginal birth with a breech presentation and understand that these risks are higher than if a cesarean delivery is planned. The experience of your health care provider in delivering breech babies vaginally is an important factor. You also may need to meet certain guidelines developed by your hospital before planning to deliver your baby vaginally.

# RESOURCES

The following resources offer more information about operative vaginal delivery and breech presentation:

**Breech Babies: What Can I Do if My Baby is Breech?**
American Academy of Family Physicians.
www.afp.org/1998/0902/p744
*Provides a detailed explanation of all aspects of breech presentation.*

**Breech Birth**
National Library of Medicine.
www.nlm.nih.gov/medlineplus/ency/patientinstructions/000623.htm
*Gives easy-to-understand overview of breech presentation and external cephalic version.*

**Forceps or Vacuum Delivery**
National Health Service.
www.nhs.uk/conditions/pregnancy-and-baby/pages/ventouse-forceps-delivery.aspx
*Description of operative delivery from the National Health Service, which provides health care in the United Kingdom. Includes a video.*

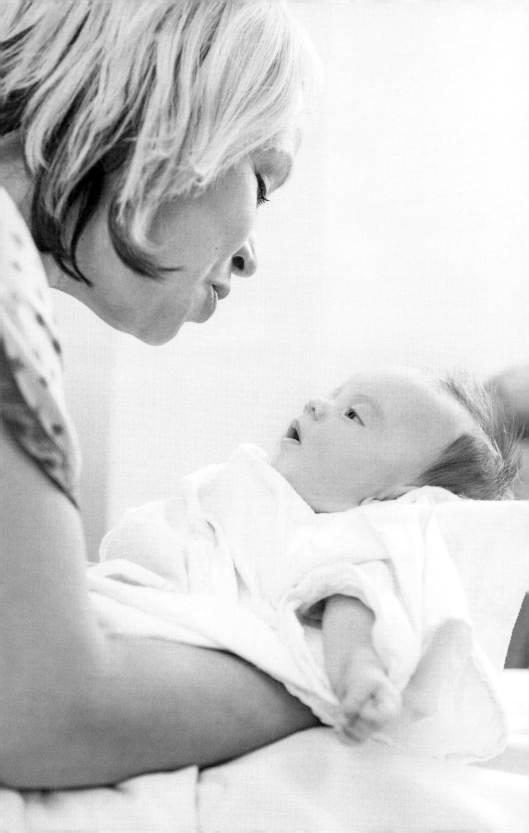

Chapter 15

# Cesarean Delivery and Vaginal Birth After Cesarean Delivery

Most babies are born through the vagina. However, in many pregnancies, a baby is delivered through incisions in the woman's abdomen and uterus. This is known as a ***cesarean delivery***. Cesarean deliveries are very common. In fact, one in three babies born in the United States is delivered this way.

It once was thought that if a woman had one cesarean delivery, all other babies she had in the future also should be born by cesarean delivery. Today, it is known that many women can undergo a ***trial of labor after cesarean delivery (TOLAC)***. After a successful TOLAC, many women will be able to give birth through the vagina (called a ***vaginal birth after cesarean delivery [VBAC]***).

## Why You May Need a Cesarean Delivery

A cesarean delivery may be needed if circumstances occur during labor that make a cesarean delivery a safer choice than a vaginal delivery for either the pregnant woman or the baby. A cesarean delivery also may be planned ahead of time because of certain problems or conditions. Some examples include the following:

- Labor fails to progress—One of the most common reasons why cesarean deliveries are performed is because labor slows down or stops. About one in three cesarean deliveries is done for this reason. For example, you may be experiencing contractions that are too weak or too infrequent to dilate the ***cervix*** wide enough for the baby to move through the vagina. Sometimes, even if your cervix dilates enough, the baby may be too big for your pelvis or the baby's position may not allow passage in a safe and timely manner.

- The fetal heart rate is abnormal—An abnormal fetal heart rate may mean that labor is too stressful for the baby.

- There is a problem with the **umbilical cord**—If the umbilical cord becomes pinched or compressed, the baby may not get enough **oxygen**.

A cesarean delivery also may need to be scheduled before you go into labor. Reasons for a scheduled cesarean delivery include the following:

- You had a previous cesarean delivery—A previous cesarean delivery may mean that you'll need to have a cesarean delivery again depending on the way the prior incision in your uterus was made. After discussing options with your health care provider, you may choose to have a repeat cesarean delivery even if you are a candidate for TOLAC.

- You're having more than one baby—If you are having two or more babies, you may need to have a cesarean delivery. Many women having twins are able to have a vaginal delivery. However, if the babies are being born too early or if the "presenting twin" (the twin who is in a position to be born first) is not in a head-down position, a cesarean delivery is preferred. The likelihood of having a cesarean delivery increases with the number of babies you are carrying.

- You have a large baby (a condition called **macrosomia**) or a small pelvis— Sometimes a baby is too big to pass safely through a woman's pelvis and vagina. This condition is called **cephalopelvic disproportion**.

- Your baby is in a **breech presentation** or is lying in an abnormal position— If your baby is in a breech presentation (with buttocks or feet closest to the vagina), a planned cesarean delivery is the safest and most common method of delivery. A planned vaginal delivery may be possible in some situations. If the baby is transverse (lying sideways in the uterus rather than head down), a cesarean delivery is the only choice for delivery.

- There are problems with the placenta—**Placenta previa** is a condition in which the placenta is below the baby and covers part or all of the cervix, blocking the baby's exit from the uterus. This may be associated with heavy bleeding if vaginal delivery is attempted.

- You have a medical condition that may make vaginal birth risky—For example, a cesarean delivery may be done if a woman has an active herpes infection during labor.

- You request it—Some pregnant women prefer to undergo a cesarean delivery even when there is no medical reason why it must be done. This is known as "cesarean delivery on maternal request." If you are interested in requesting a cesarean delivery, you and your health care provider will need to discuss this option in advance. Cesarean birth is major surgery, and there is a risk of serious complications for both you and your baby. When there is no medical reason for a cesarean delivery, the risks of having a cesarean delivery often outweigh the benefits. This issue is discussed in more detail in the section "Cesarean Delivery on Request" in Chapter 6, "Month 6 (Weeks 21–24)."

## What Happens During a Cesarean Delivery

The process of cesarean delivery can vary depending on the reason why it is being done. However, in most cases, cesarean deliveries follow a similar procedure.

### Anesthesia

Different types of **anesthesia** are used for pain relief during a cesarean delivery. They include **epidural block**, **spinal block**, **combined spinal–epidural block**, or **general anesthesia**. The type of anesthesia chosen depends on several factors, including your health and that of your baby as well as why the cesarean delivery is being done. An **anesthesiologist** will talk with you about the benefits and risks of each type of anesthesia and suggest the best option for you.

If you are given an epidural during labor and then need to have a cesarean delivery, usually your anesthesiologist will be able to inject more medication or a different medication through the same **catheter** to increase your pain relief. The **anesthetic** will numb you completely for the surgery. Although you will not feel any pain, there may be a feeling of pressure.

### Preparing You for Surgery

Before the cesarean delivery starts, a few steps are taken to prepare you for surgery:

- Your blood pressure, heart rate, and breathing will be monitored during the surgery. An oxygen mask will be placed over your nose and mouth or a tube will be placed under your nose to make sure you and your baby get plenty of oxygen during surgery.

- You will receive **antibiotics** through your **intravenous (IV) line**. This is done to prevent infection.

- Your abdomen will be washed and then swabbed with an antiseptic. If needed, pubic hair may be trimmed with clippers before washing the abdomen. If your cesarean delivery is planned, it is important not to remove pubic hair with a razor the night or morning before surgery. Using a razor increases the risk of surgical-site infections.

- Sterile drapes will be placed around the area of the incision.

- A catheter will be inserted into your **bladder**. The catheter keeps the bladder empty so that it's not injured during surgery.

- Special devices will be applied to your legs to reduce the risk of **deep vein thrombosis (DVT)** during surgery. These devices encircle your legs and periodically fill with air to encourage blood circulation in your veins. If you have risk factors for DVT, you may receive medication instead of having the devices.

   In cesarean deliveries that are not being done for an emergency situation, most hospitals allow you to have a support person with you in the operating room. Your support person will be given a surgical gown, mask, hat, and gloves to wear. He or she can stay with you throughout the surgery.

### Making the Incisions

Two incisions are made: one in your abdomen and one in your uterus. Once your abdomen is cleaned and you are numb from the anesthetic, your doctor will make the abdominal incision:

- The incision is made through the skin and the wall of the abdomen and goes from side to side, just above the pubic hairline (transverse) or, in some cases, up and down (vertical).

- The abdominal muscles are separated, and an incision is made through the lining of the abdominal cavity. The abdominal muscles usually are not cut.

- When your doctor reaches the uterus, another cut is made in the uterine wall. This incision also can be transverse (side to side) or vertical (up and down). In most cases, a transverse incision is made. This type of cut is done in the lower, thinner part of the uterus. It causes less bleeding and heals with a stronger scar. A vertical incision may need to be done if

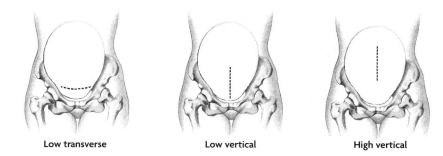

| Low transverse | Low vertical | High vertical |

**Types of uterine incisions for a cesarean birth.** The type of incision made in the skin for a cesarean birth may not be the same type of incision made in the uterus.

you have placenta previa, if the baby is in an unusual position, or if your baby is extremely **preterm** or smaller than average.

An important point to remember is that the incision made in your abdomen may be different from the incision made in your uterus. Although this information should be entered into your medical record, make sure that you also know the type of incision that was made in your uterus. This is a major factor in determining whether you can have a vaginal birth in the future. The type of incision most favorable for a vaginal birth after a cesarean delivery is a low transverse incision.

## Delivering the Baby

The baby is delivered through the incisions. The umbilical cord then is cut, and the baby is passed to the nurse.

## Afterbirth and Closing the Incisions

After the baby is delivered, the placenta is removed from the uterus. The incisions made in the uterus and abdominal wall are closed. The incision in the uterus usually is closed with sutures that absorb into the body. Different materials, including surgical thread, staples, or surgical glue, may be used to close the abdominal incision. Depending on what is used, you may need to have the stitches removed at a later date. Other types of closures are absorbed into the body and do not need to be removed.

## Risks

Like any major surgery, cesarean delivery involves risks. Problems occur in a small number of women. They usually can be treated, but, in very rare cases, complications can be serious or even fatal:

- The uterus, nearby pelvic organs, or skin incision can get infected.

- You can bleed too much. This is called a **hemorrhage**. A blood **transfusion** may be needed in a few cases. In very rare cases, a **hysterectomy** (surgical removal of the uterus) may need to be done if bleeding cannot be controlled.

- You can develop blood clots in the legs (DVT) that can travel to the lungs. For this reason, it's standard practice to place air-filled devices on your legs to help prevent this complication.

- Your bowel or bladder can be injured.

- You can have a reaction to the medications or anesthetics that are used.

There also are long-term risks associated with cesarean delivery. Some of these risks may affect future pregnancies. With each cesarean delivery, the risk of problems with the placenta—such as placenta previa and **placenta accreta**—increases. Placenta accreta is a serious condition in which the placenta grows into the muscular walls of the uterus. Placenta accreta can cause hemorrhage and can be life threatening.

Because of these risks, cesarean birth usually is done only when the benefits of the surgery outweigh the risks. In some situations, **cesarean birth** is the best option. In other situations, vaginal birth is best. You should understand the risks and benefits of both options for your particular situation.

## Recovery

If you are awake for the surgery, you probably can hold your baby after the surgery is completed. You will be taken to a recovery room or directly to your hospital room. Your blood pressure, pulse rate, breathing rate, and abdomen will be checked regularly.

If you plan on breastfeeding, be sure to let your health care provider know. Having a cesarean delivery does not mean you won't be able to breastfeed your baby. If all is going well for you and your baby, you should be able to begin breastfeeding soon after delivery.

You will receive fluids intravenously after your delivery until you are able to eat and drink. You will be able to eat and drink as soon as you would like to. The abdominal incision will be sore for the first few days. Pain medication can be given after the anesthesia wears off. There are many different ways to control pain. Talk to your health care provider about your options.

Soon after surgery, the catheter is removed from the bladder. A nurse will help you get out of bed and sit in a chair. Walking soon after a cesarean delivery helps to decrease the risk of developing blood clots, so you will be encouraged to walk a short distance as soon as you feel able to do so. You can shower as soon as you would like to. Most women are able to walk on their own and to eat and drink within 24 hours after surgery. The usual hospital stay after a cesarean delivery is 2–4 days. How many days you will have to stay depends on why you needed the cesarean delivery and how long it takes for your body to recover.

## Back at Home

Once you are permitted to go home, you will need to take special care of yourself and limit your activities. Your health care provider will give you specific instructions about what you can and can't do. The bottom line is that you need to take it easy. You just had major surgery, and it will take a few weeks for your abdomen to heal. During the weeks you are recovering from the surgery, you may experience the following:

• Mild cramping, especially when you are breastfeeding
• Bleeding or discharge for about 4–6 weeks
• Bleeding with clots and cramps
• Pain in the incision

Your health care provider will tell you not to place anything in your vagina (such as tampons) or have sex for a few weeks in order to prevent infection. Give yourself time to heal before doing any strenuous activity. If you have a fever, chills, leg pain, draining or leakage from your abdominal incision, heavy bleeding, or worsening pain, call your health care provider right away.

## Vaginal Birth After Cesarean Delivery

It once was thought that if a woman had one cesarean delivery, she should give birth to all her other babies the same way in the future. This thinking, however, has changed in recent years. Many women now can try to give birth through the vagina (vaginally) after a cesarean delivery. This is known as having a trial of labor after cesarean, or TOLAC. Many women attempting a trial of labor will be able to give birth through the vagina—what's known as a vaginal birth after cesarean delivery, or VBAC.

Between 60% and 80% of women are successful with TOLAC and are able to give birth vaginally. Sometimes, though, problems may arise. One of the most serious is *uterine rupture*, in which the scar on your uterus from your previous cesarean delivery opens. If this happens, your health care provider may need to perform an emergency cesarean delivery.

The decision of whether to try a vaginal delivery or to have a repeat cesarean delivery can be complex. There are a few factors that help determine if TOLAC is a good choice for your next delivery.

### Is It Right for You?

Trial of labor after cesarean birth is considered a safe option for many women. In deciding whether you are an appropriate candidate for a TOLAC, your health care provider will consider the following factors:

- Type of uterine incision—The incision made in your uterus (not the one in your skin) for your previous cesarean delivery is a key factor in deciding whether you should attempt to have a VBAC. This information should be in your medical records. A low transverse (sideways) incision is the most common type used in cesarean birth and the least likely to rupture (tear).

- Previous deliveries—A VBAC is more likely to be successful if you have had at least one vaginal delivery in addition to a previous cesarean delivery. A VBAC can be considered in women who have had up to two previous cesarean deliveries.

- Future deliveries—Multiple cesarean deliveries are associated with additional potential risks. If you know that you want more children, you should keep these risks in mind when making your decision.

- A pregnancy problem or medical condition—Vaginal delivery is riskier if there is a problem with the placenta, problems with the baby, or certain (but not all) medical conditions during pregnancy.

- Type of hospital—The hospital in which a woman has a TOLAC should be prepared to deal with emergencies that may arise. Some hospitals may not offer TOLAC because hospital staff does not feel they can provide needed emergency care. If the hospital you have chosen does not have the appropriate resources, you often can be referred to one that does.

Let your health care provider know if you're interested in trying to have a VBAC early in your pregnancy. Together, you and your health care provider can consider this option. Discussing VBAC early on allows you to consider all of the benefits and risks that apply to your individual situation and to think about all of the options. Many of the factors that go into the decision are known early in pregnancy. Also, if the type of incision used in the previous cesarean delivery is not known, an attempt can be made to find this information.

## Benefits

There are many benefits to VBAC. With a VBAC, you avoid the risks and discomfort of major abdominal surgery. There is less blood loss and a lower risk of infection. There is also less risk of blood clots. With a vaginal birth, there also is a shorter recovery time after giving birth compared with a cesarean delivery. You'll be back on your feet much quicker.

For women planning to have more children, having a VBAC may help prevent some of the potential future complications of multiple cesarean deliveries. These complications include bowel or bladder injury, hysterectomy, and problems with the placenta.

## Risks

Vaginal birth after cesarean delivery is not the right choice for every woman. There are some risks involved, including infection, injury, and blood loss. The most serious risk is the possible rupture of the cesarean scar on the uterus or rupture of the uterus itself. Although a rupture of the uterus is rare, it may harm the pregnant woman and her baby if it does occur. Women who had a vertical incision that was made on the upper part of the uterus (called a "high vertical" or "classical" incision) have the highest risk of rupture. For this reason, VBACs are not recommended for women with a high vertical incision. If a vertical incision was made in the lower part of the uterus, a VBAC still can be considered.

### Best Chances for Success

Although your health care provider will not be able to predict whether TOLAC and VBAC will be successful, there are several factors that are known to play a role in the chances of it turning out as planned. Women with the highest chance of a successful VBAC are those who have given birth vaginally and whose labor progressed naturally without needing to be induced. On the other hand, women with the following conditions have a lower chance of success:

- Recurrent indication for first cesarean delivery
- Being obese
- Being older
- Being a race other than white
- Having a baby weighing more than 9 pounds
- Having a pregnancy lasting beyond 40 weeks
- Having a short time between pregnancies
- Having *preeclampsia*

### Be Prepared for Changes

Although you may have decided on a certain plan for your delivery, things can happen during your pregnancy and labor that change your plan. For example, you may need to have your labor induced, which can reduce your chances of having a successful VBAC. If circumstances change, you and your health care provider may want to reconsider your decision. Keep in mind that your health care team is there to help guide you in making the best decision for you and your baby.

# RESOURCES

The following resources offer more information about cesarean birth and VBAC:

**Cesarean Delivery**
Medline Plus
www.nlm.nih.gov/medlineplus/cesareansection.html
*A great place to start learning about all things related to cesarean birth.*

**Cesarean Delivery: Resource Overview**

*The American College of Obstetricians and Gynecologists (ACOG)*

https://www.acog.org/Womens-Health/Cesarean-Delivery

*Lists ACOG's articles and patient education resources about cesarean delivery.*

**Vaginal Birth After Cesarean (VBAC): Resource Overview**

*The American College of Obstetricians and Gynecologists (ACOG)*

https://www.acog.org/Womens-Health/Vaginal-Birth-After-Cesarean-VBAC

*Lists ACOG's articles and patient education resources about VBAC.*

**VBAC Calculator**

*Eunice Kennedy Shriver* National Institute of Child Health and Human Development

https://mfmu.bsc.gwu.edu/PublicBSC/MFMU/VGBirthCalc/vagbirth.html

*This interactive calculator can help predict the chance of a VBAC. Note that it is designed for educational use and should not be used by itself to predict your individual chance of success.*

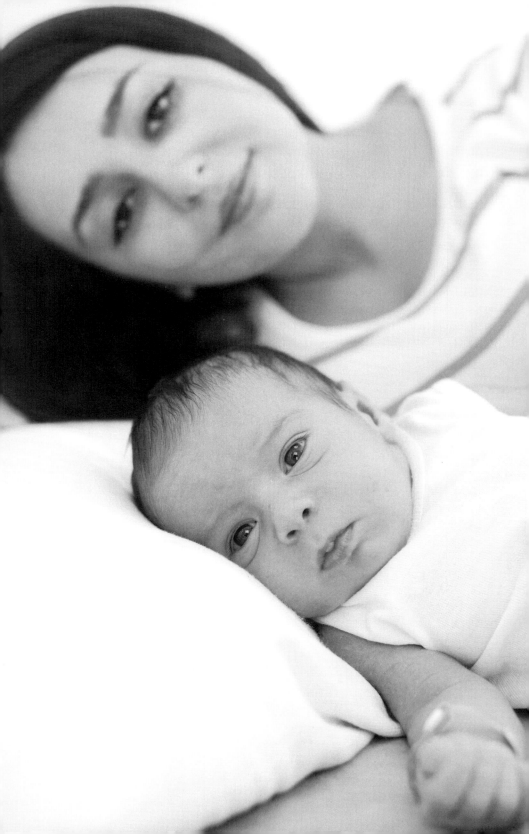

Chapter 16

# The Postpartum Period

It may be hard to believe that childbirth is over and that this baby is really yours. The postpartum period can be a time of joy and happiness, but it also can bring fatigue and sometimes sadness. If you know what's happening to your body and emotions, you can better face the ups and downs of the first few months of being a mom.

## Right After the Baby Is Born

In the moments after birth, if you both are doing well, you most likely will be able to hold and cuddle your baby. Over the next few hours, your caregivers will be busy assessing your newborn's health as well as checking on your condition to make sure all is well.

### Your Baby's Apgar Score

Your baby's health will be assessed with the Apgar test 1 minute after birth and then again 5 minutes after birth. The *Apgar score* rates five newborn features: 1) heart rate, 2) breathing, 3) muscle tone, 4) reflexes, and 5) skin color. Each of these features is given a score of 0, 1, or 2. Then all of the scores are added up, with a maximum possible score of 10. Most babies have an Apgar score of 7 or more at 5 minutes after birth. Few babies score a perfect 10 (see Table 16-1).

The Apgar score is used to check the baby's condition right after delivery. It also is a good way to measure how well the baby adjusts to the outside world in the minutes after birth. The Apgar score does not show how healthy

## Table 16-1 The Apgar Score

| Component | Score | | |
|---|---|---|---|
| | 0 | 1 | 2 |
| Heart rate | Absent | Fewer than 100 beats per minute | More than 100 beats per minute |
| Respiration | Absent | Weak cry or hyperventilation | Good, strong cry |
| Muscle tone | Limp | Some flexing of arms and legs | Active motion |
| Reflexes (response to airway being suctioned) | No response | Grimace | Cries or withdraws; coughs; sneezes |
| Color* | Blue or pale | Body is pink; hands and feet are blue | Pink all over |

*In babies with dark skin, the mouth, lips, palms, and soles are examined.*

your baby was before birth, nor does it predict how healthy your baby will be in the future.

### Your Baby's First Breath

During pregnancy, your baby received oxygen through the **placenta** and **umbilical cord**. In the moments after birth, your newborn takes his or her first breath of air. It's not just the lungs that must be working and able to fill with air seconds after delivery. All the related body parts, such as muscles around the lungs and airways leading from the mouth and nose, also must be ready to start working.

After birth, there's more pressure outside the lungs than there is inside them. This pressure causes the lungs to expand and fill with air. As a result, the baby may start crying. Many babies cry on their own at birth. Others don't cry right away. Instead, they simply start breathing.

After birth, your baby's breathing is monitored closely. If the baby isn't breathing well, steps may be taken to help him or her. Often, this simply means rubbing the baby's body. Sometimes the baby may be given oxygen.

### Maintaining the Baby's Temperature

Before birth, your baby was kept warm by your body. After the baby is born, he or she has to adjust to an environment that's much cooler. The baby's skin is wet with **amniotic fluid**, and a lot of heat can be lost as the moisture on the skin evaporates. Although newborns have built-in controls to keep their body temperature even, they do not work as well as adults' do. Holding your baby on your bare chest and abdomen immediately after birth can help keep the baby warm and helps encourage breastfeeding. In the coming days, it also will be important to monitor the baby's environment and make sure that the baby is dressed appropriately. As a general rule, the baby should be dressed in one more layer than what you are wearing.

## Getting to Know Your Baby

You'll never forget the first time you see your new baby. As a new mom, you may have lots of questions about the way your newborn looks and acts. Knowing what's normal and what to expect at this time in your baby's life will help you relax and enjoy watching your baby grow.

**Your Baby's Weight.** One of the first questions people ask after a baby arrives is how much he or she weighs. In fact, that's one of the first things your health care provider wants to know too. There is a range that is thought to be normal for most babies. Most full-term babies weigh between 5½ pounds and 9½ pounds. The average weight is 7½ pounds.

The weight often depends on how close to the due date the baby is born. Babies born early tend to weigh less than those born at **full term** (from 39 and 0/7 weeks to 40 and 6/7 weeks after your **last menstrual period**). Babies born late tend to weigh more. In the first 3 days after birth, it is normal for a baby to lose a very small amount of weight before beginning to gain weight.

**How Your Baby Looks.** If you're used to seeing newborns on television, you may be surprised to know that most shows use babies who are a few months old to portray newborns. Real newborns look very different in the first few days after birth:

• The body may seem scrunched up because a new baby draws his or her arms and legs up close, into the so-called fetal position. This is the way babies fit into the close confines of the uterus. Even though there's more room now, it'll take a few weeks for the baby to stretch out a bit.

• The face may be slightly swollen, and the area around the eyes may be a little puffy for a few days.

• The baby's head may be long and pointy for a few days or weeks. Why? Babies have two soft spots on the top of their heads where the skull bones haven't joined yet. These soft spots make the head flexible enough to fit through the birth canal.

• Right after birth, the baby's genitals may be swollen. The swelling usually is caused by extra fluid that has built up in the baby's body. In girls, the **labia** may be swollen because of the high levels of maternal hormones that she was exposed to in the uterus. Boys may have extra fluid around their testicles that may make the **scrotum** appear swollen. This swelling usually resolves within days.

**How Your Baby Acts.** Most newborns' basic needs and responses to the outside world are the same. Even so, each baby has a unique personality right from the start.

The way one baby behaves and interacts with people can be very different from the way another newborn acts. Some babies are quiet and calm. Other babies are bundles of energy from the start. They cry and kick with vigor and demand around-the-clock attention.

After the stress of birth, most newborns are very alert for the first hour or so. This is a good time to attempt to breastfeed, talk to, or just hold your new son or daughter.

When this alertness fades, the baby will get sleepy. Don't worry if your newborn seems very drowsy or sleeps a lot for the next few hours or even days. After all, you are not the only one who needs to recover from the birth.

Many babies do little else besides sleep at first. Most newborns spend 14–18 hours a day sleeping, although not all at once. Short stretches of sleep broken up by brief alert periods are normal. But again, it depends on the baby. Some newborns sleep less and are fussy when they wake up. Others sleep for long stretches and are quiet and calm when they are awake.

## What Happens to Your Baby Next

When you both are ready, nurses will weigh and measure the baby, give him or her a bath, slip identification bands around the baby's ankle and wrist, and perhaps take handprints and footprints. For the next few hours, both you and your baby will be monitored to make sure you're doing well.

Your baby can stay with you in your room the entire time you are in the hospital. This is called "rooming in." It makes it easier for you to breastfeed and allows you and your family to bond with the baby. In most hospitals, you can do this even if you have had a **cesarean delivery**. You may need to have someone with you throughout your stay to help you take care of the baby. If you wish, the baby also can stay in the hospital's nursery. The baby does not have to stay there all the time. You can have your baby with you whenever you want.

**Medical Care.** Your baby will receive a complete physical exam in the hospital. A health care provider will examine your baby from head to toe, listen to the breathing and heartbeat, check the pulse, feel the belly, and look for normal newborn reflexes. Other steps will be taken to help prevent health problems:

- Vitamin K shot—A newborn's body can't make vitamin K on its own for a few days, so vitamin K routinely is given by an injection. Vitamin K is needed for the blood to clot after a cut. The vitamin K shot also helps protect against a rare but severe bleeding disorder that can cause permanent brain injury.

- *Antibiotic* ointment or solution in the baby's eyes—This treatment protects against a serious infection from germs that can get into the eyes during birth. It can be done after you've had time to hold and breastfeed your baby.

- Immunization against *hepatitis B virus (HBV)*—The hepatitis B vaccine is a series of three shots. Babies receive the first dose of HBV vaccine before discharge from the hospital. The second dose should be administered at 1–2 months of age. The third dose should be administered by 6–18 months of age. Infants who did not receive a birth dose should receive 3 doses of a hepatitis B-containing vaccine on a schedule of 0, 1–2 months, and 6 months starting as soon as feasible. If you have tested positive for the HBV surface *antigen*, your baby should be given the HBV vaccine and a dose of *hepatitis B immune globulin* within 12 hours of birth. At approximately 1–3 months after completion of the three-dose vaccine series, the baby should be tested for HBV infection.

**Newborn Screening Tests.** By law, your baby must be screened for a number of medical conditions before he or she leaves the hospital. A second round of testing also may be required in some states. Which conditions the baby is screened for depends on the state you live in, but they are usually those for which early diagnosis and treatment can have an important effect on the baby's long-term health.

Newborn screening usually involves a hearing test and a blood test and may include a pulse oximetry test. The pulse oximetry test checks for different forms of congenital heart disease. It is done by placing a small sensor on the baby's skin.

The hearing test checks for certain congenital hearing problems. It can be done in two different ways. In one test, a tiny speaker and microphone are put in the baby's ear. The speaker makes soft clicking sounds. The ear's response to the sounds is measured by the microphone. In the other test, soft earphones are placed over your baby's ears. Then three special sensors are attached to the baby's head. The earphones play soft clicks. The sensors measure brainwave responses to the sounds. If the hearing test shows there might be hearing loss, your baby will be referred to a hearing specialist for further testing.

For the blood test, a few drops of blood are taken from the baby's heel and placed on a special card. The blood is sent to a lab and tested for various medical conditions. Some of these conditions affect a baby's **metabolism** or **immune system**. Others affect the baby's blood. Screening for various infections may be done, such as **human immunodeficiency virus (HIV)** infection and **toxoplasmosis**. You and your pediatrician also can request tests for additional conditions, but these tests may not be covered by your insurance. Your pediatrician will be notified of the results of the screening tests and will discuss the results with you at a pediatric office visit. If your baby has a positive screening test result for any condition, further testing usually is recommended. It is important to get this follow-up testing as soon as possible.

**Circumcision.** If you and your partner have decided to have your baby boy circumcised, it will be done by your **obstetrician–gynecologist**, pediatrician, or family medicine practitioner soon after birth, before the baby leaves the hospital. The procedure is performed with **local anesthesia**. Circumcision for religious reasons can be done outside the hospital (see Chapter 8, "Month 8 [Weeks 29–32]" for more discussion).

## Postpartum: The First Week

If you had a normal vaginal delivery, you will be discharged from the hospital soon after the baby is born, once it is established that your condition is stable. How long you stay depends on your health. However, your insurance policy may have limits as to how long they will cover hospitalization postpartum. How long you stay after a cesarean delivery can depend on why the cesarean delivery was done and how much time you need to resume normal functions.

Before you are discharged, you will be given instructions to follow in case of problems or an emergency. You should arrange for a follow-up exam for you and your newborn. Your health care provider will want to check you about 2–6 weeks after the birth. Your baby generally should be evaluated within 1–2 weeks unless there are issues that need to be addressed sooner. Monthly visits with a health care provider usually are done for the first 3 months of a baby's life.

## Bleeding

Once your baby is born, your body sheds the blood and tissue that lined your uterus. This vaginal discharge is called *lochia*. For the first few days after delivery, lochia is heavy and bright red. It may have a few small clots. You should wear sanitary pads during this time, not tampons.

As time goes on, the flow gets lighter in volume and color. A week or so after birth, lochia often is pink or brown. Bright red discharge can come back, though. You may feel a gush of blood from your vagina during breastfeeding, when your uterus contracts. By 2 weeks postpartum, lochia often is light brown or yellow. After that, it slowly goes away. How long the discharge lasts differs for each woman. Some women have discharge for just a couple of weeks after their babies are born. Others have it for a month or longer. If bleeding is heavy—you are soaking through two maxipads an hour for more than an hour or two—call your health care provider.

## Uterine Contractions

Right after birth, your uterus starts the process of returning to normal size. Over the coming days, your uterus will get smaller and firmer and descend from the level of your navel back below the pubic bone. By about 10 days after birth, you will no longer be able to feel your uterus in your abdomen.

You will feel your uterus contract and then relax as it shrinks back to its normal size. These cramps sometimes are called afterbirth pains. If you need to, you can take an over-the-counter pain reliever. Check with your baby's health care provider before taking any over-the-counter medications while you are breastfeeding.

## Perineal Pain

Your *perineum* is the area between your vagina and *anus*. During childbirth, the skin of the perineum stretches to accommodate the baby's head. Sometimes, the skin and tissues of the perineum tear. There are different degrees of perineal tears (or lacerations, as they sometimes are called). Minor tears may heal on their own without stitches. Some tears can be repaired with a few stitches that are done by your health care provider in the delivery room right after birth. You will receive a local anesthetic if you did not have epidural or spinal **anesthesia** during childbirth. You also can hold your baby while these repairs are being done. If you have a tear that involves the **anal sphincter** and rectal muscles, it usually requires a more extensive surgical repair.

If you have had a perineal tear, you'll likely have a few weeks of swelling and pain as the perineum heals. To help ease the pain and heal quicker, try these tips:

- Apply cold packs or chilled witch-hazel pads to the area.

- Ask your health care provider about using a numbing spray or cream to ease pain.

- If sitting is uncomfortable, sit on a pillow. There also are special cushions that may be helpful.

- Sit in warm water that's just deep enough to cover your buttocks and hips (called a sitz bath). Special basins that can be filled with clean, warm water from the faucet and then placed on a toilet seat are made for this purpose.

## Painful Urination

In the first days after delivery, you may feel the urge to urinate but not be able to pass any urine. You may feel pain and burning when you urinate. That's because during birth, the baby's head put a lot of pressure on your **bladder**, your **urethra** (the opening where urine comes out), and the muscles that control urine flow. This pressure can cause swelling and stretching that gets in the way of urination.

To lessen swelling or pain, try a warm sitz bath. When you are on the toilet, spray warm water over your genitals with a squeeze bottle. This can help trigger the flow of urine. Running the tap while you are in the bathroom may help too. Be sure to drink plenty of fluids as well. This pain usually goes away within days of delivery.

Many new mothers have another problem: involuntary leakage of urine, or urinary **incontinence**. With time, the tone of your pelvic muscles will return and the incontinence will go away in most cases. You may feel more comfortable wearing a sanitary pad until the problem goes away. Doing Kegel exercises (see Chapter 2, "Months 1 and 2 [Weeks 1–8]) also will help tighten these muscles sooner.

## Abdomen

Right after delivery, you still will look like you are pregnant. During pregnancy, the abdominal muscles stretched out little by little. They won't just snap back into place the minute your baby is born.

Give your body time to go back to normal. Exercise will help. Ask your health care provider when it is safe to start exercising. Doing a few exercises at least three times per week will get you started. The exercises in the box "Exercises for the Postpartum Period" are designed to gently tone stretched muscles and prepare you for more rigorous exercise when you are ready.

## Hemorrhoids

If you had **varicose veins** in your **vulva** or hemorrhoids during pregnancy, they may get worse after delivery. These sore, swollen veins also can show up for the first time now because of the intense straining you did during labor. In time, hemorrhoids and vulvar varicosities will get smaller or go away. For relief, try medicated sprays or ointments, dry heat (from a heat lamp or hair dryer turned on low), sitz baths, and cold witch-hazel compresses. Also, try not to strain when you have a bowel movement because this can make hemorrhoids worse. See the suggestions in the "Bowel Problems" section for avoiding constipation.

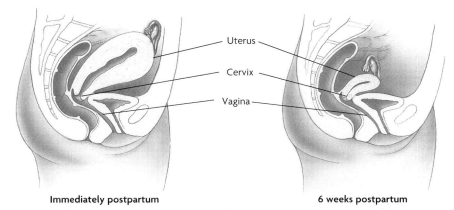

Uterus
Cervix
Vagina

Immediately postpartum        6 weeks postpartum

**The uterus after birth.** Just after birth, the uterus measures about 7 inches long and weighs about 2 pounds (*left*). In 6 weeks, it has returned to normal size (*right*). The normal size is about 3 inches long, weighing about 2 ounces.

## Exercises for the Postpartum Period

During pregnancy, the growing uterus stretches the muscles in your abdomen and your lower back—your "core" muscles. The following exercises are designed to be done in order to gradually help tone and strengthen these muscles. When you master one exercise—you can do 20 repetitions without stopping—move on to the next one. Make sure you get your health care provider's approval before starting any exercise program after pregnancy.

1. **4-Point Kneeling**
   - Kneel on all fours. Make sure your hips are positioned directly over your knees and your shoulders are positioned directly over your hands. Your back should be straight, not curved upward or downward.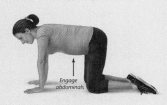
   - Inhale deeply. Then, exhale—do not hold your breath. As you exhale, pull your abdominal muscles in. Imagine that you are pulling your belly button inward up to your spine. Make sure your back stays straight. This is called "engaging" your abdominal muscles.
   - Return to the starting position.

2. **Leg Slides**
   - Lie flat on your back, bending your knees slightly, with your feet flat on the floor. Engage your abdominal muscles by pulling your navel in toward your spine and not moving your back.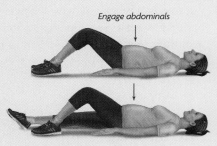
   - Inhale, and slide one leg from a bent to a straight position.
   - Exhale, and bend it back again. Do not hold your breath.
   - Be sure to keep both feet on the floor and keep them relaxed.
   - Repeat with your other leg.

3. **Knee Raises**
   - Start from the same position as the leg slide: Lie flat on your back, bending your knees slightly, with your feet flat on the floor.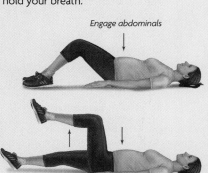

- Raise one leg with the knee bent so that your knee is above your hip. Slide the other leg from a bent to a straight position.
- Keep your abdominal muscles engaged. Focus on drawing your belly button inward. Do not move your back. Remember to breathe.
- Return to starting position. Repeat with opposite leg.

## 4. Heel Touches

- Start out in the same position as the leg slide and knee raises: Lie flat on your back, bending your knees slightly, with your feet flat on the floor.
- Raise both legs with knees bent. Your knees should be at a 90-degree angle above your hips. The lower part of your legs should be parallel to the floor.
- Lower one leg to the floor, keeping the knee bent, and touch your heel to the floor. Make sure that the knee stays bent at a 90-degree angle.
- Keep your abdominal muscles engaged. Focus on drawing your belly button inward. Do not move your back. Remember to breathe.
- Bring the leg back up to the starting position.
- Repeat with the opposite leg.

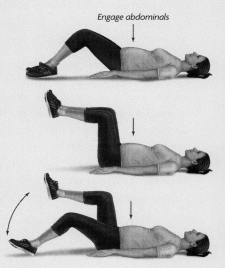

*Engage abdominals*

## 5. Leg Extensions

- Start out in the same position as the leg slide, knee raises, and heel touches: Lie flat on your back, bending your knees slightly, with your feet flat on the floor.
- Raise both legs with knees bent at a 90-degree angle above the hips. The lower part of your legs should be parallel to the floor.
- Extend one leg out with the foot 12–24 inches off the floor. Remember to breathe.
- Return your extended leg to the starting position. Repeat with the opposite leg.

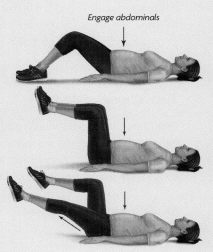

*Engage abdominals*

### Bowel Problems

It may be hard to have bowel movements for a few days after delivery. There are lots of reasons for this: stretched abdominal muscles, sluggish bowels as a result of surgery or pain medication, and an empty stomach after not eating during labor. You also may be afraid to move your bowels because of pain from a perineal tear or hemorrhoids. If you have constipation or painful gas, try these tips to help the problem:

• Take short walks as soon as you can.
• Eat foods high in fiber and drink plenty of fluids.
• Ask your health care provider about taking a stool softener.

You may find that the urge to have a bowel movement may not feel the way it used to. In some cases, you may not be able to control your bowel movements or you may pass gas when you do not mean to or do not expect it. Loss of normal control of the bowels is called fecal incontinence or ***accidental bowel leakage***. It can be caused by damage to the muscles and nerves of the ***rectum*** and anus during childbirth. If you have lost the normal control of your bowels, tell your health care provider about your symptoms. A variety of treatment options are available, including lifestyle changes, physical therapy, medications, and surgical procedures.

## Postpartum: Weeks 2–12

In the weeks after your baby's birth, your body will change as it adjusts to not being pregnant. You also will be caring for a newborn. It can be a very stressful time. Taking care of your physical and mental well-being is key. Having people nearby for support also may help ease your transition into your new role.

### Your Changing Body

While you were pregnant, your body worked round-the-clock to help your baby grow. Now that your baby is here, there's more work to be done as your body recovers from pregnancy, labor, and delivery. It will take time for things to get back to normal.

**Swollen Breasts.** Your breasts fill with milk about 2–4 days after delivery. When this happens, they may feel very full, hard, and tender. The best relief for this engorgement is breastfeeding. Once you and your baby settle into a regular nursing pattern, the discomfort usually goes away. Severe engorgement should not last more than about 36 hours.

Women who do not breastfeed may experience discomfort from engorgement. When the breasts are not stimulated to produce more milk, this feeling will subside gradually, but it often takes about 7–10 days. In the meantime, try the following measures:

• Wear a well-fitting support bra or sports bra. Do not bind your breasts, which can make your pain worse.

• Apply ice packs to your breasts to reduce swelling.

• Don't express any milk. This sends a signal to your breasts to make more.

• Take pain medication, such as ibuprofen, if you need it.

**Fatigue.** You are going to be tired. You just finished a very hard task—childbirth. Your new baby will cause you and your partner many sleepless nights for a while until he or she gets into a regular sleeping schedule. You can't really avoid fatigue, but there are steps you can take to make sure you're not totally exhausted from the job of being a new mom:

• Ask for help—Your family and friends are more than likely eager to pitch in. Let them. Be specific when others want to know what they can do. Ask a friend to bring something for dinner, stop at the grocery store, start a load of laundry, or watch the baby or an older child for a couple of hours so you can take a nap.

• Sleep when your baby sleeps—Use your baby's nap time to rest—not to tackle household chores.

• Suggest quiet play—If you have an older child, set him or her up with a few puzzles, picture books, or other quiet activities so you and the baby can rest.

• Take it easy—Only do what must be done and keep trips out of the house short.

• Limit visitors—If you are feeling tired, it's perfectly fine to say no to family and friends who want to stop by. Don't feel guilty. There will be plenty of time for people to meet your new baby when you are feeling rested.

• Eat a healthy diet—It may be hard to find time to eat when you are caring for a new baby. Even so, it's vital that you do. Foods rich in protein and iron help fight fatigue.

**Sweating.** In the weeks after childbirth, many new mothers find themselves drenched with sweat. This happens most often at night. Your body is adjusting to changing hormone levels. To keep your sheets and pillow dry at night, you can sleep on a towel until the sweating eases.

**Return of Menstrual Periods.** If you are not breastfeeding, your period may return about 6–8 weeks after giving birth. It could start even sooner. If you are breastfeeding, your menstrual periods may not start again for months. Some breastfeeding mothers don't have a menstrual period until their babies are fully weaned.

After birth, your *ovaries* may release an egg before you have your first menstrual period. This means you can get pregnant before you even know you are fertile again. If you don't want another baby right way, start using a birth control method, such as a condom, as soon as you resume having sex.

Once your menstrual period returns, it may not be the same as before you were pregnant. Menstrual periods may be shorter or longer, for instance. Chances are, they'll slowly return to normal. Some women notice that menstrual cramps are less painful than they were before they got pregnant.

## Postpartum Danger Signs

Postpartum discomforts are normal. However, some discomforts may be a sign that there is a problem. Call your health care provider if you have any of these signs or symptoms:

- Fever more than 100.4°F

- Nausea and vomiting

- Pain or burning during urination

- Bleeding that's heavier than a normal menstrual period or that increases

- Severe pain in your lower abdomen

- Pain, swelling, and tenderness in your legs

- Chest pain and coughing or gasping for air

- Red streaks on your breasts or painful new lumps in your breasts

- Pain that doesn't go away or that gets worse from an episiotomy, perineal tear, or abdominal incision

- Redness or discharge from an *episiotomy*, perineal tear, or abdominal incision

- Vaginal discharge that smells bad

- Feelings of hopelessness that last more than 10 days after delivery

## Postpartum Sadness and Depression

Feeling sad after having a baby is actually very common. In fact, about 70–80% of new mothers have feelings of sadness that are known as the "baby blues" or "maternity blues." But for about 10–15% of women, these feelings are more intense and don't go away in a few weeks. This can signal a more serious condition called *postpartum depression*.

**Baby Blues.** The baby blues usually start within a few days of giving birth. Many new mothers feel depressed, anxious, and upset after the birth of a child. These feelings don't seem to match their expectations. They wonder, "What have I got to be depressed about?" Also, they fear that having these feelings means they are bad mothers. These emotions, however, are very normal. Many women feel sad after giving birth. Most often, the baby blues go away on their own within a couple of days.

When you feel blue, remind yourself that you have just taken on a huge job. Feeling sad, anxious, or even angry doesn't mean you are a failure as a mother. It also doesn't mean you are mentally ill. It simply means that your body is adjusting to the normal changes that follow the birth of a child.

It can be helpful to talk to your health care provider about your feelings. The following also may help you feel better:

- Talk to your partner or a good friend about how you feel.

- Get plenty of rest.

- Ask your partner, friends, and family for help.

- Take time for yourself. Get out of the house each day, even if it's only for a short while.

**Postpartum Depression.** Postpartum depression is marked by feelings of despair, severe anxiety, or hopelessness that get in the way of daily life. It can occur up to 1 year after having a baby, but it most commonly happens about 1–3 weeks after childbirth.

Some women are more likely to have postpartum depression than others. Risk factors for postpartum depression include the following:

- History of *depression* before, after, or during pregnancy

- History of premenstrual syndrome or premenstrual dysphoric disorder

- Recent stress, such as losing a loved one, a family illness, or moving to a new city

- Lack of support from others

If you have the signs and symptoms of postpartum depression, or if your partner or family members are concerned that you do, it is important to see your health care provider as soon as possible. Do not wait until your postpartum checkup. The sooner you get help, the sooner you will feel better and be able to enjoy your new family. Your health care provider most likely will ask questions about your signs and symptoms (see the "Edinburgh Postnatal Depression Scale" in Chapter 7, "Month 7 [Weeks 25–28]"). If your health care provider determines that you have postpartum depression, you will work together to find the best treatment options to relieve your symptoms. Depression can be treated with medications called ***antidepressants***. Talk therapy also is used to treat depression, often in combination with medication.

If you are breastfeeding and need to take an antidepressant, you should be aware that these medications can be transferred to babies during breastfeeding, although the amounts generally are very low. Breastfeeding has many benefits for both you and your baby. Deciding to take an antidepressant while breastfeeding involves weighing these benefits against the potential risks of your baby being exposed to the medication in your breast milk. It is best to discuss this decision with your health care provider and with your baby's pediatrician or health care provider.

### Exercise

The demands of being a mother may leave you feeling too tired to exercise. The extra effort is worth it, though. Working out boosts your energy level and your sense of well-being. It also restores muscle strength and helps you get back in shape.

Most women can start exercising as soon as they feel up to it. However, you should talk to your health care provider about when you can get started. If you had a cesarean delivery or problems after delivery, it may take a little longer to feel ready for exercise. For safety's sake, follow the same guidelines you did for a healthy lifestyle when you were pregnant.

If you stayed fit during pregnancy, you'll have a head start. Even so, don't attempt hard workouts right away. If you didn't do much exercise before, take it slowly now. Start with easy exercises and work up to harder ones.

Walking is a very good way to ease back into fitness. Take brisk walks as often as you can—every day if possible. This will help prepare you for more intense exercise when you feel up to it. Walking is a great activity. It's easy to do, and you don't need anything except comfortable shoes. You can even take the baby with you in a stroller or carrier, so you don't need to hire a babysitter. It may do you both good to get fresh air and see other people.

Swimming is another great postpartum exercise. There also are exercise classes designed just for new mothers. To find one, check with local health and fitness clubs, community centers, and hospitals.

No matter what sort of exercise you do, design a program that meets your needs. You may want to strengthen your heart and lungs, tone your muscles, lose weight, or do all three.

Also try to choose a program you'll keep doing. Staying fit over the long haul is more important than getting into shape right after birth. Your health care provider can suggest forms of exercise that will help you meet your fitness goals.

## Nutrition

It's common to lose as many as 20 pounds in the month after delivery. Although it may be tempting to follow up this weight loss with a crash diet so you can squeeze back into your old clothes, don't do it. Dieting can deny your body vital **nutrients** and delay healing after birth. Instead, try to be patient. Keep up the good eating habits you began in pregnancy. If you do, you'll be close to your normal weight within a few months. Combining healthy eating with exercise will help the process.

## Lifestyle Changes

The healthy lifestyle habits you developed while you were pregnant shouldn't stop once the baby is born. If you smoked but stopped during pregnancy, don't start up again. If you need help quitting, see your health care provider. Secondhand smoke has been linked to an increased risk of **sudden infant death syndrome** in newborns. Babies exposed to secondhand smoke also are more likely to develop lung problems (such as asthma), allergies, and ear infections than babies who are not exposed to secondhand smoke. If you are breastfeeding, be aware that the nicotine and other chemicals in cigarettes can be passed along to your baby (although there is no conclusive evidence that these chemicals can harm the baby). Not smoking is one of the best things that you can do for your own health as well as your baby's.

## Life With Your New Baby

Having a baby will change the way you live your life. Your relationship with your partner will be affected. Your old routines may no longer work. If you know this in advance and try to accept these changes, you'll be a lot more relaxed as you start your life with the new baby.

Keep in mind, too, that a new baby touches the lives of the whole family. Each person has a role and should take part in the baby's care. There will be some tension as you all adjust to having a baby around. Talk about it. Share your feelings with your partner, your parents, and your children. Listen to their concerns as well.

Talk to other new moms, too. Just hearing that your family isn't the only one feeling the effects of the birth of a baby can help you cope during this stressful time. The support of other mothers also can make you feel more comfortable in your new role.

If the stress of parenting seems like too much to handle, get some help. Talk to your doctor or call a local crisis hotline. All new parents reach the end of their rope from time to time. This is even truer if you don't have a lot of support or if your baby is fussy.

No matter what triggers them, never take out your emotions on your child. A baby can get injured easily, even if you don't intend to hurt him or her. Shaking a baby for just a few seconds, for instance, can do enough harm to cause lifelong brain damage or even death.

If you ever fear that you are going to lose control and hurt your baby, hand him or her to your partner or another loved one and walk away. If you are alone, put your baby in a safe place, such as the crib. Then go into another room (if you can, choose one that's out of earshot of your baby's cries) until you calm down.

Once the episode has passed, ask yourself what you can do to prevent it from happening again. Tell your partner you need more help, for instance. Ask friends and relatives for help when you have been on baby duty for too long without a break. Find out what sort of community services, such as counseling or financial help, are available to you.

## Postpartum Check-Up

Arrange a visit to see your health care provider 4–6 weeks after your baby's birth. (If you had a cesarean delivery, you may be seen about 2 weeks after surgery to check the incision.) The goal of this checkup is to make sure that your body has recovered from pregnancy and birth and that you are not having any problems. It also allows you and your health care provider to discuss your birth control use, breastfeeding concerns, lifestyle changes that you should make to optimize your health, whether your immunizations are up to date, and your future reproductive plans.

During the visit, your health care provider will check your weight, blood pressure, breasts, and abdomen. He or she also will do a **pelvic exam** to make sure a perineal tear or episiotomy has healed and that your vagina, cervix, and uterus have returned to their normal state. If you had **gestational diabetes mellitus**, you may need to have a blood **glucose** test at this visit (see Chapter 23, "Diabetes Mellitus").

Use this time to bring up any questions or concerns you have about the healing process, breastfeeding, birth control, weight loss, exercise, sex, or your emotions. To help you remember everything you want to talk about, jot down any questions you have and bring them with you to this visit.

## Sex After Childbirth

There is no set time for when you can resume having sex after childbirth. After about 2 weeks postpartum, bleeding and infection are not likely to occur. Many health care providers recommend waiting until 6 weeks after childbirth, but there is no scientific evidence to back this up. Just make sure that before you and your partner resume **sexual intercourse**, you have started using a reliable birth control method.

It's normal to be apprehensive about having sex for the first time after childbirth. Discomfort is common. The following suggestions may help lessen discomfort and increase your and your partner's enjoyment:

- Find a time for sex when you are not rushed. Wait until the baby is sound asleep or you can drop him or her off with a friend or a relative for a couple of hours.

- If you are breastfeeding, vaginal dryness can be a problem. This is caused by low levels of **estrogen**. Use a lubricant to help with vaginal dryness. Many types of lubricants are available. Water-soluble lubricants are less sticky than other types. They are easily absorbed into the skin and may have to be reapplied frequently. Silicone-based lubricants last longer and tend to be more slippery than water-soluble lubricants. Avoid oil-based lubricants, which include petroleum jelly, baby oil, and mineral oil. Oil-based lubricants may cause vaginal irritation. They also should not be used with latex condoms. They can dissolve the latex and cause the condom to break. You also should avoid "warming" lubricants that claim to enhance sexual response. They contain chili pepper oil or menthol that can cause burning or stinging of inflamed vaginal tissues.

• Try different positions to take pressure off of a sore area and to control penetration. Being on top of your partner may be more comfortable for you.

However, it is perfectly normal to find that you don't have much interest in sex even after these weeks have passed. There are many reasons for this:

• Fatigue—Once you get your baby to sleep, all you or your partner may want to do is sleep too.

• Stress—Coping with your baby's demands can leave you with little desire for sex.

• Fear of pain—Your breasts may be tender and your perineum may be sore. If you are breastfeeding, your vagina may be dry. This can make sex uncomfortable.

• Lack of desire—Hormone levels decrease after birth. As a result, so does your desire for sex.

• Lack of opportunity—Sex takes energy, time, and focus. When you are a new parent, these all tend to be in short supply.

During the weeks that you may not feel up to sexual intercourse, you can be intimate with your partner in other ways, such as hugging and kissing. When you do feel comfortable and ready to have sex again, it's a good idea to keep the following things in mind:

• Spend private time with your partner when you talk only about each other—not the baby or household problems.

• If sex isn't comfortable yet, there are many other ways to give and receive sexual pleasure, such as mutual masturbation or oral sex.

• If you have concerns about sexual problems, be honest and discuss them with your partner.

If you continue to feel pain during sexual intercourse, it is a good idea to talk with your health care provider. He or she may have additional suggestions about how to ease discomfort. If you have vaginal dryness or are healing from a perineal tear, estrogen cream that is applied to the vagina may be prescribed.

This form of estrogen can be used while you are breastfeeding because very little estrogen is absorbed into the bloodstream.

## Birth Control

When you and your partner are ready to start having sex again, it is important to use birth control. Using birth control can allow your body time to heal before having another baby and gives you the opportunity to plan your family. Even if you want your children to be close in age, it's best to wait at least 12 months before getting pregnant again. Getting pregnant less than 6 months after you give birth increases the risk that your baby will be born **preterm**. Babies born soon after their siblings also are more likely to be smaller than average. These problems may be because the mother's body has not had time to replace nutritional stores. Postpartum stress also is a factor. Of course, each family has different needs and desires when it comes to child spacing. Discuss the issue with your partner and your health care provider.

If you are not breastfeeding, **ovulation** may return soon after you have your baby. Once ovulation occurs, you are able to become pregnant again. If you are breastfeeding, ovulation returns by about 6 months. You can get pregnant even if you are not yet having periods. Keep in mind, too, that if you used fertility drugs to get pregnant the first time, it doesn't mean you can't get pregnant without them.

Many birth control options are available for both women and men. Before choosing one, talk about it with your health care provider. You may find that the birth control method you used before you had a baby is no longer the best option for you after you've had a baby. Also, if you want to have more children, make sure the method you choose is easily reversible.

Some birth control methods can be started immediately after childbirth. With others, you need to wait for a few weeks to start the method. To prevent an unintended pregnancy, it is important to keep these waiting periods in mind. In addition, some forms of birth control are not effective right away, so you need to use an additional method of birth control for a number of days after starting the method. Table 16-2 gives information about the effectiveness of each method, when each method can be started after childbirth and whether an additional method of birth control is needed, whether you can breastfeed while using the method, and whether the method protects against **sexually transmitted infections**.

## Table 16-2 Birth Control Methods

| MOST EFFECTIVE | | | |
|---|---|---|---|
| | **Method** | **Protects Against STIs?** | **OK With Breastfeeding?** |
| Less than 1 pregnancy per 100 women per year | Sterilization | No | Yes |
| | Implant | No | Yes |
| | Intrauterine Device | No | Yes |
| 6–12 pregnancies per 100 women per year | Injection | No | Yes |
| | Combined Hormonal Methods | No | Yes, after breast-feeding is established (usually 30–42 days after childbirth) |
| | Progestin-Only Pills | No | Yes |
| | Diaphragm | No | Yes |
| 18 or more pregnancies per 100 women per year | Condom | Yes | Yes |
| | Cervical Cap* | No | Yes |
| | Sponge* | No | Yes |
| | Spermicide | No | Yes |
| LEAST EFFECTIVE | | | |

Abbreviations: DVT, deep vein thrombosis; IUD, intrauterine device; STIs, sexually transmitted infections.

*These methods are much less effective in women who have given birth (24 pregnancies per 100 women in 1 year) than in women who have not had children (12 pregnancies per 100 women in 1 year).

| How to Start After Pregnancy |
| --- |
| Surgical methods of sterilization: Can be done immediately after childbirth. Hysteroscopic sterilization: Need to wait for 3 months after childbirth to have the procedure and need to use another method until a hysterosalpingogram confirms that tubes are blocked, which typically takes 3 months after having the procedure. Therefore, you will need to use another form of birth control for at least 6 months until you can rely on the procedure for birth control. |
| Can be inserted immediately after childbirth; use another form of birth control for the next 7 days if<br>• you have had a menstrual period and it has been more than 5 days since bleeding started.<br>• it has been 21 days or more since you gave birth and your menstrual period has not returned. |
| Can be inserted immediately after childbirth. There is no need to use another birth control method after insertion of the copper IUD. For the hormonal IUD, use another form of birth control for the next 7 days if<br>• you have had a menstrual period and it has been more than 7 days since bleeding started.<br>• it has been 21 days or more since you gave birth and your menstrual period has not returned. |
| Can be started immediately after childbirth; use another form of birth control for the next 7 days if<br>• you have had a menstrual period and it has been more than 7 days since bleeding started.<br>• it has been 21 days or more since you gave birth and your menstrual period has not returned. |
| Can be started 21 days after childbirth if you are not breastfeeding and if you do not have additional risk factors for DVT; can be started 30–42 days after childbirth if you are breastfeeding and if you do not have additional risk factors for DVT. |
| Can be started immediately after childbirth; use another form of birth control for the next 2 days if<br>• you have had a menstrual period and it has been more than 5 days since bleeding started.<br>• it has been 21 days or more since you gave birth and your menstrual period has not returned. |
| You should wait 6 weeks after giving birth to use the diaphragm until the uterus and cervix return to normal size. If you used a diaphragm before, you must be refitted after giving birth. |
| Can be used at any time following childbirth. |
| You should wait 6 weeks after giving birth to use the cervical cap until the uterus and cervix return to normal size. If you used a cervical cap before, it needs to be refitted after giving birth. |
| Can be used at any time following childbirth. |
| Can be used at any time following childbirth. |

### Intrauterine Devices

The **intrauterine device (IUD)** is a small, T-shaped device that is inserted into the uterus by a health care provider. There are two types of IUDs available in the United States: hormonal IUDs and the copper IUD. Both types prevent pregnancy mainly by preventing **fertilization** of the egg by the **sperm**. Hormonal IUDs release a small amount of **progestin** into the uterus. One brand is approved for use for up 5 years; another brand is approved for use for up to 3 years. The copper IUD releases a small amount of copper and is approved for use for up to 10 years.

IUDs have many benefits. They are highly effective in preventing pregnancy, with effective rates that are the same as those for permanent **sterilization**—fewer than 1 in 100 women (less than 1%) will become pregnant in the first year of typical use of the IUD. It can be inserted immediately after childbirth or a few weeks after childbirth, even if you are breastfeeding. You do not need to do anything else to prevent pregnancy once it is inserted. If you want to get pregnant, you can have the IUD removed, and your fertility returns right away.

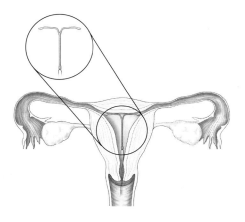

Intrauterine device

### Implant

The **birth control implant** is a single rod about the size of a matchstick that is inserted under the skin in the upper arm. It releases progestin into the body and works mainly by preventing ovulation. It protects against pregnancy for up to 3 years and is highly effective: fewer than 1 in 100 women using an implant will become pregnant in the first year of typical use. The implant can be inserted immediately after childbirth, even if you are breastfeeding. Once your

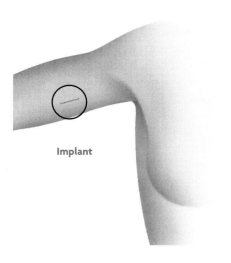

Implant

health care provider inserts the implant, you do not need to do anything else to prevent pregnancy. If you wish to become pregnant, the implant can be removed easily by your health care provider, and fertility returns quickly. The most common side effect of the implant is unpredictable bleeding, especially in the first 3 months of use.

## Injection

The birth control injection contains **_depot medroxy-progesterone acetate (DMPA)_**, a type of progestin. It works mainly by preventing ovulation. The birth control injection is given by your health care provider in your arm or buttock every 3 months. With typical use, 6 women out of 100 (6%) will become pregnant during the first year of use of the injection. Other than getting your injections on time, you don't have to do anything else to prevent pregnancy. You can be as much as 2 weeks late for an injection with no decrease in effec-

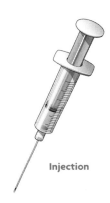

Injection

tiveness. The injections can be started immediately after childbirth, even if you are breastfeeding. If you want to get pregnant again, there may be a delay in the return of your fertility after stopping injections. It takes an average of 10 months for pregnancy to occur after stopping the injection. For some women, it takes longer.

## Combined Hormonal Methods

Combined hormonal birth control methods contain estrogen and progestin and include pills, the vaginal ring, and the patch. These methods work mainly by preventing ovulation. With typical use, 9 women out of 100 (9%) will become pregnant during the first year of using these methods.

Combined hormonal methods should not be used during the first 21 days after delivery. During pregnancy and the postpartum period, there is an increased risk of blood clots developing in veins located deep in the body. This condition, called **_deep vein thrombosis (DVT)_**, can cause serious complications if a piece of a clot breaks free and moves through the blood vessels to the lungs. The risk of DVT is highest in the first 21 days after delivery. Using combined hormonal methods during this time may increase this risk even more. For this reason, if you have additional risk factors for DVT—for example, you have had a previous DVT, you had a cesarean delivery, or you are obese—you generally should not use combined hormonal contraceptives during the first 21–42 days after delivery.

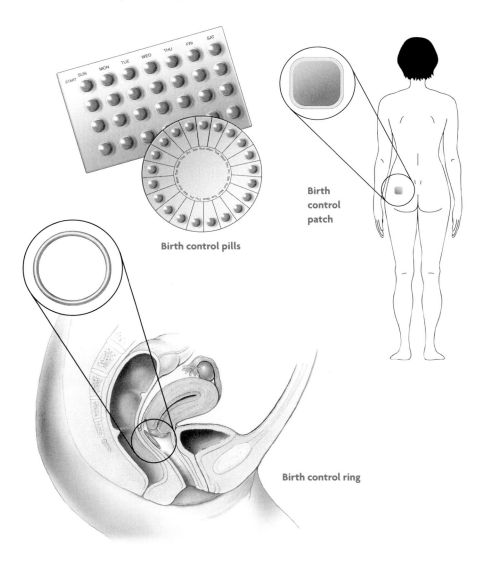

**Birth control pills**

**Birth control patch**

**Birth control ring**

If you are breastfeeding, a short additional waiting period is recommended beyond the waiting period to avoid DVTs. There is a theoretical risk that combined hormonal methods can affect milk supply, especially when you first start breastfeeding. For this reason, experts suggest starting these methods 30–42 days after delivery, when breastfeeding usually is well established.

### Progestin-Only Pills

These pills contain only progestin and work mainly by preventing fertilization of the egg by the sperm. With typical use, 9 women out of 100 (9%) will become pregnant during the first year of use of the progestin-only pill. These pills do not increase the risk of DVT, so you can start taking these pills immediately after childbirth, even if you are breastfeeding. Progestin-only pills need to be taken at the same time each day. If a pill is taken more than 3 hours late, the missed pill should be taken as soon as possible, even if it means taking two pills on the same day. You also need to avoid sexual intercourse or use an additional method, such as a condom, until you have taken a pill at the same time for two days in a row.

### Barrier Methods

Barrier methods work by keeping sperm from reaching the egg. If you choose a barrier method, it must be used each time you have sex to be effective. The following barrier methods are available:

- Condoms—The male condom is a thin latex sheath worn over a man's penis, which blocks his ejaculate from entering the vagina. The female condom is a plastic pouch that lines the vagina. It is held in place by a closed inner ring at the cervix and an open outer ring at the entrance of the vagina. The male condom provides the best protection against sexually transmitted infections. With typical use, 18 women out of 100 (18%) will become pregnant in the first year of use of the male condom and

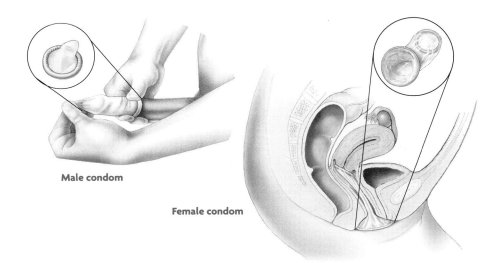

Male condom

Female condom

21 women out of 100 (21%) will become pregnant in the first year of use of the female condom.

- Diaphragm—A diaphragm is a dome-shaped device that fits inside the vagina and covers the cervix. It can be inserted 1–2 hours before you have sex and is used with a spermicide. The diaphragm must be fitted and pre-scribed by a health care provider. If you used a diaphragm before, you must be refitted after giving birth. You should wait 6 weeks after giving birth to use the diaphragm when the uterus and cervix have returned to normal size. With typical use, 12 women out of 100 (12%) will become pregnant in the first year of using the diaphragm.

- Cervical cap—The cervical cap is smaller than a diaphragm and fits more tightly over the cervix. It stays in place by suction. It is used with spermi-cide. Like the diaphragm, it must be fitted and prescribed by a health care provider. Also like the diaphragm, you should wait 6 weeks after giving birth to use the cervical cap when the uterus and cervix have returned to normal size, and it needs to be refitted after you have had a baby. It is less effective in women who have given birth than in women who haven't. With typical use, 24 women out of 100 who gave birth previously (24%) will become pregnant in the first year of using the cervical cap; 12 women out of 100 (12%) who have not given birth previously will become preg-nant in the first year.

- Sponge—The sponge is a doughnut-shaped device made of soft foam with spermicide. It is inserted into the vagina and covers the cervix. The sponge is convenient because it's available over the counter. However, it is less effective in women who have given birth—the effectiveness rates are the same as those for the cervical cap.

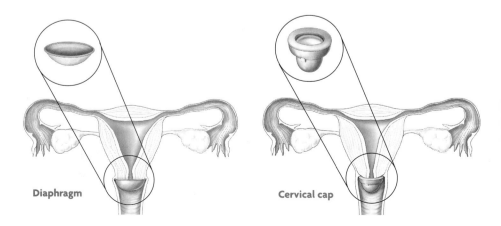

Diaphragm

Cervical cap

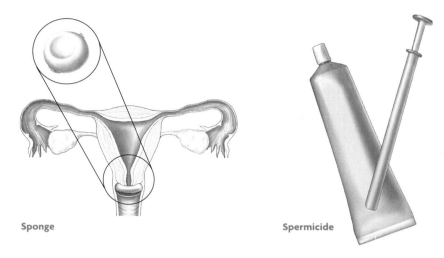

Sponge

Spermicide

- Spermicides—Spermicides are chemicals that destroy sperm before they can fertilize the egg. Spermicides come in various forms, including creams, gels, foams, and vaginal suppositories. Spermicides are placed in the vagina, close to the cervix, before sex. With typical use, 28 women out of 100 (28%) will become pregnant in the first year of using spermicides.

## Lactational Amenorrhea Method

The *lactational amenorrhea method (LAM)* is a temporary method of birth control that is based on the natural way the body prevents ovulation when a woman is breastfeeding. If a woman does not ovulate, she cannot become pregnant. The method is 98% effective if used correctly.

For this method to work, three conditions must be met:

1. Your menstrual period has not returned.
2. You are fully or nearly fully breastfeeding.
3. Your baby is 6 months of age or younger.

Full or nearly full breastfeeding means that the infant receives no other liquid or food, not even water, in addition to breast milk. Although giving other liquids or formula on occasion may be fine, it may make ovulation and, therefore, unintended pregnancy more likely. Also, the time between feedings should not be longer than 4 hours during the day or 6 hours at night. LAM may be more effective when the baby directly suckles from the breast rather than feeds from a bottle with expressed (pumped) breast milk.

An important part of LAM is knowing when to start using another form of birth control to prevent pregnancy. To determine this time, you should ask yourself three questions:

1. Has my period returned?
2. Am I supplementing regularly with formula or other food or liquids or going long periods without breastfeeding, either during the day or at night?
3. Is my baby more than 6 months old?

If you answer yes to any of these questions, your risk of pregnancy is increased, and you should use another form of birth control. However, you still can continue to breastfeed your baby.

### Emergency Contraception

If you and your partner have unprotected sex or your birth control method fails during sex, you can use emergency contraception to prevent pregnancy. There are three types of emergency contraception: 1) the copper IUD, 2) progestin-only pills, and 3) the ulipristal pill. The pills must be taken as soon as possible within 120 hours (5 days) of unprotected sex. Likewise, the IUD must be inserted within 120 hours of unprotected sex. The copper IUD is the most effective form of emergency contraception and can be kept in place for continued use as a birth control method for up to 10 years. A health care provider must insert the copper IUD.

Some progestin-only emergency contraception products are available on regular store shelves (with other over-the-counter drugs) without a prescription to people of any age. Ulipristal is available only by prescription.

## Permanent Birth Control

Sterilization is an option if you and your partner are sure you don't want more children. Sterilization is more than 99% effective. It is a permanent form of birth control. Although there is surgery to reverse sterilization, it doesn't always result in pregnancy. **In vitro fertilization** may be an option, but there are no guarantees about whether you will conceive.

### Female Sterilization

Female sterilization closes off or removes the **fallopian tubes**. This prevents the **egg** from moving down the fallopian tube to the uterus and keeps the sperm from reaching the egg. It can be performed during a surgical procedure or with a procedure called a **hysteroscopy**.

A risk common to all female sterilization methods is that if pregnancy does occur, there is an increased chance that it will be an **ectopic pregnancy**. However, the risk of ectopic pregnancy occurring in women who have had **tubal sterilization** is lower than in women who do not use any birth control.

**Surgical Methods.** There are several ways that sterilization surgery can be performed. **Postpartum sterilization** usually is done within a few hours or days after delivery. The surgery is easier to perform then because the uterus still is enlarged and pushes the fallopian tubes up in the abdomen. It's also convenient because you don't have to return to the hospital to have it done and it is effective right away. How the surgery is performed depends on whether you had a vaginal delivery or a cesarean delivery:

- If you had a vaginal delivery, a small incision is made in the abdomen. The fallopian tubes are brought up through the incision. The tubes are then closed off with clips or, more commonly, a small section of each tube or the entire tube is removed. If you had an **epidural block** for the delivery, it often can be used for the sterilization procedure. If you did not have anesthesia for the delivery, you will receive **regional anesthesia** or **general anesthesia** for sterilization.

- If you had a cesarean delivery, the operation can be done immediately afterward through the same incision that was made for delivery of the baby.

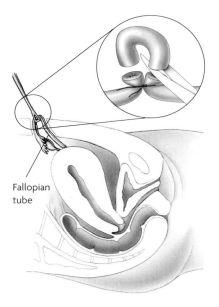

Fallopian tube

As with any type of surgery, there is a risk of bleeding, problems with wound healing, infection, and complications from the anesthesia used. Other organs in the pelvis can be injured during the surgery.

If you are interested in having postpartum sterilization, talk to your health care provider about it well before you

**Postpartum sterilization.** Right after childbirth, the uterus is still enlarged and the fallopian tubes are pushed up, making them more accessible. The tubes are brought up through the incision. The tubes are closed off with clips or bands, or a small section or the entire tube is removed.

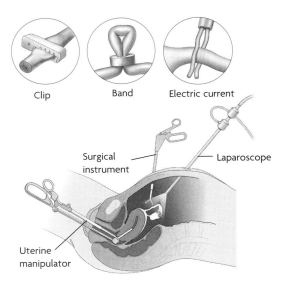

Clip　　　　Band　　　Electric current

Surgical instrument — — Laparoscope

Uterine manipulator

**Laparoscopic sterilization.** This method of sterilization requires a few small incisions in the abdomen.

have the baby. There may be certain waiting periods or other restrictions that need to be addressed before you can have sterilization. Check with your health insurance provider to see if the procedure is covered. You also need to check whether the hospital where you give birth offers sterilization.

You also can choose to have sterilization surgery later as a separate procedure. The method usually used is a surgical procedure called *laparoscopy*, which typically is done with general anesthesia. A device called a *laparoscope* is inserted through a small incision made in or near the navel. The laparoscope allows the pelvic organs to be seen. The fallopian tubes are closed off using instruments passed through the laparoscope or with another instrument inserted through a second small incision. The tubes can be closed with bands, clips, or an electric current. Alternatively, a small section of each tube or the entire tube can be removed. Laparoscopy can be performed as outpatient surgery, so you can go home the same day if there are no problems.

**Hysteroscopic Sterilization.** Another method of sterilization, called *hysteroscopic sterilization*, also is available. This procedure can be performed in a health care provider's office, a clinic, or a surgery center with *local anesthesia* and it does not require an abdominal incision. It can be done beginning 3 months after childbirth. Hysteroscopic sterilization involves inserting

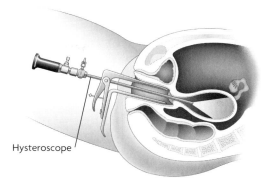

Hysteroscope

**Hysteroscopic sterilization.** With the hysteroscopic method, a small device is inserted through the vagina into each fallopian tube. This device causes scar tissue to grow in the tubes. The scar tissue blocks the fallopian tubes and prevents the sperm from reaching the egg.

an instrument called a *hysteroscope* into the uterus though the vagina and placing a small device into each fallopian tube. The devices cause scar tissue to form, which blocks the fallopian tubes and prevents the egg from being fertilized. It takes about 3 months after the procedure for the tubes to become completely blocked. During this time, you can become pregnant, and you will need to use another form of birth control. At the 3-month mark, you will have a *hysterosalpingogram*, an X-ray procedure, to make sure that the fallopian tubes are blocked. Hysteroscopic sterilization should not be solely relied upon for birth control until this test shows that the tubes are blocked. It may take more than 3 months for this to happen. In a few cases, the tubes do not become completely blocked, or it's not possible to place the devices into one or both fallopian tubes.

## Male Sterilization

Male sterilization is called *vasectomy*. It involves cutting or tying the *vas deferens* (tubes through which sperm travel) so that no sperm is released when a man ejaculates. Vasectomy does not affect a man's ability to get erections or have *orgasms*. A vasectomy may be done in a doctor's office, clinic, or hospital. The man can go home the same day if there are no complications. Vasectomy generally is considered to be safer than female sterilization and requires only local anesthesia. Also, there is no increased risk of ectopic pregnancy if the vasectomy fails.

A vasectomy is not effective right away because some sperm still may be in the tubes at the time of procedure. It takes about 2–4 months for the semen to become totally free of sperm. A couple must use another method

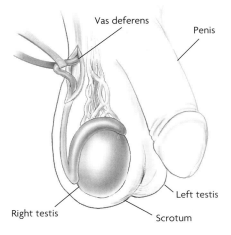

**Vasectomy.** One or two small cuts are made in the skin of the scrotum. Each vas is pulled through the opening until it forms a loop. A small section is cut out of the loop and removed.

of birth control or avoid sexual intercourse until a sperm count confirms that no sperm are present. In this test, the number of sperm in a semen sample is counted.

## Returning to Work

If, when, and how you go back to work after having a baby are personal choices. Paid maternity leave policies vary from state to state and from employer to employer. The federal Family and Medical Leave Act guarantees women up to 12 weeks of unpaid leave after giving birth.

Beyond your recovery from birth, there are other factors to take into account. You have to think about how much money you make and how long your family can do without it. You have to look at the costs of and options for child care too. If you are breastfeeding, you should give yourself time to establish a good nursing relationship with your baby. You also will want to consider how to continue breastfeeding when you go back to work. The Affordable Care Act now requires employers to provide reasonable break time for an employee to express breast milk for 1 year after a child's birth. The employer also must provide a place other than a bathroom for the employee to express breast milk.

Be careful to build in some leeway for yourself. In other words, you can't predict for sure what will happen. You may not know how you'll feel about work until after your baby is born.

Moms who work outside the home have a number of options these days. A growing number of employers let new mothers work part-time, work from home 1 or 2 days a week, job share, condense their work weeks, or work flexible hours. Asking an employer about some of these flexible work schedule opportunities can make some of these options possible for you, even if it hasn't been done before at your place of work. Also, some companies offer on-site child care, which is a real bonus for new mothers. They can bring their babies to work with them, visit them during breaks and lunch hours, and continue to breastfeed.

If your partner is not staying at home to care for the baby, you will need to find child care. There are many things to consider when searching for good child care for your newborn. Will you use a day care center, in-home day care, or a nanny? Finding child care for a young infant can be an anxious time for any couple. But be patient and make your selection only when you're most at ease.

# RESOURCES

The following resources offer more information about the postpartum period, including newborn screening, contraception, nutrition, and more:

**Birth Control (Contraception): Resource Overview**
The American College of Obstetricians and Gynecologists (ACOG)
http://www.acog.org/Womens-Health/Birth-Control-Contraception
*Lists ACOG's articles and patient education resources about birth control methods.*

**Newborn Screening Tests**
Medline Plus
www.nlm.nih.gov/medlineplus/ency/article/007257.htm
*Provides a general description of newborn screening tests, how they are done, and what the results may mean.*

**Recovering From Birth**
The Office on Women's Health
http://womenshealth.gov/pregnancy/childbirth-beyond/recovering-from-birth.html
*Gives practical advice about the postpartum recovery process and offers tips about navigating the first few weeks after childbirth.*

**Special Supplemental Nutrition Program for Women, Infants, and Children (WIC)**
www.fns.usda.gov/wic/women-infants-and-children-wic
*The WIC program provides nutritional help for low-income women and children.*

# Part III
## Nutrition

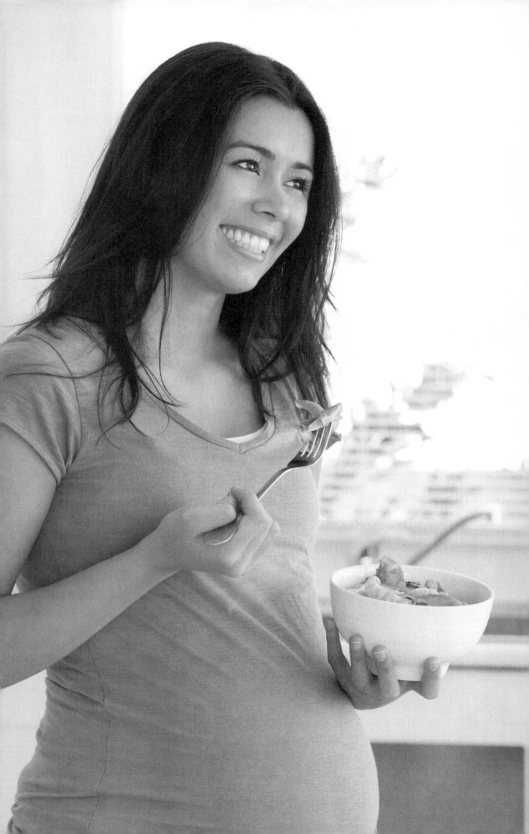

Chapter 17

# Nutrition During Pregnancy

Healthy eating is important during pregnancy. Good nutrition is needed to meet the added demands on your body as well as those of your growing baby. Eating healthy while you're pregnant may take a little extra effort, but it will have major benefits for you and your baby. If you already eat a balanced diet, all you have to do is add a few extra well-chosen **calories**. If you have not been eating a healthy diet, pregnancy is a great time to change old habits and develop healthy new ones. Breastfeeding mothers need to pay careful attention to their diets as well (see Chapter 18, "Breastfeeding and Formula-Feeding Your Baby").

Healthy eating also includes knowing how much you should eat. Pregnant women used to be told to "eat for two." This is still true—to a point. We now know that you can't just eat twice as much as you normally do. Finding a balance between getting enough **nutrients** to fuel the baby's growth and maintaining a healthy weight is important for your and your baby's future health. A pregnant woman who has a **body mass index (BMI)** in the normal range before pregnancy needs, on average, only about 300 extra calories a day—the amount in a glass of skim milk and half a sandwich. If you are pregnant with twins, you'll need 600 extra calories per day. You can calculate your BMI using an online calculator (you can find one at www.nhlbi.nih.gov/health/educational/lose_wt/BMI/) or use the chart in Appendix A.

## Balancing Your Diet

Nutrients are the building blocks of the body. Important nutrients include proteins, carbohydrates, and fats. When you're pregnant, you not only need to maintain your own body with nutrients, you also need to support the growth of your baby. Getting enough nutrients during pregnancy safeguards your own health and contributes to your baby's normal development.

### *Protein*

Protein provides the nutrients your body needs to grow and repair muscles and other tissues. Protein is found in the following foods:

- Beef, pork, and fish
- Poultry
- Eggs
- Milk, cheese, and other dairy foods
- Beans and peas
- Nuts and seeds

For vegetarians, protein can be found in nuts, seeds, nut butters, and soy products such as tempeh and tofu. Vegetarians who include dairy products in their diets also can get needed protein from milk and eggs.

### *Carbohydrates*

All carbohydrates are broken down into **glucose**, the body's main fuel that powers all of its activities. There are two types of carbohydrates: simple carbohydrates and complex carbohydrates. Simple carbohydrates provide a quick energy boost because they are digested and absorbed rapidly. They are found in naturally sweet foods like fruits and also can be added to foods in the form of table sugar, honey, and maple syrup. Simple carbohydrates often are high in calories. It is best to limit your intake of simple carbohydrates to those found naturally in food. Stay away from sugary drinks and foods with added sugar.

Complex carbohydrates include dietary fiber and starches. It takes your body longer to process them, so complex carbohydrates provide longer-lasting energy than simple carbohydrates. Complex carbohydrates are found in bread, rice, pasta, some fruits, and starchy vegetables such as potatoes and corn.

Fiber is found in plant foods. It is the part of the plant that your body cannot digest. Fiber passes relatively unchanged through your digestive system. It can help prevent constipation by adding bulk to the stool, making it easier to pass. You should eat about 25 grams of fiber daily. The following foods are good sources of fiber:

- Fruits (especially dried fruits, berries, oranges, apples, and peaches with the skin)

- Vegetables (such as dried beans, peas, and leafy vegetables like spinach and kale)

- Whole-grain products (such as whole-wheat bread or brown rice)

Fiber also helps maintain a stable blood glucose level because it passes slowly through the digestive tract. Foods that do this are described as "low glycemic" because they do not cause the blood glucose level to spike. Eating low-glycemic foods can help you feel full and reduce the feeling of hunger. Low-glycemic foods also may help reduce **cholesterol** levels and prevent diabetes.

## Fats

The body needs a certain amount of fat to function normally. Some types of fats, called omega-3 fatty acids, play an important role in brain development. Fats also are essential to the function of the **immune system**, aid in blood clotting, and help your body use vitamins A, D, E, and K.

The fat in the foods you eat is digested and sent to the liver. The liver then assembles the fat into lipoproteins. Lipoproteins are made of cholesterol, fats, and protein. Lipoproteins carry fat through your bloodstream for use by or storage in other parts of the body.

There are different types of fat found in foods. You should be aware of these different types of fat in your diet:

- Saturated fats come mainly from meat and dairy products. They tend to be solid when chilled. Examples include butter and lard. There also are two plant-based saturated fats: 1) palm oil and 2) coconut oil.

- Unsaturated fats tend to be liquid and come mostly from plants and vegetables. Olive, canola, peanut, sunflower, and fish oils are all unsaturated fats.

- Trans fats are unsaturated fats that have been chemically processed to be solid at room temperature. This is done to make foods last longer and give them better flavor. Vegetable shortenings, margarines, crackers, cookies, and snack foods like potato chips often contain trans fats.

Oils and fats give you important nutrients. During pregnancy, the fats you eat provide energy and help build many fetal organs and the **placenta**. However, too much saturated fat and trans fat can lead to health problems, including heart disease. Fats should make up about 20–35% of your total food intake—that's about 6 tablespoons per day. Most of the fats and oils in your diet should be unsaturated fats, such as olive oil and peanut oil. Limit saturated fats, such as butter and fatty red meats, and avoid trans fats, which have no nutritional value.

## Planning Healthy Meals

It's not hard to plan healthy meals while you are pregnant, and the U.S. Department of Agriculture has made it even easier by creating www.choosemyplate.gov. The "MyPlate" web site helps everyone from dieters and children to pregnant women learn how to make healthy food choices at every meal.

With MyPlate, you can get a personalized nutrition and physical activity plan by using the "SuperTracker" program. This program shows you the foods and amounts that you need to eat each day during each trimester of pregnancy. The amounts are calculated according to your height, prepregnancy BMI, due date, and how much you exercise during the week. The amounts of food are given in standard sizes that most people are familiar with, such as cups and ounces.

## The Five Food Groups

To get an idea of how MyPlate works, Table 17-1 shows the foods and amounts that a pregnant woman with a normal BMI before pregnancy should eat for each trimester of pregnancy. You'll notice that food is broken down into the following five food groups:

1. Grains—Bread, pasta, oatmeal, cereal, and tortillas are all grains. Make one half of the grains you eat whole grains. Whole grains are those that have not been processed and include the whole grain kernel. They include oats, barley, quinoa, and brown rice. Look for the words "whole grain" on the product label.

2. Fruits—Fruits can be fresh, frozen, canned, or dried. Juice that is 100% fruit juice also counts.

## Table 17-1 Daily Food Choices

Recommended daily food intake for a pregnant woman who is a normal weight and who gets less than 30 minutes of exercise each day.

| | First Trimester | Second Trimester | Third Trimester | Comments |
|---|---|---|---|---|
| Total calories per day | 1,800 | 2,200 | 2,400 | |
| Grains | 6 ounces | 7 ounces | 8 ounces | 1 ounce is one slice of bread, ½ cup of cooked rice, ½ cup of cooked pasta, 3 cups of popped popcorn, or five whole wheat crackers |
| Vegetables | 2 ½ cups | 3 cups | 3 cups | 2 cups of raw leafy vegetables count as 1 cup |
| Fruits | 1 ½ cup | 2 cups | 2 cups | One large orange, one small apple, eight large strawberries, or ½ cup of dried fruit count as 1 cup |
| Dairy | 3 cups | 3 cups | 3 cups | Two small slices of swiss cheese or ⅓ cup of shredded cheese count as 1 cup |
| Protein foods | 5 ounces | 6 ounces | 6 ½ ounces | 1 ounce lean meat or poultry, one egg, 1 tablespoon peanut butter, or ½ ounce of nuts or seeds count as 1 ounce |
| Fats and oils | 5 teaspoons | 7 teaspoons | 8 teaspoons | Olives, some fish, avocados, and nuts |

3. Vegetables—Vegetables can be raw or cooked, frozen, canned, dried, or 100% vegetable juice. Make sure that you get a mixture of dark green, orange, starchy, and other vegetables, including dry beans and peas.

4. Dairy—Milk and products made from milk, such as cheese, yogurt, and ice cream, make up the dairy group. Make sure any dairy foods you eat are pasteurized (see the section "Food Safety" in this chapter for information about foodborne illnesses) and choose fat-free or low-fat (1%) varieties.

5. Protein Foods—Protein foods include meat, poultry, seafood, beans and peas, eggs, nuts, and seeds. Include a variety of proteins in your diet and choose lean or low-fat meat and poultry.

## Key Vitamins and Minerals

Vitamins and minerals play important roles in all parts of your body. During pregnancy, you need more *folic acid* and iron than a woman who is not pregnant (see Table 17-2). Taking a prenatal vitamin supplement can ensure that you are getting these extra amounts. A well-rounded diet should supply all of the other vitamins and minerals you need during pregnancy.

### Table 17-2  Key Vitamins and Minerals During Pregnancy

| Nutrient (Daily Recommended Amount) | Why You and Your Baby Need It | Best Sources |
|---|---|---|
| Calcium (1,300 mg for ages 14–18 years; 1,000 mg for ages 19–50 years) | Builds strong bones and teeth | Milk, cheese, yogurt, sardines, green leafy vegetables |
| Iron (27 mg) | Helps red blood cells deliver oxygen to your baby | Lean red meat, poultry, fish, dried beans and peas, iron-fortified cereals, prune juice |
| Vitamin A (750 micrograms for ages 14–18 years; 770 micrograms for ages 19–50 years) | Forms healthy skin and eyesight; helps with bone growth | Carrots, green leafy vegetables, sweet potatoes |
| Vitamin C (80 mg for ages 14–18 years; 85 mg for ages 19–50 years) | Promotes healthy gums, teeth, and bones | Citrus fruit, broccoli, tomatoes, strawberries |
| Vitamin D (600 international units) | Builds your baby's bones and teeth; helps promote healthy eyesight and skin | Sunlight, fortified milk, fatty fish such as salmon and sardines |
| Vitamin B$_6$ (1.9 mg) | Helps form red blood cells; helps body use protein, fat, and carbohydrates | Beef, liver, pork, ham, whole-grain cereals, bananas |
| Vitamin B$_{12}$ (2.6 micrograms) | Maintains nervous system; needed to form red blood cells | Meat, fish, poultry, milk (vegetarians should take a supplement) |
| Folic acid (600 micrograms) | Helps prevent birth defects of the brain and spine and supports the general growth and development of the fetus and placenta | Green leafy vegetables, orange juice, beans, fortified cereals, enriched bread and pasta, nuts |

## Folic Acid

Folic acid, also known as folate, is a B vitamin that is important for pregnant women. Taking 400 micrograms (0.4 mg) of folic acid daily for at least 1 month before pregnancy and during pregnancy may help prevent major **birth defects** of the baby's brain and spine called **neural tube defects**.

Current dietary guidelines recommend that pregnant women get at least 600 micrograms of folic acid each day from all sources, including food and vitamin supplements. Many foods contain folic acid, such as fortified cereal, enriched bread and pasta, peanuts, dark green leafy vegetables, orange juice, and beans. However, it may be hard to get all of the folic acid you need from food alone. To ensure they are getting enough, pregnant women should take a daily vitamin supplement that contains folic acid. Most prenatal multivitamin supplements contain 600–800 micrograms of folic acid.

Some women may need a higher amount of folic acid each day. If you have already had a pregnancy affected by a neural tube defect or if you are taking an antiseizure medication, talk with your health care provider to make sure you get the right amount.

## Iron

Iron is used by your body to make a substance in red blood **cells** that carries **oxygen** to your organs and tissues. During pregnancy, you need more iron than you did before pregnancy. This extra iron helps your body make more blood to supply oxygen to your baby. Not having enough iron is called iron-deficiency **anemia**. Anemia increases the risk of certain problems, including **preterm** delivery and having a low-birth-weight baby.

The recommended daily intake for iron during pregnancy is 27 mg, which is found in most prenatal vitamin supplements. You also can eat foods rich in a certain type of iron called heme iron. Heme iron is absorbed more easily by the body and is found in animal foods, such as red meat, poultry, and fish. Your blood will be tested during pregnancy to check for anemia. If you are found to be anemic, your health care provider may recommend additional iron supplements.

## Calcium

Calcium is used to build your baby's bones and teeth. All women aged 19 years and older should get 1,000 mg of calcium each day. For those aged 14–18 years, the recommended amount is 1,300 mg a day. Milk and other dairy products, such as cheese and yogurt, are the best sources of calcium. If you have trouble digesting milk products, you can get calcium from other sources, such as broccoli, fortified orange juice, sardines or anchovies with the bones, or a calcium supplement.

### Vitamin D

Vitamin D works with calcium to help build your baby's bones and teeth. It also is key for healthy skin and eyesight. While you're pregnant or breast-feeding, you need 600 international units of vitamin D each day. Most prenatal vitamins have about 400 international units of vitamin D per tablet.

You can get the extra amounts of vitamin D from your diet. Good sources are vitamin D–fortified milk and breakfast cereal, salmon, and egg yolks. Also, exposure to sunlight converts a chemical in the skin to vitamin D. Many women, however, still do not get enough vitamin D every day. If your health care provider thinks you may have low levels of vitamin D, a test can be done to check the level in your blood. If it is below normal, you may need to take a vitamin D supplement.

## Putting It All Together

All of this advice can seem overwhelming. The following tips can help guide you when you are making food choices and ensure that you're eating in a healthy way:

- Make one half of your plate fruits and vegetables.

- Switch to skim milk or 1% milk.

- Make one half of your grains whole grains.

- Vary your protein sources. Eat fish 2–3 times a week (see the section "Fish and Shellfish" later in this chapter for information about the types of fish to choose), and choose lean meats and poultry. Vegetarians can get protein from a wide variety of plant-based foods such as nuts, seeds, and soy products.

- Limit foods with "empty" calories. These are foods that have a lot of calories but little nutritional value, such as candy, chips, and sugary drinks.

- Take a vitamin supplement that contains 600 micrograms of folic acid and 27 mg of iron.

When planning your meals, remember to add snacks, which are a good way to get needed nutrition and extra calories. Pick snacks that have the right nutrients and that are low in fat and sugar. Fruit, cereal, and yogurt are healthy snack choices.

You may find it easier to eat six smaller meals spread out over the day than to try to consume your necessary nutrients and calories in three larger meals, especially later on in pregnancy when you may be experiencing indigestion after eating larger meals. To make these mini meals, just divide the daily recommended amount of foods from each of the food groups into small portions. Milk and half a sandwich made with meat, fish, peanut butter, or cheese with lettuce and tomato make an excellent mini meal. Other ideas are low-fat milk and fresh fruits, cheese and crackers, and soups.

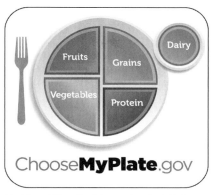

**My Plate.** What should your plate look like? Half of your plate should be fruits and vegetables. The other half should be lean protein and whole grains. You also should take a prenatal vitamin supplement containing folic acid and iron each day. Courtesy of United States Department of Agriculture Center for Nutrition Policy and Promotion.

## Weight Gain During Pregnancy

The amount of weight you should gain depends on your health and your BMI before pregnancy. Recommendations for weight gain for women who are pregnant with twins are somewhat higher (see Table 17-3).

Weight gain during pregnancy should be gradual. During your first 12 weeks of pregnancy—the first trimester—you may gain only 1–5 pounds or no weight at all. In your second and third trimesters, if you were a healthy weight before pregnancy, you should gain between ½ pound and 1 pound per week.

The key to gradual weight gain is to slowly increase the number of calories you consume throughout your pregnancy. In the first trimester, when weight gain is minimal, no extra calories usually are needed. In the second trimester, you need an extra 340 calories a day, and in the third trimester, about 450 extra calories a day. Keep in mind that these amounts are for women who were a normal weight before pregnancy. If you were overweight or obese, you may need fewer extra calories.

## Table 17-3 Weight Gain During Pregnancy

| Prepregnancy Body Mass Index | Recommended Total Weight Gain During Pregnancy With a Single Baby (in Pounds) | Rate of Weight Gain in the Second and Third Trimesters* (Pounds per Week) | Recommended Weight Gain During Pregnancy With Twins (in Pounds) |
|---|---|---|---|
| Underweight (BMI less than 18.5) | 28–40 | 1.0–1.3 | — |
| Normal weight (BMI 18.5–24.9) | 25–35 | 0.8–1.0 | 37–54 |
| Overweight (BMI 25–29.9) | 15–25 | 0.5–0.7 | 31–50 |
| Obese (BMI more than 30) | 11–20 | 0.4–0.6 | 25–42 |

Abbreviation: BMI, body mass index.

*Assumes a first-trimester weight gain between 1.1 pounds and 4.4 pounds.

Data from Institute of Medicine. Weight gain during pregnancy: reexamining the guidelines. Washington, DC: National Academies Press; 2009.

You will have your weight checked at each **prenatal care visit**, and your health care provider will keep track of how much weight you have gained. A woman who gains too few pounds is more likely to have a small baby (less than 5½ pounds). These babies often have health problems after birth. Women who gain too much weight also are at risk of health problems. These problems include **gestational diabetes mellitus**, **high blood pressure**, and a baby that's too large (**macrosomia**).

If you are overweight or gaining weight too quickly, it may be necessary to adjust your nutrition and exercise plan. Talk to your health care provider first before making any major changes. Usually, you can start by cutting down on the "extra" calories that you consume from extra fats and sugars. Watch your portion size, and avoid second helpings. Focus on eating foods that have lots of nutrients, such as beans, leafy greens, and nuts.

## Special Concerns

Certain foods, diets, or health conditions often cause some pregnant women to be concerned about their diets. Being aware of these concerns is important.

### Fish and Shellfish

Fish and shellfish are excellent sources of omega-3 fatty acids. Three of these fatty acids—DHA, EPA, and ALA—are considered "essential," meaning that they are not manufactured by the body and are supplied by diet alone. There is strong scientific evidence to suggest that these fats are important in the development of the fetal nervous system. Fish are also a good source of protein and other nutrients. To gain these benefits, women who are or who may become pregnant or who are breastfeeding should eat at least 8 ounces and up to 12 ounces (about two to three servings) of fish or shellfish per week.

Some types of fish have higher levels of a metal called mercury than others. Mercury has been linked to birth defects. To limit your exposure to mercury, follow a few simple rules. Choose fish that are lower in mercury, such as shrimp, salmon, catfish, canned light tuna (not albacore, which has a higher level of mercury), and sardines. Do not eat shark, swordfish, king mackerel, or tilefish, which have the highest levels of mercury. If you want to eat albacore tuna, limit the amount to 6 ounces a week. If you eat fish caught in local waters, check any advisories about mercury or other pollutants (see the "Resources" section in this chapter). If no information is available, limit your intake of such fish to 6 ounces a week, and do not eat any other fish that week.

## Caffeine

Although there have been many studies on whether caffeine increases the risk of *miscarriage*, the results are unclear. Most experts believe that consuming less than 200 mg of caffeine a day during pregnancy is safe. That is equal to one 12-ounce cup of coffee.

Remember that caffeine also is found in teas, colas, and chocolate. Make sure you count these sources in your total caffeine for the day.

## Vegetarian Diets

There are different types of vegetarians—some include dairy products in their diets and others strictly avoid all products that come from animals. If you are a vegetarian, it still is possible to get all of the nutrients you and your baby need during pregnancy. It just takes extra planning. It's a good idea to tell your health care provider at your first prenatal care visit that you are a vegetarian and ask for a recommended diet plan you can follow. The following tips can help you maximize the key nutrients you need while still eating a vegetarian diet:

- Make sure you get enough protein from foods such as soy milk, tofu, and beans. Eggs, milk, and cheese also are good protein sources if you eat some animal foods.

- Eat lots of iron-rich vegetables and legumes, such as spinach, white beans, kidney beans, and chickpeas. You can increase the amount of iron that your body absorbs if you also eat foods high in vitamin C, like oranges or tomatoes, at the same time that you eat an iron-rich food.

- To get the recommended amount of calcium if you don't eat dairy foods, eat dark leafy greens, calcium-enriched tofu, and other calcium-enriched products (soy milk, rice milk, and orange juice).

- Vitamin $B_{12}$ can be obtained by eating cereals that are fortified with this vitamin or by drinking milk.

### Lactose Intolerance

Women who have trouble digesting dairy products can get calcium from other foods, including seeds, nuts, and soy. Lactose-free milk, cheese, and other dairy products also are available in grocery stores. Talk with your health care provider if you are having trouble consuming the recommended 1,000 mg each day. You may be advised to take a calcium supplement.

### Celiac Disease

Women who have celiac disease are unable to eat foods containing gluten, which is found in wheat, barley, and rye. There are many foods that are gluten free, so pregnant women with celiac disease can choose fruits, vegetables, meats, potatoes, poultry, and beans. There also are many gluten-free products sold in grocery and natural food stores or online.

### Food Safety

Pregnant women can get food poisoning just like anyone else. However, food poisoning in a pregnant woman can cause serious problems for both her and her baby. Vomiting and diarrhea can cause your body to lose too much water and can disrupt your body's chemical balance. Several types of **bacteria** can cause food poisoning. It's important to contact your health care provider as soon as you have these signs and symptoms.

**Listeriosis** is a type of food-borne illness caused by bacteria. Pregnant women are 13 times more likely to get listeriosis than the general population. Listeriosis can cause mild, flu-like symptoms such as fever, muscle aches, and diarrhea, but it also may not cause any symptoms at all. However, it can lead to serious complications for your baby, including miscarriage, **stillbirth**, and premature delivery. If you think you have eaten food contaminated with this bacteria or if you have any of the symptoms of listeriosis, call your health care provider. ***Antibiotics*** can be given to treat the infection and protect your baby. To help prevent getting the bacteria, avoid eating the following foods while you're pregnant:

- Unpasteurized milk and foods made with unpasteurized milk, including soft cheeses such as feta, queso blanco, queso fresco, Camembert, Brie, or blue-veined cheeses unless the label says "made with pasteurized milk."

- Hot dogs, luncheon meats, and cold cuts unless they are heated until steaming hot just before serving.

- Refrigerated pâté and meat spreads

- Refrigerated smoked seafood

While you are pregnant, avoid all raw and undercooked seafood, eggs, and meat. Do not eat sushi made with raw fish (cooked sushi is safe). In addition, follow these four steps for food safety:

1. **Clean.**
   - Wash your hands with soap and water before and after handing raw food.
   - Wash fruits and vegetables under running tap water before eating, cutting, or cooking.
   - Keep your kitchen clean. Wash your utensils, countertops, and cutting boards with soap and hot water after handling and preparing uncooked foods. You can sanitize them by applying a solution of 1 teaspoon of liquid chlorine bleach per gallon of water. Allow the surface to air dry.

2. **Separate.**
   - Keep raw meat, poultry, eggs, and seafood and their juices away from ready-to-eat food.
   - Separate raw meat, poultry, and seafood from produce in your shopping cart by placing them into plastic bags.
   - Keep raw meat, poultry, and seafood on a plate, in a container, or in a sealed plastic bag in the refrigerator.
   - Use a separate cutting board for raw meat, poultry, and seafood.
   - Never put cooked food back on the same plate that previously held raw food unless the plate has been washed in hot, soapy water. Do not use sauce used to marinate raw food on cooked food unless it is boiled first.

3. **Cook.**

- Use a food thermometer to check doneness of meat, poultry, seafood, and egg products. These items should be cooked to a safe minimum temperature (see www.foodsafety.gov/keep/charts/mintemp.html).
- Place the food thermometer in the thickest part of the food, away from bone, fat, and gristle.

4. **Chill.**

- Keep your refrigerator at 40°F or below and the freezer at 0°F or below.
- Thaw food in the refrigerator, microwave, or in cold (not hot) water.
- Do not leave food at room temperature for more than 2 hours (1 hour when the temperature is above 90°F).
- Meat and poultry defrosted in the refrigerator may be refrozen before or after cooking. If thawed in the microwave or cold water, cook before refreezing.
- Only buy eggs from a refrigerator or refrigerated case. Store eggs in the refrigerator in their original carton and use within 3–5 weeks.
- When selecting precut produce, choose only those items that are refrigerated or surrounded by ice and keep them refrigerated at home to maintain both quality and safety.

Eating well during your pregnancy is one of the best things you can do for yourself and your baby. Start now on balancing healthy eating with maintaining a healthy weight to give your baby the best start in life.

---

# RESOURCES

To help you plan a healthy diet during pregnancy, check out the following resources:

**Choose Fish and Shellfish Wisely**
Environmental Protection Agency
www.epa.gov/choose-fish-and-shellfish-wisely/fish-and-shellfish-advisories-and-safe-eating-guidelines
*Information from the Environmental Protection Agency about safe fish consumption.*

**Food Don'ts**

The Office on Women's Health

www.womenshealth.gov/publications/our-publications/pregnancy_food_donts.pdf

*Short, easy-to-read guide about food safety during pregnancy.*

**Food Safety for Pregnant Women**

U.S. Food and Drug Administration

www.fda.gov/Food/FoodborneIllnessContaminants/PeopleAtRisk/ucm312704.htm

*Booklet that you can download that gives details about food safety specifically for pregnant women.*

**MyPlate**

U.S. Department of Agriculture

www.choosemyplate.gov/pregnancy-breastfeeding.html

*Site of the Department of Agriculture that can help you plan, analyze, and track your diet and exercise. Includes tools such as daily food plans, calorie burn chart, and BMI calculator for people of all ages.*

**Nutrition During Pregnancy**

The American College of Obstetricians and Gynecologists (ACOG)

www.acog.org/Patients/FAQs/Nutrition-During-Pregnancy

*Answers to frequently asked questions about healthy eating during pregnancy.*

**Special Supplemental Nutrition Program for Women, Infants, and Children (WIC)**

www.fns.usda.gov/wic/women-infants-and-children-wic

*The WIC program provides nutritional help for low-income women and children.*

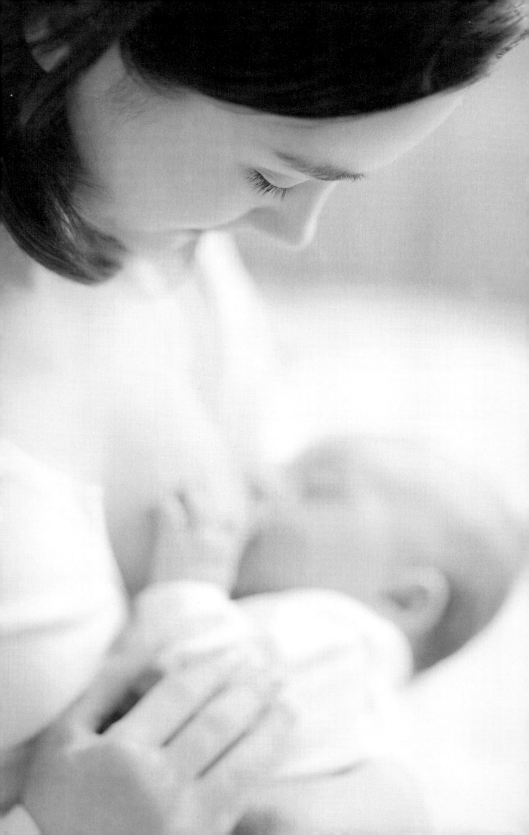

Chapter 18

# Breastfeeding and Formula-Feeding Your Baby

Deciding how to feed your baby is an important decision all parents-to-be must make. The purpose of this chapter is to give you the information that you need in order to make the decision that is right for you, your baby, and your family.

Breastfeeding—feeding an infant from your breast—is the recommended way to feed your baby. Expressing breast milk and feeding it to your baby with a bottle is another option that provides important health benefits for mother and child. Some women cannot or choose not to breastfeed their babies and feed their babies formula.

If you are having a difficult time deciding which method is best for you, it may help to talk to your or your baby's health care provider and to educate yourself about each of the options (see the "Resources" section in this chapter). Remember, though, that the decision is a personal one. Feeding your baby should be an enjoyable and comfortable experience for both of you. Whichever option you choose, you should receive support and guidance from your health care provider, your partner, and your family.

## The Benefits of Breastfeeding

More and more women are choosing to breastfeed their babies, and for good reason. Breast milk provides the perfect mix of vitamins, protein, and fat that your baby needs to grow. It also protects your baby against certain diseases. Some of the benefits that breastfeeding has for babies include the following:

- Human milk is the most complete form of nutrition for infants. It has the right amount of fat, sugar, water, and protein that is needed for a baby's growth and development. And as your baby grows, your breast milk changes to adapt to the baby's changing nutritional needs.

- Human milk is easier than formula for babies to digest. Infants who are breastfed have less gas, fewer feeding problems, and often less constipation than those given formula.

- Human milk contains **antibodies** that protect infants from infections. Studies show that breastfed infants have a reduced risk of digestive tract infections and ear infections. Infants who are breastfed also tend to get sick less often and recover from certain illnesses more quickly than infants who are not breastfed.

- Breastfed infants have a lower risk of **sudden infant death syndrome**. Any amount of breastfeeding appears to help lower this risk.

- For premature babies, mother's milk can be especially beneficial. **Preterm** infants fed human milk are less likely to develop some of the health problems of being born too early. It also has been shown to improve preterm babies' development of thinking and reasoning skills in the long term.

Breastfeeding also may contribute to a child's future health by reducing the risk of **obesity**, type 2 **diabetes mellitus**, and heart disease. However, the research on these benefits is less clear. Some of the benefits attributed to breastfeeding also may be related to the fact that children in general are born healthier than in generations past.

Breastfeeding also has benefits for you—the breastfeeding mom—as well:

- Breastfeeding burns **calories**, which may make it easier to lose the weight you gained during pregnancy. This may explain why mothers who breastfeed longer have lower rates of type 2 diabetes, **high blood pressure**, and heart disease.

- Breastfeeding stimulates the release of **oxytocin**, a hormone that makes the uterus contract. This helps the uterus return to its original size and decreases the amount of bleeding you may have after giving birth.

- Breastfeeding may reduce the risk of certain types of cancer. There is some research that shows an association between breastfeeding and reduced risk of breast cancer. Breastfeeding also may result in a small reduced risk of ovarian cancer. However, more research needs to be done to clarify these associations.

- Breastfeeding delays the return of normal *ovulation* and menstrual cycles and can prevent pregnancy in the first 6 months after delivery. This birth control method, called the *lactational amenorrhea method (LAM)*, can provide greater than 98% protection from pregnancy when breastfeeding rules are followed. See Chapter 16, "The Postpartum Period," for a detailed discussion of LAM. If you're not certain about the extent to which you're going to breastfeed, it's a good idea to talk with your health care provider about other birth control options that are compatible with breastfeeding.

## Who Should Not Breastfeed

As good as breastfeeding is, it is not the best choice for every woman. There are some situations in which a woman should not breastfeed:

- Infections—Certain infections can be passed to your baby through breast-feeding. However, not all infections prevent you from breastfeeding—only some (see box "You Can Still Breastfeed If You Have . . ."). Mothers with *human immunodeficiency virus (HIV)* should not breastfeed. Moms with

### You Can Still Breastfeed If You Have . . .

- *Hepatitis B* infection (a positive test result for hepatitis B surface *antigen*) provided that your baby gets the hepatitis B vaccine and *hepatitis B immune globulin* within the first few hours after birth.
- Hepatitis C infection (a positive test result for *hepatitis C virus* antibody or hepatitis C virus-RNA)
- Herpes simplex virus infection (cold sores or *genital herpes*) as long as the breast or nipple is not affected and any active sores are covered
- *Chorioamnionitis* before delivery or *endometritis* after delivery
- *Cytomegalovirus (CMV)* infection (a positive blood test result for CMV, not recent conversion; however, if the baby is preterm, talk with your health care provider)
- *Mastitis* (breast infection)

certain other infections may need to be separated from their babies or express and discard their milk until there's no longer a risk of infecting the baby. These infections include active *tuberculosis*, *chickenpox* contracted within 5 days before delivery through 2 days after delivery, or a herpes outbreak that affects the breast. If you have tuberculosis that is being treated and you are no longer contagious, you can breastfeed your baby. If you have a herpes outbreak affecting the breast, you can breastfeed once the sores heal. It's OK to breastfeed at any time if you have genital herpes or a herpes sore anywhere else. You should wash your hands with soap and water thoroughly before and after breastfeeding and keep any active sores that could come into contact with the baby covered while you are breastfeeding. If you have chickenpox, you can express your milk and give it to your baby and resume breastfeeding when you are well.

- Substance abuse—If you are abusing illegal substances, seek professional help. Until you are able to stop using these substances, formula-feeding is best for your baby.

- Certain medications—Most medications are safe for use if you are breastfeeding. If there is concern about a medication that you are taking, you often may be able to switch to a drug that is considered to be safer. See the discussion about taking medications later in this chapter.

## Deciding to Breastfeed

If you've decided to breastfeed, it is a good idea to find information and resources while you are still pregnant. Many hospitals and parents' centers offer breastfeeding classes taught by international board-certified lactation consultants (IBCLCs). These consultants can teach you what you need to know to get started. IBCLCs also can help you navigate some common problems many mothers face when they first start to breastfeed. You can find an IBCLC near you through the International Lactation Consultant Association web site (see the "Resources" section in this chapter). You also may want to check out whether your hospital has been designated as "Baby Friendly" (see box "Is Your Hospital Baby Friendly?").

If you aren't able to take a class, there is plenty of information available on the Internet or just a phone call away. La Leche League International and Best for Babes are two organizations that provide support and education to mothers who wish to breastfeed and can answer any of your questions and concerns (see the "Resources" section in this chapter).

## Is Your Hospital Baby Friendly?

Did you know that hospital routines—such as whether your baby stays in your room and how often babies are fed—can affect breastfeeding rates? In 1991, a team of global experts working with the World Health Organization came up with 10 steps that hospitals can take to help moms and babies get off to a good start with breastfeeding. Hospitals that adopt all 10 steps and that have been assessed by the Baby-Friendly Hospital Initiative are certified as Baby Friendly. The "Ten Steps to Successful Breastfeeding" are as follows:

1. Have a written breastfeeding policy that is routinely communicated to all health care staff.

2. Train all health care staff in the skills necessary to implement this policy.

3. Inform all pregnant women about the benefits and management of breastfeeding.

4. Help mothers initiate breastfeeding within 1 hour of birth.

5. Show mothers how to breastfeed and how to maintain lactation, even if they are separated from their infants.

6. Give infants no food or drinks other than breast milk, unless medically indicated.

7. Practice rooming in—allow mothers and infants to remain together 24 hours a day.

8. Encourage breastfeeding on demand.

9. Give no pacifiers or artificial nipples to breastfeeding infants.

10. Foster the establishment of breastfeeding support groups and refer mothers to them on discharge from the hospital or birth center.

You can find out whether your hospital is certified as Baby Friendly by going to www.babyfriendlyusa.org/find-facilities. If your hospital is not certified, it does not mean that it does not support breastfeeding; it may just mean that your hospital has not met all of the criteria for certification but still has breastfeeding-friendly policies in place. You can contact your hospital directly to ask about their breast-feeding policies and whether they are pursuing Baby-Friendly certification.

### After the Baby Is Born

Most healthy newborns are ready to breastfeed within the first hour after birth. Those who are breastfed soon after birth may have an easier time breastfeeding than babies who are not. To help give you and the baby a good start, tell your health care provider during pregnancy that you want to breastfeed. When you are admitted to the hospital in labor, remind your health care team that you plan to breastfeed.

Holding your baby directly against your bare skin immediately after the birth helps encourage your baby to start breastfeeding. Maintaining skin-to-skin contact also helps stabilize the baby's body temperature, heart rate, breathing, and **glucose** levels. Babies who have skin-to-skin contact seek out your breast and can latch on themselves. Skin-to-skin contact may be possible after a **cesarean delivery**. Ask your health provider whether this is an option at your hospital.

During the first few days after birth, your breasts initially produce **colostrum**, a thick, yellowish fluid. Colostrum is the same fluid that leaks from some women's breasts during pregnancy. The colostrum that your breasts produce for the first few days after birth helps your newborn's digestive system grow and mature. It is rich in protein and is all your baby needs for the first few days of life. It is especially high in antibodies that help make your baby **immune** to diseases.

About 40–72 hours after birth, your breasts begin to make a larger amount of milk. You may hear this referred to as your milk "coming in." You will probably notice a change in the size of your breasts 2–5 days after childbirth.

Milk is made continuously in the breast and stored in the breast tissues. When your baby starts to breastfeed, the nerves in your nipples send a message to your brain. In response, your brain releases hormones that signal the milk lobules to contract (squeeze) and expel milk so that it flows through your nipples. This is called the let-down reflex. Some women barely notice let-down. Others have a pins-and-needles feeling or even sharp pain in their breasts 2–3 minutes after their babies start nursing. For most women, pain during let-down gradually eases as their bodies adjust to breastfeeding.

Let-down also can be triggered simply by looking at your baby, thinking about your baby, or hearing your baby cry. Hearing any baby cry will trigger the let-down reflex in some women.

When your baby starts feeding from your breast, the milk that is released first is thin, watery, and sweet. It quenches the baby's thirst and provides sugar, proteins, minerals, and fluid the baby needs. Once the baby gets this "foremilk," the milk then becomes thick and creamy. This milk will satisfy

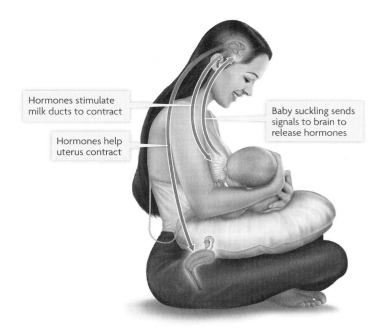

Hormones stimulate milk ducts to contract

Hormones help uterus contract

Baby suckling sends signals to brain to release hormones

**The "let-down" reflex.** The baby's mouth on the mother's nipple signals the brain to release hormones. These hormones cause the milk ducts to contract and expel milk and stimulate the uterus to contract.

hunger and give your baby the **nutrients** he or she needs to grow. The more milk your baby removes from your breast, the more milk you will produce, so your milk production will keep up with the baby's demand. If your baby needs more milk—during a growth spurt, for example—the baby's increased suckling leads to increased emptying of your breast, which in turn stimulates increased milk production. If you give the baby other foods, milk production is reduced proportionately.

### Get the Baby Latched On

To begin breastfeeding, the baby needs to attach to or "latch on" to your breast. A nurse or lactation specialist can help you find a good position (see box "Good Breastfeeding Positions"). Cup your breast in your hand and stroke your baby's lower lip with your nipple. This stimulates the baby's rooting reflex. The rooting reflex is a baby's natural instinct to turn toward the nipple, open his or her mouth, and suck. The baby will open his or her mouth wide (like a yawn). Pull the baby close to you, aiming the nipple toward the roof of the baby's mouth. Remember to bring your baby to your breast—not your breast to your baby.

## Good Breastfeeding Positions

Finding a good position will help the baby latch on. It also will help you relax and be comfortable. Use pillows or folded blankets to help support the baby.

- *Cradle Hold*—Sit up as straight as you can and cradle your baby in the crook of your arm. The baby's body should be turned toward you and his or her belly should be against yours. Support the baby's head in the bend of your elbow so that he or she is facing your breast.

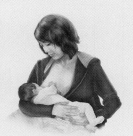

- *Cross-Cradle Hold*—As in the cradle hold, nuzzle your baby's belly against yours. Hold the baby in the arm opposite the one you are using to nurse. For instance, if the baby is nursing from your right breast, hold him or her with your left arm. Place the baby's bottom in the crook of your left arm and support the baby's head and neck with your left hand. This position gives you more control of the baby's head. It's a good position for a newborn who is having trouble nursing.

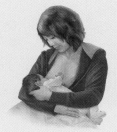

- *Football Hold*—Tuck your baby under your arm like a football. Hold the baby at your side, level with your waist, so he or she is facing you. Support the baby's back with your upper arm and hold his or her head level with your breast.

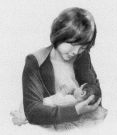

- *Side-Lying Position*—Lie on your side and nestle your baby next to you. Place your fingers beneath your breast and lift it up to help your baby reach your nipple. Rest your head on your lower arm. You may want to tuck a pillow behind your back to help hold yourself up. This position is good for night feedings. It's also good for women who had a cesarean delivery because it keeps the baby's weight off your abdomen and incision.

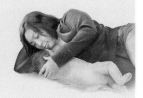

Another way to get the baby to latch on is to use a technique called "baby-led latch." Babies are born with a set of reflexes that help guide them to the breast to latch. The baby-led latch technique helps babies tap into these reflexes. To initiate the baby-led latch, lie back on a bed or couch with your back and shoulders supported. Place your baby belly-down onto your chest, with the baby's cheek close to your bare breast. Over a few minutes, your baby will explore your breast, find the nipple, and latch.

## Check the Baby's Technique

The baby should have all of your nipple and a good deal of the areola in his or her mouth. The baby's nose will be touching your breast. The baby's lips also will be curled out on your breast. The baby's sucking should be smooth and even. You should hear the baby swallow. You may feel a slight tugging. You may feel a little discomfort for the first few days. If you feel severe pain, talk to your health care provider or an IBCLC.

If you feel discomfort or notice that your baby's mouth is not wide open, gently break the suction by inserting a clean finger between your breast and your baby's gums. When you hear or feel a soft pop, pull your nipple out of the baby's mouth.

## Watch Your Baby, Not the Clock

Let your baby set his or her own nursing pattern. In the first few weeks, it's normal for babies to feed 10–12 times a day. Newborns usually nurse for at least 10–15 minutes on each breast. They also can nurse for much longer periods, sometimes 60–120 minutes at a time. These long breastfeeding sessions, called cluster feeds, may occur during a growth spurt and happen most often towards the end of the day.

Some babies feed from one breast per feeding, while others feed from both breasts. When your baby releases one breast, offer the other. If he or she is not interested, plan to start on the other side for the next feeding. You may want to put a safety pin on your bra strap to mark the side your baby nursed from last. At the next feeding, offer the other breast first.

## Nurse on Demand

When babies are hungry, they will nuzzle against your breast, suck on their hands, or flex their fingers and arms. Crying usually is a late sign of hunger. When babies are full, they relax their arms and legs and close their eyes.

The baby's stomach is very small at first—it holds only a little more than half an ounce at birth. Also, human milk is emptied from a baby's stomach faster than formula. For these reasons, you will typically breastfeed at least 8–12 times in 24 hours, or at least every 2–3 hours (timed from the start time of one feeding to the start time of the next feeding) during the first weeks of your baby's life. If it has been more than 4 hours since the last feeding, you may need to wake your infant up to feed him or her. Some newborns are happy to go 3 hours between feedings. Others need to nurse once an hour for the first few weeks. Over time, you and your baby will set your own schedule.

### Give a Vitamin D Supplement

Whether you feed your baby human milk or formula, it is recommended that all babies get 400 international units of vitamin D a day to ensure strong, healthy bone growth. Vitamin D is available in liquid form that you give your baby with a dropper. Starting at about 4 months of age, babies who get more than half of their nutritional needs from human milk should be given a supplement containing 1 mg of iron each day.

## Breastfeeding Challenges

Some new mothers breastfeed without any problems. For others, breastfeeding can be a challenge. It's perfectly normal for problems to arise at first, especially if it is your first time breastfeeding. Many problems can be overcome with help and support. If you need help, don't hesitate to call your health care provider or consult an IBCLC.

### Sore Nipples

Many women experience nipple tenderness or pain in the first few weeks of breastfeeding. As you continue to breastfeed, the initial tenderness usually goes away. If it does not, there are things that you can try to be more comfortable.

The first thing to try is to make sure that your baby is latched on well. Poor latch-on and positioning are the major causes of sore nipples because the baby is probably not getting enough of the areola into his or her mouth and is sucking mostly on the nipple. Check the positioning of your baby's body and the way he or she latches on and sucks. To minimize soreness, make sure that your baby's mouth is open wide, with as much of the areola in his or her mouth as possible. If it hurts, break the baby's suction with your finger and try again. You may find that it feels better right away once the baby is positioned correctly. After breastfeeding, you can apply a little expressed milk to your nipple, which may provide better relief of nipple pain than any type of ointment or cream. If the pain is severe, see a health care provider with expertise in breastfeeding or an IBCLC.

Some women describe shooting, burning pain that radiates from the nipple out to the rest of the breast after feeding their babies. It is thought that this pain is due to spasms of the blood vessels in the breast (vasospasm). Some women report this type of pain when they are exposed to cold temperatures (like the frozen food section of a grocery store or when stepping out of a warm shower). A heating paid or warm gel pack applied after breastfeeding may be helpful. See your health care provider if the pain continues for more than a few days.

## Engorgement

Engorgement can occur when your milk comes in a few days after delivery. Engorged breasts feel full and tender. You even may run a low fever. If the fever exceeds 101°F or if you are in severe pain, call your health care provider. If your breasts are very engorged, it can be hard for your baby to latch on. Once your body figures out how much milk your baby needs, the problem should go away. This often takes a week or so. The following things can help relieve engorgement:

- Feed the baby more often to help drain your breasts.

- Express a little milk with a pump or by hand to soften your breasts before nursing.

- To help your milk flow, massage your breasts, take warm showers, or apply warm packs to your breasts before feedings.

- After feedings, apply cold packs to your breasts to relieve discomfort and reduce swelling.

If you still are not able to express milk or the baby is unable to latch on after trying these measures, contact your health care provider or an IBCLC for assistance.

## Delayed Milk Production

A woman's milk usually "comes in" within 72 hours of birth. For some women, milk production can be delayed. If it takes more than 3 days for milk to be produced, this condition is called "delayed lactogenesis." It's not known what causes this condition, but it can be related to hormonal factors, a long or difficult labor, breast injury or other abnormalities, or medications. Whatever the cause, delayed lactogenesis can be distressing. Hungry babies aren't shy about expressing their feelings. And the more stressed and anxious you become, the more it can affect the natural let-down reflex. Delayed milk production is probably one of the number one reasons why women stop trying to breastfeed exclusively.

If milk production is delayed, work with a health care provider with expertise in breastfeeding or an IBCLC. Increasing the number of breastfeeding sessions and using a breast pump to express milk after breastfeeding can be helpful. In some situations, if a baby has lost more than 8–10% of his or her birth weight, small supplemental feedings with expressed breast milk, donor milk, or formula may be recommended. An IBCLC can help you to give these supplements with a feeding syringe at the breast, so that the baby continues to stimulate milk-making hormones during feeding.

### Low Milk Supply

Some women have difficulty making enough milk to meet their baby's needs. The most common cause of low milk supply is not removing milk often enough. Healthy newborns feed 10–12 times a day, and for some women, less frequent feeding or pumping sends a signal to the breast to make less milk. Another cause of low milk supply is preterm birth. If the baby is born early, he or she may tire easily and not remove enough milk to stimulate milk production. To sort out these possibilities, work with a health care provider with breastfeeding expertise or an IBCLC.

Even with frequent feedings and skilled support, some women are not able to make enough milk to feed their babies only breast milk. It is not true that "every mother can breastfeed." The fact is that breastfeeding, like any other body function, may not work for some women because of various medical conditions. If supplements are needed, know that you still can nurture your baby at the breast, regardless of how much milk is transferred.

### Inverted or Flat Nipples

It is common for one or both nipples not to protrude fully. In most cases, women with flat or inverted nipples can breastfeed.

Flat or inverted nipples are most likely to present problems during the first feedings after birth, when the baby is learning to latch on. It may be hard for the baby to latch on at first, but breastfeeding will be easier as the baby grows bigger and stronger. Nipple shields can be helpful for flat nipples. A nipple shield is a nipple-shaped piece of plastic with holes in the end that can be placed over your nipple. The baby latches directly onto the nipple shield and your nipple will be sucked into the shield while the baby nurses. After using the shield for a period of time, your nipple may begin to protrude better and the baby can latch directly onto your nipple. Talk with an IBCLC or a health care provider with breastfeeding expertise about whether a nipple shield might be helpful. They can show you and your baby how to latch with a shield in place, and they can work with you to wean your baby from the shield as he or she gets used to breastfeeding. Using a manual or electric breast pump just before feeding also may be helpful in getting flat nipples to protrude. If you have any concerns about the shape of your nipples, be sure to ask your health care provider or a lactation specialist.

## Blocked Ducts

If a duct gets clogged with unused milk, a hard, tender knot will form in your breast. Call your health care provider if the knot doesn't go away within a few days or if you run a fever. In the meantime, try these tips:

- Take a warm shower or apply a warm pack to the lump before nursing.

- Offer the breast with the blocked duct first.

- Let your baby nurse long and often on the breast that is blocked.

- Massage the lump while your baby nurses to help the milk drain.

- If there's any milk left in your breast after a feeding, pump it out or hand-express it.

## Mastitis

If a blocked duct doesn't drain, it may become inflamed and a breast infection—called mastitis—can result. If you have this condition, you may have flu-like symptoms, such as fever, aches, and fatigue. Your breasts also will be swollen, painful, feel hot to the touch, and may be streaked with red.

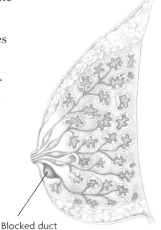

Blocked duct

**Blocked duct.** This condition occurs when a duct becomes clogged with milk.

If you think you have mastitis, call your health care provider right away. He or she will prescribe an **antibiotic** to treat the infection that's safe to take while breastfeeding. You should feel better within a day or two of starting treatment, but keep taking the treatment for the full prescription.

Until then, do the same things you'd do to treat a blocked duct. Get plenty of rest and drink lots of fluids. Your health care provider may suggest taking ibuprofen to ease your discomfort. In the meantime, make sure to continue breastfeeding—your baby will help drain your breast and unclog the blocked area. The baby won't get sick from the infection. If you do not empty the infected breast, the clogged duct will become more inflamed, your milk supply will go down, and recovery will take longer.

## Common Questions About Breastfeeding

The following are some of the most common questions asked about breastfeeding:

### How long should I breastfeed my baby?

The American College of Obstetricians and Gynecologists recommends exclusive breastfeeding for the first 6 months of the baby's life and continuing as new foods are introduced up to the baby's first birthday or beyond if both mother and baby are willing. According to the Centers for Disease Control and Prevention (CDC), about 79% of new mothers start breastfeeding their babies, and 49% still are breastfeeding when the baby is 6 months of age.

Any amount of breastfeeding is good for you and your baby, and the longer you stick with it, the better off you and your baby will be. Start out with short-term goals, like breastfeeding for the next week, and see how it goes. Check in with yourself each time you reach a goal, and think about how the benefits of breastfeeding balance with challenges you might be experiencing. You're the one person who knows whether continuing to breastfeed is best for you and your baby.

When you want to stop breastfeeding or pumping, there are a few ways to do it. Some moms and babies gradually reduce feedings as the baby eats more food and starts drinking from a cup. This can be a long process. It's a gradual change for both of you.

Other women decide to wean their baby when he or she reaches a certain age. In this case, it's still best to take it slow. A sudden stop in breastfeeding or pumping can cause you physical pain or mastitis as your breasts fill with unused milk. It also can be hard for your baby.

One approach is to replace one nursing session with a bottle or cup feeding every few days. Start by cutting out the feedings your baby seems to enjoy the least. Slowly work your way up to the more important ones. Most often, the feeding before bedtime is the last to go and the hardest to give up. As you reduce the amount you nurse, your milk supply will decrease slowly.

## What is "exclusive" breastfeeding?

**Exclusive breastfeeding** means that human milk is the only food provided to the baby. Medicines and vitamin supplements can be given, but no other food, water, juice, or other substances are given. Exclusively fed babies also include those who are fed only expressed human milk from you or from a donor. Exclusive breastfeeding is recommended for the first 6 months of a baby's life.

## Is my baby getting enough milk?

When an infant is fed with a bottle, you can see how much he or she is eating by looking at the side of the bottle. Breasts don't have ounces marked on the sides, but babies are smart, and they use cues to tell their caregivers when they are satisfied:

- Your baby tells you. Babies use cues to communicate their needs, and a full baby's arms are typically relaxed, with palms outstretched, and the baby is drowsy and content. When the baby is ready to eat again, arms will be flexed with hands in a fist, and the baby will try to suck on his or her fingers. Watch for these early feeding cues, not the clock, to know when to offer the breast.

- Your baby nurses often. Healthy newborns nurse at least 8–12 times in 24 hours. As babies grow, their stomachs are able to hold more at each feeding, and they will need to nurse less often. Even so, healthy newborns don't go more than about 3–4 hours without nursing, even at night. Each nursing session should last 10–45 minutes. Newborn feeding schedules can be unpredictable. Babies may eat for a brief time and then want to eat again a short time later. Sometimes, a newborn may eat for an extended period of time (1–2 hours) and then fall into a deep sleep.

- Your breasts soften with feedings. Your breasts are never really empty; they are always making milk. However, your breasts may feel more full and firm before feedings. Afterwards, they may feel softer. As your baby gets older, these changes may be less noticeable.

- The baby goes through lots of diapers. Once your breasts transition from colostrum to mature milk, your baby should soak at least six diapers per day. The baby's urine should be light in color rather than dark yellow. During the first month of life, your baby should have at least three bowel movements per day. In fact, most breastfed newborns pass a stool after each feeding. The stool should be soft and yellow.

- Your baby is gaining weight. All newborns lose a little weight in the first few days of life—a loss of up to 7% of birth weight is normal. For example, a healthy 8-pound baby might lose up to 9 ounces in the first few days of life. After 10 days, your baby should be back up to his or her weight at birth. The baby's health care provider will weigh your baby at each visit and keep track of his or her weight. If you are worried that your baby isn't getting enough milk, tell your health care provider.

## What should I eat and how much?

When you are pregnant, your body stores extra nutrients and fat to prepare for breastfeeding. Even so, once your baby is born, you need more food and nutrients than normal to fuel milk production. While you are breastfeeding, your body uses an additional 500–600 calories per day. You'll also need to drink lots of liquids during the day because breastfeeding uses up lots of fluid. You need at least eight glasses of liquid per day. If you get dehydrated, it can affect your milk supply.

Breastfeeding moms need 1,000 mg of calcium per day. You can get this amount by eating plenty of dairy products like milk, yogurt, and cheese. If you can't digest milk products, ask your health care provider about taking a calcium supplement. Be sure to get at least 400 micrograms (0.4 mg) of *folic acid* each day, too. This will help you maintain good health and ensure that you have plenty of folic acid stores. Your health care provider may suggest that you keep taking a daily prenatal vitamin supplement until your baby is weaned.

Fish and shellfish are great sources of protein and provide beneficial vitamins and minerals for you and your baby. While you're breastfeeding, try to eat fish at least 2–3 times a week (about 8–12 ounces total). It's recommended that you continue to follow the same fish consumption guidelines that you did during pregnancy (see Chapter 17, "Nutrition During Pregnancy") to avoid eating fish containing high levels of mercury.

Some nursing infants are sensitive to certain foods in their mothers' diets. About 1 in 100 exclusively breastfed babies develop eczema and blood in their stools due to an allergy to something in the mom's diet. If your baby has blood in his or her stools, let his or her health care provider know. This can signal a food allergy. In about one half of cases, the cause is milk protein from foods made from cow's milk (cheese, yogurt). In other cases, babies are sensitive to peanuts, soy, wheat, eggs, and corn. Work with your baby's health care provider to try eliminating one food at a time from your diet for about 2 weeks and see if your baby seems better. You also may want to keep a food diary to help spot links between what you eat and how your baby reacts.

### Now that I'm no longer pregnant, is it OK for me to smoke cigarettes and drink alcohol again?

It's important to keep in mind that when you breastfeed, what you put into your body can still go to your baby, just like when you were pregnant. If you smoke, pregnancy and breastfeeding are very good motivators to help you quit successfully. Quitting smoking is the best thing you can do for your health and your baby's health; however, it's better for your baby to breastfeed than to formula feed, even if you continue to smoke.

Whether it's OK to drink alcohol and breastfeed depends on how much and when you drink. Alcohol enters breast milk, but it leaves the breast at the same time that it is cleared from your body. That means you do not need to express and discard breast milk after having a drink—you just need to wait about 2 hours per serving for the alcohol to leave your body. If you drink alcohol heavily (more than two drinks per day on a regular basis), however, research shows it can harm your baby, including causing drowsiness, weakness, and abnormal weight gain.

### Can I give my baby a pacifier?

In the first few weeks, it's ideal for babies to suckle at the breast for comfort rather than use a pacifier. Suckling at the breast stimulates milk-making hormones and helps to establish a milk supply, while sucking a pacifier does not help moms make milk. That's why some experts recommend that until your baby gets the hang of breastfeeding, pacifier use should be limited to only a few instances. You may only want to give a pacifier to help with pain relief (while getting a shot, for instance). Allowing your baby to suck on your clean pinky finger also can help with pain relief. However, some women find that a pacifier can be helpful in soothing a fussy baby. If your nipples are sore or cracked, a pacifier can help comfort your baby while your nipples heal.

### *I'm expecting twins. Can I breastfeed them?*

Twins and even triplets can be breastfed successfully, often without the need for supplementation. It does take more time to breastfeed multiples, and you will need to take in extra calories—for each baby, your body will use an extra 500–600 calories per day. You also will have to decide whether to feed the babies simultaneously or separately (see box "Positions for Breastfeeding Twins"). If you choose to feed them separately, you'll also need to decide whether you will feed both on demand or one on demand and the other one immediately afterward. However, it's best to start out breastfeeding each baby individually. Multiples do not necessarily have the same sucking abilities, and feeding them one at a time at first can be less stressful (and less tiring) for you.

As breastfeeding is established, you can adapt your breastfeeding schedule to your and your babies' needs. Some moms breastfeed exclusively, while others use a combination of breastfeeding and formula-feeding. Expressing milk into bottles allows your partner and others to help out with feeding duties.

### *I've had breast surgery. Can I still breastfeed?*

Surgery to remove cysts and other benign breast lumps rarely causes problems with future breastfeeding. If you have had surgery on your breasts, talk to your health care provider or surgeon before your delivery date to help plan for breastfeeding. Make sure to tell your baby's health care provider as well so that your baby's weight gain can be monitored in the first few weeks of life.

Many women who have had their breasts enlarged are able to nurse their babies, especially if the implant is placed behind the chest muscles. If the implant is very large, however, it can limit the amount of milk that the mother can store. A large implant also can restrict blood flow in the breast and decrease the amount of milk that can be produced. If there was very little breast tissue before the implants were in place, it may not be possible for a woman to make enough milk to meet all of her baby's needs.

Women who have had surgery to reduce the size of their breasts and whose nipples have been repositioned may have breastfeeding problems. Breast-reduction surgery can cut into milk ducts and prevent a nursing mother from making enough milk. It also can limit milk storage capacity. If you have had this surgery, you may want to talk with your surgeon about what type of surgery was done and whether your nipples, areolas, and ducts were left intact. Many mothers enjoy nursing their babies, even if they aren't able to make 100% of the milk that their babies need.

## Positions for Breastfeeding Twins

- *Football or double-clutch hold*—Hold one baby under each arm, elbows bent, like you are holding two footballs. Hold the babies at your sides, level with your waist, so they are facing you. Support the babies' backs with your upper arms and hold their heads level with your breasts. Or, use a pillow or other support device on your lap to support the babies' backs and heads. This hold is good for newborns and for moms who have had a cesarean delivery.

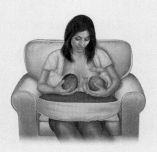

- *Parallel or "spoons" hold*—One baby is held in a cradle hold (head cradled in the crook of your arm). The second baby lies parallel to the first baby. The babies both face in the same direction on the same side. Pillows are helpful for this hold.

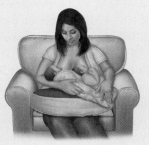

- *Criss-cross or double-cradle hold*—Sit up as straight as you can and cradle each baby in the crook of each arm. The babies' bodies should be turned toward you and their bellies should be against yours. The babies' legs should be criss-crossed in front of you. Support the babies' heads in the bends of your elbows so that they are facing your breasts.

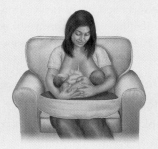

- *Front V-Hold*—This position is useful when the babies are able to sit up and their heads don't require as much support. In this hold, you sit on a chair with the babies kneeling or sitting on your lap. Each baby faces you while you support their upper bodies in the bends of your elbows. The babies do not recline, so their legs do not criss-cross in front of you.

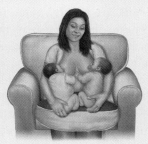

### I've heard about human milk banks. What are they?

Human milk banks collect donated milk from nursing mothers and make it available to premature and critically ill babies in hospitals across the country. Some hospitals also provide donor milk for healthy newborns that need a little extra milk in the first few days of life. The Human Milk Banking Association of North America (HMBANA) is a voluntary association that issues guidelines about screening milk donors and collecting, processing, handling, testing, and storing the milk.

Milk for these milk banks is donated by breastfeeding mothers who have an abundant milk supply. Donors who are part of the HMBANA are asked detailed questions about their past and current diseases, use of drugs and medications, and other factors that may affect the quality or safety of their milk. They also are tested for certain infectious diseases and for illegal drug use. These tests are repeated periodically. The milk is tested and pasteurized by the milk bank. Once a mother becomes a donor, she sends frozen milk to the local human milk bank to help babies in need. If you're interested in donating milk or using human milk from a bank, your health care provider or lactation specialist may be able to give you information about banks in your area.

You should only use human milk from a source such as a milk bank that has screened its donors and taken other precautions to ensure safety. Some women have set up informal networks to share breast milk. These networks are not regulated. For this reason, use of these networks is not recommended.

### What do I need to know about taking medications while breastfeeding?

Most drugs are safe to take while you are breastfeeding. Although medications taken by a breastfeeding mom can pass into her breast milk, levels in the milk are usually much lower than levels in the mom's bloodstream. Exceptions include cancer medications and radioactive drugs. The latest information about medications and their effects on breastfed babies can be found at LactMed, a database of scientific information that is updated frequently and can be downloaded as a free app on your smart phone (see the "Resources" section in this chapter).

If you need to take a prescription medication to manage a health condition and want to breastfeed, discuss this with your health care provider and with the baby's health care provider. Your health care provider can help determine whether you still need to take the drug and, if so, whether a safer drug is available. Sometimes, the amount of the drug that reaches a breastfeeding infant can be reduced if a woman takes her medication after feedings. If a woman needs to take a medication that is known to pose a risk to a breastfeeding infant, the baby should be monitored for any unusual health effects. Your baby's health care provider may periodically perform blood tests on the infant to measure how much of the drug is in his or her system.

## Going Back to Work

You can continue feeding your baby your milk by expressing and storing it even after you return to work. It does take extra time and planning. Some women use this option as the primary way to feed their babies. See the box "Expressing and Bottle-Feeding" for more information.

### Tell Your Employer

Employers must provide reasonable break time and a safe, clean place that is not a bathroom for hourly workers and some salaried workers to express milk for a baby for up to 1 year after birth. Businesses with 50 employees or fewer may apply for an exemption from this law. If you will be breastfeeding, it's ideal to discuss the details of how you will be expressing your milk and how to store it with your supervisor before you go on maternity leave. Before returning to work, contact your supervisor (as well as your human resources department, if there is one) and tell them that you will need to take breaks throughout the day to express your milk to give to your baby later. If you have on-site day care, you can simply breastfeed your baby at regular intervals.

When you return to work, make sure that the area where you will be expressing your milk is clean and private. You'll need a chair, a small table, and an outlet if you are using an electric pump. Also make sure you have somewhere to store the milk (see box "Storing Breast Milk").

You can plan to express your milk during lunch or other breaks. If you use a breast pump, you should be able to pump enough milk during morning, lunch, and afternoon breaks. Using a double breast pump—which pumps both breasts at the same time—is even quicker. By double pumping, you may be able to pump in 10–15 minutes rather than 20–30 minutes. A hands-free pumping bra makes double pumping easier.

## Expressing Breast Milk and Bottle-Feeding

Some women decide to express breast milk and feed their babies from a bottle. This option often is used when an infant is preterm or sick and is being cared for in a *neonatal intensive care unit*. Women who breastfeed their babies from birth also use this option if they return to work outside the home. In the past 20 years, more and more women are choosing this option as the primary way to feed their babies. Women who choose this option have cited the following reasons for their decision:

• Difficulties establishing breastfeeding, which can have a variety of causes

• Breastfeeding problems, such as recurrent mastitis

• Concerns about feeding the baby in public

• Ability to share feeding duties (eg, someone else can feed the baby expressed breast milk)

There have been no studies to date that directly compare the benefits of breast-feeding from the breast and feeding expressed breast milk. It also is not known exactly how many women are using this option primarily. You may wonder whether feeding your baby expressed milk has the same benefits for you and your baby that breastfeeding from the breast offers. Feeding expressed breast milk likely has the same benefits as breastfeeding in terms of protecting your baby against disease and providing nutrients he or she needs to grow. Your baby will get the same antibodies and the same nutrients no matter how the breast milk is given.

One difference between feeding from the breast and feeding from a bottle is that bottle-feeding may not teach your baby to self-regulate the amount of milk he or she consumes. Some research suggests that breastfed babies learn this concept by feeding from the breast. Self-regulation may help prevent overeating and obesity later on in life. Also, expressing your milk may not offer you the same level of protection against pregnancy as full or nearly full breastfeeding can (although more research into this issue is needed).

There are some challenges that you may encounter if you choose to express and bottle-feed. It may be more difficult for your body to regulate milk production when you express milk than when the baby feeds from your breasts. Milk is produced in response to the baby's suckling and how fast the baby empties the breast. If the baby is experiencing a growth spurt, he or she will empty the breast more quickly, and the mother's body responds by making more milk. A mom who expresses her milk will need to increase the number of pumping or hand-expressing sessions in order to keep up with these growth spurts.

**Expressing Breast Milk and Bottle-Feeding,** *continued*

Expressing and storing breast milk also may not be as convenient as breast-feeding. In addition to expressing your breast milk, you will need to maintain the pump (if you use one), get bottles ready, and store the milk at appropriate temperatures. However, many moms like the flexibility that sharing feeding duties offers with this option and feel that this more than makes up for the time required to prepare bottles.

If you are interested in this option as the primary way of feeding your baby, talk to your health care provider or a lactation specialist. If you feel that this option is right for you, you should be supported in your decision.

## Expressing Breast Milk

There are two ways to express milk from your breast: 1) by hand or 2) with a pump. Whichever method you choose, stimulating the let-down reflex is important in order to express a good amount of milk. It may help to have a picture of your baby nearby. You also can try other things to stimulate the let-down reflex, like applying a warm, moist compress to the breast, gently massaging the breast, or just sitting quietly and thinking about your baby.

**By Hand.** Expressing milk by hand is a good solution if you are away from your baby for a short time or to relieve engorgement. It takes about 20–30 minutes to express milk from both breasts using this technique. The hand-expressing technique takes a little practice, but it's not difficult. If you are interested in learning this technique, an educational video can be helpful (a good one can be found at http://newborns.stanford.edu/Breastfeeding/HandExpression.html). To start, first wash your hands with soap and water, and make sure the container into which you are expressing your milk is clean and placed on a clean surface. Place your hand with the fingers below and your thumb about 3 centimeters above the nipple, forming a "C" around the areola. Press inward toward your chest and then roll your thumb and fingers toward the nipple. Reposition your hand periodically so you go all around the areola while you press and roll. Don't squeeze the nipple. To get the most milk, massage your breast, starting from the outside and moving inward, with your other hand.

**Pumping.** Health insurance providers under the Affordable Care Act are required to pay for a breast pump or the rental cost of one as well as breast-feeding counseling. You should check with your individual insurance carrier for details about what kinds of pumps are covered and how to obtain them. You may need to have your health care provider write a prescription for a breast pump. See the "Resources" section in this chapter for links to useful information about this provision of the Affordable Care Act.

There are many types of breast pumps that are available, but they fall into three broad categories:

1. Manual pumps—You provide the suction for these pumps by squeezing a lever or handle. Manual breast pumps are inexpensive (ranging in price from $14 to $50) and also have the advantage of being useable during a power outage. Even if you purchase an electric pump, you may want to have a manual pump on hand in case the electricity goes out.

2. Battery-operated pumps—These pumps run on batteries. If you decide to get a battery-operated pump, think about purchasing a back-up manual pump in case you run out of batteries.

3. Electric pumps—These pumps are plugged into an electrical outlet. You can buy a single electric pump that pumps one breast at a time or a double pump that pumps both breasts at the same time. Double pumps can save you time and are especially useful if you need to pump milk during your workday. Electric pumps also can be operated by batteries.

You also can rent a pump from a hospital, doctor's office, or breastfeeding center. Rental costs may be covered by your health insurance, but be sure to check your individual plan. The types of pumps that are rented are designed for multiple users because the parts that come into contact with your milk are disposable. These pumps are designated as "multiple-user" or "hospital-grade" pumps. If you rent a pump, you will need to purchase a new pump kit that includes the breast shield and tubing that only you will use. Pumps that are made for one user only are called "single-user" pumps. Borrowing or sharing a single-user breast pump is not recommended because of the risk of contamination.

No matter what type of pump you choose, you need to maintain a clean environment before, during, and after pumping. Wash your hands before pumping your breast milk and make sure the table or area where you are pumping also is clean. After pumping, wash your equipment with soap and water, or use a microwave-sterilization bag. This helps prevent germs from getting into the milk. If there's not an easy way to wash your pump

## Storing Breast Milk

- Store your breast milk in clean glass or plastic bottles or special milk-collection bags. Store it in small amounts (2–4 ounces) to avoid wasting it. Mark the bottles or bags with the date the milk was pumped. If you are going to freeze it, leave a 1-inch space at the top of the container because the milk may expand when frozen.

- Breast milk can be stored at room temperature for 3–4 hours (optimal) or 6–8 hours under very clean conditions. You can keep your milk in the refrigerator (39°F or below) for up to 3 days (optimal) or for 5–8 days under very clean conditions. Do not store milk in the door of the refrigerator because the temperature there can vary.

- Breast milk can be frozen (0°F or below) for up 6 months (optimal) or 12 months under very clean conditions.

- Never thaw frozen milk at room temperature. To thaw frozen milk, hold it under cool running water. Once it has begun to thaw, use warm running water to finish. You also can let frozen milk slowly thaw in the fridge. Once milk is thawed, use it within 24 hours. Never refreeze milk that has been thawed.

- You can add freshly expressed milk to breast milk that was pumped before. Always cool the fresh milk first.

- Warm previously chilled breast milk by placing it in a bowl of very warm water. Don't heat bottles on the stove or in the microwave. This destroys breast milk's disease-fighting qualities and creates hot spots.

equipment at work, you may want to pack several sets and wash them all when you get home.

## Choosing to Formula-Feed

If you are unable to breastfeed or express your milk, or if you do not wish to, formula-feeding is an option. Formula-feeding can be convenient for the following reasons:

- Babies who are fed commercially prepared infant formula mostly likely are getting the recommended amount of vitamin D per day and do not need additional vitamin D supplements by dropper, but check the label on your baby's formula to make sure.

- Because formula digests more slowly than human milk, formula-fed babies usually need to eat less often than breastfed babies do. However, mothers who formula-feed do not get more sleep than mothers who breastfeed.

- Women who formula-feed don't have to worry about possible effects of alcoholic beverages or medications that they are taking that could affect their babies.

- Either parent (or another caregiver) can feed the baby a bottle at any time. But keep in mind that babies also can be bottle-fed with expressed breast milk that you pump and store.

### Picking a Formula

If you have decided that formula-feeding is a better option for you, rest assured that formulas on the market today will give your baby the right nutrients he or she needs to grow. There are different types of infant formula to choose from, so talk to your baby's pediatrician for recommendations on picking the best one. There are three major types available:

1. Cow's milk formulas—Most infant formula is made with cow's milk that has been changed to give it the right balance of nutrients for an infant. You should not give your infant regular cow's milk until he or she is 1 year old.

2. Soy-based formulas—Soy-based infant formulas are an option for babies who can't digest or are allergic to cow's milk formula or to lactose, a sugar naturally found in cow's milk. However, babies who are allergic to cow's milk also may be allergic to soy milk.

3. Protein hydrolysate formulas—These are meant for babies who have a family history of milk or soy allergies. Protein hydrolysate formulas are easier to digest and less likely to cause allergic reactions than are other types of formula. They also are called hypoallergenic formulas.

Once you choose the type of formula to feed your baby, you'll have to decide which form to buy as well. Infant formulas come in three forms:

1. Powdered formula is the least expensive. Each scoop of powdered formula must be mixed with water, and it does not need to be refrigerated until it is mixed with water.

2. Liquid concentrated formula also must be mixed with water and must be refrigerated once the container is opened.

3. Ready-to-use formulas do not need to be mixed with water but are the most expensive and must be refrigerated once the container is opened.

## Bottles

A wide variety of bottle and nipple systems are available for formula-feeding. Your baby may take to just about any bottle, or he or she may be more particular. It's a good idea to start with the least expensive bottles and see if they work first before moving on to the deluxe models.

You may have heard about a chemical called bisphenol-A (BPA) that is used in some plastic bottles and in the lining of canned foods. Results of some research suggest that BPA can disrupt the body's hormones and may lead to problems such as infertility and cancer. Research results also suggest that BPA can have toxic effects on infants and children who are exposed to it. Because BPA crosses the *placenta*, infants can be exposed to BPA indirectly before birth. After birth, infants can be exposed through eating food stored or given in plastic bottles. BPA also has been found in human milk.

In 2012, the U.S. Food and Drug Administration banned the use of BPA in all baby bottles, children's dishes and cups, and infant food packaging. BPA is not banned for use in other types of food and beverage containers or in the lining of canned foods. Keep this in mind when transitioning your baby to cup-feeding or solid foods.

## The Challenges

As with breastfeeding, families who formula-feed their babies have to cope with a few challenges. Dealing with these challenges requires time and planning.

**Preparation.** You will have to have enough formula on hand at all times, and you must prepare the bottles. The powdered and condensed formulas must be prepared with sterile water, which needs to be boiled until the baby is at least 6 months old. You also can purchase sterile water at most drugstores or baby supply stores, but even with sterile water, the CDC recommends heating water to at least 158°F when preparing powdered formula.

Some parents warm bottles up before feeding the baby, although this often isn't necessary. Never microwave a baby's bottle because it can create dangerous hot spots. Instead, run refrigerated bottles under warm water for a few minutes if the baby prefers a warm bottle to a cold one. Another option is to put the baby's bottles in a pan of hot water (away from the heat of the stove) and test the temperature by squirting a drop or two of formula on the inside of your wrist.

**Sterilization.** Bottles and nipples need to be sterilized before they are used the first time. You then must wash them after each time you use them. Bottles and nipples can transmit **bacteria** if they aren't cleaned properly, as can formula if it isn't stored in sterile containers.

**Refrigeration.** If bottles are left out of the refrigerator longer than 1 hour, the formula must be thrown out. Prepared bottles of formula should be stored in the refrigerator for no longer than 24–48 hours (check the formula's label for complete information).

*Remember:* Never use a microwave to warm a baby's bottled milk or formula.

## Final Thoughts on Feeding Your Baby

If you choose to breastfeed your baby, there are plenty of resources and support available. More and more women are choosing this option, so you will have lots of company. But if you can't or choose not to breastfeed, it doesn't mean that you're not a good mom. You should choose the method that benefits your baby, you, and your family.

# RESOURCES

If you have questions about feeding your baby, you're in luck—there are lots of resources available to answer your questions.

**Affordable Care Act Breastfeeding Benefits**
Healthcare.gov
www.healthcare.gov/coverage/breast-feeding-benefits/
*Explains the various benefits breastfeeding moms and infants are entitled to under the Affordable Care Act.*

**Best for Babes**
www.bestforbabes.org
*Provides information and support to help all mothers meet their personal breastfeeding goals.*

**Human Milk Banking Association of North America (HMBANA)**

www.hmbana.org

*This professional association for human milk banks issues safety guidelines for member banks on screening human milk donors and collecting, processing, handling, testing, and storing milk.*

**International Lactation Consultant Association**

www.ilca.org

*Provides a directory of lactation consultants as well as information about breastfeeding.*

**LactMed**

http://toxnet.nlm.nih.gov/newtoxnet/lactmed.htm

*Provides a searchable database of drugs to which breastfeeding mothers may be exposed and gives information about the possible effects on breastfed infants as well as alternative drugs to consider. There is also a free app that you can download onto your smartphone.*

**La Leche League International**

www.llli.org

*Provides information and support for breastfeeding moms and offers referrals to local support groups.*

# Part IV
# Special Considerations

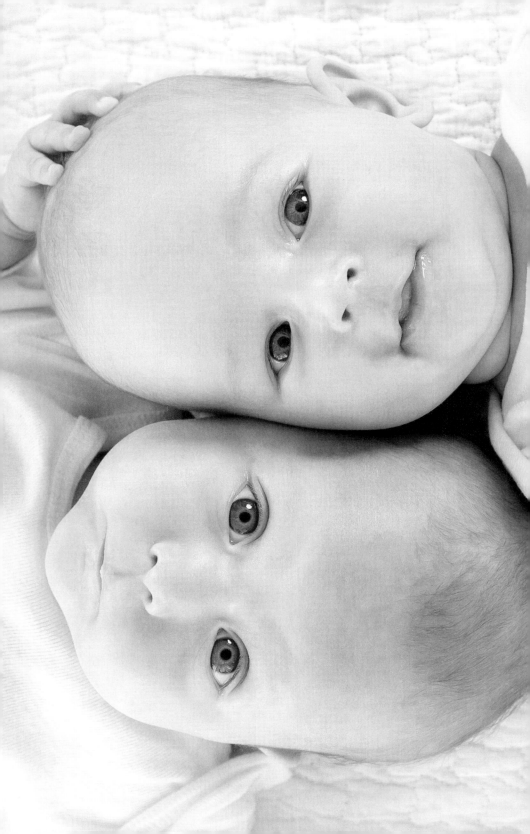

Chapter 19

# Multiples: When It's Twins, Triplets, or More

When a woman is carrying more than one baby, it is called a ***multiple pregnancy***. In the past 20 years, multiple pregnancies have become more common in the United States. In 2012, 1 in every 30 babies born in the United States was a twin, compared with 1 in every 53 babies in 1980. According to the National Center for Health Statistics, between 1980 and 2009, the number of twin births increased more than 75%. The number of triplet and higher-order multiple births (four or more babies) increased 400% between 1980 and 2000, but it has declined by about 30% in the past decade.

Some of the increase in multiple pregnancies is because more women older than 35 years are having babies; women in this age group are at higher risk of having twins. Another reason for the increase is that more women are undergoing fertility treatments to become pregnant. These treatments increase the risk of multiple pregnancy. It is important to discuss the risks of multiple pregnancy, and possible ways to prevent it, with your health care provider if you are having fertility treatments (see box "Fertility Treatments and Multiple Pregnancy").

## Making Multiples

Multiple births occur when more than one ***embryo*** grows in the uterus. This process can occur naturally, or it can occur artificially during fertility treatments.

# Fertility Treatments and Multiple Pregnancy

Fertility treatments are a major factor in the increase in multiple pregnancies over the past 20 years. Although all fertility treatments increase the risk of multiple pregnancy, it is most common in women who use fertility drugs to induce **ovulation**. Several drugs can be used to stimulate ovulation. When a drug called clomiphene citrate is used, about 10% of the pregnancies that are achieved are twins and less than 1% are triplets or greater. When drugs called gonadotropins are used, 30% of the pregnancies achieved are multiple pregnancies. Most of these are twin pregnancies, but up to one third are triplets or greater.

With **assisted reproductive technologies (ART)**, **eggs** are fertilized outside of the body. The eggs can be from a donor, or they can be generated by the woman herself with fertility drugs. The resulting embryo or embryos are transferred to a woman's uterus. The risk of multiple pregnancy increases as the number of transferred embryos increases. About 45% percent of pregnancies aided by ART result in twins and about 7% in triplets or more when two embryos are transferred.

Because of the risks associated with multiple pregnancy, the American Society for Reproductive Medicine recommends taking a preventive approach when fertility treatments are used. If you and your partner are considering fertility treatments, your fertility specialist will talk with you about the risks of having a multiple pregnancy and how you may avoid having more than one baby. For example, with ART you may choose to limit the number of embryos that are transferred to the uterus. The chance for a successful outcome with transferring a single embryo is increased for women who meet certain criteria, such as those who are younger than 35 years, are participating in their first ART cycle, and have generated a relatively large number of high-quality embryos.

With ovulation induction, **ultrasound exams** can be used to monitor the number of eggs that are developing in the **ovaries**, and blood tests can measure hormone levels. If an ultrasound exam reveals a large number of developing eggs, or if the blood test results show a high level of hormones, it may be recommended that you do not attempt pregnancy during that cycle to avoid the risk of multiple pregnancy.

If a triplet or higher-order pregnancy occurs, a procedure called **multifetal pregnancy reduction** may be considered. This procedure reduces by one or more the total number of babies in a multifetal pregnancy. There are risks associated with this procedure, including the risk of loss of all of the babies. However, with higher-order multiple pregnancies, these risks are generally believed to be outweighed by the potential benefits of this procedure, including a decrease in the risks associated with **preterm** delivery. Reducing a pregnancy also decreases maternal risks, including **hypertension**, **preeclampsia**, and **gestational diabetes mellitus**.

### Fraternal or Identical Twins?

The most common kind of multiple pregnancy is twins, and twins come in two types—fraternal and identical:

*   ***Fraternal twins***—Most twins are fraternal. Each fraternal twin grows from a separate fertilized egg and **sperm**. Because each twin grows from the union of a different egg and a different sperm, these twins are similar only in the way any siblings are similar. The twins can be both boys, both girls, or one of each.

*   ***Identical twins***—When one fertilized egg splits early in pregnancy and grows into two embryos, identical twins are formed. Identical twins are the same sex and have the same blood type, hair color, and eye color. They usually look very much alike.

### Three or More Babies

A pregnancy with three or more babies can be formed by more than one egg being fertilized, a single fertilized egg splitting, or both processes occurring

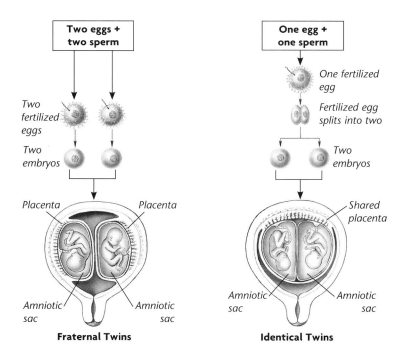

**Types of twins.** Fraternal twins are formed from two eggs and each has a placenta. Identical twins are formed from one egg that splits into two.

in the same pregnancy. This higher-order pregnancy rarely happens naturally and is most often the result of fertility treatments.

## How to Know When It's More Than One Baby

There are signs that can indicate to your health care provider that you are pregnant with more than one baby:

- Rapid weight gain during the first trimester
- Severe morning sickness
- Hearing more than one heartbeat during a prenatal exam
- Your uterus being larger than expected during a prenatal exam

Most women learn they're carrying multiples fairly early in their pregnancies. An ultrasound exam can detect most multiples by week 12 of pregnancy. When a twin or higher-order multiple pregnancy is diagnosed, the *chorionicity* (whether the babies share a *chorion* and *placenta*) and *amnionicity* (the number of *amniotic sacs*) also are determined with an ultrasound exam.

## Risks

A multiple pregnancy can affect your health as well as your babies' health. However, with proper *prenatal care*, your health care provider can diagnose and manage any complications that may arise and help protect you and the babies from more serious problems (see box "What Kind of Health Care Provider Should You See?"). You should be aware of the complications that are more likely with a multiple pregnancy.

The risk of problems during pregnancy increases with the number of babies. This means that there is a higher risk of problems with twins than with a single baby and a higher risk of problems with triplets than with twins.

### Preterm Birth

Preterm birth—birth before 37 weeks of gestation—is the most common problem of multiple pregnancies. More than 50% of twins and more than 90% of triplets are born preterm. The number of weeks at which you are likely to give birth decreases with each additional baby (see Table 19-1).

Preterm babies are more likely to have health problems than babies born at term because they may not have finished growing and developing. They

## What Kind of Health Care Provider Should You See?

Many women who are expecting multiples wonder if they need to see a *maternal–fetal medicine subspecialist* during pregnancy. These subspecialists, also called perinatologists, are obstetricians who specialize in caring for pregnant women who may be at high risk of special health problems. But having a multiple pregnancy does not necessarily mean you need a subspecialist. If you are healthy, you can choose to see an obstetrician who has experience caring for women with multiple pregnancies. If you have other conditions that put you at risk of complications or if you have a history of pregnancy problems, your obstetrician may refer you to a subspecialist. The maternal–fetal medicine subspecialist usually will help take care of you and your babies along with your regular obstetrician.

Keep in mind that being referred to a maternal–fetal medicine subspecialist does not mean that your pregnancy is expected to be difficult. Usually, the referral is done to give extra protection for you and the babies and to put your mind at ease.

## Table 19-1 Duration of Multiple Pregnancies

| Type of Pregnancy | Average Gestational Age at Time of Delivery | Average Birth Weight |
|---|---|---|
| Singleton | 38.6 weeks | 7.3 lb (3,300 grams) |
| Twin | 35.0 weeks | 5.1 lb (2,300 grams) |
| Triplet | 32.0 weeks | 3.7 lb (1,660 grams) |
| Quadruplet | 30.0 weeks | 2.9 lb (1,300 grams) |

*Data from Multiple pregnancy and birth: twins, triplets, and higher order multiples: a guide for patients. Patient Information Series. Birmingham, AL: American Society for Reproductive Medicine; 2004.*

may be born with serious health problems, some of which can last a lifetime. Some problems, such as learning disabilities, appear later in childhood or even in adulthood. Preterm multiples are at increased risk of brain damage and bleeding in the brain than preterm single babies. *Cerebral palsy* is more prevalent in preterm multiples than in preterm single babies.

There is no treatment that can be given to prevent preterm birth from happening in multiple pregnancies. Because prematurity is so common in multiple pregnancies, the best thing is to be prepared for the possibility that your babies may be born preterm. If your labor does start early, certain things can be done to prolong the pregnancy for a short time. If you go into labor and are likely to give birth between 24 weeks and 34 weeks of pregnancy, you may be given **corticosteroids**. These medications help the babies' lungs and other organs mature. In many cases, you also may be given a medication called a **tocolytic**. Tocolytics are drugs used to delay delivery for a short time (up to 48 hours). They are given to allow time for corticosteroids to do their job or to transport you to a hospital that offers high-level care for infants who are born preterm or with other complications. A tocolytic called **magnesium sulfate** may be given. In addition to delaying preterm birth, it has been shown to reduce the risk and severity of cerebral palsy in preterm infants if it is given before 32 weeks of pregnancy.

Tocolytics can have side effects for the mother, some of which can be serious and life threatening. The risk of these side effects occurring is greater in women with multiple pregnancies than in women with single pregnancies. For this reason, they are not recommended to prevent preterm labor. Tocolytics and corticosteroids are given to a woman with a multiple pregnancy only when preterm labor is diagnosed.

It's important to be able to recognize preterm labor if you are pregnant with more than one baby and to call your health care provider if you have any of these signs or symptoms:

• Change in vaginal discharge (becomes watery, mucus-like, or bloody)

• Increase in amount of vaginal discharge

• Pelvic or lower-abdominal pressure

• Constant low, dull backache

• Mild abdominal cramps, with or without diarrhea

• Regular or frequent contractions or uterine tightening, often painless (four times every 20 minutes or eight times an hour for more than 1 hour)

• Ruptured membranes (your water breaks, with a gush or a trickle of fluid)

For more information about preterm birth, see Chapter 27, "Preterm Labor, Premature Rupture of Membranes, and Preterm Birth."

## Chorionicity and Amnionicity

Early in a multiple pregnancy, an ultrasound exam is done to find out whether each baby has its own placenta, amniotic sac, and chorion (the outermost membrane that surrounds the developing babies). Types of twins are as follows:

• **Diamniotic–dichorionic**—Twins who have their own chorions and amniotic sacs. They may or may not share a placenta.

- *Diamniotic–monochorionic*—Twins who share a chorion and placenta but have separate amniotic sacs

- *Monoamniotic–monochorionic*—Twins who share a chorion, placenta, and amniotic sac

Triplets can all have their own placentas and amniotic sacs or two of the triplets may share a sac, a placenta, or both. Rarely, triplets may share one placenta and one amniotic sac.

Monochorionic babies have a higher risk of complications than those with separate placentas. One problem that can occur in monochorionic-diamniotic babies is ***twin–twin transfusion syndrome (TTTS)***. In TTTS, the blood flow between the twins becomes unbalanced because of a problem with the placenta. One twin donates blood to the other twin. The donor

Chorion
Amnion
Placenta

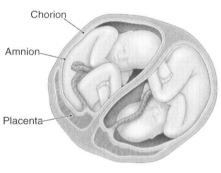

**Diamniotic–dichorionic, two placentas**

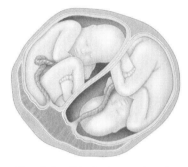

**Diamniotic–dichorionic, one placenta**

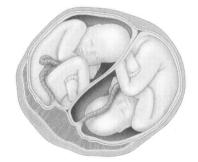

**Diamniotic–monochorionic, one placenta**

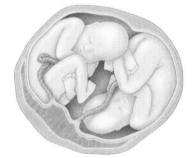

**Monoamniotic–monochorionic, one placenta**

**Chorionicity and amnionicity.** Reproduced from Beckman RBC, Ling FW, Herbert WNP, Laube DW, Smith RP, Casanova R, et al. *Obstetrics and gynecology.* 7th ed. Philadelphia (PA): Lippincott Williams & Wilkins; 2014.

twin has too little blood, and the recipient twin has too much blood. This condition can lead to problems for both babies. Treatment is available for TTTS if it is diagnosed during pregnancy. One treatment that can be done is to periodically remove extra fluid from the recipient's twin amniotic sac. This needs to be done every few days or weekly. Severe cases of TTTS that are diagnosed early may be treated with laser surgery on the placenta. This surgery should be performed in a hospital by a health care provider with experience in performing these procedures.

Although monochorionic–monoamniotic babies are rare, this type of pregnancy is very risky. The most common problem is an **umbilical cord** complication. If the babies get tangled in their cords, they may not be able to move and grow. Women with a monoamniotic pregnancy are monitored more frequently and will need to have their babies by **cesarean delivery**.

### Gestational Diabetes Mellitus

Women carrying multiple babies are at increased risk of gestational diabetes mellitus—a pregnancy-related form of **diabetes mellitus**. In a multiple pregnancy, gestational diabetes mellitus can increase the risk of breathing difficulties and other problems during the newborn period. Managing diabetes through diet, exercise, and sometimes medication can reduce the risk of these complications occurring (see Chapter 23, "Diabetes Mellitus," for more information).

### High Blood Pressure and Preeclampsia

Women with multiple pregnancies have a higher risk of developing **high blood pressure** conditions during pregnancy than women carrying singleton pregnancies. Preeclampsia is a blood pressure disorder that usually starts after 20 weeks of pregnancy. It also can occur in the postpartum period. It occurs more frequently in women pregnant with twins than in women pregnant with one baby. It also tends to occur earlier in multiple pregnancies. Preeclampsia can lead to long-term damage to the mother's **kidneys** and liver and can increase the risk of heart disease later in life. Preeclampsia that worsens and causes seizures in the woman is called **eclampsia**. When symptoms of preeclampsia become severe and if they occur during pregnancy, the babies may need to be delivered right away, even if they are not fully grown. Preeclampsia is discussed in greater detail in Chapter 22, "Hypertension and Preeclampsia."

### Growth Problems

Multiples generally grow at a slower rate during pregnancy than singletons. For example, about 25% of twins and 60% of triplets are born at a smaller-than-average size. One reason that multiples may be born smaller than average is that the placenta of one or more than one baby may not be in the best place or the umbilical cord may not be formed normally. These problems can limit the amount of **nutrients** the babies receive.

Twins are called **discordant** if one is much smaller than the other. Discordant twins are more likely to have problems during pregnancy and after birth. Twins may be discordant because of poor functioning of the placenta, genetic problems, or TTTS.

Beginning at about 24 weeks of pregnancy, ultrasound exams typically are used to check the growth of each baby and the amount of **amniotic fluid** every 4–6 weeks. If a growth problem is suspected, ultrasound exams are done more frequently. If a problem is found, special tests also may be done.

## What to Expect

If you are carrying more than one baby, you may need to adjust your diet and exercise routine. You may see your health care provider more often than a woman carrying one baby. You also may need special care during pregnancy, labor, and delivery.

### Nutritional Considerations

When pregnant with multiple babies, you will need to eat more than if you were carrying one baby. Eating well is important for your health and the health of your babies. If you are pregnant with twins, you need to eat about 600 extra calories per day—that's double the number of extra calories that's recommended for a single pregnancy. For triplets, you should triple the number of calories needed for a single pregnancy. These calories should come from healthy foods to meet your body's nutritional needs. Some women with twins may have more nausea and vomiting, which may make getting the right amount of calories difficult. It may be easier to eat smaller, more frequent meals.

All pregnant women need to get extra amounts of iron (27 mg a day) and **folic acid** (600 micrograms a day). Taking a prenatal multivitamin supplement will ensure you are getting these recommended amounts.

## Weight Gain

Along with eating well, gaining the right amount of weight is very important for the health of your babies. You will need to gain more weight when carrying more than one baby than if you were carrying only one.

If you're expecting twins and you were a normal weight before pregnancy, it is suggested that you gain between 37 pounds and 54 pounds. If you were overweight before pregnancy, however, you should gain between 31 pounds and 50 pounds. If you were obese (a body mass index of 30 or greater), you should gain between 25 pounds and 42 pounds (see Table 19-2). Gaining the necessary pounds during your pregnancy should be done gradually. With twins, you should gain about 1 pound per week in the first half of pregnancy. In the second half of pregnancy, you should aim to gain a little more than 1 pound each week.

## Exercise

Getting regular exercise is important in every pregnancy. When you're carrying multiple babies, however, most health care providers recommend some caution. Your health care provider may advise you to avoid strenuous activity and high-impact exercise, such as aerobics and running. Better choices for you to remain active during your pregnancy are sports that are lower impact, such as swimming, prenatal yoga, and walking.

## Prenatal Genetic Screening and Diagnosis

Having a multiple pregnancy means that there are special considerations for routine screening and diagnosis of **birth defects**. Because each baby is at risk of having a birth defect, the chance of a birth defect in one or more babies is increased. The risk of a birth defect occurring is therefore higher in a multiple

### Table 19-2 Weight Gain Recommendations for a Twin Pregnancy

| Prepregnancy Body Mass Index | Category | Recommended Weight Gain for a Twin Pregnancy (in Pounds) |
|---|---|---|
| Less than 18.5 | Underweight | Not known |
| 18.5–24.9 | Normal weight | 37–54 |
| 25.0–29.9 | Overweight | 31–50 |
| 30.0 and above | Obese | 25–42 |

Data from Institute of Medicine. Weight gain during pregnancy: reexamining the guidelines. Washington, DC: National Academies Press; 2009.

pregnancy. Standard **screening tests** for chromosomal disorders, such as **Down syndrome**, involve taking a sample of your blood and measuring the level of certain substances. If the results of a screening test indicate that there is a possibility of a disorder, it's not possible to tell from the test results how many of the babies are affected.

Another type of screening test uses **cell-free DNA** that circulates in the mother's blood. This test is used to screen for some chromosomal disorders. However, more information is needed about the use of this test in women with multiple pregnancies.

Because of the increased risk of birth defects and the limitations of screening tests in a multiple pregnancy, your health care provider may recommend **diagnostic testing** for birth defects. These tests include **chorionic villus sampling** and **amniocentesis**. These tests are invasive, meaning that a small amount of amniotic fluid or a piece of the placenta needs to be obtained. Before having one of these tests, you should know that

- a sample usually needs to be taken from each baby
- the risks of the procedures are increased with more than one baby
- results may show that one baby is normal and the other baby has a defect

In addition, these tests are more technically difficult to perform in multiple pregnancies. To reduce the risk of complications, it is recommended that only experienced health care providers perform these tests if you are carrying more than one baby.

## Monitoring

You will need special prenatal care if you are pregnant with multiples. You will visit your health care provider more frequently if you are carrying twins. Your health care provider will monitor the health of your babies during your pregnancy with exams and special tests. Some tests are routine. Others may be done only when a problem is suspected. You may have some or all of these tests, depending on the status of your pregnancy:

- Assessment of the **cervix** for signs associated with preterm labor
- More frequent ultrasound exams to check the babies' growth
- **Nonstress test**, in which the babies' heart rates are measured
- **Biophysical profile**, which includes checking the babies' body movements, breathing movements, muscle tone, and the amount of amniotic fluid. The babies' heart rates may be checked as well.

### Bed Rest and Hospitalization

Bed rest with or without hospitalization has been commonly recommended to women pregnant with multiple babies. Recent studies, however, have concluded that routine hospitalization or bed rest for women with uncomplicated twin pregnancies does not result in healthier babies or healthier moms. In fact, bed rest can actually increase the risk of a woman developing ***deep vein thrombosis***, a condition in which a blood clot forms in the deep veins in the body. For these reasons, routine bed rest and hospitalization are not recommended for women with multiple pregnancies.

## Delivery

When and how your babies are born depends on certain factors, including the following:

- Position of each baby
- Weight of each baby
- Your health
- Health of the babies

You and your health care provider will discuss the best time for you to give birth to the babies. After about 38 weeks of pregnancy, the placenta does not function as efficiently in women carrying twins compared with women carrying one baby, and there is a slightly increased risk of ***stillbirth***. However, delivering the babies too early may increase the risk of problems associated with being born preterm. Most experts agree that if there are no complications, twins can be delivered at 38 weeks of pregnancy.

The chance of needing a cesarean delivery is higher when you're pregnant with twins than when you're pregnant with one baby. However, you have a good chance of having a normal vaginal delivery if the presenting twin (the one nearest to the cervix) is in a head-down position, there are no other complications, and you are at least 32 weeks pregnant. If you're carrying three or more babies, a cesarean delivery is recommended because it is safer for the babies.

If you are able to give birth vaginally, be prepared for a longer labor. Labor, especially the pushing stage, may take longer with twins. Babies usually are born several minutes apart in a vaginal delivery, but it can take longer.

## Getting Ready

Having more than one baby can be both exciting and overwhelming. It is important for you and your partner to be as prepared as possible for the coming adventure of being new parents to more than one baby. It may be helpful to talk with other parents who have multiple babies. Having help and support will make life with multiples go much smoother.

Although it's impossible to be prepared for every contingency, the following challenges are those that many families of multiple babies encounter:

- High health care costs—Because multiple babies often are born with health problems, they may require short-term and long-term specialized health care. Have a financial plan in place to deal with these health care costs. If you have health insurance, make sure that it will cover the costs of this specialized care.

- Breastfeeding—Many women wonder if they can breastfeed more than one baby. Breastfeeding any baby takes practice, and the same goes for multiples. Mother's milk has the right amount of all the nutrients the babies need and adapts as your babies' needs change. When you breastfeed, your milk supply will increase to the right amount. You will need to eat healthy foods and drink plenty of liquids. Lactation specialists, nurses, and your health care provider can help you get started and work out any problems you may have. If your babies are premature, you can express and store your milk until they are strong enough to feed from the breast. See Chapter 18, "Breastfeeding and Formula-Feeding Your Baby," for more information on breastfeeding multiples.

- Extra help—You will need some extra hands to help care for your babies, so be sure to line up your volunteers well before your due date. Also, make sure that at least some of your helpers are in for the long haul. You most likely will need helpers for several weeks or months, depending on how many babies you have.

- Stress and fatigue—Caring for multiples is stressful. Preterm babies need smaller, more frequent feedings, and sleep can be in short supply for the parents. One parent most likely will need to stay at home to care for multiple infants.

- *Postpartum depression*—The "baby blues" are very common after pregnancy. About 2–3 days after childbirth, some women begin to feel depressed, anxious, and upset. These feelings usually go away after a week or two. If they do not, or if they get worse, it may be a sign of a more serious condition called postpartum depression. Having multiples might increase your risk of this condition. If you have intense feelings of sadness, anxiety, or despair that prevent you from being able to do your daily tasks, let your health care provider know.

It's a good idea to enroll in a childbirth class especially designed for parents expecting twins or more. Plan to take the classes during your fourth month to sixth month of pregnancy, when you are likely to be most comfortable. Your health care provider should be able to help you find a class.

# RESOURCES

The following resources offer more information about multiple pregnancy:

**Challenges of Parenting Multiples**
American Society for Reproductive Medicine
www.asrm.org/FACTSHEET_Challenges_of_Parenting_Multiples/
*Addresses the social, economic, and psychological issues of multiple pregnancy.*

**Mothers of Supertwins (MOST)**
www.mostonline.org
*Nonprofit national organization that provides information and support for parents of multiples. A comprehensive site that covers all aspects of having multiples—not just twins.*

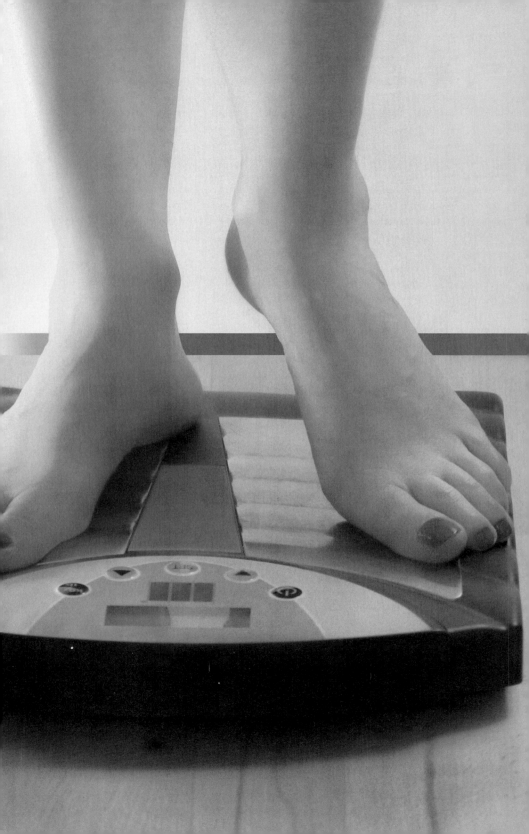

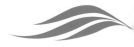

Chapter 20

# Obesity and Eating Disorders

*Obesity* and eating disorders are common in women. Both can affect pregnancy. If you have either of these conditions, you need to be aware of the risks that they pose. You and your health care provider can work together to manage your pregnancy and avoid some of these risks.

## Obesity and Pregnancy

Obesity is a major health problem in the United States. The number of obese men and women in the United States has increased a great deal during the past 25 years, and it is one of the country's fastest-growing health problems. About one half of pregnant women are now obese.

When a pregnant woman is obese, it can have serious effects on her health and the health of her baby. If you are already pregnant, good prenatal care, healthy eating, and regular exercise can help decrease your risk and your baby's risk of problems. If you are planning a pregnancy, the best way to prevent problems caused by obesity is to lose weight before you become pregnant.

### Defining Obesity

You are considered obese if your **body mass index (BMI)** before pregnancy is 30 or higher (use the chart in Appendix A to determine your BMI or go to www.nhlbi.nih.gov/health/educational/lose_wt/BMI/). Body mass index measures your body fat based on your height and weight. There are four different categories of weight that are based on BMI. These categories are as follows:

1. Underweight—BMI of less than 18.5
2. Normal weight—BMI of 18.5–24.9
3. Overweight—BMI of 25–29.9
4. Obese—BMI of 30 or greater

Within the general category of obesity, there are three subcategories that also are based on BMI. With increasing BMI, the risk of life-threatening disease also increases:

- Obesity category I—30–34.9
- Obesity category II—35–39.9
- Obesity category III—40 or greater

### Risks of Obesity During Pregnancy

As with any other time in your life, being obese during pregnancy poses extra health risks. Problems that can affect you during pregnancy if you are obese include the following:

- **High blood pressure**—High blood pressure that starts during the second half of pregnancy is called **gestational hypertension**. It can lead to serious complications. Obese women have a higher risk of developing this condition than nonobese women.

- **Preeclampsia**—Preeclampsia is a serious high blood pressure disorder that can occur during pregnancy (usually in the second half of pregnancy) or soon after childbirth. This condition can cause the mother's **kidneys** and liver to fail. Seizures can occur if the condition is not managed. In rare cases, stroke can occur. The baby is at risk of growth problems and problems with the **placenta**. It may require early delivery, even if the baby is not fully grown. In severe cases, the woman, baby, or both may die if the condition is not recognized and managed.

- **Gestational diabetes mellitus**—High blood **glucose** (sugar) levels during pregnancy increase the risk of having a very large baby and a **cesarean delivery**. Women who have had gestational diabetes have a higher risk of having diabetes in the future, as do their children (see Chapter 23, "Diabetes Mellitus").

Being obese during pregnancy also increases the risk of the following problems for your baby:

- Birth defects—Babies born to obese women have an increased risk of having birth defects, such as heart defects and **neural tube defects**.

- Problems with tests—Having too much body fat can make it difficult to see certain problems with the baby's anatomy on an **ultrasound exam**. Checking the baby's heart rate during labor also may be more difficult if you are obese.

- **Macrosomia**—In this condition, the baby is larger than normal. This can increase the risk of the baby being injured during birth. For example, the baby's shoulder can become entrapped after the head is delivered. Macrosomia also increases the risk of **cesarean birth**.

- **Preterm** birth—Problems associated with a woman's obesity may mean that her baby will need to be delivered early. Preterm infants have an increased risk of health problems, including breathing problems, eating problems, and developmental and learning difficulties later in life.

- **Stillbirth**—The higher the mother's BMI, the greater the risk of stillbirth.

### Risks of Obesity During Childbirth

Obesity increases the risks of several complications during childbirth. Being obese can make the chance of a successful vaginal delivery less likely. It can be harder to monitor the baby during labor. For these reasons, obesity during pregnancy increases the risk of having a cesarean delivery.

If a cesarean delivery is required, it is riskier for an obese woman than for a woman of normal weight. In general, the time it takes to perform the operation may be longer. The longer the operation, the greater the risk of complications. These complications include infection, problems with the **anesthesia** used for the procedure, and excessive blood loss. Surgery increases the risk of **deep vein thrombosis**, especially in obese women. Healing may take longer, and you are more likely to have problems with the wound opening and becoming infected.

### Managing Obesity During Pregnancy

Despite the risks, you can have a safe pregnancy and a healthy baby if you are obese. You will need to work with your health care provider to monitor your weight, get regular **prenatal care**, and take steps to be as healthy as possible during your pregnancy.

**Nutrition and Exercise.** Good nutrition and regular exercise are keys to a healthy pregnancy. Eating well and exercising regularly during pregnancy also can start you on the right track for a healthier lifestyle after pregnancy.

While you are pregnant, the food you eat fuels your body's activities and also helps your baby grow. Finding a balance between eating healthy foods while maintaining a healthy weight is important for your health as well as your baby's health. The rate at which you gain weight is important, too. Experts recommend that after an initial weight gain of 2–4 pounds in the first trimester, overweight women should gain a little over one half of a pound each week and obese women should gain a little under one half of a pound each week during the second and third trimesters of pregnancy. If you need help planning a healthy diet, your health care provider may recommend nutrition counseling.

If you have never exercised before, pregnancy is a great time to start. Discuss your exercise plan with your health care provider to make sure that you do not have any health conditions that would prevent you from exercising. Begin with as little as 5 minutes of exercise a day and add 5 minutes per day each week. Your goal is to stay active for 30 minutes each day. Walking is a good choice if you are new to exercise. Brisk walking gives a total body workout and is easy on the joints. Swimming is another good exercise for pregnant women. The water supports your weight so you can avoid injury and muscle strain. It also helps you stay cool.

**Monitoring Your Weight.** At your first prenatal visit, you and your health care provider should discuss how much weight you should gain. The Institute of Medicine has published guidelines for weight gain during pregnancy. These weight gain ranges are based on extensive research and are associated with the best possible outcomes for pregnant women and their babies (see Table 20-1).

You and your health care provider will keep track of how much weight you gain at each prenatal visit. The growth of your baby also will be checked. Keep in mind that even for obese women, pregnancy is not the time to

## Table 20-1 Weight Gain Recommendations for Pregnancy

| Weight Before Pregnancy | BMI | Total Weight Gain Range (Pounds) |
| --- | --- | --- |
| Underweight | 18.5 or less | 28–40 |
| Normal weight | 18.5–24.9 | 25–35 |
| Overweight | 25.0–29.9 | 15–25 |
| Obese | 30.0 or greater | 11–20 |

*Modified from Institute of Medicine (US). Weight gain during pregnancy: reexamining the guidelines. Washington, DC. National Academies Press; 2009. ©2009 National Academy of Sciences.*

actively try to lose weight. However, if you are overweight or obese and are gaining less than what the guidelines suggest, and if your baby is growing well, gaining less than the recommended amount can have benefits, such as decreased risks of needing a cesarean delivery and of having a very large baby. If your baby is not growing well, changes may need to be made to your diet and exercise plan.

**Testing for Gestational Diabetes.** Your health care provider may test you for gestational diabetes during the first 3 months of your pregnancy. Overweight and obese women have a higher risk of this complication than women who are a normal weight. You also may be given the test again in the later months of your pregnancy.

**Labor and Delivery.** As you get closer to your due date, you may be referred to health care providers with expertise in certain areas who will provide specialized care during delivery. For example, you may see an ***anesthesiologist*** who will discuss with you your options for managing pain during labor and delivery.

Steps usually will be taken to reduce the chance of complications. As your due date approaches, your health care provider may explain that you need special care if you have a cesarean delivery. Obese women may need extra attention before, during, and after the procedure to decrease the risk of certain problems, such as deep vein thrombosis. For example, you may be given a medication to prevent deep vein thrombosis or special stockings or boots to wear before, during, and after surgery. Although all pregnant women receive ***antibiotics*** to prevent infection during a cesarean birth, you may receive a higher dose.

**After the Baby Is Born.** Once you are home with your new baby, continue your healthy eating and exercise habits to reach a normal weight. Not only is breastfeeding the best way to feed your baby, it also may help with postpartum weight loss. Overall, women who breastfeed their babies for at least a few months tend to lose pregnancy weight more quickly than women who do not breastfeed.

If you had gestational diabetes during your pregnancy, you have an increased risk of developing diabetes after pregnancy. You will need to have a follow-up test of your glucose level between 6 weeks and 12 weeks after you give birth. If your test result is normal, you should be retested for diabetes every 3 years. Maintaining a healthy weight, eating a balanced diet, and staying active may decrease your risk of getting diabetes in the future.

## Losing Weight After Pregnancy

Many women find it hard to lose the weight they gain during pregnancy. If you are overweight or obese and planning another pregnancy in the future, talk to your health care provider about weight loss and achieving a healthier weight beforehand. Losing excess weight before getting pregnant again is especially important if you had complications in your previous pregnancy. It also is recommended because the weight can add up with each pregnancy. Give yourself enough time to get into shape between pregnancies. Choose a birth control option and start using it before you and your partner begin having sex again.

**Losing Weight Safely.** Losing weight involves using up more *calories* than you take in. You can do this by getting regular exercise and eating healthy foods. An added benefit of these changes is that you will reduce your risk of serious medical problems, such as diabetes and high blood pressure.

Exercise should be an important part of your weight loss plan. Most people who have lost weight and kept it off get 60–90 minutes of moderate-intensity activity on most days of the week. Moderate intensity activities include biking, brisk walking, and yard work. You do not have to do this amount all at once. For instance, you can exercise for 20–30 minutes three times a day.

**Medications.** If you have tried to lose weight through diet changes and exercise and you still have a BMI above 30 or a BMI of at least 27 with certain medical conditions, such as diabetes or heart disease, your health care provider may suggest medications to help with weight loss. These medications should not be taken once you become pregnant.

**Surgery.** If diet and exercise or medications do not work, a special type of surgery, *bariatric surgery*, may be an option for people who are very obese (a BMI of 40 or greater or a BMI between 35 and 39 with major health problems caused by obesity). Bariatric surgery can be divided into two main types: 1) those that reduce the amount of food the stomach can hold (called restrictive surgery) and 2) those that change the way food is absorbed through the intestines (called malabsorptive surgery). Each type of surgery has different benefits, risks, and success rates, which you should discuss in detail with your health care provider. Weight loss with restrictive surgery tends to be slow and steady, whereas weight loss with malabsorptive surgery may be more rapid and significant.

If you have weight-loss surgery, you should delay getting pregnant for 12–24 months after surgery, when you will have the most rapid weight loss. If you have had fertility problems, they may resolve on their own as you rapidly lose the excess weight. It is important to be aware of this possibility because the increase in fertility can lead to an unintended pregnancy. Some types of weight-loss surgery may affect how the body absorbs medications taken by mouth, including birth control pills. You may need to switch to another form of birth control.

Most women who have had bariatric surgery in the past do well during pregnancy. Nevertheless, you may need to pay attention to a few special issues:

- You may be monitored for vitamin deficiencies, especially if you have had malabsorptive surgery. If deficiencies are found, it may be necessary for you to take extra amounts of iron, vitamin $B_{12}$, folic acid, vitamin D, and calcium in addition to the amounts provided in your prenatal multivitamin supplement. It is recommended that you get these vitamins as separate supplements rather than taking an additional multivitamin supplement. An excess of the other vitamins in multivitamin supplements, such as vitamin A, can be harmful during pregnancy.

- Nutritional counseling may be recommended to ensure that you are getting adequate *nutrients* and to help you cope with the nutritional demands of pregnancy.

- Your health care provider may recommend that you visit your bariatric surgeon for an evaluation after you become pregnant. If you've had gastric band surgery (a type of restrictive surgery), adjustments may need to be made to the band during pregnancy. Problems related to the surgery may be more difficult to diagnose during pregnancy because signs and symptoms of these problems are the same as those that commonly occur during pregnancy (abdominal pain, nausea, and vomiting). Involving your surgeon early if you have any of these problems may lead to earlier diagnosis of possible problems with your surgery.

- If you've had malabsorptive surgery, you may not be able to tolerate the test commonly used to screen for gestational diabetes, which involves drinking a sugary mixture. It's important that you tell your health care provider about your surgery because you may need to have a different type of test to screen for gestational diabetes.

## Eating Disorders and Pregnancy

Each year in the United States, 10 million women struggle with eating disorders. Some women with eating disorders may experience a temporary remission of their symptoms when they become pregnant. For other women, eating disorders that were under control before pregnancy may start again during pregnancy. However, sometimes an eating disorder may begin during pregnancy.

### *Types of Eating Disorders*

*Anorexia nervosa* and *bulimia nervosa* are two types of eating disorders. They often have different warning signs and result in different health problems.

**Anorexia Nervosa.** A person with anorexia nervosa diets to extremes because she feels she is overweight even when she is not. Most women with anorexia nervosa have an intense fear of being overweight. They want to be thin so badly that they may starve themselves—sometimes to death.

You should be aware of the symptoms of anorexia nervosa and tell your health care provider if you have them:

- You diet nonstop (even when you are a normal weight or are underweight), refuse to eat except in small portions, or want to eat alone.

- You have lost a lot of weight and still think you are overweight.

- Your menstrual periods stop.

- You exercise excessively.

- You have fine hair growing on your face and arms.

- You are losing hair from your head.

- Your skin is dry, pale, and yellowed.

**Bulimia Nervosa.** Women with bulimia nervosa binge eat, which means they eat large amounts of food in a short time. They then purge the excess food by vomiting; using *laxatives*, diuretics (water pills), or emetics (pills that cause vomiting); or fasting.

Signs that you may have bulimia include the following:

- Swelling around the jaw
- Bloating
- Bloodshot eyes

- Problems with teeth and gums
- Weakness and fatigue
- Mood swings and a feeling of being out of control

## How Eating Disorders Can Harm You and Your Baby

Having an eating disorder can affect your pregnancy in many ways. If you do not gain enough weight while you're pregnant, it can lead to a number of problems for you and your baby. Some of these problems include the following:

- Miscarriage
- Preterm birth
- *Low birth weight*
- *Depression*
- Slow growth of the baby
- Preeclampsia

The laxatives, diuretics, and other medications you take to purge your meals also can harm your baby. These substances take away nutrients and fluids before your body is able to absorb them and pass them on to your baby.

## Getting Help

If you are living with an eating disorder, tell your health care provider right away. The sooner you can address and resolve the problem, the better. The good news is that many women with eating disorders can have healthy babies. Also, it is not uncommon for women with eating disorders who are underweight to have problems conceiving. With a return to normal weight, fertility often returns as well.

Have your health care provider refer you to a trained professional who can help treat your disorder and deal with any other concerns. It's a good idea to try both individual and group therapy. You may need medication as well.

As you work to overcome the negative effects of anorexia nervosa or bulimia nervosa, there are steps you can take to get on a path to a healthy pregnancy. First, ask your health care provider to refer you to a nutritionist who can help you learn about healthy eating. Once you have an eating plan in place, try to gain the recommended amount of weight during your pregnancy. Gaining the right amount of weight is crucial to having a healthy baby. If you need more support, ask for it.

### If You Have a History of Eating Disorders

Some women who have had an eating disorder and have received treatment may experience a return of the signs and symptoms of their eating disorder during pregnancy. Pregnancy raises body image issues for just about every woman. For a woman with a past eating disorder, these issues can trigger the return of the disorder.

If you have a history of an eating disorder, it is important to tell your health care provider early in pregnancy. Together, you can monitor your feelings and be alert to any signs that the disorder has returned. It may be a good idea to continue counseling or seek out a counselor when you become pregnant.

# RESOURCES

The following resources offer more information about some of the topics discussed in this chapter:

**Healthy Weight Gain During Pregnancy**
Institute of Medicine
http://resources.iom.edu/Pregnancy/WhatToGain.html
*Web site with an interactive calculator that gives you the recommended amount of weight you should gain during pregnancy based on your BMI.*

**National Eating Disorders Association**
www.nationaleatingdisorders.org/pregnancy-and-eating-disorders
*Presents an overview of the risks that eating disorders pose during pregnancy and maintains an extensive list of resources to find help and support.*

**Overweight and Obesity During Pregnancy**
March of Dimes
www.marchofdimes.com/pregnancy/overweight-and-obesity-during-pregnancy.aspx
*Provides useful information and advice about managing obesity before, during, and after pregnancy.*

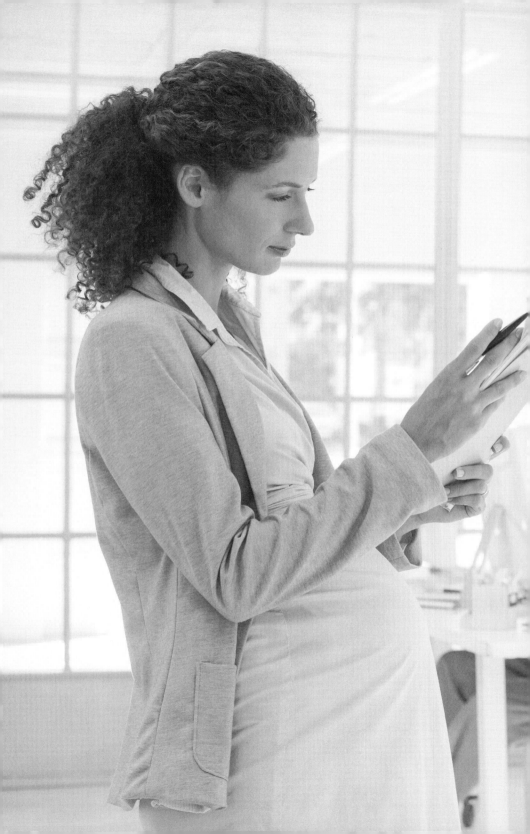

Chapter 21

# Reducing Risks of Birth Defects

Some of the most common questions that pregnant women ask their health care providers are about whether a certain substance has the potential to cause **birth defects**. A birth defect is a change in your baby that may be identified before or after birth and affects how your baby looks, functions, or both. From hair dye and nail polish to microwave ovens and food additives, many parents-to-be worry about the effects that certain items have on a developing baby.

All pregnant women have a 3–5% chance of having a baby with a birth defect. This risk is called the "background risk." A **teratogen** is an agent that increases the risk of having a baby with a birth defect above that of the background risk.

Teratogens can potentially be found in the home, workplace, and environment. They can take several forms:

• Chemicals and **toxins** such as mercury, a metal used in industry

• Alcohol and some illicit drugs

• Vitamins and minerals, such as excessive amounts of vitamin A

• Medications, including warfarin, a medication used to keep blood from clotting

• Maternal infections, such as **chickenpox** (see Chapter 30, "Protecting Yourself From Infections")

• Maternal medical conditions, such as uncontrolled **diabetes mellitus**

Although it is natural to be concerned about the possible effects that medications and environmental agents may have on your pregnancy, there is very little scientific evidence with which to form a risk estimate to human pregnancy from exposure to these agents. Only a few agents have been identified that are known to cause birth defects in infants whose mothers were exposed during pregnancy. One of the most common teratogens is alcohol (discussed later in this chapter). Another common teratogen is high blood glucose levels caused by uncontrolled diabetes (discussed in Chapter 23, "Diabetes Mellitus"). It also is thought that relatively few women come into contact with agents known to be associated with an increased risk of physical or mental disabilities.

The scientific community continues to gather information about the effects of environmental agents, medications, and other agents on reproductive health and fetal development. For now, it makes sense to take stock of your environment and lifestyle and learn about how to take practical steps for minimizing your risk of exposure to known teratogens before and during pregnancy (see box "A Checklist for Reducing Risks of Birth Defects").

## A Checklist for Reducing Risks of Birth Defects

- See your health care provider before becoming pregnant. If you are thinking about getting pregnant, visit your health care provider first for a **preconception care** checkup. The goal of this checkup is to find things that could affect your pregnancy. Along with advice about diet, exercise, and other healthy behaviors, you can make sure that your vaccinations are up to date for your age and risk factors. If you have a medical condition, seeing your health care provider gives you the chance to get in the best possible health before you try to get pregnant. This may involve making changes to your diet, medication, or other areas to bring your condition under control. See Chapter 1, "Getting Ready for Pregnancy."

- Know your genetic risk factors. Some people have **genetic disorders** in their families that can increase their risk of having children with birth defects. Chapter 25, "Screening and Diagnostic Testing for Genetic Disorders," gives detailed information about assessing your baby's risk of genetic disorders and recommendations for screening and diagnostic testing.

- Take a daily vitamin supplement containing at least 400 micrograms (0.4 mg) of **folic acid** before and during pregnancy. Folic acid—a form of a B vitamin—can help prevent **neural tube defects** in your baby. To be effective, you must have enough folic acid in your body at least 1 month before pregnancy and

**A Checklist for Reducing Risks of Birth Defects,** *continued*

during pregnancy. Taking a supplement containing folic acid every day ensures that you get this important vitamin. Women who have previously had a baby with a neural tube defect should take 4 mg of folic acid beginning 1 month before trying to conceive and continuing through the first 3 months of pregnancy.

• Use medications wisely. Tell anyone who prescribes drugs for you that you are pregnant or thinking of becoming pregnant. Do not stop taking a medicine prescribed for you without talking to your health care provider because not taking your medication could cause harm to you or your unborn baby. Also, check with your health care provider before taking any over-the-counter drug, such as pain relievers, *laxatives*, cold or allergy remedies, vitamins, herbal products, and skin treatments.

• Maintain a healthy weight. Being at a healthy weight before becoming pregnant benefits both mother and baby. Women who are obese (have a body mass index of 30 or greater) before becoming pregnant are at increased risk of having babies with birth defects, including neural tube defects, heart defects, and abdominal wall defects. It also may be more difficult to diagnose fetal defects during *ultrasound exams* when the mother is obese. In addition to birth defects, *obesity* is linked to many pregnancy problems, including *gestational diabetes*, *preeclampsia*, *cesarean deliveries*, and infections. See Chapter 20, "Obesity and Eating Disorders."

• Do not use alcohol. Alcohol use during pregnancy is a leading cause of intellectual disability and other birth defects. It is not clear how much, if any, alcohol is safe to drink during pregnancy. For this reason, pregnant women should avoid drinking any alcohol.

• Prevent infections. Several infections, including *toxoplasmosis*, *cytomegalovirus* infection, and German measles, can cause birth defects. See Chapter 30, "Protecting Yourself From Infections," for recommendations on how to prevent infections, including vaccine recommendations.

• Assess your environment for potentially harmful agents. Exposure to toxic agents, such as lead, mercury, or radiation, can cause birth defects. Learn the practical steps you can take—such as the ones mentioned in this chapter—to lessen your risk.

## Teratogens and Pregnancy

Scientists use the word "exposure" to describe when a person comes into contact with something. You can be exposed to toxic agents in the air; in food, water, and medications; through skin contact; or by having a medical condition such as diabetes. Exactly how teratogens may affect your health and the health of your unborn baby depends on the amount you are exposed to, how long you were exposed, how far along you are in your pregnancy, and how your body reacts to the exposures. Many, but not all, agents can be passed from your bloodstream to the baby through the **placenta**. In some cases, such as with lead, chemicals can build up in the tissues of the *fetus*. This can result in a much higher exposure for the fetus than for the mother.

Being exposed to toxic agents at certain times during pregnancy may do more harm than at other times. For example, during the first 8 weeks of pregnancy, major organs and body systems of the fetus are being formed. Exposures that occur very early in pregnancy can happen even before you know that you are pregnant. It is during these weeks that the fetus may be most vulnerable to being harmed by toxic agents. Another vulnerable time is during breastfeeding. Agents that you are exposed to can be transferred to the baby through breast milk.

One reason why we have so little scientific information concerning teratogens is that it is difficult to study how chemicals affect pregnancy. The only way to find out what effects a chemical may have during pregnancy is to observe what happens in children born to women who are known to have been exposed to the chemical while pregnant. Although this information is helpful, it cannot specify the exact amounts and the length of time of exposure that can cause problems.

## What Is an Exposure History?

Before you become pregnant or as soon as you learn you are pregnant, talk with your health care provider about the medications, chemicals, and other agents that you may be exposed to at work or at home. This is called an environmental exposure history (see Table 21-1). This process asks you to think about places and situations in which you may be exposed to toxic substances. Think about things such as the foods you eat, the pesticides you use for your garden, personal care products, household cleaners or building materials, and materials that you use to do crafts or hobbies or ones that are in your workplace. Your health care provider can assist you with the environmental exposure history, or he or she may refer you to other health

## Table 21-1 Environmental Exposure History Form

| Assessment | Yes | No |
|---|---|---|
| Have you or anyone living in your house ever been treated for lead poisoning? | | |
| Do you live in a house built before 1978? | | |
| Are there any plans to remodel your home? | | |
| Have you ever lived outside the United States? | | |
| Do you or your family members use imported pottery, ceramics, china, or crystal for cooking, eating, or drinking? | | |
| Have you ever used any home remedies such as azarcon, greta, or pay-loo-ah? | | |
| Have you ever eaten candy or canned food imported from foreign countries, especially Mexico? | | |
| Have you ever eaten any of the following? | | |
|   Clay | | |
|   Soil or dirt | | |
|   Pottery | | |
|   Paint chips | | |
| Do you wear jewelry that may contain lead (eg, purchased from large-volume stores or from vending machines)? | | |
| Is there a mercury thermometer in your home? | | |
| Do you eat any of the following types of fish? | | |
|   Shark | | |
|   King mackerel | | |
|   Swordfish | | |
|   Tilefish | | |
|   Albacore tuna ("white" tuna) | | |
| Do you eat any locally caught fish? | | |
| Do you eat at least two meals per week of the fish listed? | | |
|   Anchovies, herring, and shad | | |
|   Catfish | | |
|   Clams | | |
|   Cod (Atlantic and Pacific) | | |
|   Crab (blue, king, snow, queen, dungeness) | | |
|   Crayfish | | |
|   Croaker | | |
|   Flounder, plaice, and sole | | |
|   Haddock and hake | | |
|   Lobster (American) | | |
|   Mackerel (Atlantic and Pacific—not king) | | |
|   Marlin | | |
|   Oysters | | |

**Table 21-1 Environmental Exposure History Form,** *continued*

| Assessment | Yes | No |
|---|---|---|
| Perch | | |
| Pollock (Atlantic and walleye) | | |
| Salmon (Atlantic, Chinook, coho) | | |
| Sardines (Atlantic and Pacific) | | |
| Shrimp | | |
| Squid | | |
| Tilapia | | |
| Trout (freshwater) | | |
| Tuna (light canned) | | |
| Whitefish | | |
| Whiting | | |
| Do you use insecticides (insect sprays and powders), herbicides (weed killer), or rodenticides (rat or mouse poison)? | | |
| Inside your home? | | |
| Outside your home? | | |
| On your pets? | | |
| Are you exposed to any of the following at work? | | |
| Metals | | |
| Solvents | | |
| Chemicals | | |
| Radiation | | |
| Fumes | | |
| Do you have any of the following hobbies? | | |
| Stained glass | | |
| Ceramics | | |
| Furniture refinishing | | |

*Adapted from Chicago Consortium for Reproductive Environmental Health in Minority Communities, Chicago, Illinois.*

care professionals with special knowledge and experience in this area. Once you have determined the agents you may have contact with, you can devise strategies to minimize your exposure or to avoid them altogether.

## Medications

Taking a medication during pregnancy is common. In fact, about 90% of pregnant women take at least one medication and about 70% take at least one prescription medication. Not all medications, however, are safe to take when you are pregnant. For this reason, it's very important to know which medications are safe to use and which ones should be avoided both during pregnancy and as you prepare to become pregnant.

In the past, the U.S. Food and Drug Administration (FDA) assigned a letter category (eg, A, B, C, etc.) to each drug that reflected any known and potential risks of taking the drug during pregnancy and while breastfeeding. These categories often overly simplified the available information about a drug. The FDA has eliminated these categories and is now requiring manufacturers of prescription medications to supply more detailed information about these risks. This information should allow health care providers and patients to make more informed decisions about the known and potential risks of taking a drug for both the woman and her baby. If new information becomes available about a drug, the drug label must be revised to include it.

It will take some time to implement the new labeling. For now, it's best to discuss all of the medications that you take with your health care provider. Do not make any decisions on your own about what to take and what not to take. Some women need to continue to take their medications during pregnancy to safeguard their health as well as that of their babies. How much of the medicine you take during pregnancy may need to be increased or decreased. It may be advised that you take a different drug altogether. All decisions should be made in consultation with your health care provider.

## Prescription Medications

Most medications are considered to be safe for use during pregnancy. Only a small number of medications are known to cause birth defects. They include (but are not limited to) the oral form of **isotretinoin**, a medication used to treat serious, cystic acne; warfarin, a drug used to manage certain blood conditions; the antiseizure drugs valproic acid and carbamazepine; and angiotensin-converting enzyme inhibitors, which are used to treat some heart conditions and high blood pressure. For other prescription medications, the evidence about their effects during pregnancy is conflicting or not powerful enough to draw a clear conclusion. The web site Organization of Teratology Information Specialists (OTIS) as well as other organizations have information about the teratogenic potential of many common prescription medications (see the "Resources" section in this chapter).

It's important to tell your health care provider about any medications you are taking as soon as you find out you're pregnant. Even better, discuss your medications with your health care provider before you become pregnant so they can be adjusted or changed if needed. Take all containers of your prescription medications with you to your appointment.

If you are taking a medication to treat a health condition, do not stop taking it until you have talked with your health care provider. Although some medications may increase the risk of birth defects, the benefits of continuing to take the medication during pregnancy may outweigh any risk to your baby. For example, asthma is a long-lasting condition that can decrease the level of *oxygen* in your body as well as the amount of oxygen that reaches your baby. Uncontrolled asthma can lead to fetal growth problems and a smaller-than-normal baby. Problems with fetal growth also increase the risk of *preterm* birth, which in turn can lead to serious, sometimes lifelong, health problems for the baby. If you have severe, uncontrolled asthma, taking an oral **corticosteroid** may be the best course of action for you if other medications do not work.

These considerations also apply to mental illnesses, such as *depression*, and the medications used to treat them. If you are taking an *antidepressant* medication to manage depression and you become pregnant (or are thinking of becoming pregnant), you and your health care provider will need to discuss whether you should stop or continue your medication while you are pregnant. Sometimes, not taking an antidepressant can cause more problems during pregnancy than taking the medication. If your depression recurs, you may have trouble eating, sleeping, and getting exercise, all of which could affect your pregnancy.

As you can see by these examples, the decision to continue or stop taking a medication is a complex one and depends on several factors, such as the severity of your illness, whether you currently are having symptoms, and the information that is known about your medication's risk of causing birth defects. You and your health care provider should discuss all of these factors and weigh the risks and benefits. In some cases, it may be possible to decrease your dosage or to switch to another medication that is considered to be safer. In other cases, it may be recommended that you stop taking your medication. The most important point to remember is to consult your health care provider and not make these decisions on your own. The benefits of continuing to take the medication during pregnancy may outweigh any risk to your baby.

Pregnancy exposure registries are research studies that collect information from women who take prescription medications or vaccines while they're pregnant. If you do end up taking a prescription drug during pregnancy, you may want to enroll in one of these studies. By joining a registry, you can help researchers expand their knowledge about the safety of certain medications during pregnancy. See the "Resources" section in this chapter for more information. Registries also can provide you with information about the medications you need to take or may take before and during pregnancy.

### Over-the-Counter Medications

There are many medications that are available over the counter: pain relievers, laxatives, antacids, cold and allergy remedies, skin treatments, patches (heat wraps for pain relief), nasal sprays, and smoking cessation aids. Herbal medications and vitamin supplements also are available over the counter. Some over-the-counter drugs can cause problems during pregnancy. In addition, some over-the-counter medications can affect how your prescription medications work. Some of these interactions may have as-yet unknown effects on a developing baby.

Some of the concerns about herbal remedies and vitamins are related to the fact that the FDA considers them to be dietary supplements, not drugs. Manufacturers are required to conduct their own safety studies, but the FDA does not oversee this process. There also are no standards for purity or regulation of the ingredient amounts. For these reasons, it is best to avoid taking herbal supplements during pregnancy. However, you should take a daily prenatal vitamin supplement as recommended by your health care provider. If an additional amount of a vitamin or mineral has been recommended for you, such as iron or folic acid, take it as a single supplement; do not try to get these extra amounts by taking additional multivitamin supplements.

What should you do if you have a cold or indigestion and want to take an over-the-counter drug? Always talk to your health care provider before taking any over-the-counter medication. You may want to try relieving your symptoms without taking medicine. For example, drinking lots of water, putting a warm washcloth on your face, and using a humidifier to put moisture in the air can help with nasal congestion. For heartburn, try sitting up or standing to direct the acidic contents of your stomach downward. Your health care provider may suggest other ideas for you to try depending on your specific symptoms.

## Alcohol

Drinking alcohol during pregnancy is a leading cause of birth defects. There is no established safe level of alcohol use during pregnancy. Alcohol can affect a baby throughout pregnancy, including the first weeks of pregnancy, before many women even know they are pregnant.

"Fetal alcohol spectrum disorders" is a term that describes the different effects that can occur in the fetus when a woman drinks during pregnancy. These effects may include physical, mental, behavioral, and learning disabilities that can last a lifetime. The most severe disorder is **_fetal alcohol syndrome (FAS)_**. FAS causes growth problems, intellectual and behavioral problems, and abnormal facial features. Women at highest risk of giving birth to a child with FAS are those who drink heavily and who continue to drink heavily throughout pregnancy. But even moderate alcohol use during pregnancy can adversely affect a child's growth and development and lead to behavioral and learning problems.

All of these alcohol-related effects are 100% preventable by not drinking during pregnancy or before pregnancy. However, if you drank alcohol before you knew you were pregnant, there is no need to panic. Just stop consuming alcohol as soon as you realize that you are pregnant. It is unlikely that inadvertently drinking a small amount of alcohol very early in pregnancy will cause serious birth defects.

## Environmental Toxins

Current research suggests that almost every pregnant woman in the United States is exposed to at least 43 different chemicals. There is increasing evidence that exposure to some of these toxic agents in the environment before and during pregnancy may have lasting effects on reproductive health. Despite this growing body of evidence, there still is not much concrete information on which to base recommendations about what things to avoid and how to minimize your risk.

### Toxins in the Workplace

Workplace exposure to chemicals and other toxins may be a key concern for many women. Women who work in farming, factories, dry cleaners, electronics, or printing should be sure to talk about possible harmful agents with their health care providers. Some women who work in the health care field may be exposed to bloodborne **_pathogens_**, such as **_human immunodeficiency virus_** and **_hepatitis B virus (HBV)_**.

If you think you may be exposed to a harmful agent at work, also talk to your employer. The Occupational Safety and Health Act was enacted in 1970 to protect workers from unsafe and unhealthy conditions in the workplace. To oversee this effort, the law also created the Occupational Safety and Health Administration within the U.S. Department of Labor. Employers are responsible for placing warning labels on all potentially hazardous materials and for training workers who are at risk of occupational exposure to these materials. Employees are responsible for learning about the hazards in their workplace and for following the established guidelines for protecting themselves. Employers must issue appropriate protective equipment at no cost to employees whose job duties put them in contact with workplace hazards.

If you work in an environment that may expose you to HBV, your employer is required to provide the HBV vaccination free of charge. If a pregnant woman is infected with HBV, the fetus also can become infected (see Chapter 30, "Protecting Yourself From Infections," for more information about hepatitis B infection during pregnancy). The Centers for Disease Control and Prevention (CDC) and the American College of Obstetricians and Gynecologists recommend that pregnant women at risk of HBV infection during pregnancy be vaccinated. The vaccine does not contain a live virus and there is no risk that the fetus will become infected if you are vaccinated.

## Avoiding Known Environmental Toxins

There are steps that you can take to reduce your exposure to some of the known chemical teratogens during pregnancy. The federal government and other safety organizations have worked together to determine the best ways you can avoid the risks that the following agents might pose to your health and that of your unborn baby.

**Lead.** Although lead has been removed from paint and gasoline during the past 30 years, 1% of women who are of childbearing age still have unsafe levels of lead in their blood. Lead can be found in older homes, lead-glazed pottery, and imported cosmetics, and it still is used in some manufacturing jobs. Lead exposure during pregnancy has been linked to several pregnancy complications, including high blood pressure and preterm delivery. Prenatal lead exposure can interfere with the baby's normal brain development. It is not known how much lead is necessary to cause these effects.

The CDC has issued guidelines about testing for lead exposure in pregnant women (see the "Resources" section in this chapter). If you are at risk of lead exposure, the CDC recommends that you have a blood test to measure the level of lead in your body. This testing is not recommended for women who are not at risk of lead exposure. If you are found to high have levels of lead, the source of the exposure should be found so that you can avoid further contact. Often, avoidance of the lead source is enough to decrease the lead levels in your blood to a safe threshold. If you have a very high level of lead in your body, treatment with medication may be recommended.

Most women will not be exposed to high levels of lead. However, follow a few common-sense tips. Never eat nonfood items such as clay, paint, or soil because they could be contaminated with lead. Stay away from repair or remodeling work in homes built before 1978, and avoid hobbies that use lead glaze.

**Mercury.** Mercury can adversely affect the development of the nervous system in the fetus. Some of the effects linked to mercury exposure during pregnancy include learning difficulties, problems with thinking and reasoning, and language and motor skill problems. Fetal exposure to mercury can result from a pregnant woman eating certain fish, using alternative or traditional remedies containing mercury, or inhaling mercury vapors at work. The amount of mercury in fish varies, with some fish containing higher levels than others. Fish is a healthy food, and you should eat 8–12 ounces (two to three servings) per week to get the benefits of omega-3 fatty acids, which may help your baby's brain development. To decrease your exposure to mercury in fish, follow these guidelines:

- Avoid eating fish that are known to have high mercury levels, such as shark, swordfish, king mackerel, and tilefish. Instead, plan meals that use healthy fish, such as salmon, tilapia, and shrimp, at least twice a week.

- Albacore tuna has higher levels of mercury than canned light tuna and should be limited to no more than 6 ounces a week.

- Check local advisories about the safety of fish caught in local waters. If there is no information available, limit your intake of fish from these waters to no more than 6 ounces a week (and do not eat any other fish during that week).

For more information about mercury and fish, see the web sites listed in the "Resources" section in this chapter.

**Pesticides.** Pesticides are chemicals used to kill bugs, weeds, rodents, and mold. More than 1 billion pounds of pesticides are used in the United States each year. You can be exposed to pesticides from eating fruits or vegetables and from using chemicals in your home or on your pets. Exposure during pregnancy can cause poor brain development in the baby, low IQ, and childhood leukemia. Do not use pesticides in your home and don't buy chemical tick and flea collars or dips for your pets. Wash all fruits and vegetables before you eat them.

## Other Potential Hazards

Many women have questions about other potential hazards. A few of these concerns are addressed in this section. The "Resources" section in this chapter gives recommendations about additional sources of information for other agents not covered in this chapter.

### X-Rays

Ionizing radiation is the type of radiation used in X-rays. There is a mistaken belief that any exposure to ionizing radiation will cause birth defects. This is not true. The risk of birth defects caused by radiation is related to the dose. The higher the dose of radiation, the higher the risk of birth defects. The amount of radiation used in a standard X-ray is well below the level needed to threaten the well-being of a developing fetus. If you do need an X-ray or other type of imaging test while you are pregnant, it is safe to do so provided that certain guidelines are followed:

- The lowest dose of radiation is used (this guideline applies to everyone, not just pregnant women).

- If you need an X-ray that doesn't involve your pelvis, your uterus will be shielded from radiation with a special cover.

- If you have a condition for which multiple X-rays are needed, **magnetic resonance imaging (MRI)** may be preferable to X-ray imaging because it does not use radiation.

- Radioisotopes—chemicals that give off radiation—are not hazardous to the fetus when used in certain diagnostic tests. Radioisotope imaging often is used to diagnose thyroid disease. The amount of radiation given off by radioisotopes in these diagnostic tests is low. However, the use of iodine-131 for the treatment of Graves disease, a thyroid disorder, should be avoided. High doses of iodine 131 can cause defects in the fetal thyroid gland.

- **Contrast agents** (substances that are injected into the body during some X-ray or MRI procedures to make certain organs or other structures more visible) are not likely to be harmful to the fetus. There is some concern about contrast agents that contain iodine. In theory, these agents can damage the fetus's thyroid gland. It's recommended that these agents be used during pregnancy only if the potential benefit justifies the potential risk to the fetus. All infants are screened for thyroid problems soon after birth.

### Elevated Core Body Temperature

There is some evidence that an increase in body temperature during pregnancy is associated with birth defects. For this reason, it is reasonable to try to avoid prolonged exposure to saunas (no more than 15 minutes) and hot tubs (no more than 10 minutes). In addition, it is best to ensure that your head, arms, shoulders, and upper chest are not under the water while you are in a hot tub so that less of your body surface area is exposed to heat.

## If You Have Questions

If you have questions that pertain to your specific situation, don't hesitate to ask your health care provider. If he or she does not know the answer, you can be referred to someone who does. Remember, though, that not all birth defects can be prevented. Still, it makes sense to do all that you can to maximize your chances for a healthy pregnancy by avoiding known risks.

---

# RESOURCES

The following resources offer more information about medications, toxins, and other agents and their potential effects on pregnancy:

**Food and Drug Administration Pregnancy Registries**
Food and Drug Administration Office of Women's Health
www.fda.gov/ScienceResearch/SpecialTopics/WomensHealthResearch/ucm251314.htm
10903 New Hampshire Avenue
WO32-2333
Silver Spring, MD 20993
301-796-9440
Fax: 301-847-8604

*Provides information about the various pregnancy registries being conducted throughout the United States and gives guidelines for joining a registry.*

**Lead and Pregnancy**
Centers for Disease Control and Prevention
www.cdc.gov/nceh/lead/publications/leadandpregnancy2010.pdf
*Discusses guidelines for testing for lead exposure in pregnant women.*

**Motherisk**
The Hospital for Sick Children—Toronto
www.motherisk.org
1-877-439-2744
*Provides information about the risk or safety of prescription and over-the-counter drugs, herbal products, chemicals, X-rays, chronic disease and infections, and everyday exposures during pregnancy and while breastfeeding and maintains helplines for you to call and ask Motherisk counselors specific questions.*

**MotherToBaby**
Organization of Teratology Information Specialists (OTIS)
www.mothertobaby.org
(866) 626-6847
*MotherToBaby is dedicated to providing the latest information to mothers, health care professionals, and the general public about medications and other exposures during pregnancy and while breastfeeding.*

**Occupational Safety and Health Administration (OSHA)**
www.osha.gov
200 Constitution Avenue NW
Washington, DC 20210
800-321-6742
877-889-5627 (TTY)
*Prevents work-related injuries, illnesses, and deaths by enforcing laws designed to protect workers' health and safety.*

# Part V
# Medical Problems
# During Pregnancy

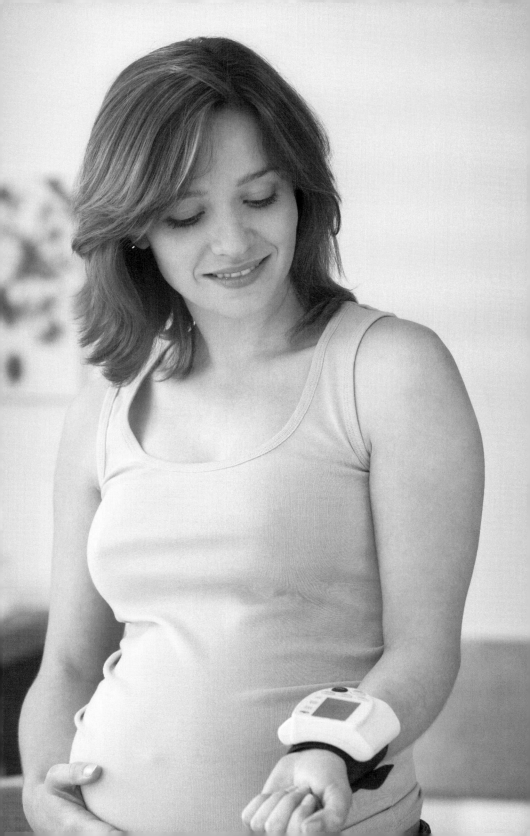

# Chapter 22

# Hypertension and Preeclampsia

**Hypertension**, or **high blood pressure**, can lead to health problems at any time in life. Hypertension is a "silent disease" because it does not in itself cause symptoms. During pregnancy, severe or uncontrolled hypertension can cause complications for both you and your baby. Some women already have hypertension when they become pregnant. Others develop it for the first time during pregnancy. A serious high blood pressure disorder called **preeclampsia** also can occur during pregnancy or soon after childbirth.

High blood pressure that occurs during pregnancy is classified as either **chronic hypertension** or **gestational hypertension**. The type you have depends on whether the high blood pressure was present before pregnancy and whether it goes away after pregnancy. No matter when high blood pressure occurs, it usually happens without causing any signs or symptoms. Having your blood pressure checked regularly is one reason why seeing your health care provider during pregnancy is so important.

## Blood Pressure

Each time the heart contracts (squeezes), it pumps blood into blood vessels called arteries. The arteries carry the blood to the body's organs. Other blood vessels called veins return the blood to the heart. Blood pressure is the pressure of the blood against the vessel walls.

To measure your blood pressure, a cuff with a balloon inside is wrapped around your upper arm. Air is pumped into the balloon and the cuff tightens.

Blood pressure is expressed in "millimeters of mercury" (mm Hg) because the original blood pressure meters used a column of mercury to measure pressure.

A blood pressure reading has two numbers separated by a slash. A blood pressure reading of 110/80 mm Hg, for instance, is referred to as "110 over 80." The first number is the pressure against the artery walls when the heart contracts. This is called the *systolic blood pressure*. The second number is the pressure against the artery walls when the heart relaxes between contractions. This is called the *diastolic blood pressure*.

Your health care provider will check your blood pressure at each prenatal care visit. Blood pressure changes often during the day. It can increase if you are excited or when you exercise. It can decrease when you are resting. These short-term changes in blood pressure are normal. Because of the normal ups and downs in blood pressure, if you have one high reading, another reading may be taken a little later to confirm the result.

## Chronic Hypertension

Chronic hypertension is hypertension that was present before a woman became pregnant or that occurs in the first half of pregnancy (before 20 weeks of pregnancy). If you were taking blood pressure medication before you became pregnant—even if your blood pressure is normal—you have chronic hypertension. Chronic hypertension can be mild to moderate or severe. Mild-to-moderate hypertension is defined as a systolic blood pressure of 140–159, a diastolic blood pressure of 90–109, or both. Severe hypertension is defined as a systolic blood pressure of 160 or greater, a diastolic blood pressure of 110 or greater, or both.

### Risks

Chronic hypertension increases the risks of complications for both the woman and her baby. With mild hypertension, the risk of complications is small. With severe hypertension, the risk is greater.

During pregnancy, a woman's body makes more blood to help the baby grow. If blood pressure increases, it can place extra stress on her heart and *kidneys*. This can lead to heart disease, *kidney disease*, and stroke.

High blood pressure can reduce blood flow to the *placenta*. As a result, the baby may receive fewer of the *nutrients* and less of the *oxygen* he or she needs to grow and function. This can lead to a condition called fetal growth restriction, in which the baby does not grow normally.

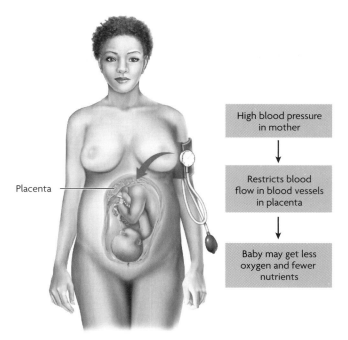

Placenta

High blood pressure in mother

↓

Restricts blood flow in blood vessels in placenta

↓

Baby may get less oxygen and fewer nutrients

**Hypertension.** Hypertension during pregnancy can decrease the amount of oxygen and nutrients the baby receives.

Other risks of high blood pressure during pregnancy include the following:

- Preeclampsia—This condition is more likely to occur in women with chronic high blood pressure than in women with normal blood pressure.

- *Preterm* delivery—If the placenta is not providing enough nutrients and oxygen to the baby, it may be decided that early delivery is better for the baby than allowing the pregnancy to continue. Early delivery also may be needed to prevent further complications for the pregnant woman.

- *Placental abruption*—This condition, in which the placenta prematurely detaches from the wall of the uterus, is a medical emergency that requires immediate treatment.

- *Cesarean delivery*—Women with hypertension are more likely to have a cesarean delivery than women with normal blood pressure. A cesarean delivery may be needed if the baby is very small or if there are other complications. Cesarean delivery carries risks of infection, injury to internal organs, and bleeding. It also can affect the way that a woman gives birth later on if she decides to have more children.

## Treatment

Treatment depends on whether your hypertension is mild or severe. In the first half of pregnancy, blood pressure normally decreases as your body's circulatory system expands to supply the developing baby with oxygen and nutrients. If your hypertension is mild, your blood pressure may stay that way or even return to normal during pregnancy. Your health care provider may decide to decrease your medication dosage or advise you to stop taking your medication during pregnancy. If you have severe hypertension or have health problems related to your hypertension, you may need to start or continue taking blood pressure medication during pregnancy.

Whether your hypertension is mild or severe, your blood pressure will be monitored closely throughout pregnancy. You may need to monitor your blood pressure at home. **Ultrasound exams** may be done throughout pregnancy to track fetal growth. If fetal growth problems are suspected, you may have additional tests that monitor the health of the baby. This testing usually begins in the third trimester of pregnancy.

If your condition remains stable, early delivery of the baby (before 39 weeks of pregnancy) usually is not necessary. If complications develop, it may be necessary to deliver the baby early. After delivery, you will need to continue to monitor your blood pressure. Blood pressure often increases in the weeks after childbirth. You may need to go back to taking your medication, or your medication dosage may need to be adjusted. Many blood pressure medications are safe for women who are breastfeeding.

## Gestational Hypertension

When high blood pressure first occurs in the second half (after 20 weeks) of pregnancy, it is called gestational hypertension. Most women with gestational hypertension have only a mild increase in blood pressure. Some women, however, develop severe hypertension and are at risk of serious complications. All women with gestational hypertension are monitored frequently for signs of preeclampsia and to make sure that their blood pressure does not go too high.

Although gestational hypertension usually goes away after childbirth, it may increase the risk of developing hypertension in the future. If you had gestational hypertension, it is important to keep this risk in mind as you make decisions about your health. Healthy eating, weight loss, and exercise all have been shown to be helpful in preventing high blood pressure.

## Preeclampsia

Preeclampsia is a serious blood pressure disorder that can affect all of the organs in a woman's body. It usually occurs after 20 weeks of pregnancy, typically in the third trimester. When it occurs before 32 weeks of pregnancy, it is called early-onset preeclampsia. It also can occur in the postpartum period. Rarely, it can occur before 20 weeks of pregnancy.

It is not clear why some women develop preeclampsia. The risk of developing preeclampsia is increased in women who

- are pregnant for the first time
- have had preeclampsia in a previous pregnancy or have a family history of preeclampsia
- have a history of chronic hypertension, kidney disease, or both
- are 40 years or older
- are carrying more than one baby
- have certain medical conditions, such as *diabetes mellitus*, thrombophilia, or *lupus*
- are obese
- had *in vitro fertilization*

### Risks

Preeclampsia is a leading cause of death worldwide for women and infants. Preeclampsia that causes seizures is a condition called *eclampsia*. It also can cause *HELLP syndrome*. HELLP stands for *hemolysis*, elevated *liver enzymes*, and low *platelet* count. In this condition, red blood cells are damaged or destroyed, blood clotting is impaired, and the liver can bleed internally, causing chest or abdominal pain. HELLP syndrome is a medical emergency. Women can die from HELLP or have lifelong health problems as a result of the condition.

When preeclampsia occurs during pregnancy, the baby may need to be delivered right away, even if he or she is not fully grown. Preterm babies have an increased risk of serious complications, such as breathing problems, problems with eating or staying warm, or vision or hearing problems. Some preterm complications last a lifetime and require ongoing medical care. Babies born very early also may die.

Women who have had preeclampsia—especially those whose babies were born preterm—have an increased risk later in life of cardiovascular disease and kidney disease, including heart attack, stroke, and high blood pressure. Also, having preeclampsia once increases the risk of having it again in a future pregnancy.

## Signs and Symptoms

Preeclampsia can develop quietly without you being aware of it. When symptoms do occur, they can be confused with normal symptoms of pregnancy (see box "Signs and Symptoms of Preeclampsia"). A woman has preeclampsia when she has high blood pressure and other signs that her organ systems are not working normally. One of these signs is **proteinuria** (an abnormal amount of protein in the urine). A woman with preeclampsia whose condition is worsening will develop other signs and symptoms known as "severe features." These include a low number of platelets in the blood, abnormal kidney or liver function, pain over the upper abdomen, changes in vision, fluid in the lungs, or a severe headache. If the systolic blood pressure is 160 mm Hg or higher or the diastolic blood pressure 110 mm Hg or higher, this also is considered a severe feature.

## Diagnosis

A high blood pressure reading may be the first sign of preeclampsia. If your blood pressure measurement reading is high, a repeat blood pressure measurement may be done to confirm the results. You will have a urine test to

## Signs and Symptoms of Preeclampsia

If you have any of the following symptoms, especially if they occur in the second half of pregnancy, you should contact your health care provider right away:

- Swelling of face or hands
- A headache that will not go away
- Seeing spots or changes in eyesight
- Pain in the upper abdomen or shoulder
- Nausea and vomiting (in the second half of pregnancy)
- Sudden weight gain
- Difficulty breathing

check for protein. If you are diagnosed with preeclampsia, you may have tests to check how your liver and kidneys are working and to measure the number of platelets in your blood. You also will be asked whether you have any of the symptoms of preeclampsia.

## Treatment

Based on your test results, your health care provider will discuss a course of treatment with you. The goal of treatment is to limit complications for you and to deliver the healthiest baby possible.

**Management of Mild Gestational Hypertension or Preeclampsia Without Severe Features.** Treatment of mild gestational hypertension or preeclampsia without severe features may take place either in a hospital or on an outpatient basis (you can stay at home with close monitoring by your health care provider). If you are treated at home, strict bed rest usually is not necessary, but you may be advised to limit heavy physical or other stressful activities. You may be asked to keep track of fetal movement by doing a daily kick count and to measure your blood pressure at home. You will need to see your health care provider at least weekly and sometimes twice weekly. At these visits, the following tests may be done:

- Blood pressure measurement

- Blood tests to check your liver and kidney function and platelet counts

- **Nonstress test** to check the baby's general well-being

- Ultrasound exam to track fetal growth and to measure the amount of **amniotic fluid**

Once you reach 37 weeks of pregnancy, it may be recommended that you have your baby. Labor may need to be induced (started with medications). If test results show that the baby is not doing well, you may need to have the baby earlier. Preeclampsia does not mean that you cannot have a vaginal delivery. If you have problems during labor or if there are problems with the baby, you may have a cesarean delivery.

**Management of Preeclampsia With Severe Features.** If you have preeclampsia with severe features, you most likely will be treated in the hospital. If you are at least 34 weeks pregnant, it often is recommended that you have your baby as soon as your condition is stable. If you are fewer than 34 weeks pregnant and your condition is stable, it may be possible to wait to deliver your baby. Delaying delivery for just a few days can be helpful in some cases because it allows time for certain medications to be given and other arrangements to be made that may reduce your baby's risk of some of the complications of being born preterm. You may be transferred to a hospital with a special high-risk maternity unit and a high-level *neonatal intensive care unit*. These units are specially equipped and have doctors and nurses with advanced training and experience in caring for complicated pregnancies and preterm babies. *Corticosteroids* may be given to help the baby's lungs mature, and you most likely will be given medications to help reduce your blood pressure and to help prevent seizures. If your or the baby's condition worsens, prompt delivery is needed.

## Prevention

Currently, there is no screening test that can predict whether a woman will develop preeclampsia during pregnancy. For now, prevention involves identifying whether you have risk factors for preeclampsia and taking steps to address these factors.

### Preconception Care

Ideally, if you have had chronic hypertension for several years, you should see your health care provider before becoming pregnant. The purpose of this prepregnancy evaluation is to determine whether your hypertension is under control and whether it has affected your health. You also should learn about the signs and symptoms of preeclampsia so that you can watch out for them.

Because hypertension may affect the heart and kidneys, you may be given tests to check the function of these organs. The information gained from these tests is used to assess the risks of pregnancy on your future health. If you have severe hypertension, you may be at risk of serious complications during pregnancy, such as kidney or heart failure. However, most pregnant women with mild chronic hypertension have perfectly normal pregnancies without any long-term problems.

In addition to tests, you and your health care provider can discuss steps that you can take to help make your pregnancy safer. The goal of these actions is to lower your blood pressure before pregnancy:

- If you are overweight, lose weight through diet and exercise.
- Take your blood pressure medication as prescribed.
- Stop smoking.

If you have had preeclampsia in a prior pregnancy, a ***preconception care*** visit allows you and your health care provider to identify factors that may increase the risk of recurrence and to discuss a plan to achieve the best possible health before pregnancy. If you are overweight, weight loss usually is advised before pregnancy. If you have a medical condition such as diabetes, it usually is recommended that your condition be well controlled before you become pregnant.

### Aspirin Therapy

Low-dose aspirin therapy has shown some promise in reducing the risk of preeclampsia in women at high risk. Taking low doses of aspirin beginning late in the first trimester may be recommended if you had preeclampsia in more than one pregnancy or if you have had early-onset preeclampsia and a preterm delivery at less than 34 weeks of pregnancy. Although no immediate safety concerns have been found with this type of aspirin therapy, information about its long-term safety is lacking. It is best to follow the standard advice to talk with your health care provider before taking any medication during pregnancy.

# RESOURCES

The following resources offer more information about hypertension and preeclampsia:

**High Blood Pressure During Pregnancy**
National Heart, Lung, and Blood Institute
www.nhlbi.nih.gov/health/resources/heart/hbp-pregnancy
*Information about the diagnosis and management of high blood pressure during pregnancy.*

**Preeclampsia and Hypertension in Pregnancy: Resource Overview**
The American College of Obstetricians and Gynecologists
http://www.acog.org.Womens-Health/Preeclampsia-and-Hypertension-in-Pregnancy
*Lists ACOG's articles and patient education resources on high blood pressure disorders that occur during pregnancy.*

**Preeclampsia Foundation**
www.preeclampsia.org
*National organization dedicated to preeclampsia education, advocacy, and research.*

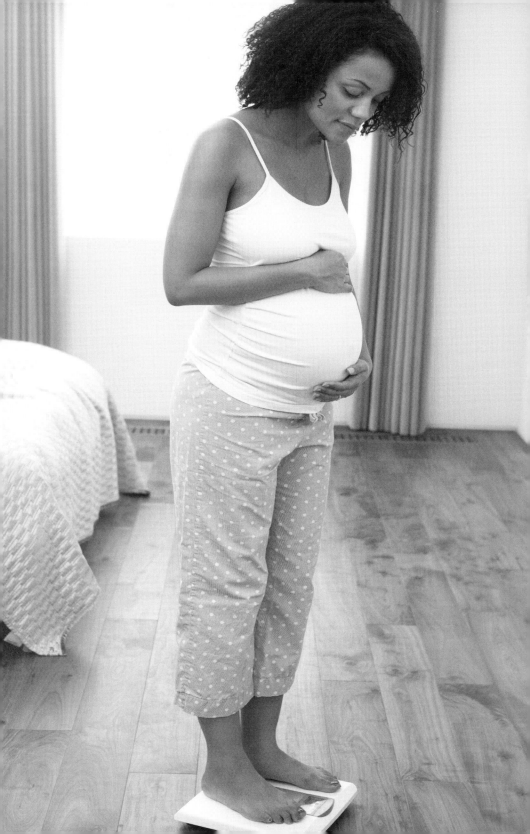

# Chapter 23

# Diabetes Mellitus

***Diabetes mellitus*** is a disease in which the body either does not make enough ***insulin*** or is not able use insulin properly. Insulin is a hormone that is made by the pancreas. It moves ***glucose***, the body's main type of fuel, into ***cells*** where it can be turned into energy. When the body does not make enough insulin or when the body's cells are resistant to its effects, glucose cannot get into cells and instead stays in the blood. This causes higher than normal blood glucose levels. Over time, high glucose levels can damage the heart, eyes, ***kidneys***, and other organs.

There are three types of diabetes mellitus: type 1 diabetes mellitus, type 2 diabetes mellitus, and ***gestational diabetes mellitus***. In type 1 diabetes mellitus, the body makes little or no insulin on its own. In type 2 diabetes mellitus, the body makes enough insulin but the body's cells are insulin resistant. It takes more than the normal amount of insulin to manage the blood glucose level. Gestational diabetes mellitus is diabetes mellitus that is diagnosed during pregnancy.

## Gestational Diabetes Mellitus

During pregnancy, a woman's cells naturally become more resistant to insulin's effects. This change increases the mother's blood glucose level to make more ***nutrients*** available to the baby. To keep the blood glucose level in the normal range, the mother's body needs to make more insulin. About 5% of women are unable to produce enough insulin to maintain a normal blood glucose level. These women develop gestational diabetes.

For most women, gestational diabetes goes away after childbirth, but they remain at increased risk of having diabetes later in life. Some women with gestational diabetes may have had mild diabetes before pregnancy that was not diagnosed. For these women, diabetes will be a lifelong condition.

### Risk Factors

Several risk factors are linked to gestational diabetes. It also can occur in women who have no risk factors. But it is more likely in women who

- are older than 25 years

- are overweight

- have had gestational diabetes before

- have had a very large baby

- have a close relative with diabetes

- have had a **stillbirth** in a previous pregnancy

- are African American, American Indian, Asian American, Hispanic, Latina, or Pacific Islander

### How Gestational Diabetes Can Affect You and Your Baby

If gestational diabetes is not treated, it can increase the risk of certain problems for mother and baby. It increases the risk of having a very large baby (a condition called **macrosomia**) and **cesarean birth**. High blood pressure and **preeclampsia** are more common in women with gestational diabetes. Babies born to mothers with gestational diabetes may have problems with breathing, low glucose levels, and **jaundice**.

Women who have had gestational diabetes are at higher risk of having diabetes in the future, as are their children. Regular testing for diabetes after pregnancy is recommended for these women. Their children also will need to be monitored for diabetes risks (see "Care After Pregnancy" later in this section).

### Testing for Gestational Diabetes

All pregnant women should be screened for gestational diabetes. Your health care provider may perform this screening by asking about your medical history, determining whether you have risk factors, or testing your blood

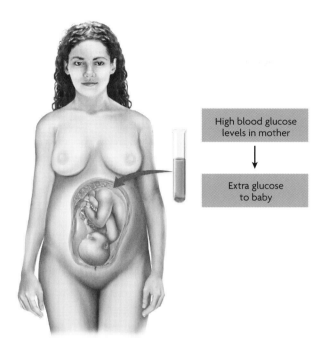

High blood glucose
levels in mother

↓

Extra glucose
to baby

**Diabetes during pregnancy.** During pregnancy, high blood glucose levels can cause the developing baby to receive too much glucose. As a result, the baby can grow too large.

glucose levels. If you have certain risk factors for gestational diabetes, such as gestational diabetes in a previous pregnancy, obesity, or prediabetes (a higher than normal blood glucose level that has not yet reached the range for diabetes), your blood glucose level is measured early in pregnancy. If you do not have risk factors, your blood glucose level may be measured between 24 weeks and 28 weeks of pregnancy.

The test is safe and simple. In the most commonly used test, you first drink a sugary drink. A blood sample is taken 1 hour later. If the level of glucose is high, you will have another, similar test in which several blood samples are taken to confirm the result.

## Controlling Gestational Diabetes

Studies show that treating gestational diabetes can greatly reduce the risk of complications for you and your baby. Treatment can reduce the risk of macrosomia and the birth injuries that can result from it. The rates of ***preeclampsia*** and other ***high blood pressure*** disorders also decrease when women keep their blood glucose levels under control.

Treatment involves several things. If you are diagnosed with gestational diabetes, you will need more frequent *prenatal care* visits to monitor your health and your baby's health. You will need to keep your blood glucose level under control. This may require eating healthy foods, exercising regularly, daily testing of glucose levels, and sometimes, taking medications.

Your health care provider may recommend that you see a diabetes educator or a dietitian. A diabetes educator is a health care provider who teaches people how to live with diabetes. A dietitian (nutritionist) is an expert in nutrition and meal planning. Later in pregnancy, special tests of the baby's growth and well-being may be done. You are more likely to have these tests if your gestational diabetes is not well controlled, you need to take medications, or you develop problems.

**Tracking Glucose Levels.** Checking your glucose level is an important part of keeping it within the normal range. For the best results, follow the schedule your health care provider gives you.

A glucose meter is used to test glucose levels. This device tests a small drop of blood. Keep a glucose level log and bring it with you to each prenatal visit. In some cases, glucose logs also can be kept online and e-mailed to your health care provider.

**Healthy Eating.** A balanced diet is a key part of any pregnancy. Your baby depends on the food you eat for growth and nourishment. Healthy eating is even more important if you have diabetes. Women with gestational diabetes have special dietary needs. Not eating properly can cause glucose levels to go too high or too low.

If you have gestational diabetes, you will need to eat regular meals throughout the day. You may need to eat small snacks as well, especially in the evening. Eating regularly helps avoid blood glucose levels that are too high or too low. So does limiting the amount of carbohydrates you eat and avoiding certain foods that are high in sugars. Carbohydrates are sugars and starches. Eating a lot of carbohydrates can increase the level of glucose in the blood. Some experts recommend limiting carbohydrates to 33–40% of your total calories, with the balance divided between protein (20%) and fat (40%). Eating more complex carbohydrates (foods that are high in starch or fiber) rather than simple carbohydrates (sugary foods) also may help you control your blood glucose levels.

The number of calories needed daily during pregnancy depends on your prepregnancy weight, stage of pregnancy, and level of activity. It is important to gain the recommended amount of weight but not gain too much. Gaining too much weight during pregnancy may be especially problematic for a woman with gestational diabetes. Excess weight or weight gained too quickly can make the body even less responsive to insulin and make it harder to keep blood glucose levels under control.

A dietitian can help you plan your meals to make sure you are getting the recommended amounts of nutrients. You will be asked to keep a log of what you eat. Changes may be made to your diet to improve glucose control or to meet the needs of your growing baby.

**Exercise.** For all pregnant women, but especially for those with diabetes, exercise is important. Exercise helps keep glucose levels in the normal range. In general, 30 minutes of moderate exercise on most days of the week is recommended. Examples of moderate exercise include brisk walking, swimming, or stationary biking. If you have never exercised before, you should not begin an exercise program without discussing it with your health care provider.

**Medications.** Gestational diabetes often can be controlled with diet and exercise. If diet and exercise are not enough, medication may be needed to control blood glucose levels. Some women may take oral medications; others may need insulin. Insulin is a drug that is injected. Your health care provider or diabetes educator will teach you how to give yourself insulin shots if you need them.

If you are prescribed medications, you need to keep monitoring your blood glucose level as recommended by your health care provider. Your health care provider will review your glucose log to make sure that the medication is working. Because your body becomes more resistant to insulin as your pregnancy grows, changes to your medications likely will be needed to help keep your blood glucose level in the normal range.

Insulin is considered a very safe drug to use during pregnancy because it does not cross the *placenta*. Most oral diabetes medications also are considered safe, although there is some evidence that they can cross the placenta. No short-term effects on babies have been noted, but long-term effects have not been studied.

## Special Tests

If you have diabetes during your pregnancy, you may need special tests to check the well-being of the baby. These tests can help your health care provider detect possible problems and take steps to manage them. They may include fetal movement counting (sometimes called "kick counts"), *nonstress test*, *biophysical profile*, and *contraction stress test*. These tests are discussed in detail in Chapter 26, "Testing to Monitor Fetal Well-Being."

Your baby's growth and the amniotic fluid level around the baby also may be tracked throughout your pregnancy with **ultrasound exams**.

### Labor and Delivery

Most women with gestational diabetes are able to have a vaginal birth, but they are more likely to have a cesarean birth to prevent delivery problems than women without diabetes. Labor also may be induced (started by drugs or other means) earlier than the due date.

### Care After Pregnancy

Gestational diabetes is not just a problem during pregnancy. It greatly increases your risk of developing diabetes after you have your baby. One third of women who had gestational diabetes will have diabetes or a milder form called insulin resistance soon after giving birth. Within 25 years of giving birth, about one half of women who had gestational diabetes will develop diabetes. Children of women who had gestational diabetes may be at risk of becoming overweight or obese during childhood. They also have a higher risk of developing diabetes.

If you have had gestational diabetes, you should get regular tests for diabetes after pregnancy. You should have a test for diabetes 6–12 weeks after you give birth. If your postpartum glucose test result is normal, you need to be tested for diabetes every 3 years. Be sure to tell all of your health care providers that you have had gestational diabetes so that you continue your regularly scheduled tests. Your baby also should be checked throughout childhood for insulin resistance and other risk factors for diabetes, such as obesity.

Breastfeeding is the best way to feed your baby. It also can help with postpartum weight loss. As your child gets older, a healthy lifestyle may be helpful in preventing diabetes. Maintaining a healthy weight, eating a balanced diet, and staying active may decrease your risk of getting diabetes in the future.

## Pregestational Diabetes Mellitus

If you have type 1 or type 2 diabetes mellitus before you become pregnant, it is known as pregestational diabetes mellitus. About 1 in 100 pregnant women have this condition.

## Risks to Your Pregnancy

Women with poorly controlled pregestational diabetes are at risk of several pregnancy complications. However, the risk of developing the following complications can be reduced significantly if a woman controls her blood glucose levels before and during pregnancy:

- *Birth defects*—High blood glucose levels early in pregnancy increase the risk of birth defects, most often involving the heart, brain, and skeleton.

- *Miscarriage* and stillbirth—Both miscarriage and stillbirth are more common in pregnant women with poorly controlled diabetes.

- *Hydramnios*—Hydramnios is a condition in which there is too much *amniotic fluid* in the *amniotic sac* that surrounds the baby. It can lead to *preterm* labor and delivery.

- Preeclampsia

- Macrosomia

- *Respiratory distress syndrome*—This syndrome can make it harder for the baby to breathe after birth. The risk of respiratory distress syndrome is greater in babies whose mothers have diabetes.

## Preconception Care

If you have diabetes and are planning to become pregnant, it is important to see your health care provider for a *preconception* visit. It is recommended that you get your blood glucose level under control before you become pregnant (if it is not already under control). Having a stable glucose level is important because some of the birth defects caused by high glucose levels happen when the baby's organs are developing in the first 8 weeks of pregnancy— before you may know you are pregnant. Getting your glucose level under control may require changing your medications, diet, and exercise program.

In addition to keeping your glucose level in the normal range, preconception care also allows you to do the following:

- Get treatment for any medical problems that you may have because of your diabetes, such as high blood pressure, heart disease, *kidney disease*, and eye problems.

- Learn how to lose weight before pregnancy, if necessary, through a healthy diet and exercise.

- Start taking a multivitamin or prenatal vitamin supplement containing at least 400 micrograms of folic acid to help prevent neural tube defects.

## Controlling Your Diabetes During Pregnancy

Managing your diabetes while you are pregnant is a must. You can control your glucose levels with a combination of eating right, exercising, and taking medications as directed by your health care provider.

Women with diabetes need to see their health care providers more often than other pregnant women. Your health care provider will schedule frequent prenatal visits to check your glucose level and for other tests.

**Tracking Glucose Levels.** Many women with diabetes who have never been pregnant are surprised at how low the recommended blood glucose level is for pregnancy. Your health care provider likely will recommend that you check your blood glucose level several times a day to make sure it is in the normal range. Keep a log that lists your glucose levels with the time of day and share your log with your health care provider at each prenatal visit.

A blood test that measures hemoglobin $A_{1C}$ may be used to track your progress. This test result gives an estimate of how well your blood glucose level has been controlled during the past 4–6 weeks. Your hemoglobin $A_{1C}$ should not be higher than 6%.

Be aware that even with careful monitoring, women with diabetes are more likely to have low blood glucose levels, known as hypoglycemia, when they are pregnant. Hypoglycemia can occur if you do not eat enough food, skip a meal, do not eat at the right time of day, or exercise too much. Signs and symptoms of hypoglycemia include the following:

- Dizziness
- Feeling shaky
- Sudden hunger
- Sweating
- Weakness

If you think you are having symptoms of hypoglycemia, check your blood glucose level right away. If it is below 60 mg/dL, eat or drink something, such as a glass of milk, a few crackers, or special glucose tablets. Make sure your family members know what to give you as well. If you have repeated low glucose values, your caregiver may prescribe a glucagon pen. This device allows you to inject yourself with glucagon, a substance that causes glucose to be released into the bloodstream.

Your blood glucose level also can go too high despite treatment, which is called hyperglycemia. When your glucose level is too high, your body might make substances called ketones that can be harmful to your baby. Hyperglycemia can happen if you don't take your medicine at the recommended times, eat more food than usual or eat at irregular times, are sick, or are less active than normal. If you have hyperglycemia, talk to your health care provider. You may need to change your diet, exercise routine, or medications.

**Healthy Eating.** Eating a well-balanced, healthy diet is a critical part of any pregnancy because your baby depends on the food you eat for its growth and nourishment. In women with diabetes, diet is even more important. Not eating properly can cause your glucose level to go too high or too low. Your health care provider may recommend that you see a dietitian or diabetes educator to help with planning your meals. In most cases, your meal plan will include eating several small meals and snacks throughout the day and before bedtime.

**Exercise.** Another key part of a healthy pregnancy is exercise. Exercise helps keep your glucose level in the normal range and has many other benefits, including controlling your weight; boosting your energy; aiding sleep; and reducing backaches, constipation, and bloating. Work with your health care provider to decide what type and how much exercise is right for you. It is best to aim for at least 30 minutes of exercise on most days of the week.

**Medications.** If you took insulin before pregnancy to control your diabetes, your insulin dosage usually will increase while you are pregnant. Insulin is safe to use during pregnancy and does not cause birth defects. If you used an insulin pump before you became pregnant, you probably will be able to continue using the pump. Sometimes, however, you may need to switch to insulin shots. If you normally manage your diabetes with oral medications, your health care provider may suggest a change in your dosage or that you take insulin while you are pregnant.

## Special Tests

As your pregnancy progresses, your health care provider will likely order special tests to check the size and well-being of the baby, and the amniotic fluid around the baby. These tests can help your health care provider detect possible problems and take steps to manage them. See Chapter 26,

"Testing to Monitor Fetal Well-Being," for more information about these special tests.

## Labor and Delivery

Your health care provider will discuss the timing of your delivery with you. You may go into labor naturally. If problems with the pregnancy arise, labor may be induced (started by drugs or other means) earlier than the due date. A cesarean delivery may be necessary if the baby is very large.

While you are in labor, your glucose level will be monitored closely—typically every hour initially. If needed, you may receive insulin through an **intravenous (IV) line**. If you use an insulin pump, you might use it during labor. Women who use insulin pumps will need to work with their medical team throughout labor to monitor glucose levels and adjust the pump settings.

## Care After Pregnancy

Experts highly recommend breastfeeding for women with diabetes. Breast-feeding gives the baby the best nutrition to stay healthy, and it is good for the mother as well. It helps new mothers shed the extra weight that they may have gained during pregnancy and causes the uterus to return to its prepregnancy size more quickly.

If you breastfeed, you will need to eat extra calories every day. Talk to your health care provider about the amount and types of foods that can give you these extra calories. Eating small snacks during the day may be helpful.

You will need to closely monitor your blood glucose level after delivery. This is essential in determining your ongoing need for medication or deciding the best medication dosage. Most women who took insulin before pregnancy are able to go back to their prepregnancy insulin dosage soon after birth.

Before you and your partner start having sex again, it is important to choose a birth control method to avoid an unplanned pregnancy. Talk with your health care provider—preferably before you have your baby—about which method of birth control you plan to use after the baby is born. You also should discuss how long to plan between pregnancies.

# RESOURCES

The following resources offer more information about gestational diabetes and pregestational diabetes:

**Gestational Diabetes: Resource Overview**
The American College of Obstetricians and Gynecologists (ACOG)
http://www.acog.org/Womens-Health/Gestational-Diabetes
*Lists ACOG's articles and patient education resources on gestational diabetes.*

**Pregnancy for Women With Diabetes**
www.diabetes.org/living-with-diabetes/complications/pregnancy/
American Diabetes Association
1701 North Beauregard Street
Alexandria, VA 22311
Phone: 800-DIABETES (800-342-2383)
*Main web site for diabetes information; provides basic facts as well as information about pregestational diabetes and gestational diabetes.*

**What I Need to Know About Preparing for Pregnancy if I Have Diabetes**
National Diabetes Information Clearinghouse/National Institute of Diabetes and Digestive and Kidney Diseases
http://diabetes.niddk.nih.gov/dm/pubs/pregnancy/
*Preconception information for women with preexisting diabetes.*

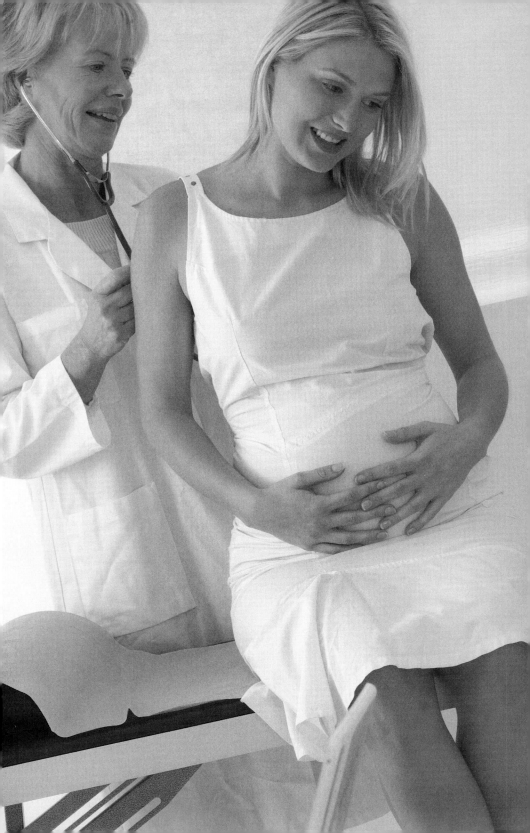

Chapter 24

# Other Chronic Conditions

Pregnancy puts many new demands on your body. For women with a medical condition, becoming pregnant may change the way their condition is managed. Most women with medical problems can have healthy babies. It just takes special care and more effort. Women with some medical conditions may need closer monitoring during pregnancy in order to prevent problems for both themselves and their babies.

If you have a medical problem, you may need to have extra tests, see your health care provider more often, or get special treatment. You may be able to monitor your condition from home; in some cases, you may need to stay in a hospital for part of your pregnancy.

Often, a team of health care providers will work together to make sure that both you and your baby get the care you need. Your health care provider may recommend that you see a *maternal–fetal medicine subspecialist*, a physician who has specialized training in caring for pregnant women with medical problems.

## Heart Disease

If you have a history of heart disease, heart murmur, or rheumatic fever, you should talk with your health care provider before you try to become pregnant. The risk of problems during pregnancy depends on the type of heart disease you have and how serious it is. A woman who has congenital heart disease (meaning that it was present at birth) has a higher risk of having a baby with some type of heart defect. Testing to determine whether your baby has a heart defect may be needed.

Pregnancy brings about major changes in the circulatory system. The blood volume (the amount of blood in your body) increases by 40–50%. This increased amount of blood makes the heart work harder. Before you become pregnant, it is recommended that you see your cardiologist or maternal–fetal medicine subspecialist to talk about how your specific condition may affect your heart during pregnancy. In some cases, pregnancy may not be recommended. In other cases, pregnancy can be attempted as long as you follow certain guidelines and see your health care providers frequently.

It's important to know that some medications that are safe to take before pregnancy should not be used once you become pregnant because they may harm your baby. If you have heart disease and need to take medications during your pregnancy, your doctor may switch you to medications that are considered safer.

## Kidney Disease

Your **kidneys** work almost 50% harder during pregnancy. The kidneys not only need to filter the wastes that your own body makes, but they also must process the baby's waste products. Because of this increased burden, the kidneys need to be working efficiently during pregnancy. If the kidneys are not working well, serious medical problems can arise that may affect both the woman and the baby:

- *Miscarriage*
- *Hypertension* (*high blood pressure*)
- *Preeclampsia*
- *Preterm* birth

In addition to these complications, pregnancy also can worsen any existing damage to your kidneys. This can greatly affect your future quality of life as well as your life expectancy.

*Kidney disease* can be mild, intermediate, or severe. If you have mild kidney disease, it is likely that you can have a healthy pregnancy. It is strongly recommended that you see a maternal–fetal medicine subspecialist or kidney specialist for *preconception care*. These specialists will evaluate your condition and explain any health risks of pregnancy. They also will review your medications and suggest substitutions, if possible, if you are taking drugs that are known to cause harm to a developing baby. For example, angiotensin II receptor blockers and angiotensin-converting enzyme inhibitors should be stopped before pregnancy or as early as possible after pregnancy is confirmed. Throughout your pregnancy, your health care providers will monitor your kidney function carefully. Tests of fetal well-being also may be performed later in pregnancy.

If you have intermediate or severe kidney disease, you may have difficulty becoming pregnant or sustaining a pregnancy. If pregnancy does occur, you have an increased risk of serious pregnancy complications. The risk of long-term kidney damage also is increased.

## Asthma

Asthma is a common condition that affects about 5% of pregnancies. For most women, asthma symptoms stay the same or even improve during pregnancy. But for one third of pregnant women, asthma symptoms worsen. During an asthma episode, the amount of *oxygen* in the blood decreases. In a pregnant woman, this also decreases the amount of oxygen the baby receives through the *placenta*. Asthma symptoms that are severe and uncontrolled can increase the risk of certain pregnancy complications, including preeclampsia, *fetal growth restriction*, need for *cesarean delivery*, preterm

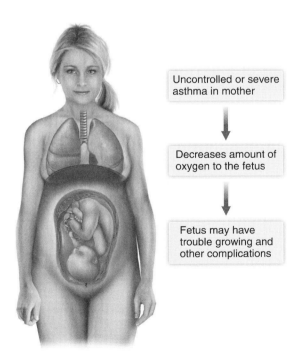

Uncontrolled or severe asthma in mother

↓

Decreases amount of oxygen to the fetus

↓

Fetus may have trouble growing and other complications

**Asthma during pregnancy.** If you have asthma episodes during pregnancy, it can decrease the amount of oxygen that goes to your baby.

birth, and maternal health risks. For these reasons, control of asthma symptoms during pregnancy is essential.

If you have a history of asthma, your health care provider will assess your current condition and perform tests of your lung function. If you have been pregnant before, how your asthma affected your previous pregnancies may give some clues about how your asthma will affect your current pregnancy. With this information, you and your health care provider will come up with a treatment plan for you to follow throughout pregnancy. Treatment plans for asthma include the following steps:

• Seeing your health care provider for tests to monitor your lung function
• Avoiding or controlling asthma triggers
• Taking medications as recommended by your health care provider

If your asthma is mild and you have only occasional episodes, you may not need medication during pregnancy. If you have more frequent episodes and your symptoms are more severe, medications may be recommended (see box "Medical Management of Asthma During Pregnancy"). The types and dosages of medications should be individualized for your particular situation.

## Medical Management of Asthma During Pregnancy

### Mild Intermittent Asthma
• No daily medications, albuterol as needed

### Mild Persistent Asthma
• Preferred—Low-dose inhaled corticosteroid
• Alternative—Cromolyn, leukotriene receptor antagonist, or theophylline

### Moderate Persistent Asthma
• Preferred—Low-dose inhaled corticosteroid and salmeterol or medium-dose inhaled corticosteroid or (if needed) medium-dose inhaled corticosteroid and salmeterol
• Alternative—Low-dose or (if needed) medium-dose inhaled corticosteroid and either leukotriene receptor antagonist or theophylline

### Severe Persistent Asthma
• Preferred—High-dose inhaled corticosteroid and salmeterol and (if needed) oral corticosteroid
• Alternative—High-dose inhaled corticosteroid and theophylline and oral corticosteroid if needed

Working closely with your health care provider to monitor your lung function can give a better picture of how well your medications are working. If you have moderate or severe asthma, your symptoms are not well controlled, or you have just had a severe asthma episode, your baby's growth and well-being may be tracked closely.

Most asthma medications have not been shown to be harmful to the developing baby. Inhaled drugs, such as albuterol and inhaled corticosteroids, are the preferred medications for use during pregnancy. Lower dosages of these drugs are needed to control symptoms, so less of the drug reaches the baby.

## Thyroid Disease

Certain disorders cause the body's thyroid gland to release too much or too little *thyroid hormone*. *Hypothyroidism* means the thyroid isn't as active as it should be. *Hyperthyroidism* means the thyroid is too active. Either condition can harm you or your baby during pregnancy. With treatment, however, most pregnant women with thyroid disease can have healthy babies. The chance of problems during pregnancy is greatest when thyroid disease is not under control.

Uncontrolled hyperthyroidism is associated with a greater risk of preterm delivery, preeclampsia, and heart failure. These complications may make it necessary to deliver the baby early, which increases the risk of serious health problems for the baby. Mothers with hypothyroidism are at increased risk of excessive bleeding after delivery. Uncontrolled hypothyroidism can lead to a rare condition called myxedema. Myxedema can cause coma and in some cases can be life threatening. Severe hypothyroidism also is associated with a condition called infantile myxedema. This condition can cause dwarfism, intellectual disabilities, and other serious health problems.

If you have hyperthyroidism, medications (eg, methimazole, propylthiouracil) usually are prescribed to keep the level of thyroid hormone in the normal range. The lowest possible dosage of the medication is used in order to minimize exposure of the baby to the drug. If you have hypothyroidism, you most likely will be prescribed thyroxine, a drug that works to increase the levels of thyroid hormone in your body. This treatment is the same as the treatment you would receive if you were not pregnant. In both cases, blood tests to check your thyroid function will be performed at regular intervals during your pregnancy to be sure your thyroid is functioning within the normal range. Radioactive iodine, which sometimes is used to treat hyperthyroidism, cannot be taken during pregnancy. It may injure the thyroid gland of the baby and increase the risk of hypothyroidism in the baby.

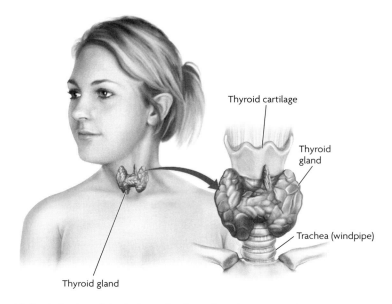

Thyroid cartilage

Thyroid gland

Trachea (windpipe)

Thyroid gland

**Thyroid gland.** The thyroid gland is located in the neck. It releases thyroid hormone. Thyroid hormone plays many roles in the body, including maintaining heart rate and regulating body temperature.

Some women have a condition called subclinical hypothyroidism in which the level of thyroid hormone is normal but the level of thyroid-stimulating hormone is elevated. At this time, there is little information about the risks of subclinical hypothyroidism during pregnancy or whether treatment has any benefit.

Some women who do not have thyroid problems during pregnancy may develop a thyroid condition called postpartum thyroiditis after childbirth. It often is a short-term problem and hormone levels quickly return to normal. Sometimes this condition can lead to long-term hypothyroidism, which will require treatment.

Testing the function of the thyroid gland is not a routine part of prenatal care. But, if you have a history or symptoms of thyroid disease and are thinking of becoming pregnant or are pregnant already, talk to your health care provider so that he or she can decide the best way to evaluate you and manage your pregnancy.

## Digestive Diseases

If you have a digestive disease that affects how your body digests food, you'll have to work closely with your health care provider throughout your pregnancy. You will need to make sure you and your developing baby are getting enough of the crucial vitamins and *nutrients* you both need for a healthy pregnancy.

## Inflammatory Bowel Disease

Inflammatory bowel disease (IBD) is a condition in which chronic inflammation occurs in the digestive tract. Researchers believe that IBD is an *autoimmune disorder* caused by a misdirected *immune system* attack against the normal bacteria found in the digestive system. There are two kinds of IBD: 1) Crohn disease and 2) ulcerative colitis. Both cause similar symptoms of diarrhea, abdominal pain, fever, and rectal bleeding. Like the symptoms of many autoimmune disorders, IBD symptoms may come and go. A person with IBD may experience periods of intense symptoms (flares) followed by periods of mild or no symptoms (remission).

If you have IBD, it probably is difficult for you to get the nutrients you need from the foods you eat. Your body may not be able to absorb enough protein, vitamins, or calories. You also may have intestinal damage. Before you become pregnant, it is important to see your health care provider to discuss your condition and how you will manage it during your pregnancy. It is recommended that pregnancy be attempted when you are not experiencing a symptom flare-up. You and your health care provider should discuss the medications that you are taking and whether you should continue to use the same drugs while you are pregnant. Consulting with a nutritionist or dietitian also may be helpful.

## Irritable Bowel Syndrome

Irritable bowel syndrome (IBS) mainly affects women between the ages of 30 years and 50 years. For some people, it is only mildly annoying. For others, it can be serious. It is not clear what causes IBS. Symptoms may include cramps, gas, bloating, and alternating diarrhea and constipation.

Stress, eating large meals, or travel may trigger the symptoms. Certain medicines or foods also can cause symptoms to flare up. When you're pregnant, you will have to become more aware of what triggers your symptoms. This will help make it easier to cope with the body changes that you will experience throughout your pregnancy.

Although there is no cure for irritable bowel syndrome, it can be managed to reduce the symptoms. Your health care provider or a dietitian can suggest changes in your diet, such as eating more fiber or eating more frequent, smaller meals, to help manage your symptoms. Some medications also can be used to relieve symptoms.

### Celiac Disease

People with celiac disease cannot tolerate gluten, a protein found naturally in wheat, rye, and barley. It also is added to certain food products. When gluten is eaten, the immune system reacts by damaging the lining of the small intestine. As a result of this damage, nutrients cannot be absorbed properly. Symptoms of celiac disease vary. Some people have no symptoms. Others may have diarrhea, constipation, fatigue, or abdominal pain and bloating. If celiac disease is not managed, it can cause serious health problems and may affect your ability to become pregnant. Some studies also have found links between celiac disease that is not managed and increased risk of repeated miscarriage.

It is entirely possible to have a healthy pregnancy if you have celiac disease. The key is to maintain a gluten-free diet before, during, and after pregnancy. It is a good idea to review your gluten-free diet with your health care provider and a dietitian to make sure that it gives you and the baby enough nutrients to grow and stay healthy. You may need to make adjustments in your diet if you are not gaining enough weight or if you develop complications, such as *anemia*.

## Other Autoimmune Diseases

Autoimmune diseases are those caused by a mistaken attack of the immune system against the body's own tissues. It is not clear what causes the immune system to go on the attack, but some autoimmune diseases are thought to be at least partly inherited (passed down through a person's *genes*). Although these disorders often cannot be cured, they can be managed. Pregnancy has certain effects on the course of many autoimmune diseases. For some autoimmune diseases, pregnancy can increase the signs and symptoms associated with the disease and can lead to certain complications. For others, pregnancy actually causes symptoms to become less severe. If you have an autoimmune disorder, it is recommended that you, your pregnancy health care provider, and other health care professionals work as a team to maintain adequate control of your condition and to increase your chances of having a healthy pregnancy.

### Antiphospholipid Syndrome

*Antiphospholipid syndrome (APS)* is caused by the presence of certain *antibodies* that attack substances called phospholipids. Phospholipids are found in the membranes of *cells*. When these antibodies bind to phospholipids, it damages the cells and can cause blood clots to form in the body's blood vessels. A common location where the blood clots develop is in the deep veins of the lower leg, which is called ***deep vein thrombosis (DVT)***. If a piece of a clot breaks free and moves through the blood vessels to the lungs, it is very serious. This condition, called pulmonary embolism (PE), can be fatal. Blood clots also can form in organs such as the kidneys, eyes, or brain, leading to kidney disease, vision problems, heart attack, and stroke. During pregnancy, APS can have serious effects on you and your baby, including miscarriage, preeclampsia, problems with fetal growth, and preterm delivery.

APS occurs more frequently in women with certain other disorders, including ***lupus*** and rheumatoid arthritis. Women who have had an unexplained DVT, a blood clot during pregnancy, a heart attack or stroke, or unexplained miscarriages usually are tested for APS.

If you have APS and are pregnant, you will receive special care throughout your pregnancy. Beginning in the third trimester, you may have special tests of fetal well-being or serial ***ultrasound exams*** to track the growth of the baby. Depending on your history of blood clots, you may need to take a medication called heparin, sometimes along with low-dose aspirin. Heparin and aspirin are drugs that help prevent the blood from clotting abnormally. You also may need to continue taking medication for several weeks after you have your baby.

## Lupus

Lupus is an autoimmune disorder that affects various parts of the body, including the skin, joints, blood vessels, and organs such as the kidneys or brain. Lupus is associated with an increased risk of miscarriage and stillbirth. The risks of preeclampsia, preterm birth, and fetal growth problems also are increased. Women with lupus, especially those with antiphospholipid antibodies, are more likely to develop DVT than women who do not have the disease. Lupus also can affect the baby after he or she is born. Babies born to women with lupus may have symptoms of the disease and have an increased risk of certain heart problems.

Today, more than one half of women with lupus have uncomplicated pregnancies. One way to increase the chances of a healthy pregnancy is to make sure your lupus is under control for at least 6 months before attempting pregnancy. However, pregnancy for a woman with lupus is considered high risk. If you have lupus, you should be cared for by a maternal–fetal medicine subspecialist or an internal medicine specialist who is experienced in treating lupus during pregnancy. You'll need to see your health care provider frequently because many problems that may happen during pregnancy can be treated more easily if found early. You may need special tests later in pregnancy to see how the baby is growing and to monitor your condition. You may need to continue to take medications to control your condition throughout pregnancy. Your health care provider will review your medications and determine whether they are acceptably safe to use during pregnancy. In some cases, you may need to take a different medication or adjust the dosage.

### Multiple Sclerosis

Multiple sclerosis is a disease that affects the central nervous system. The symptoms of the disease are different for every person but mostly include extreme fatigue, vision problems, loss of balance and muscle control, and stiffness. A person can have relapses or flare-ups when symptoms get worse and also can have periods with no symptoms.

Women with multiple sclerosis are able to have healthy pregnancies. Pregnancy does not make the disease worse, and the baby will grow normally. In fact, some women report that their symptoms get better when they are pregnant. If you have multiple sclerosis, the best therapy is to follow a healthy lifestyle of good nutrition, exercise, rest, and prenatal care. However, the risk of having a flare-up increases in the weeks after pregnancy. If you do have a relapse in the postpartum period, it does not appear to change the course of the disease or worsen your prognosis.

### Rheumatoid Arthritis

Rheumatoid arthritis causes pain and swelling in the joints. It also can cause stiffness in the morning and a general feeling of fatigue and discomfort. Rheumatoid arthritis can flare up and then lessen for a time, or it can get worse and damage the joints. During pregnancy, rheumatoid arthritis greatly improves for many women.

Rheumatoid arthritis often is treated with antiinflammatory medications, which can cause complications in pregnant women. You will have to make sure your health care provider tells you which pain relief medications you can use while you are pregnant. There are some drugs used to treat rheumatoid arthritis, including methotrexate and cyclophosphamide, that you should avoid during pregnancy.

## Thrombophilias

People with a thrombophilia tend to form blood clots too easily because they have either too much or too little of certain proteins in their blood. Many of these diseases are inherited (passed down from parents to children in genes). In some cases, blood clots can lead to serious problems, including PE, stroke, and heart attacks.

Some of these diseases are known by the name of the defective gene and whether the person has one defective copy or two defective copies of the gene. For example, **Factor V Leiden** is a protein that helps in blood clotting. If Factor V Leiden is not working correctly, the blood tends to clot more easily. Factor V Leiden heterozygote means that a person has one defective Factor V Leiden gene. Factor V Leiden homozygote means that a person has two defective Factor V Leiden genes. Other factors in which defective genes can result in a thrombophilia include the following:

- Prothrombin G20210A
- Protein C deficiency
- Protein S deficiency
- Antithrombin deficiency

Thrombophilias are classified as low risk and high risk. Low-risk thrombophilias carry a small chance of causing a blood clot. Low-risk thrombophilias include Factor V Leiden heterozygous, prothrombin G20210A heterozygous, and protein C or protein S deficiencies. High-risk thrombophilias carry a higher risk of causing a blood clot. High-risk thrombophilias include antithrombin deficiency, double heterozygous for prothrombin G20210A mutation and factor V Leiden, factor V Leiden homozygous, and prothrombin G20210A mutation homozygous.

Most women who have a thrombophilia have healthy pregnancies. However, there may be an association between thrombophilias and some pregnancy complications, including miscarriage, **placental abruption**, and **stillbirth**. The risk of these complications occurring during pregnancy depends on the type of thrombophilia that you have, whether you have ever had a blood clot or if you have a close relative who has had a blood clot, and whether you are taking anticoagulant medication. Your health care provider will assess your individual history to decide whether you should receive treatment during pregnancy and, if so, the type of medication and dosage. Women with low-risk thrombophilias may just need careful monitoring during pregnancy. Women with high-risk thrombophilias, a personal or family history of blood clots, or both, may need to take medication during pregnancy. Treatment with medication may need to continue after pregnancy as well. The anticoagulant drugs warfarin and heparin do not accumulate in breast milk and can be used by women who are breastfeeding.

If you have never been diagnosed with a thrombophilia but have a history of blood clots, or if you have a parent or sibling with a thrombophilia, let your health care provider know, preferably before you become pregnant. You may need to have screening tests for certain thrombophilias. Although you can have these tests while you are pregnant, the screening tests ideally should take place when you are not pregnant.

## Von Willebrand Disease

Von Willebrand disease is the most common inheritable bleeding disorder that affects women. It is caused by a deficiency in von Willebrand factor (vWF), a protein that helps the blood to clot. Von Willebrand disease is an inherited disorder that is passed down from either parent to a child. The most common symptom in women is heavy menstrual bleeding that occurs with the first menstrual period. Other symptoms may include nosebleeds, bleeding gums, and bleeding problems during surgery.

There are multiple concerns for a pregnant woman with von Willebrand disease. The disease can lead to miscarriage and postpartum *hemorrhage*. Special care needs to be taken when administering epidural or spinal anesthesia, as the needle used for placement of these types of anesthesia can cause swelling and bruising of the spinal cord. In addition, because von Willebrand disease is an inherited disorder, the baby can have up to a 50% risk of being affected. For this reason, certain tests, such as fetal scalp electrode or fetal scalp sampling, should be avoided, and circumcision should be postponed until the newborn can be tested for the disease. Operative vaginal deliveries, in which there may be an increased risk of trauma to the newborn, should be avoided because of the potential risk of bleeding in the baby's brain.

In many women, pregnancy causes levels of vWF to increase, and the risk of bleeding is lower than when they are not pregnant. Levels of vWF and other blood clotting proteins will be measured throughout pregnancy, especially later in pregnancy as delivery gets closer. Your health care provider may consult with a blood specialist to plan the best way for the baby to be delivered with the least risk of bleeding and hemorrhage.

## Seizure Disorders

Epilepsy and certain other disorders cause seizures. *Seizure disorders* can affect pregnancy in several ways. Some of these effects are related to antiepilepsy drugs (AEDs). Others are caused by the condition itself. Some of the ways that seizure disorders can affect pregnancy include the following:

- Higher risk of birth defects, most commonly cleft lip, cleft palate, **neural tube defects**, and heart defects. The increased risk of birth defects may be related to the disorder itself or to the effects of AEDs.

- Injury and complications resulting from seizures, such as injuries from falls, decreased oxygen to the baby during a seizure, and preterm birth

- Increase in seizure frequency during pregnancy, which occurs in about one third of women

With good medical care before and during pregnancy, many of these effects can be avoided.

Preparing for pregnancy is vital if you have a seizure disorder. Use of AEDs can decrease the levels of **folic acid** in the body. Low levels of folic acid before pregnancy and during early pregnancy have been linked to an increased risk of having a baby with a neural tube defect. Taking extra folic acid before and during the first weeks of pregnancy may decrease the risk of this problem. If you are taking AEDs and you can become pregnant, it is recommended that you take 4 mg of folic acid daily and continue taking this amount for the first trimester of pregnancy. This amount of folic acid is 10 times higher than the amount recommended for women who do not take AEDs. To get the extra amount, you should take a separate folic acid supplement in addition to a single multivitamin pill—not extra multivitamin pills. While it has not been proved that taking extra folic acid can prevent drug-related birth defects, this treatment is considered safe and may be beneficial for women taking AEDs.

Another important way to prepare for pregnancy is to review your medications with your health care provider. During pregnancy, the type, amount, or number of AEDs that you take may need to change. Ideally, any changes in medication should be made before pregnancy. This allows you and your health care provider to see how the medication changes affect you without putting the baby at risk. The changes that are made depend on your individual situation:

- If you have not had a seizure in at least 2 years, it may be possible for you to stop the medication gradually.

- The type of medication may be changed. Some AEDs are considered to be safer for the baby than others.

- If you take more than one medication to control your seizures, it may be recommended that you take only one medication. Taking only one medication may decrease the risk of birth defects. There also may be fewer drug interactions and fewer side effects than if you took multiple medications.

During pregnancy, you will see your health care provider frequently. Blood tests may be done regularly to be sure that medication levels are constant. Levels that are too high can lead to side effects. Levels that are too low can lead to seizures. Keep in mind that after you have your baby, your medications may need to be adjusted again.

Having a seizure disorder does not affect how you will have your baby. Like most women, women with a seizure disorder are able to give birth to their babies vaginally unless a problem arises during labor or delivery. In these cases, a cesarean delivery may be needed.

## Mental Illness

Millions of women are affected by mental illness in the United States. Some mental illnesses are more common in women than in men:

- *Depression*

- Bipolar disorder

- Schizophrenia

- Anxiety disorders (panic disorder, obsessive–compulsive disorder, and phobias)

- Personality disorders

Although most women with a mental illness can have successful pregnancies, these conditions can affect pregnancy in a number of ways. If you have a mental illness or had one in the past, be sure to tell your health care provider. Being pregnant can cause some mental illnesses to worsen. Pregnancy may cause a recurrence of a mental illness. This may be a result of hormonal changes or stress. If a mental illness is not treated, you may not be able to take care of yourself properly. For example, you could have trouble eating well or getting enough rest. You also may be less likely to get regular prenatal care.

Your pregnancy care provider needs to know about any medications you are taking to control your mental illness. Some medications are safe during pregnancy, but there are some that can harm a growing baby. If you are currently taking a medication, your pregnancy care provider and mental health care provider can discuss with you whether you should stop or continue taking this medication while you are pregnant. This decision is based on several factors, such as the severity of your illness, whether the illness has recurred, and whether you currently have symptoms. Use of a single medication at a higher dose may be recommended over the use of multiple medications for the treatment of mental illness during pregnancy. You and your health care providers will need to decide if the benefit of using a drug to control your mental condition outweighs any possible risks. If your medication is stopped, alternative therapies, such as psychotherapy, may be an option.

Some women will have mental health problems after delivery. Women with preexisting mental health problems are 20 times more likely to be admitted to a hospital for a psychiatric illness in the month after giving birth than they are in the 2 years that led up to it. They also are more likely to have *postpartum depression*.

The first weeks after a newborn arrives are stressful for any new mother. During the early weeks, help and support are important to help you adjust to being a new mother or a mother to more than one child.

## Physical Disability

For women who are physically disabled, pregnancy and being a parent pose special challenges. That doesn't mean they can't—or shouldn't—become mothers. Few, if any, physical disabilities directly limit a woman's ability to become pregnant.

If you have a physical disability, it's recommended that you meet with your health care provider before getting pregnant. Preconception care will help reduce the odds of medical problems during pregnancy. You also can receive specific screening for medical conditions that may affect you during pregnancy. If your disability is an inherited condition (meaning that it is caused by a defective gene that is passed down from one generation to the next), you may want to have genetic counseling.

Special care also will be needed after pregnancy begins. Your pregnancy care provider may work closely with your primary health care provider or other specialists. He or she also may suggest occupational or physical therapy to help you cope with the stresses pregnancy puts on the body.

Before the baby arrives, special equipment may need to be installed or modified at home to help in caring for the baby. Leaving the hospital may require postpartum home care for you and the baby.

# RESOURCES

For many medical conditions, organizations exist that provide patient education and address patient concerns. The following organizations offer information for pregnant women about how pregnancy affects the course of the condition, whether the condition may affect the developing baby, and how the condition is managed during pregnancy:

**American College of Allergy, Asthma, and Immunology**
www.acaai.org/allergies/who-has-allergies/pregnancy-allergies
85 West Algonquin Road, Suite 550
Arlington Heights, IL 60005
Phone: (847) 427-1200
Fax: (847) 427-1294
E-mail: mail@acaai.org

**American Heart Association**
www.heart.org
7272 Greenville Ave.
Dallas, TX 75231
Phone: 1-800-AHA-USA-1

**Arthritis Foundation**
www.arthritis.org
1330 W. Peachtree Street, Suite 100
Atlanta, GA 30309
Phone: 404-872-7100

**Crohn's and Colitis Foundation of America**
www.ccfa.org/resources/pregnancy-and-ibd.html
733 Third Avenue, Suite 510
New York, NY 10017
Phone: 800-932-2423
E-mail: info@ccfa.org

**Epilepsy Foundation**
www.epilepsy.com/learn/gender-issues/women-and-epilepsy
8301 Professional Place
Landover, MD 20785
Phone: 800-332-1000
Fax: 301-577-2684

**Irritable Bowel Syndrome Self Help and Support Group**
www.ibsgroup.org
24 Dixwell Avenue, #118
New Haven, CT 06511
Phone: 203-424-0660

**Lupus Foundation of America**
www.lupus.org/tag/pregnancy
2000 L Street, N.W., Suite 410
Washington, DC 20036
Phone: 800-558-0121

**National Alliance on Mental Illness**
www.nami.org
3803 N. Fairfax Drive, Suite 100
Arlington, VA 22203
Phone: 703-524-7600
Fax: 703-524-9094
Information Helpline: 800-950-NAMI (6264)

**National Endocrine and Metabolic Diseases Information Service**
www.endocrine.niddk.nih.gov/pubs/pregnancy/
6 Information Way
Bethesda, MD 20892–3569
Phone: 888-828-0904
TTY: 866-569-1162
Fax: 703-738-4929
E-mail: endoandmeta@info.niddk.nih.gov

**National Foundation for Celiac Awareness (NFCA)**
www.celiaccentral.org
PO Box 544
Ambler, PA 19002-0544
Phone: 215-325-1306
E-mail: info@celiaccentral.org

**National Kidney Foundation**
www.kidney.org/atoz/content/pregnancy.cfm
30 East 33rd Street
New York, NY 10016
Phone: (800) 622-9010
E-mail: info@kidney.org

**National Multiple Sclerosis Society**
www.nationalmssociety.org/Living-well-with-MS/Family-and-Relationships/pregnancy
733 Third Avenue, 3rd Floor
New York, NY 10017
Phone: 800-344-4867

# Part VI
# Testing

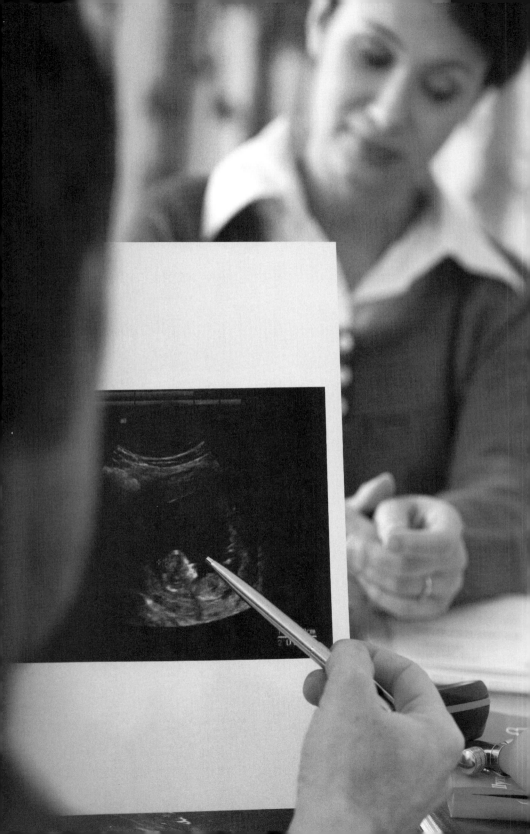

# Chapter 25

# Screening and Diagnostic Testing for Genetic Disorders

Although most babies are born healthy, parents-to-be often worry about the possibility that their baby will be born with a medical condition or physical disability. A **birth defect** is a physical problem or intellectual disability that is present at birth, although some birth defects may not be noticed until the child is older. About 3 in 100 babies in the United States are born with a major birth defect.

Many birth defects are caused by problems with a person's **chromosomes** or **genes**. These types of disorders are called **genetic disorders**. Genetic disorders can range from mild, such as **color blindness**, to severe, such as some forms of **hemophilia** or **Tay–Sachs** disease. Some genetic disorders are not harmful and no special treatment is needed. For many genetic disorders, medical treatment and specialized care can greatly improve a child's quality of life. However, for some genetic disorders, there is no effective treatment. Table 25-1 lists some of the more common genetic disorders.

There are many ways to assess the risk of having a child with certain disorders. These tests are called **screening tests**. Other tests are available that can find out for sure if there are specific problems in the baby. These tests are called **diagnostic tests**. Both screening and diagnostic testing are offered to all pregnant women. You don't have to be a certain age or have a family history of a disorder to have these tests.

Whether you want to be tested is a personal choice. Some couples would rather not know if they are at risk or whether their child will have a disorder, but others want to know in advance. Knowing beforehand gives you and your family time to learn about a particular disorder and organize any special care that your child may need. For a very small number of disorders, it may be

**Table 25-1 Common Genetic Disorders**

| Disorder | What It Means | Who Is at Highest Risk? |
|---|---|---|
| **Dominant Disorders** | | |
| Neurofibromatosis | Disorder that causes growth of tumors in the nervous system | Those with a family history of the disorder |
| Isolated polydactyly | Having extra fingers or toes | Those with a family history of the disorder, African Americans; commonly occurs without risk factors |
| **Recessive Disorders** | | |
| Thalassemia | Causes anemia; there are different types of the disorder, and some are more severe than others. | Depends on the type of disorder; Mediterranean (especially Greek or Italian), Middle Eastern, African, or Asian descent |
| Sickle cell anemia | A blood disorder in which the red blood cells have a crescent, or "sickle," shape rather than the normal doughnut shape. Because of their odd shape, these cells get caught in the blood vessels. This prevents oxygen from reaching organs and tissues, which causes pain. | African Americans |
| Tay–Sachs disease | A disease in which harmful amounts of a fatty substance called ganglioside GM2 collect in the nerve cells in the brain. It causes severe intellectual disability, blindness, and seizures. Symptoms first occur at about 6 months of age. | Ashkenazi Jews, French Canadians |

possible to treat the condition during pregnancy (with fetal surgery, for example). You also may have the option of not continuing the pregnancy. Your health care provider or a ***genetic counselor*** can discuss all of the testing options with you and help you decide.

## Genes and Chromosomes

Genes are the coded instructions that direct every process that takes place in your body and provide the "blueprints" for all of your physical traits. A gene is a short segment of a chemical called ***DNA***. DNA consists of two strands of four different kinds of building blocks called nucleotides. The order in which

**Table 25-1 Common Genetic Disorders,** *continued*

| Disorder | What It Means | Who Is at Highest Risk? |
|---|---|---|
| Cystic fibrosis | Causes problems with digestion and breathing. Symptoms appear in child-hood—sometimes right after birth. Some individuals have milder symptoms than others. Over time, the problems tend to become worse and harder to treat. | White individuals of Northern European descent |
| *X-Linked Disorders* | | |
| Duchenne muscular dystrophy | Causes progressive muscle weakness, loss of muscle tissue, and abnormal bone development. The muscle problems cause problems with move-ment, especially walking, and breathing problems. Heart defects usually are present. Most affected individuals do not live beyond age 30 years. | Males |
| Color blindness | A condition in which a person cannot see certain colors | Males |
| Hemophilia | A disorder caused by the lack of a substance in the blood that helps it clot. Affected individuals are at risk of bleeding to death if they are injured. | Males |

these building blocks occur along the strands of DNA is the genetic code that tells cells how to function.

Genes usually come in pairs. Each member of a gene pair is called an *allele*. Some traits, such as blood type, are determined by a single gene pair. Other traits, including skin color, hair color, and height, are the result of many genes working together.

DNA is packaged into structures called *chromosomes*. Chromosomes also come in pairs. One allele of a gene pair is located on one chromosome in a pair, and the other allele of the gene pair is located on the other chromosome in the pair. Every *cell* in your body except *eggs* and *sperm* contains 23 pairs of chromosomes (46 chromosomes). The egg and the sperm each contain half that amount—23 chromosomes (not pairs). Chromosome pairs 1–22 are called *autosomes*. The 23rd pair of chromosomes are the *sex chromosomes*, which are called X and Y.

Genes are inherited—they are passed down from parents to children. During fertilization, when an egg and sperm join, the cell that is formed contains the full set of 46 chromosomes (or 23 pairs of chromosomes). In this way, a baby receives one half of its genes from the mother and one half from the father.

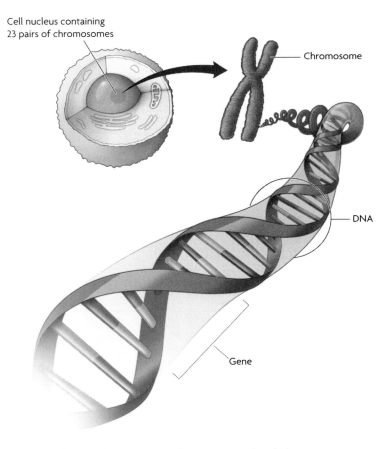

Cell nucleus containing
23 pairs of chromosomes

Chromosome

DNA

Gene

**Chromosomes and genes.** Chromosomes are the structures inside cells that carry a person's genes. Each person has 22 pairs of autosomes and one pair of sex chromosomes. A single gene is a segment of a large molecule called DNA.

A baby's sex is determined by the sex chromosomes it receives. The egg always has an X chromosome, but the sperm can have either an X or a Y chromosome. A combination of XX results in a female and XY results in a male.

## Inherited Disorders

Some genetic disorders are caused by a change in a gene. These changes are called **mutations**. Most mutations are harmless. Some mutations, however, can cause disease or can affect a child's appearance or physical function. Mutations can be passed down from parents to their children, or they can appear for the first time in a child. If a parent has a mutation, there is a chance that his or her child will receive the mutation and inherit the disease or disability. The chance of a child inheriting a mutation depends on whether the gene is dominant or recessive (see Table 25-1).

## Autosomal Dominant Disorders

With a dominant gene disorder, just one gene inherited from either parent can cause the disorder. A disorder is called **autosomal dominant** when the mutation is located on any of the 44 chromosomes that are not the sex chromosomes. If one parent has the gene that causes an autosomal dominant condition, each child of the couple has a 50% chance of inheriting the disorder. An example of an autosomal dominant disorder is **neurofibromatosis**. This is a group of disorders that causes growth of tumors in the nervous system.

## Autosomal Recessive Disorders

With an **autosomal recessive** gene disorder, two genes inherited from both parents are needed to cause the disorder. If only one parent has the

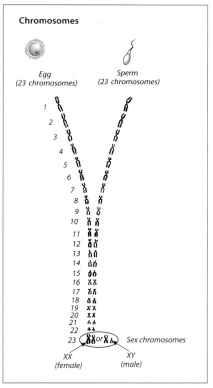

**How genes are inherited.** Every cell in the body, except for eggs and sperm, has 46 chromosomes. The chromosomes carry all of a person's genes. During fertilization, when an egg and sperm join, the cell that is formed contains the full set of 46 chromosomes (or, 23 pairs of chromosomes). In this way, a baby receives one half of its genes from the mother and one half from the father. A baby's sex is determined by the sex chromosomes it receives. The egg always has an X chromosome, but the sperm can have either an X or a Y chromosome. A combination of XX results in a female and XY results in a male.

gene, then the child cannot have the recessive disorder. If a child inherits a recessive gene for a disorder, he or she is known as a **carrier** of the disorder. Carriers often do not know that they have a recessive gene for a disorder. They usually do not have any symptoms of the disorder, but they are able to pass the gene to their children. If both parents are carriers, there is a 25% chance that the child will get the gene from each parent and will have the disorder. There is a 50% chance that the child will be a carrier of the disorder—just like the carrier parents. If only one parent is a carrier, there is a 50% chance that the child will be a carrier of the disorder.

Some recessive disorders are known to occur more often in certain races and ethnic groups. The following are examples of recessive disorders:

- *Sickle cell disease*—In this disorder, red blood cells have a crescent shape that causes them to block the blood vessels. This cuts off the flow of *oxygen* to organs, causing variable episodes of severe pain and organ damage. It occurs most often in African Americans.

- *Tay–Sachs disease*—This disorder causes blindness, seizures, and death, usually by age 5 years. It occurs most often in people of Eastern European Jewish descent (Ashkenazi Jews) and among French Canadians and Cajuns.

- *Cystic fibrosis*—This disorder causes severe problems with breathing and digestion and can lead to early death. It is most common in non-Hispanic white individuals.

## Sex-Linked Disorders

Disorders that are caused by genes on the sex chromosomes (the X chromosome or Y chromosome) are called *sex-linked disorders*. An example of a sex-linked disorder is color blindness. In this condition, a gene that controls how the eye sees color does not function properly. The gene is located on the X chromosome. Boys can be affected by color blindness if they inherit one of the mutations. Girls usually are not affected if they inherit one of the mutations because the other X chromosome has a normal gene. This normal gene "cancels out" the abnormal gene.

## Multifactorial Disorders

Multifactorial disorders are caused by a number of different factors working together. Some factors are genetic, whereas others are environmental. These disorders can run in families, but the way they are inherited is not completely understood. *Neural tube defects*, heart defects, and cleft palate are examples of multifactorial disorders. Many people are born with genes that give them a higher chance of developing cancer or *diabetes mellitus* but never develop these diseases. This may be because an environmental factor, such as exposure to a cancer-causing chemical, smoking, a high-fat diet, or being overweight, is needed to trigger the disease.

Researchers have been able to identify some of the environmental factors that trigger a few of these disorders. Neural tube defects are a group of

## Types of Genetic Disorders

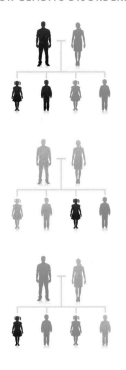

**Dominant Disorder**
If one parent has a dominant gene disorder, there is a 50% chance that it will be passed to each child.

**Recessive Disorder**
If both parents carry the recessive gene for a disorder, there is a 25% chance that a child they have will have the disorder, a 50% chance that a child will be a carrier, and a 25% chance that a child will not get the gene at all.

**X-linked Disorder**
If a woman is a carrier of an X-linked disorder and she has a son, there is a 50% chance that he will have the disorder. If she has a daughter, there is a 50% chance the daughter will be a carrier. If the father has an X-linked disorder, all the daughters will be carriers and none of the sons will be affected.

■ Affected person      ▦ Carrier      ▧ Unaffected person

disorders that can happen when the fetal spine does not form correctly. They have been linked in some cases to a woman not getting enough *folic acid*, a B vitamin, in the weeks before pregnancy and during early pregnancy. For this reason, it is recommended that all women of childbearing age take a vitamin supplement containing 400 micrograms of folic acid daily to help prevent neural tube defects if a pregnancy should occur (see the section "Take Folic Acid" in Chapter 1, "Getting Ready for Pregnancy"). However, for most multifactorial disorders, the causes are not known.

## Chromosomal Disorders

Some genetic disorders are caused by having too many or too few chromosomes. Having an abnormal number of chromosomes is called *aneuploidy*. Another type of genetic disorder is caused by problems with the structure of chromosomes. These disorders sometimes are called "structural chromosomal disorders."

## Aneuploidy

Most children with aneuploidy have physical defects and intellectual disabilities. The most common aneuploidy is a **trisomy**, in which there is an extra chromosome. Examples of trisomies include **trisomy 13 (Patau syndrome)**, **trisomy 18 (Edwards syndrome)**, and **trisomy 21 (Down syndrome)**. Down syndrome is the most common trisomy in the United States. It occurs in about 1 in 700 births, and it is estimated that there are about 6,000 new cases each year. A **monosomy** is a condition in which there is a missing chromosome. Monosomies are much rarer than trisomies. An example of a monosomy is **Turner syndrome**, in which a female has a missing X chromosome.

Aneuploidy usually occurs because the mother's egg or father's sperm contains an abnormal number of chromosomes. These errors occur when the egg or sperm are formed and usually happen by chance. However, the chance of these errors occurring in a woman's eggs increases as she ages. The chance of aneuploidy therefore increases as well. For example, the risk of having a baby with Down syndrome calculated according to the mother's age when the baby is born is as follows:

- 1 in 1,250 at age 25 years
- 1 in 1,000 at age 30 years
- 1 in 400 at age 35 years
- 1 in 100 at age 40 years
- 1 in 30 at age 45 years

It's important to keep in mind that although women older than 35 years are considered most likely to have a baby with Down syndrome, about 80% of babies with Down syndrome are born to women who are younger than 35 years simply because younger women have far more babies.

## Structural Chromosomal Disorders

In these types of disorders, a part of a chromosome may be missing (deletion), a part of a chromosome may be duplicated (duplication), or a piece of a chromosome can break off and relocate to another chromosome (translocation). Some structural chromosomal disorders are inherited due to the presence of abnormal chromosomes in the eggs or sperm. Others occur during prenatal development or even later in life.

Translocations do not always cause a disease or physical disability. A translocation is called unbalanced when genetic material is lost or gained. A balanced translocation does not result in any gain or loss of genetic material. People who have a balanced translocation usually have no medical effects. However, a person with a balanced translocation can have a child with an unbalanced translocation. Unbalanced translocations also have been linked to repeated **miscarriages**.

Structural chromosomal disorders are named according to the chromosome number that is affected and sometimes by the location where the deletion, insertion, or translocation occurs. Examples of structural chromosomal disorders include the following:

- 5p deletion syndrome—Also known as cri du chat syndrome, this disorder is caused by a deletion from chromosome 5. It causes severe intellectual and physical disabilities, poor growth, and weak muscle tone. Babies with this syndrome have a high-pitched cry that has been compared to that of a cat.

- 22q11.2 deletion syndrome—Also known as DiGeorge syndrome, this disorder is caused by a deletion from chromosome 22 at a specific location called 11.2. It causes a variety of signs and symptoms. Children with this syndrome have developmental delays and learning disabilities as well as heart defects, problems with some endocrine glands, and characteristic facial features.

- 4p deletion syndrome—This condition, also known as Wolf-Hirschhorn syndrome, is caused by deletion of genetic material near the end of one of the arms of chromosome 4. It causes characteristic facial features of wide-set eyes, small head, and misshapen ears. Children with this syndrome may have intellectual and developmental disabilities as well as physical problems, including seizures, weak muscles, and dental problems.

## Assessing Your Risk

All women are offered the option of having screening and diagnostic testing during pregnancy regardless of whether they have risk factors. In the past, if the mother was aged 35 years or older at the time of delivery, she was automatically considered at high risk of having a child with Down syndrome and offered diagnostic testing. However, any woman of any age can give birth to a child with Down syndrome or another trisomy, although the risk increases with increasing age of the mother. For this reason, a woman's age is no longer used to determine whether she should have screening or invasive diagnostic testing.

To help guide the decision about which tests to have or not to have, your health care provider may ask you certain questions about your health and your family history (see box "Risk Factors for Genetic Disorders"). These questions are designed to find out whether you have risk factors that increase your chances of having a baby with a genetic disorder. Even if you have risk factors, it does not mean that your baby will have a disorder. In fact, most

## Risk Factors for Genetic Disorders

It's a good idea to review your risk factors before you see your health care provider to discuss prenatal screening and diagnostic testing. It may be helpful for you to talk with your and your partner's family members for information about diseases or conditions that run in your families.

\_\_\_\_ What is your age?

\_\_\_\_ What is the baby's father's age?

\_\_\_\_ If you or the baby's father is of Mediterranean or Asian descent, do either of you or anyone in your families have thalassemia?

\_\_\_\_ Is there a family history of neural tube defects?

\_\_\_\_ Have you or the baby's father ever had a child with a neural tube defect?

\_\_\_\_ Is there a family history of congenital heart defects?

\_\_\_\_ Is there a family history of Down syndrome?

\_\_\_\_ Have you or the baby's father ever had a child with Down syndrome?

\_\_\_\_ If you or the baby's father is of Eastern European Jewish, French Canadian, or Cajun descent, is there a family history of Tay–Sachs disease?

\_\_\_\_ If you or your partner is of Eastern European Jewish descent, is there a family history of Canavan disease or any other genetic disorders?

\_\_\_\_ If you or your partner is African American, is there a family history of sickle cell disease or sickle cell trait?

\_\_\_\_ Is there a family history of hemophilia?

\_\_\_\_ Is there a family history of muscular dystrophy?

\_\_\_\_ Is there a family history of Huntington disease?

\_\_\_\_ Does anyone in your family or the family of the baby's father have cystic fibrosis?

\_\_\_\_ Does anyone in your family or the baby's father's family have an intellectual disability? Or have they had early menopause or tremors at an early age?

\_\_\_\_ If so, was that person tested for fragile X syndrome?

\_\_\_\_ Do you, the baby's father, anyone in your families, or any of your children have any other genetic diseases, chromosomal disorders, or birth defects?

\_\_\_\_ Do you have a metabolic disorder such as diabetes mellitus or phenylketonuria?

\_\_\_\_ Do you have a history of pregnancy issues (miscarriage or *stillbirth*)?

babies with a birth defect are born to couples who have no known risk factors. Risk factors that may increase the risk of having a child with a genetic disorder include the following:

- Older age in either the father or mother

- One or both parents have a genetic disorder.

- A couple already has a child with a genetic disorder.

- There is a family history of a genetic disorder.

- One or both parents belong to an ethnic group that has a high rate of carriers of certain genetic disorders.

A genetic counselor or other health care provider with expertise in genetics can be useful in some situations. A genetic counselor can study your family health history and make recommendations about which tests are most appropriate for you. He or she also can interpret test results, provide counseling about your options, and talk about any concerns you may have.

## Types of Tests for Genetic Disorders

Many types of tests are available to help address concerns about genetic disorders:

- **Carrier screening**—Carrier screening is done on parents (or potential parents). It can show if you or your partner carries a gene for a disorder that could be passed to your children. Carrier screening can be done before pregnancy (**preconception**) or during pregnancy and involves a simple blood test. Cystic fibrosis carrier screening is offered to all women of reproductive age because it is one of the most common genetic disorders.

- Screening tests for aneuploidy and neural tube defects—These prenatal screening tests assess the risk that a baby will have Down syndrome and other trisomies as well as neural tube defects. They are done at different times during pregnancy. These tests do not tell whether the baby actually has these disorders, only the risk that the baby has the disorders. There are no risks to the unborn baby with having these screening tests.

- Diagnostic tests—Diagnostic tests can provide information about whether the baby has a genetic condition. These tests are done on cells obtained through **amniocentesis**, **chorionic villus sampling (CVS)**, or, rarely, **fetal blood sampling**. The cells can be analyzed using different techniques.

**First-trimester screening**
-Timing: 10–14 wks
-Blood test + ultrasound exam

**MSFAP**
-Timing: 16–18 wks
-Blood test

**Second-trimester screening**
-Timing: 15–22 wks
-Blood test

**Integrated and sequential screening**
-Timing: 10–22 wks
-Combines results (integrated) or uses 1st trimester result to guide further testing (sequential)

**Cell-free DNA screening**
-Timing: 10 wks and beyond
-Blood test

**Carrier screening**
-Timing: Can be performed at any time; most useful when performed before pregnancy
-Blood or tissue (from inside the cheek) test

**CVS**
-Timing: usually 10–12 wks

**Amniocentesis**
-Timing: usually 15–20 wks

Screening    Diagnostic

Preconception    1st trimester    2nd trimester

Weeks of Pregnacy

**Prenatal testing.** This chart shows the various types of prenatal testing that are available to assess the risk of having a child with a genetic disorder (screening tests) or detecting a genetic disorder in the baby (diagnostic tests). Abbreviations: CVS, chorionic villus sampling; MSFAP, maternal serum alpha fetoprotein.

## Deciding Whether to Be Tested

If you or your partner is at an increased risk of being a carrier of a genetic disorder, you may want to consider preconception carrier screening. For most disorders, carrier screening of people who are not at increased risk is not recommended. However, you still can request carrier screening for some disorders even if you do not have a family history of the disorder.

Screening tests for birth defects are offered to all pregnant women, but it is your choice whether you want to have them done. Diagnostic tests, such as amniocentesis, also are available as a first choice for all pregnant women, even for those who do not have risk factors. A first step in deciding whether to have genetic testing and what kind of testing to have is to learn the medical facts about the different kinds of testing:

• Types of results—Screening tests only give you the probability of your baby being born with a disorder. Results of prenatal screening tests often are given as a number such as 1 in 800, meaning that there is a 1 in 800 chance that your baby will have a defect. These results then are further described as being "high risk" or "low risk." Diagnostic testing tells you whether or not the baby will be born with a chromosome disorder or a specific inherited disorder.

• Risks—Diagnostic tests are invasive. A sample of tissue needs to be taken using a needle. This can pose some risks to the pregnancy, although these complications are rare. There are no risks with having screening tests, which involve a blood test and an **ultrasound exam**.

• Accuracy—If you decide to have screening tests, there is a possibility of false-positive and false-negative results. A test result that shows there is a problem when one does not exist is called a false-positive result. A test result that shows there is not a problem when one does exist is called a false-negative result. A false-positive result can cause anxiety and may lead to unnecessary testing or treatment. A false-negative result can mean that you do not get the recommended counseling or preparation for having a child who has a medical condition or disability. With diagnostic testing, false-positive results and false-negative results are rare. Information about the rates of false-positive and false-negative results for each screening test that is offered should be made available to you.

• Timing—Screening tests for birth defects can be performed in the first trimester or in the second trimester, but the accuracy of results is higher when first-trimester results and second-trimester results are combined.

Diagnostic tests also are performed in the first trimester (generally between 10 weeks and 12 weeks of pregnancy for CVS) and in the second trimester (usually between 15 weeks and 20 weeks of pregnancy for amniocentesis). Having earlier results with CVS gives greater reassurance and allows time to get more information from a health care provider or genetic counselor if a disorder is diagnosed. Also, if you want to end the pregnancy, it is generally considered safer during the first trimester rather than later in the pregnancy, and first-trimester pregnancy termination procedures are often easier to obtain than second-trimester procedures.

- Cost—You also may want to check with your insurance carrier to make sure that the tests that you and your health care provider choose are covered by your insurance carrier. Some insurance carriers cover diagnostic testing only if you have risk factors for having a baby with a genetic disorder or if you have a positive screening test result.

    Once you know the medical facts, you also need to consider how you will use the information gained from having these tests. Your answers to these questions depend on your personal beliefs, health history, and the specific disorders you are testing for. Your decision may not be clear right away and may change as you go through the testing process. These decisions often are difficult to make. Parent support networks (such as the National Down Syndrome Society, March of Dimes, and the Cystic Fibrosis Foundation), counselors, social workers, and clergy may be able to provide additional information and support.

Your health care provider or a genetic counselor can discuss all of the options with you and recommend which tests may be best for your individual situation. There also is the option of not having any testing. If you do decide to have testing, you should understand the advantages, disadvantages, and limitations of each test.

## Carrier Screening

Carrier screening detects if a person carries a gene for many, but not all, recessive disorders. If you are a carrier, it means that you can pass the gene to your children. For this test, a sample of blood or saliva is taken and sent to a lab for study. Tests performed on the sample can determine whether the person carries the specific genes.

Carrier screening has traditionally been recommended for people who are at higher risk of certain genetic disorders because of their family history, ethnicity, or race. Individuals of Eastern European (Ashkenazi) Jewish ancestry may be offered carrier screening for Tay–Sachs disease, **Canavan disease**, cystic fibrosis, and **familial dysautonomia** and may want to have tests for other diseases, including **mucolipidosis IV**, **Niemann–Pick disease type A**, **Fanconi anemia group C**, **Bloom syndrome**, and **Gaucher disease**. Individuals of African, African American, and African Caribbean descent are offered carrier screening for sickle cell disease and for the blood disorders beta-**thalassemia** and alpha-thalassemia. Specific carrier screening tests also are offered to individuals of Southeast Asian (alpha-thalassemia), French Canadian and Cajun (Tay-Sachs disease), and Mediterranean (beta-thalassemia) descent.

However, scientists are beginning to recognize the growing difficulty of assigning a person to just one particular race or ethnicity. Many people are of mixed races and come from multiple ethnic backgrounds. For this reason, all women are offered screening for cystic fibrosis, which is a common disorder affecting many different races and ethnic groups. Screening for cystic fibrosis is most effective in populations that have a high rate of carriers, such as non-Hispanic white and Ashkenazi Jewish populations.

Another carrier screening option is called **expanded carrier screening**. It is now possible with new technology to screen for a wide variety of disorders with a high degree of accuracy and at a relatively low cost. Many labs now offer expanded carrier screening. There are some concerns about expanded carrier screening, including whether the disorders a lab screens for are appropriate for carrier testing and how the results are communicated. If you are interested in this type of screening, talk to your health care provider or genetic counselor.

Once you know your carrier status for a disorder, you do not need to be tested again in a future pregnancy for that disorder. If new carrier screening tests become available for a disorder that you have not been tested for and for which you may be at risk, you may want to discuss carrier screening for these disorders with your health care provider.

## Results

As an example, let's say that you have decided to have carrier screening for cystic fibrosis. If your test result is negative, no further testing is needed. If your test result is positive, the next step is to test your partner. If results of both tests are positive, a genetic counselor or your health care provider will help you understand your risks of having a child with the disorder, as well as your options.

## Timing

Carrier screening can be done either before pregnancy or during the early weeks of your pregnancy. If the screening is done before you are pregnant, you can use the results to decide if you want to get pregnant. If it's done after you are pregnant and you screen positive for being a carrier of a disorder, diagnostic testing may be possible to see if the baby has the disorder or is a carrier of the disorder.

## Important Considerations

A negative screening test result does not necessarily mean that you do not have a gene for the disorder being tested for. For example, with cystic fibrosis, the standard test looks only for a limited number of genetic changes. There are other, less common genetic changes that can cause cystic fibrosis. Therefore, a negative carrier test result does not completely rule out the risk that a person is a carrier. Your health care provider or genetic counselor can provide information about the limitations of the screening tests that you decide to have.

## If You or Your Partner Is a Carrier

Being a carrier of a disorder doesn't usually affect your own health. It also does not mean that all of your children will be affected. Your health care provider or genetic counselor can calculate the chances that a child will have the disorder or that a child will be a carrier. Once you receive this information, you can think about several options:

- If you have had carrier screening before pregnancy, you may choose to proceed with becoming pregnant with the option of considering prenatal diagnostic testing. You may choose to use *in vitro fertilization* with donor eggs or sperm to achieve pregnancy. *Preimplantation genetic diagnosis* can be used with this option. You also may choose not to become pregnant.

- If you are already pregnant, you may want to have diagnostic testing, if it is available, to see if the baby will be born with the disorder.

You also may want to consider telling other family members if you or your partner is a carrier. They may be at risk of being carriers themselves. However, you are not obligated to do so. Your health care provider or genetic counselor can give you advice about the best way to do this. It cannot be done without your consent.

## Screening Tests for Aneuploidy and Neural Tube Defects

A variety of tests that screen your unborn baby for aneuploidy and neural tube defects are available. Screening tests can be performed in the first trimester or in the second trimester (see Table 25-2). Results of these tests also can be combined in various ways; this type of integrated or sequential screening has higher detection rates than tests performed independently.

The types of screening tests that you will be offered depend on which tests are available in your area, how far along you are in your pregnancy, and your health care provider's assessment of which tests best fit your needs. Another type of screening test called a ***cell-free DNA*** test may be offered to women who are at high risk of having a child with aneuploidy (see box "Cell-Free DNA Test").

### Table 25-2  Screening Tests for Genetic Disorders

| Screening Test | Test Type | What Does it Screen for? | Down Syndrome Detection Rate |
|---|---|---|---|
| Cell-free DNA test | Blood test that analyzes fetal DNA from the placenta that circulates in the mother's blood | • Down syndrome<br>• Trisomy 18<br>• Trisomy 13 (some labs) | 99% |
| Combined first-trimester screening | Blood test for two proteins in the mother's blood plus an ultrasound exam | • Down syndrome<br>• Trisomy 18 | 82–87% |
| Second-trimester single screen for neural tube defects | Blood test for alpha fetoprotein | • Neural tube defects | 80% |
| Second-trimester quad screen | Blood test for four proteins in the mother's blood | • Down syndrome<br>• Trisomy 18<br>• Neural tube defects | 81% |
| Integrated screening | Blood test and an ultrasound exam in the first trimester, followed by quad screen in the second trimester | • Down syndrome<br>• Trisomy 18<br>• Neural tube defects | 94–96% |
| Contingent sequential | First-trimester combined screening result:<br>• Positive: diagnostic test offered<br>• Negative: no further testing<br>• Intermediate: second-trimester screening test offered | • Down syndrome<br>• Trisomy 18<br>• Neural tube defects | 88–94% |

## Cell-Free DNA Test

A screening test called the cell-free DNA test is available for women. A small amount of fetal DNA, which comes mainly from the *placenta*, circulates in the mother's blood. The cell-free DNA in a sample of the mother's blood can be screened for Down syndrome, trisomy 13, trisomy 18, and sex chromosome abnormalities. In women who are at high risk of having a baby with a chromosome disorder, this test is 99% accurate in detecting cases of Down syndrome and has a very low rate of false-positive results. This test can be done as early as the 10th week of pregnancy in some women. Results take about 1 week to process.

The cell-free DNA test works best for women who have an increased risk of having a child with a chromosome disorder, such as women who already have a child with a chromosome disorder. For women at low risk of having a baby with a chromosome disorder, conventional screening remains the most appropriate choice. Cell-free DNA testing is not recommended for women carrying more than one baby.

The cell-free DNA test has certain limitations. It does not screen for neural tube defects. An additional screening test needs to be done to check for these disorders. In addition, although it is highly accurate in detecting chromosome problems in high-risk women, it is not as accurate as diagnostic tests. A positive cell-free DNA test result should be followed by a diagnostic test.

### First-Trimester Screening

First-trimester screening consists of a blood test combined with an ultrasound exam. This screening sometimes is called "combined first-trimester screening." It is done between 10 weeks and 14 weeks of pregnancy to assess the risk of Down syndrome and other aneuploidies. The blood test measures the levels of two different proteins in the mother's blood. An ultrasound exam, called *nuchal translucency screening*, is used to measure the thickness at the back of the neck of the baby. An increase in the thickness of this space may be a sign of Down syndrome, trisomy 18, or other problems.

### Second-Trimester Screening

If you choose to have only combined first-trimester screening for aneuploidy, a blood test that measures a substance called maternal serum alpha-fetoprotein (MSAFP) can be done to test for neural tube defects. This test generally is done in the second trimester between 16 weeks and 18 weeks of pregnancy.

In the second trimester, a test called a "quadruple" or "quad" screen can be done to detect the presence of four different proteins in the mother's blood. This test screens for Down syndrome, trisomy 18, and neural tube defects. The quad screen can be done between 15 weeks and 22 weeks of pregnancy. The stage of pregnancy at the time of the test is important because the levels of the substances measured change throughout pregnancy.

## Integrated and Sequential Screening

The results from first- and second-trimester tests can be used together to increase their ability to screen for Down syndrome. The tests can be performed in the following ways:

* Integrated screening—Results of the first-trimester and second-trimester tests are analyzed together. The results are given only after the first-trimester and second-trimester screening tests are completed. Integrated screening is highly accurate and has a low rate of false-positive results.

* Sequential screening—Results of the first-trimester screening tests are used to determine further testing. If results show that you are at high risk, you can choose to have a diagnostic test. If results show that you are at low or intermediate risk, you can choose whether or not to have second-trimester screening. Compared with integrated screening, the chance of a false-positive result with sequential screening is slightly higher and accuracy is about the same.

## Results

With any type of testing, it is important to be aware of the possibility of false-positive and false-negative results and the consequences of these results. Information about the rates of false-positive and false-negative results can be obtained from your health care provider.

Screening test results are reported as the risk that a specific defect is present and they take your age and other factors into account. For example, the risk in the general population for women aged 31 years having a baby with Down syndrome is 1 in 820. If you are aged 31 years and you have a screening test result for Down syndrome of 1 in 900, it means you have a lower risk of having a baby with Down syndrome than the general population of women the same age as you.

Results also may be described as "screen negative" if the risk is lower than a certain cut-off point and described as "screen positive" if the risk is higher than the cut-off point. Different laboratories have different cut-offs for what is considered screen positive and screen negative.

### If Screening Test Results Show an Increased Risk

In most cases, screening test results are normal. If the results of a screening test raise concerns about your pregnancy, you will need to process the information and decide how to proceed. Your health care provider or genetic counselor can help guide you through your options. Further evaluation, such as diagnostic testing, may be available for the disorder in question and can be done to provide more information. The chances that you will have a positive diagnostic test result following a positive screening test result are low. If you are thinking about having a diagnostic test, you will need to balance the small risk of pregnancy complications that are associated with a diagnostic test against the risk of having a child with the disorder. Your health care provider or genetic counselor can explain these risks to you in detail so that you can make an informed decision.

## Diagnostic Tests

The fetal cells used in diagnostic testing are obtained using different techniques. Once the cells are obtained, they can be studied in different ways depending on the disorders being tested for. Some tests may not be available in some areas or may need to be done in a special center equipped to perform them.

### Amniocentesis

Amniocentesis usually is done between 15 weeks and 20 weeks of pregnancy. The test generally is not done any earlier than 15 weeks because the risk of complications is higher.

To perform amniocentesis, a thin needle is guided through the woman's abdomen and uterus. A small sample of amniotic fluid is withdrawn. Amniotic fluid contains cells from the baby. These cells are sent to a lab, where they are grown in a special culture. This takes about 10–12 days. When the cells are ready, they are analyzed to find out whether the baby has certain disorders, such as Down syndrome or specific genetic disorders depending on family history and ultrasound exam findings (see "How the Cells Are Analyzed" later in this chapter). The amniotic fluid also can be tested to detect neural tube defects.

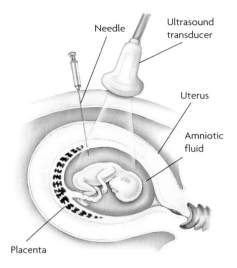

Needle

Ultrasound transducer

Uterus

Amniotic fluid

Placenta

**Amniocentesis.** In this procedure, a small sample of amniotic fluid is removed with a needle to be studied.

Complications of amniocentesis may include cramping, vaginal bleeding, infection, and leaking amniotic fluid. There is a very small chance of miscarriage (1 in 300–500).

### Chorionic Villus Sampling

Chorionic villus sampling is performed earlier than amniocentesis, generally between 10 weeks and 13 weeks of pregnancy. This earlier time frame gives you more time to think about your options and to make decisions. However, CVS is not as commonly performed as amniocentesis and may not be available at all hospitals or centers. It also is important to have CVS performed by an experienced health care provider.

To perform CVS, a small sample of tissue is taken from the placenta. The tissue contains cells with the same genetic makeup as the baby. The sample can be obtained in one of two ways. A small tube can be guided through the woman's vagina and **cervix** (transcervical CVS), or a thin needle can be guided through the abdomen and wall of the uterus (transabdominal CVS). The sample is sent to a lab. The cells are grown in a culture, which takes about 7–14 days. The cells then are analyzed.

Complications from CVS include vaginal bleeding, leakage of amniotic fluid, and infection. When CVS is performed by an experienced health care provider and in a center that performs many of these procedures, the risk of miscarriage with CVS is about the same as the risk with amniocentesis.

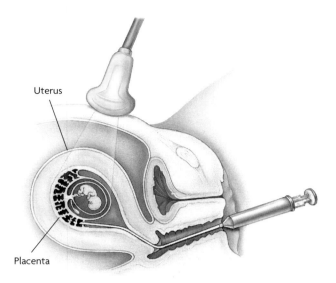

Uterus

Placenta

**Chorionic villus sampling.** In this procedure, a small sample of cells (chorionic villi) is removed from the placenta for study.

CVS cannot be used to diagnose neural tube defects prenatally. If you have CVS, you may want to have the blood test for MSAFP, a detailed ultrasound exam, or both to detect neural tube defects.

## Preimplantation Genetic Diagnosis

This test may be offered to couples who are using in vitro fertilization to become pregnant and who are at increased risk of having a baby with a genetic or chromosomal disorder. Before an **embryo** is transferred to a woman's uterus, it is tested to determine if it has a specific, known genetic disorder for which the couple is at risk.

## How the Cells Are Analyzed

A number of different technologies are used in prenatal diagnostic testing. Each one is used to detect different kinds of genetic changes. Your health care provider or genetic counselor will assess what information is being sought in the diagnostic test and select the tests that are most appropriate.

Missing, extra, or damaged chromosomes can be detected by taking a picture of the chromosomes and arranging them in order from smallest to largest. This is called a karyotype. A karyotype can show whether

• the number of chromosomes is abnormal

- the shape of one or more chromosomes is abnormal
- a chromosome is broken

A technique called *fluorescence in situ hybridization* can be used to detect the most common aneuploidies, which involve chromosomes 13, 18, 21, and the X and Y chromosomes. Results are available more quickly than with traditional karyotyping because the cells do not need to be grown in a lab. A positive test result is confirmed with a karyotype.

*Microarray analysis* can find chromosomal deletions, insertions, and translocations throughout the entire set of genes. Results may be available more quickly than with karyotyping because the cells do not need to be grown in a lab. This test can tell you a lot of information, but whether everything that is found is a cause for concern is uncertain.

Tests to find specific gene mutations also can be done. A variety of techniques for detecting gene mutations are available. Testing for gene mutations must be specifically requested. There is no one test that can find each and every gene mutation. For example, if you and your partner are carriers of the cystic fibrosis gene, you may want to request prenatal diagnostic testing for this specific mutation.

## If Your Baby Has a Disorder

If diagnostic testing shows that your baby has a disorder, you will need to think about your various options. You may choose to continue the pregnancy, or you may end the pregnancy. There is no right choice in these cases. Your health, values, beliefs, and situation all play a role in the decision.

If you decide to continue with the pregnancy, it's a good idea to learn all that you can about the condition and what it will mean for your baby's health. Some conditions are not serious or life threatening and may require only minimal special health care. With other disorders, it is helpful to prepare for caring for a child with special needs. Neonatologists are doctors who care for infants born with complex medical disorders. There also are pediatric subspecialists with expertise in specific disorders. Your health care provider or hospital staff may be able to help you find this special care. You also can seek out support groups for you and your partner. Ask whether the hospital where you are planning to deliver has pediatric doctors who can provide the best possible care for your infant. If it doesn't, consider requesting a transfer of care so that you can deliver your baby at such a facility.

Remember that educating yourself about your child's condition is crucial. You may find it helpful to find resources in your area that can put you in contact with parents of children with similar disorders (see the "Resources" section in this chapter).

# RESOURCES

The following resources give more information about the science of genetic disorders; the signs, symptoms, and treatment of different types of genetic disorders; and where to find support and counseling if you are at increased risk of having a baby with a genetic disorder or have received a diagnosis of a certain disorder in your child.

**Cystic Fibrosis Foundation**

www.cff.org

*National organization dedicated to research into cystic fibrosis and advocacy for people affected by this disorder.*

**Genetic Disorders, Genomics and Healthcare**

http://genome.gov/27527652

*Information from the National Human Genome Research Institute that covers many aspects of genetics and how it pertains to individuals and their families.*

**Genetic Science Learning Center**

http://learn.genetics.utah.edu

*Site that teaches basic information about genetics through videos, animations, and other learning aids.*

**March of Dimes**

www.marchofdimes.com

*Comprehensive site that gives information about a wide variety of birth defects, including their causes, diagnosis, and treatment. Also explains the ongoing research being done to improve the outlook for children and adults born with certain disorders.*

**National Center on Birth Defects and Developmental Disabilities (NCBDDD)**

www.cdc.gov/ncbddd/index.html

*Provides information on birth defects, developmental disabilities, and hereditary blood disorders.*

**National Down Syndrome Society**

www.ndss.org

*National society that advocates for people with Down syndrome. Provides information for new and expecting parents about the health care needs for children with Down syndrome and offers support for individuals and families.*

**National Tay-Sachs & Allied Diseases**

www.ntsad.org

*Provides services, research, and education for Tay–Sachs, Canavan and other related diseases.*

**Sickle Cell Disease Association of America**

www.sicklecelldisease.org/index.cfm

*National organization for education, awareness, and research of sickle cell disease.*

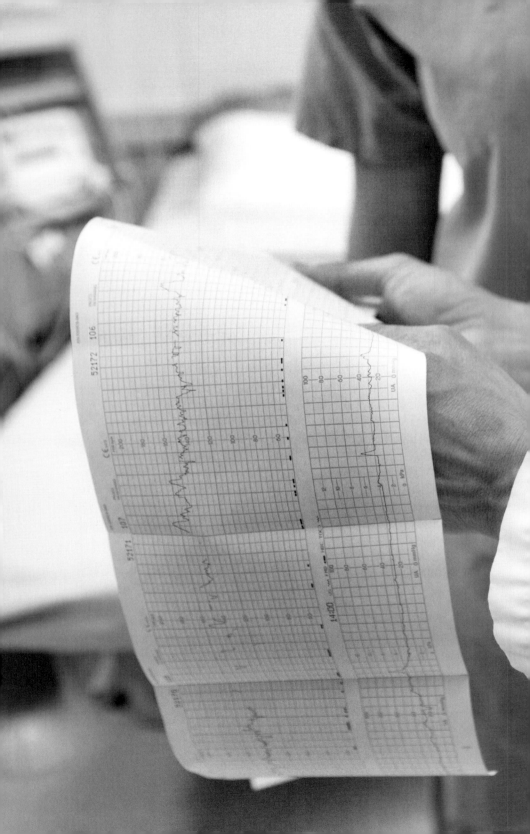

Chapter 26

# Testing to Monitor
# Fetal Well-Being

Several types of special tests can be done to check the well-being of the baby during pregnancy. These tests may be done if a problem arises during pregnancy, if you have a high-risk pregnancy, or if you go past your due date. If you need to have one of these tests, you may have questions (see box "Frequently Asked Questions"). Testing may help reassure you and your health care provider that all is going well with your pregnancy. If test results indicate a problem, more testing may be done. In some cases, the baby may need to be delivered right away. Your health care provider will carefully consider several factors when deciding how to manage an abnormal test result, including your baby's *gestational age*, your medical condition, and the condition of the baby. Each situation is different, and there is no "one size fits all" way to proceed.

## Why Testing May Be Done

Special testing during pregnancy most often is done when the baby is at increased risk of problems that could result in pregnancy complications or lead to *stillbirth*. These tests usually are done for women with high-risk pregnancies. Examples of high-risk pregnancies include those in which the woman has had a previous pregnancy in which complications occurred or has a pre-existing health condition. Some of these pre-existing health conditions include the following:

- *Diabetes mellitus*
- *High blood pressure*
- *Systemic lupus erythematosus* ("SLE" or "lupus")

## Frequently Asked Questions

### 1. Are these tests safe?

Most of these tests are noninvasive (no medical equipment has to enter your body). They pose very few risks for the baby and the woman. Sometimes, an **ultrasound exam** may be done by placing the ultrasound probe in the vagina, but this is a safe procedure when done by a trained technician or health care provider.

### 2. Will the tests hurt?

For most women, these tests are painless. Some women may feel slight discomfort from insertion of the vaginal ultrasound probe, from staying in certain positions for a while, or from the contractions that are produced during a contraction stress test.

### 3. In what order will they happen?

There is no set order for the tests. Likewise, no test has been proved to be better than another. Your health care provider will follow the best order for your situation.

### 4. Why would the same test have to be repeated?

Tests to determine the well-being of the baby may be done once or at regular intervals depending on the reason for the test. If your results are unclear or show a potential problem, tests are repeated regularly to make sure the baby continues to do well for the rest of the pregnancy. Repeat tests can show your health care provider if results were accurate. Additional care may be necessary. Repeat tests help to make sure that unnecessary steps are not taken.

- *Kidney disease*
- Certain blood disorders
- *Hyperthyroid disease* that is not well controlled
- Certain types of heart disease

A woman's pregnancy can become high risk if certain problems arise during the prenatal period. Some pregnancy-related conditions that may signal a need for special testing include the following:

- *Gestational hypertension*
- *Preeclampsia*
- Decreased fetal movement
- *Gestational diabetes*

- Too much or too little *amniotic fluid*
- Fetal growth problems
- *Late-term pregnancy* or *postterm pregnancy*
- *Rh sensitization*
- Prior fetal death
- *Multiple pregnancy* (if there are complications)

Not every complication that can happen during pregnancy can be detected with these tests. Some problems occur suddenly, such as *placental abruption* or problems with the *umbilical cord*. The tests discussed in this chapter cannot be used to predict these events.

## Interpreting Test Results

No test is 100% accurate. A test result that shows that there is no problem when one actually exists is called a false-negative result. A false-negative result from one of these special tests means that a problem has gone undetected, which could lead to further complications. The rate of false-negative results with these tests is low. If you have special testing and the result is negative, chances are good that there are no problems with the baby.

A test result that shows that there is a problem when one does not exist is called a false-positive result. A false-positive result can lead to unnecessary interventions, including early delivery. For this reason, if you have a positive test result, you most likely will have additional tests to find out whether a problem really exists.

## When Tests Are Done

Except for ultrasound exams, which can be performed at any time during pregnancy, special testing usually is started at 32 weeks of pregnancy or later. Testing may be started earlier than 32 weeks if problems are particularly serious or if there are multiple risk factors. How often the tests are done depends on the condition that prompted the testing, whether the condition remains stable, and results of the testing. If the problem that prompted the testing resolves and the test result is normal, there may be no need for further testing. Some tests are repeated weekly. In certain situations, such as diabetes in the mother, postterm pregnancy, fetal growth problems, or some chronic health conditions, tests may be done twice weekly.

## Types of Special Tests

The tests used to monitor fetal health include fetal movement counts, ultrasound, Doppler ultrasound, **nonstress test (NST)**, **biophysical profile (BPP)**, and **contraction stress test (CST)**.

### Fetal Movement Counts

Fetal movement counting (also called "kick counts") is a test that you can do at home. It does not require any special equipment.

**Why It Is Done.** Fetal movement counting may be recommended if you have felt fetal movement less often than what you think is normal. Feeling the same amount of movement from one day to the next can be a sign that the baby is doing well.

**How It Is Done.** One way to do fetal movement counting is to lie on your side and note how long it takes your baby to make 10 movements. If it takes fewer than 2 hours, the result is "reassuring" (which means that all is going well at the time). Once you have felt 10 movements, you can stop counting for that day. This test is repeated daily. Another approach is to count movements for 1 hour 3 days a week. A reassuring result is a count that is equal to or greater than previous counts.

Whichever method you use, be sure that you are counting fetal movements. Don't count the baby's hiccups, for instance. Also, when doing your kick counts, choose a time when the baby is most active, such as after you have had a meal.

**What the Results May Mean.** When you first start doing kick counts, you will receive instructions about when to call your health care provider depending on certain results. If you do not feel enough movement, it does not necessarily mean that there is a problem. It could simply mean that the baby is sleeping. Additional tests usually are needed to find out more information.

### Ultrasound Exam

Most women have at least one ultrasound exam during pregnancy. Ultrasound is a type of energy that creates pictures or sounds of the baby using sound waves. It does not cause any harm to you or the baby.

**Why It Is Done.** Some women have an ultrasound exam in the first trimester of pregnancy. Common reasons for a first-trimester ultrasound exam are to confirm the pregnancy, estimate **gestational age**, or find out whether there are multiple babies. An ultrasound exam combined with a blood test can be used during the first trimester to screen for certain chromosome problems in the baby.

If you don't have an ultrasound exam in the first trimester, you probably will have what is called a standard ultrasound exam performed between 18–20 weeks of pregnancy. This exam can provide the following information about your pregnancy:

* Estimated gestational age

* Estimated weight of the baby

* Position of the **placenta**

* Whether certain structures are developing normally, such as the heart, abdomen, face, head, and spine

* Sex of the baby

* The position, movement, breathing, and heart rate of the baby

* Amount of amniotic fluid in your uterus

* Whether you are carrying multiple babies

Other types of ultrasound exams may be performed if problems are suspected with your pregnancy. A limited ultrasound exam may be performed to check a specific issue. You may have a limited ultrasound exam if you have bleeding or pelvic pain. If a problem with fetal growth is suspected, serial ultrasound exams may be done to check how the baby is growing. Ultrasound sometimes is used to evaluate signs and symptoms of **preterm** labor. It also is used to help guide **chorionic villus sampling** and **amniocentesis** procedures.

A specialized ultrasound exam may be recommended based on your medical history, a result of a laboratory test, or the results of a standard or limited ultrasound exam. Specialized exams may use additional technology. For example, a Doppler ultrasound exam can evaluate blood flow through a blood vessel. A three-dimensional ultrasound exam can be used to show fetal anatomy in more detail.

When performed by a trained technician for medical reasons, ultrasound exams are safe during pregnancy. Having an ultrasound exam without a medical reason—such as to find out the sex of the baby or to create a "keepsake" photo—is not recommended. An ultrasound exam is a medical tool that should be used only when there is a valid medial reason.

**How It Is Done.** Your health care provider or a technician will perform the ultrasound exam using a device called a **transducer**. There are two types of transducers: one that is moved over the abdomen (**transabdominal ultrasound exam**) and one that is inserted into the vagina (**transvaginal ultrasound exam**).

For a transabdominal ultrasound exam, you will lie on your back with your abdomen exposed. A gel will be used on your abdomen to improve the contact between the transducer and the skin surface. The transducer then is moved over your abdomen and records sound waves as they bounce off of your baby. These sound waves create images that are shown on a viewing screen. For a transvaginal ultrasound exam, a vaginal transducer is inserted into the vagina to help view the pelvic organs and the baby. It delivers images in the same way as an abdominal ultrasound. Both types of ultrasound exams are shown in Chapter 3, "Month 3 (Weeks 9–12)."

**What the Results May Mean.** If something does not look normal on an ultrasound exam, you most likely will have other tests to provide more information. It is important to be aware that it is possible to have a "normal" ultrasound exam result but still have a baby with a **birth defect** or other issue. Ultrasound cannot detect every problem.

### Nonstress Test

The NST measures the fetal heart rate in response to fetal movement over a period of time. The term "nonstress" means that during the test, nothing is done to place stress on the baby.

**Why It Is Done.** The fetal heart normally beats faster (called an **acceleration**) when the baby moves. During an NST, the fetal heart rate is recorded. Your health care provider then notes the number of accelerations that occurred during the test period.

**How It Is Done.** This test may be done in the health care provider's office or in a hospital. The test is done while you are reclining or lying down and usually takes at least 20 minutes. A belt with a sensor that measures the fetal heart rate is placed around your abdomen. The fetal heart rate is recorded by a machine.

**What the Results May Mean.** If two or more accelerations occur within a 20-minute period, the result is considered reactive or "reassuring." A reactive result means that for now, it does not appear that there are any problems.

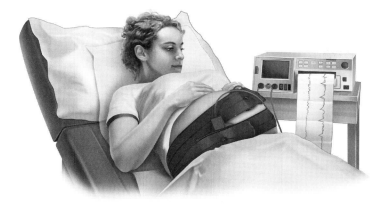

**Electronic fetal monitoring.** The fetal heart beat can be monitored continuously using a belt with special sensors. Another belt may be used to monitor the strength of contractions.

Reactive results are slightly different if the gestational age is less than 32 weeks. Sometimes, the baby may be asleep and will not move two times in 20 minutes. If this happens, the test may last for 40 minutes or longer, or the baby may be stimulated to move with sound projected over the mother's abdomen.

A nonreactive result is one in which not enough accelerations are detected in a 40-minute period. It can mean several things. It may mean that the baby is doing well but is too young for the test to be accurate. It can occur if the woman has taken certain medications. A nonreactive result also can mean that the baby is not getting enough *oxygen* or that the baby's nervous system is not functioning properly. A BPP or contraction stress test may be needed to give more information.

### Biophysical Profile

The BPP may be done when results of other tests are nonreassuring. It uses a scoring system to evaluate fetal well-being.

**Why It Is Done.** A BPP consists of an NST and an ultrasound exam that assesses the baby's well-being in four additional areas during a 30-minute period. The BPP assesses the following five areas:

1. Fetal heart rate (NST)—If the results of all four ultrasound components of the BPP are normal, the NST may not be done.

2. Breathing movements—One or more breathing movements lasting 30 seconds or more are seen.

3. Body movements—Three or more body or limb movements are seen.

4. Tone—The *fetus* opens or closes its hand or extends and retracts a limb at least once.

5. Amount of amniotic fluid—The deepest vertical pocket of amniotic fluid is greater than 2 cm.

**How It Is Done.** A BPP involves monitoring the fetal heart rate by an NST as well as an ultrasound exam. Amniotic fluid volume is assessed by measuring the depth of the single deepest amniotic fluid pocket (called the vertical pocket) in any part of the uterus.

**What the Results May Mean.** Each of the areas is given a score of 0 (not present) or 2 (present) for a possible total of 10. A score of 8 or 10 is normal. Scores that are less than normal are interpreted depending on the gestational age of the baby. A score of 6 is equivocal (neither reassuring nor non-reassuring). If you have an equivocal score, depending on how far along you are in your pregnancy, you may have another BPP within the next 12–24 hours, or it may be decided to deliver the baby. A score of 4 or less usually means that the baby should be delivered right away. If the pregnancy is less than 32 weeks, your condition may be managed until the pregnancy is further along. No matter what the score is, not enough amniotic fluid means that more frequent testing should be done or delivery may need to be considered. The decision is based on gestational age, your condition, and the baby's condition.

## Modified Biophysical Profile

The modified BPP combines an NST with an amniotic fluid assessment that is performed using ultrasound. It allows your health care provider to assess whether the baby is receiving enough oxygen and how well the placenta is working.

**Why It Is Done.** This test is done for the same reasons that a BPP is done.

**How It Is Done.** The fetal heart rate is monitored in the same way it is done for the NST. Ultrasound is used to measure the amount of amniotic fluid.

**What the Results May Mean.** If the NST results are nonreactive, it could mean that the baby is not getting enough oxygen. If the amniotic fluid level is low, it could mean that there is a problem with blood flow in the placenta. A full BPP or contraction stress test may be needed to confirm results.

### Contraction Stress Test

The CST helps your health care provider see how the fetal heart rate reacts when the uterus contracts. The heart rate of a baby that is having trouble getting oxygen will follow a characteristic pattern during a contraction. You may hear this pattern referred to as a late deceleration. A variable deceleration also can occur. This pattern can be caused by the umbilical cord becoming compressed due to a low amount of amniotic fluid.

**Why It Is Done.** The contraction stress test sometimes is used if other test results are positive or unclear.

**How It Is Done.** In this test, belts with sensors that detect the fetal heart rate and uterine contractions are placed across your abdomen, just as in a nonstress test. To make your uterus contract mildly, you may be asked to rub your nipples through your clothing or you may be given oxytocin. Your uterus may contract on its own, especially if the test is done late in pregnancy.

**What the Results May Mean.** Results are negative when there are no late or significant variable decelerations. A positive result is one in which late decelerations occur after at least one half of the contractions. Results also can be equivocal–suspicious (there are intermittent late or variable decelerations), equivocal (the results are unclear), or unsatisfactory (there were not enough contractions to produce a meaningful result).

# RESOURCES

The following resources offer more information about special fetal testing:

**Monitoring Your Baby Before Labor**
Medline Plus
www.nlm.nih.gov/medlineplus/ency/patientinstructions/000485.htm
*Describes the special tests that can be performed to assess fetal well-being before labor.*

**Obstetric Ultrasound**
American College of Radiology and Radiological Society of North America
www.radiologyinfo.org/en/info.cfm?pg=obstetricus
*Gives an overview of how ultrasound is performed during pregnancy, what it can tell you and your health care provider, and its risks and benefits.*

# Part VII
# Complications During Pregnancy and Childbirth

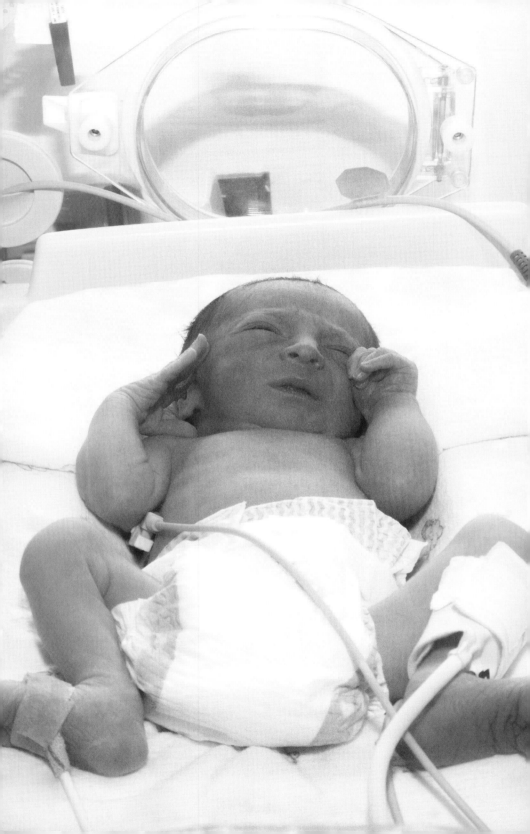

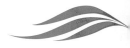

Chapter 27

# Preterm Labor, Premature Rupture of Membranes, and Preterm Birth

A normal pregnancy lasts about 40 weeks from the first day of the last menstrual period. When labor starts before 37 weeks of pregnancy, it is called *preterm* labor. *Premature rupture of membranes* (PROM) occurs when the *amniotic sac* that cushions the baby breaks before the onset of labor. When PROM happens before 37 weeks of pregnancy, it is called *preterm PROM*. Preterm PROM usually signals that there is a problem. Both preterm labor and PROM need prompt medical attention.

Preterm birth is the birth of a baby before 37 weeks of pregnancy. About one half of all the preterm births in the United States are preceded by preterm labor. But preterm birth also may be recommended in certain situations. This is called an indicated preterm birth. Indicated preterm birth may be recommended when there are medical conditions and complications during pregnancy that make preterm birth safer than continuing the pregnancy.

## Preterm Labor

Preterm labor is defined as regular contractions of the uterus resulting in changes in the *cervix* that start before 37 weeks of pregnancy. These changes include *effacement* (the cervix thins out) and *dilation* (the cervix opens so that the baby can enter the birth canal).

Preterm birth is a concern because babies who are born too early may not be fully developed. They may be born with serious health problems. The risk of health problems is greatest for babies born before 34 weeks of pregnancy. But babies born between 34 weeks and 37 weeks of pregnancy also are at risk.

Some health problems, like *cerebral palsy*, can be lifelong. Other problems, such as learning disabilities, appear later in childhood or even in adulthood.

Knowing whether you have risk factors for preterm birth, recognizing the signs and symptoms of preterm labor, and getting early care if you have signs and symptoms are important. Preterm labor may stop on its own. If it does not, treatments can be given that may help delay birth and reduce the risk of complications for the baby.

### Risk Factors

Preterm labor can happen to anyone without warning. There are some factors, however, that can increase your risk of preterm labor, including past obstetric and gynecologic conditions, current pregnancy complications, and lifestyle factors (see box "Risk Factors for Preterm Birth"). Women who have

## Risk Factors for Preterm Birth

Despite what is known about these risk factors, much remains to be learned about preterm labor and preterm birth. Many women who have preterm births have no known risk factors.

### Obstetric and Gynecologic History
- Prior preterm birth
- Short cervical length (measured during a *transvaginal ultrasound exam*)
- History of certain types of surgery on the uterus or cervix (such as a loop electrosurgical excision procedure for abnormal cervical cells)
- Short interval between pregnancies

### Pregnancy Complications
- *Multiple pregnancy*
- Vaginal bleeding during pregnancy
- Infections during pregnancy

### Lifestyle Factors
- Low prepregnancy weight
- Smoking during pregnancy
- Substance abuse during pregnancy

### Other Factors
- Age younger than 17 years or older than 35 years
- African American race
- Low socioeconomic status

had a previous preterm birth are at the greatest risk. Women with a short cervix, as measured during a transvaginal ultrasound exam, also are at increased risk.

## Diagnosis

Signs and symptoms of preterm labor are listed in the box "Warning Signs of Preterm Labor." If you have any of these signs or symptoms, do not wait. Call your health care provider's office or go immediately to the hospital.

Having regular contractions does not necessarily mean that you are in preterm labor. Preterm labor can be diagnosed only when changes in the cervix are found. Your health care provider may perform a **pelvic exam** to see if your cervix has started to change. You may need to be examined several times over a period of a few hours. Your contractions also may be monitored.

## Management

It is difficult for health care providers to predict which women with preterm labor will go on to have preterm birth. Only about 10% of women with preterm labor will give birth within the next 7 days. For about 30% of women, preterm labor stops on its own.

If you have symptoms of preterm labor, your health care provider may order certain tests. An ultrasound exam may be done to measure the length of the cervix and to estimate the **gestational age**. A vaginal swab may be used to test for the presence of a protein called **fetal fibronectin**. Fetal fibronectin is a protein that acts like a glue to help the **amniotic sac** stay connected to the inside of the uterus. The presence of this protein in the vaginal discharge

## Warning Signs of Preterm Labor

Call your health care provider right away if you notice any of these signs or symptoms:

- Mild abdominal cramps, with or without diarrhea
- Change in type (watery, mucus, or bloody) of vaginal discharge
- Increase in amount of discharge
- Pelvic or lower abdominal pressure
- Constant, low, dull backache
- Regular or frequent contractions or uterine tightening, often painless
- Ruptured membranes (your water breaks with a gush or a trickle of fluid)

puts you at higher risk of preterm birth. If your test results are positive—you are found to have fetal fibronectin in your vaginal discharge or a transvaginal ultrasound exam finds that you have a short cervix—it can help your health care provider get a better picture of what is going on. However, results of these tests are not able to predict whether you will have a preterm birth.

Management of preterm labor is based on what is thought to be best for your health and your baby's health. An important consideration is the gestational age. When there is a chance that the baby would benefit from a delay in delivery, medications can be given to help the baby's organs mature, reduce the risk of certain complications, and delay delivery for a short time. When preterm labor is too far along to be stopped or there are reasons that the baby should be born early, it may be necessary to deliver the baby.

**Corticosteroids.** *Corticosteroids* are drugs that cross the placenta and help speed up development of the baby's lungs, brain, and digestive organs. Corticosteroids are most likely to help your baby when they are given between 24 weeks of pregnancy and 34 weeks of pregnancy if you are at risk of delivering within the next 7 days. If you are likely to give birth within 1 week, two doses of corticosteroids are given over 24–48 hours or four doses every 12 hours. It takes 2 days after the first dose is given for the most benefits to occur, but some benefits occur after 24 hours.

**Magnesium Sulfate.** *Magnesium sulfate* is a tocolytic. Tocolytics are drugs used to delay delivery for a short time (up to 48 hours). Magnesium sulfate may be given if you are less than 32 weeks pregnant and are at risk of delivery within the next 24 hours. In addition to delaying delivery, this medication may help reduce the risk and severity of cerebral palsy that is associated with early preterm birth. It can cause minor side effects in the woman, including flushing, hot flashes, blurry vision, and weakness. Serious complications are rare.

**Additional Tocolytics.** Other tocolytics may allow time for corticosteroids or magnesium sulfate to be given or for you to be transferred to a hospital that offers specialized care for preterm infants.

Tocolytic drugs can have side effects, some of which can be serious. The side effects differ with each type of drug. Tocolytics are given when the benefits of the treatment are thought to outweigh the risks. Women with preterm labor symptoms but no changes in the cervix do not benefit from tocolytic treatment. There also is no benefit from continuing to give tocolytics after preterm labor has stopped.

## *Prevention*

There are treatments that can be given to help prevent preterm birth if you have risk factors. The following treatments may be recommended depending on your individual situation:

- *Progesterone* shots—If you have had a prior preterm birth with a single baby and you are now pregnant with a single baby, you may be offered progesterone shots beginning at 16 weeks–24 weeks of pregnancy. This is a hormone that may help prevent another preterm delivery. These injections will continue weekly until delivery or until 36 weeks of pregnancy.

- Vaginal progesterone—This treatment may be given if you have not had a prior preterm birth but you are found to have a very short cervix before or at 24 weeks of pregnancy. Vaginal progesterone is a gel or suppository that you place in your vagina daily until delivery or until 37 weeks of pregnancy. For women who are pregnant with a single baby, this treatment can reduce the risk of giving birth before 35 weeks of pregnancy by almost 50%.

- *Cerclage*—If you have had a prior preterm birth before 34 weeks of pregnancy and are found to have a short cervix on an ultrasound exam before 24 weeks of pregnancy, a procedure called cerclage may be considered. In cerclage, the cervix is closed with stitches. Cerclage is recommended for women with single pregnancies only. It may increase the risk of preterm birth if it is done in women with a short cervix and a multiple pregnancy.

## Premature Rupture of Membranes

When the sac that holds the amniotic fluid ruptures and your water breaks, other signs of labor usually follow. If the membranes rupture at or around the time of a woman's due date, but labor does not begin soon afterward, it is called premature rupture of membranes ("term PROM" or just "PROM"). When the membranes rupture before 37 weeks, it is called preterm premature rupture of membranes (or "preterm PROM").

Term PROM happens in about 8% of pregnancies. It is caused by the normal weakening of the amniotic sac as birth approaches as well as by the force of uterine contractions. In about 95% of cases, labor begins within 28 hours. The risks of PROM include infection of the uterus and ***umbilical cord*** problems. The likelihood of these complications occurring increases the longer labor is delayed.

Preterm PROM carries the same risks as PROM. Because it occurs before 37 weeks of pregnancy, preterm PROM also may lead to serious problems for the baby related to prematurity.

## Risk Factors

Although most cases of PROM occur in the absence of any risk factors, there are several well-established factors that do increase the chances of it occurring. The risk factors associated with PROM include infection, a low *body mass index* (less than 19), bleeding during the second or third trimesters, smoking, and dietary deficiencies. A significant risk factor is having had preterm PROM in a previous pregnancy. The risk for recurrence is between 16% and 32%.

## Diagnosis

The main symptom of PROM is leakage of fluid from your vagina. Call your health care provider if you have any fluid leakage. Your health care provider will want to determine whether your membranes have ruptured. Sometimes you may have a discharge for other reasons, including *urine* leakage, cervical mucus, vaginal bleeding, or a vaginal infection. A physical exam and lab tests may be done to find out if there is amniotic fluid in your vagina.

## Management

Once the diagnosis of PROM is confirmed, one of the first things that your health care provider will do is assess the baby's gestational age. If you have any conditions that put your or your baby's life in danger, such as *placental abruption* or infection of the uterus, your baby will be delivered right away, regardless of gestational age. But if you do not have any of these conditions, the gestational age of your baby is an important factor in determining how your condition will be managed.

If you have PROM, your baby is in the correct position for delivery, and your labor does not start on its own within a few hours, it probably will be recommended that you have your labor induced with *oxytocin*. If the baby is not in the correct position (*breech presentation*), you most likely will have a *cesarean delivery*. In either case, you also will receive *antibiotics* for *group B streptococci* based on your prior test results or risk factors if you have not been tested.

If you have preterm PROM and you have reached 34 weeks of pregnancy, delivery generally is recommended. If preterm PROM occurs after 24 weeks of pregnancy and before 34 weeks of pregnancy, your health care provider probably will try to delay birth until the baby is more developed. You may need to stay in the hospital so that you can be monitored closely. You may receive antibiotics to prevent infection and corticosteroids to help the baby's lungs mature. These measures may stop the leakage of amniotic fluid. Sometimes, preterm PROM stops on its own and the amniotic fluid level returns to normal.

If you have preterm PROM before 24 completed weeks of pregnancy, your health care provider will explain the risks of having a very preterm baby and the potential risks and benefits of trying to delay labor. You may decide to have the baby immediately. If your condition is stable and there are no signs of infection, you can opt to wait and see what happens. Your health care provider will explain the precautions you should take. You should return to the hospital if you have symptoms of infection, labor, or other complications. You may be told to take your temperature daily to check for infection. Once your pregnancy reaches about 24 weeks, you typically will need to stay in the hospital. Treatment at this point usually includes antibiotics and corticosteroids.

## Preterm Birth

Sometimes, preterm labor cannot be stopped. In some cases, it may be decided that the baby should be born early for his or her own safety or for that of the mother. If it looks like you will give birth to your baby early, your health care provider will discuss the possible health consequences for your preterm baby.

In general, infants who are born before 24 weeks of pregnancy are less likely to survive. Those that do survive are likely to have profound developmental and physical disabilities that can affect movement, speech, hearing, and vision and that will require lifelong care. By 25 completed weeks of pregnancy, survival chances increase to 75%, but one third of these babies will have severe, lifelong disabilities and one half will have moderate-to-severe disabilities.

Late preterm babies (those born from 34 and 0/7 weeks to 36 and 6/7 weeks of pregnancy) and even early term babies (those born from 37 and 0/7 weeks to 38 and 6/7 weeks of pregnancy) also may have health problems. Babies need the full 40 weeks of pregnancy to grow. Many organs, such as the brain, lungs, and liver, do not finish developing until the final weeks of pregnancy. Babies born a few weeks early may have problems breathing, eating, sleeping, and controlling their body temperature. While they are at less risk than babies born before 34 weeks, they may need to stay in the hospital longer and require more specialized care than infants born after 39 weeks of pregnancy.

### Neonatal Intensive Care

If you are likely to give birth to a preterm baby, you and the baby will be cared for by a team of health care providers. The team may include a neonatologist, a doctor who specializes in treating problems in newborns. The care your baby needs depends on how early he or she is born. High-level *neonatal intensive care units (NICUs)* provide this specialized care for preterm infants. These units are specially equipped and have doctors and nurses with advanced training and experience in caring for preterm babies.

Because of the possible need for urgent medical care for your preterm infant at birth, you may be transferred to a hospital that offers this specialized care if you go into labor early. It is safer and may provide a better outcome to give birth to a preterm baby at these hospitals than to transport the baby after birth. After the baby is born, he or she may continue to need intensive care. Some babies need to stay in the NICU for weeks or sometimes months.

### Surfactant Replacement Therapy

Babies who survive but who are at risk of breathing problems may be given *surfactant* replacement therapy. Surfactant is a substance that helps the air sacs in the lungs (called *alveoli*) stay inflated. The lungs begin making surfactant at around 23 weeks of pregnancy. Lack of surfactant is the main cause of a serious lung condition called *respiratory distress syndrome* in preterm infants.

Infants who need surfactant replacement therapy often are very sick and need highly specialized care. For this reason, surfactant therapy is offered only in hospitals where the staff is specially trained in giving this treatment and caring for very sick babies.

### Resuscitation and Breathing Support

Quick action may be needed to help the baby breathe. Your health care team will prepare for this possibility in advance. For babies who are born very early, this may involve inserting a breathing tube and using a device called a *ventilator*.

## Making Difficult Decisions

If you are likely to give birth to a preterm infant, your health care provider and NICU team will use all of the available information to give you a range of possible outcomes. This information comes from studies of infants who have been born preterm. For preterm birth that is likely to happen before 26 weeks of pregnancy, the *Eunice Kennedy Shriver* National Institute of Child Health and Human Development has an online calculator that allows you and your health care provider to see a range of possible outcomes depending on the factors that you enter (www.nichd.nih.gov/about/org/der/branches/ppb/programs/epbo/Pages/index.aspx).

As useful as the calculator is, it is important to remember that every infant is an individual and every situation is different. Also, survival and complication rates change over time and differ from state to state and even from hospital to hospital. Your health care team may provide you with local and regional information about outcomes if it is available.

Although a plan of treatment may be discussed before the baby is born, it is best to make decisions after the baby is born, when his or her condition can be assessed. Once the baby is born, the neonatologist may be able to give you a better idea of what you can expect. Decisions and expected outcomes may change based on how well the baby responds to treatment. Ask questions if any information is unclear. It is important to have support from friends, family, and your medical team in order to decide what is best for your baby.

## Caring for a Preterm Baby

Once the baby is born, your health care team will have a better idea of the baby's health and whether any problems exist. If your baby is healthy enough to overcome the challenges of being born preterm, he or she still will require special care. Neonatologists are pediatric specialists who care for preterm babies and children. Some clinics focus on follow-up care for preterm babies. Make sure you find a doctor you like and trust. The doctor will closely watch how your baby grows and check to see if any problems develop during childhood.

You also can find information for parents about caring for preterm babies. It is a good idea to become as informed as you can so you can give your baby the best care possible. For more information about preterm birth and caring for a preterm child, see the "Resources" section in this chapter.

# RESOURCES

The following resources offer more information about some of the topics discussed in this chapter:

**Preterm Birth**
www.cdc.gov/reproductivehealth/MaternalInfantHealth/PretermBirth.htm
Centers for Disease Control and Prevention
*Provides an overview of the problem of preterm birth in the United States and the warning signs to watch for.*

**Preterm Labor and Preterm Birth**
*Eunice Kennedy Shriver* National Institute of Child Health and Human Development
www.nichd.nih.gov/health/topics/preterm/Pages/default.aspx
*National institute that studies health problems of children; provides general information about preterm labor and preterm birth and details how experts are studying ways to predict and prevent it.*

**Preterm (Premature) Labor and Birth: Resource Overview**
The American College of Obstetricians and Gynecologists (ACOG)
http://www.acog.org/Womens-Health/Preterm-Premature-Labor-and-Birth
*Lists ACOG's articles and patient education resources on preterm labor and preterm birth.*

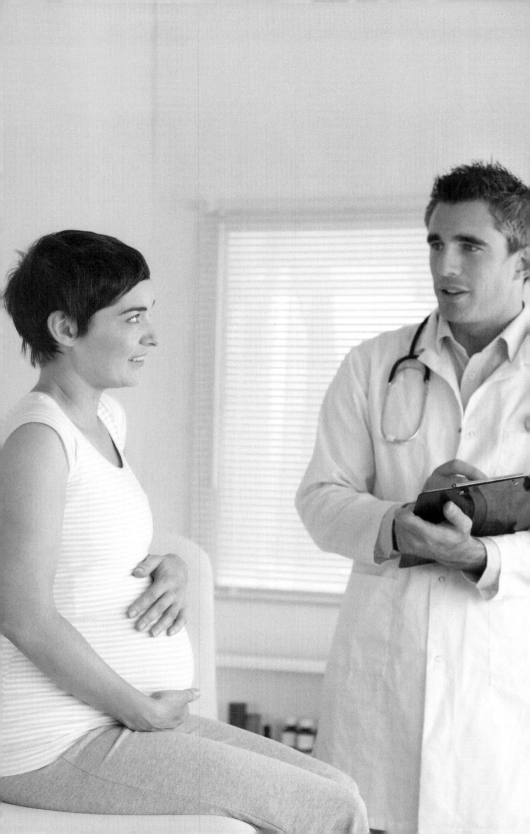

Chapter 28

# Blood Type Incompatibility

Your blood type is A, B, AB, or O. Blood types are determined by the types of *antigens*—tiny proteins—on your blood *cells*. Type A blood has only A antigens, type B has only B antigens, type AB has both A and B antigens, and type O has neither A nor B antigens. There also is an antigen called the ***Rh factor***. If your blood has the Rh factor, you are Rh positive. If it does not have the Rh factor, you are Rh negative.

As part of your ***prenatal care***, you will have blood tests to find out your blood type and to determine whether you are Rh positive or Rh negative. This information is important because complications can occur if your blood type is different from your baby's. This is called blood type incompatibility. In the past, this problem was a major cause of newborn sickness and even death. Now, with early testing and treatment, most of these complications can be prevented.

## Rh Incompatibility

The Rh factor is inherited—it is passed down through parents' ***genes*** to their children. Most people are Rh positive. If both the mother and the father are Rh positive, then the baby will be Rh positive. If both the mother and the father are Rh negative, the baby also will be Rh negative. But if the mother is Rh negative and the father is Rh positive, and the baby inherits the Rh gene from the father, the baby will be Rh positive. Problems can occur if you are Rh negative and the baby is Rh positive. This is called Rh incompatibility. Problems with Rh incompatibility usually do not occur in a first pregnancy, but they can occur in future pregnancies.

### How It Affects Your Baby

If you are Rh negative and your baby is Rh positive, and a small amount of the baby's blood mixes with your blood, it may cause your body to make **antibodies** against the Rh factor. If your body has made Rh antibodies, you are said to be "Rh sensitized." Rh antibodies attack the Rh factor as if it were a harmful substance.

**Rh sensitization** usually does not cause problems during an Rh-negative woman's first pregnancy with an Rh-positive baby. The baby often is born before the mother's body has a chance to make many antibodies. But if preventive treatment is not given during the first pregnancy and an Rh-negative woman later becomes pregnant with another Rh-positive baby, the second baby is at risk of Rh disease.

About 2 in 10 Rh-negative women will become Rh sensitized if they become pregnant with an Rh-positive baby. If both the woman and baby are Rh negative, there is no risk that the woman will become Rh sensitized.

Rh disease occurs when Rh antibodies destroy some of the baby's red blood cells. This causes **hemolytic disease of the newborn (HDN)**, in which fetal red blood cells are destroyed faster than they can be replaced. Red blood cells carry oxygen to all parts of the body. Without enough red blood cells,

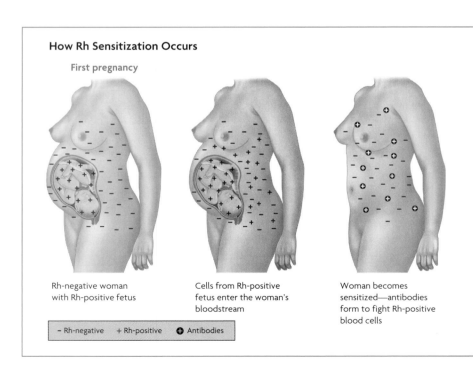

**How Rh Sensitization Occurs**

First pregnancy

Rh-negative woman with Rh-positive fetus

Cells from Rh-positive fetus enter the woman's bloodstream

Woman becomes sensitized—antibodies form to fight Rh-positive blood cells

− Rh-negative   + Rh-positive   ⊕ Antibodies

the baby will not get enough oxygen. HDN can lead to serious illness. In severe cases, HDN even may be fatal to the baby.

## How Sensitization Can Occur

During pregnancy, the woman and baby do not share blood systems. However, a small amount of blood from the baby can cross the **placenta** into the woman's system. This sometimes may happen during pregnancy, labor, or birth. It also can occur if an Rh-negative woman has had any of the following:

- *Amniocentesis*
- *Chorionic villus sampling*
- Bleeding during pregnancy
- Manual rotation of a baby in a **breech presentation** before labor
- Blunt trauma to the abdomen during pregnancy
- *Miscarriage*
- *Ectopic pregnancy*
- *Induced abortion*

If an Rh-negative woman does not receive treatment after one of these events, and she becomes pregnant with an Rh-positive baby, the baby may be at risk of Rh-related problems.

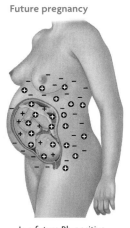

Future pregnancy

In a future Rh-positive pregnancy, antibodies attack fetal blood cells

## Prevention

The good news is that problems during pregnancy caused by Rh incompatibility can be prevented easily. The goal of preventive treatment is to stop an Rh-negative woman from making Rh antibodies in the first place. This is done by testing your blood early in pregnancy or before pregnancy. If necessary, a medication can be given to you to prevent HDN.

**Blood Testing.** A simple blood test can identify your blood type and Rh factor. During the first prenatal visit, a blood sample usually is taken in your health care provider's office and sent to a lab for analysis.

Another blood test, called an antibody screen or indirect Coombs test, can show if an Rh-negative woman has developed antibodies to Rh-positive blood and how many antibodies have been made.

If you are Rh negative and there is a possibility that your baby is Rh positive, your health care provider may request this test during your first trimester and again during week 28 of pregnancy.

**Rh Immunoglobulin.** *Rh immunoglobulin (RhIg)* is made from donated blood. When given to an Rh-negative pregnant woman who has not been sensitized, it targets and destroys any Rh-positive fetal cells that may have leaked into the mother's bloodstream. This prevents the mother from making Rh antibodies. RhIg can prevent HDN in a later pregnancy. RhIg is not helpful if the mother is already Rh sensitized. RhIg is given to Rh-negative women in the following situations:

• At around the 28th week of pregnancy to prevent Rh sensitization for the rest of the pregnancy—A small number of women may be exposed to Rh-positive blood cells from the baby in the last few months of pregnancy and may make antibodies against these cells. RhIg given at around the 28th week of pregnancy destroys these Rh-positive cells and prevents Rh-positive antibodies from being made.

• Within 72 hours after the delivery of an Rh-positive infant—RhIg prevents a woman from making antibodies that could affect future pregnancies. Each pregnancy and delivery of an Rh-positive child requires a repeat dose of RhIg.

• After a miscarriage, abortion, or ectopic pregnancy

• After amniocentesis or chorionic villus sampling

An Rh-negative woman may receive RhIg after giving birth even if she decides to have *postpartum sterilization*. In this case, RhIg treatment may be given for three reasons:

1. The woman may decide later to have the sterilization reversed.

2. There is a slight chance that the sterilization may fail to prevent another pregnancy.

3. The treatment prevents her from developing antibodies in case she ever needs to be given a blood *transfusion* in the future. The presence of antibodies makes matching blood types for transfusions more difficult.

## Treatment if Antibodies Develop

RhIg treatment does not help if an Rh-negative woman already has developed antibodies. Depending on the father's blood type, it may be necessary to assess the unborn baby's blood to determine whether the baby is Rh negative or Rh positive. This is done by **amniocentesis**. If the baby is Rh positive, special monitoring of the pregnancy is needed. This usually involves a specialized **ultrasound exam** and tests of the mother's blood to check antibody levels. If tests show that the baby has severe HDN, it may be decided to deliver the baby early (before 37 weeks of pregnancy). In some severe cases of HDN, it may be necessary to give a blood **transfusion** through the umbilical cord while the baby is still in the mother's uterus. If HDN is mild, the baby may be delivered at 37–38 weeks of pregnancy. After delivery, the baby may need a transfusion to replace the blood cells.

## ABO Incompatibility

Although it occurs very rarely, some pregnant women's blood types are incompatible with their babies' blood types. When this happens, the mother usually is type O and her baby is type A or type B. A mother with type O blood makes antibodies against the antigens that are present on type A and type B blood cells. If these antibodies cross the placenta, they can attack the baby's red blood cells. This is known as ABO incompatibility.

Unlike Rh incompatibility, the effects of ABO incompatibility occur during the first pregnancy with an incompatible baby, and they do not worsen with future pregnancies.

### How It Affects Your Baby

Newborns born with ABO incompatibility can have mild HDN and high levels of **bilirubin** in the blood. Bilirubin is a substance that forms when old red blood cells break down. **Jaundice** (yellowish skin and eyes) is a sign of high levels of bilirubin. Too much of the substance can be harmful, especially to the baby's nervous system, and can cause developmental problems.

### Treatment

There is no preventive treatment that can be given during pregnancy. ABO incompatibility usually is diagnosed after the baby is born, and it usually is mild. If your baby has jaundice caused by HDN, the level of bilirubin in the baby's blood will be measured. If it's high, special treatment, such as the use of special lights, will bring the level down. If this treatment does not decrease the bilirubin level, if the level is very high to begin with, or if the infant is showing signs of bilirubin toxicity, a blood transfusion may be needed.

# RESOURCES

The following resources offer more information about Rh and ABO incompatibility during pregnancy:

**Hemolytic Anemia**
National Institutes of Health/National Heart, Lung, and Blood Institute
www.nhlbi.nih.gov/health/health-topics/topics/ha/
*Describes hemolytic anemia, why it occurs, and how it is treated.*

**Rh Incompatibility**
National Institutes of Health/National Heart, Lung, and Blood Institute
www.nhlbi.nih.gov/health/health-topics/topics/rh/
*Provides a definition of Rh incompatibility and discusses how this condition is prevented and treated.*

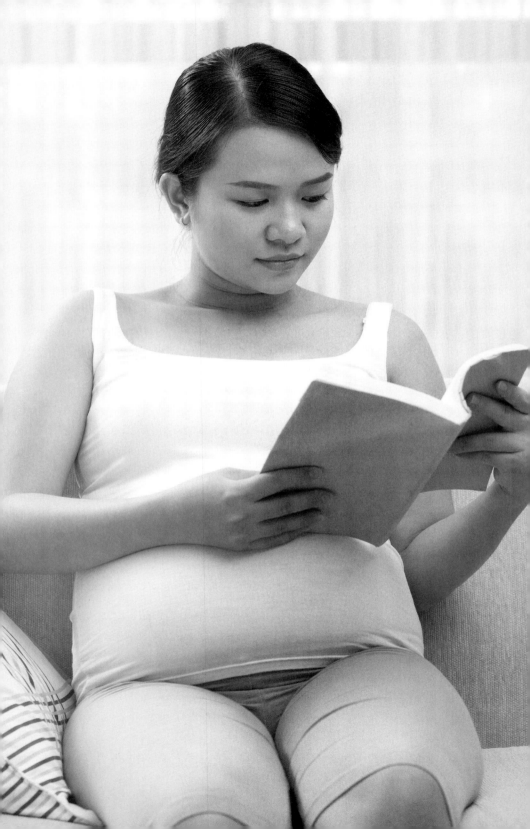

# Chapter 29
# Placental Problems

The **placenta** is a unique organ that is present only during pregnancy. It delivers **nutrients** and **oxygen** to and removes waste products from the baby. In a normal pregnancy, the placenta is attached high on the wall of the uterus away from the **cervix**. It remains attached until shortly after the baby is born, when it detaches from the wall of the uterus.

Certain problems with the placenta can occur during pregnancy. They can cause serious complications if they are not identified early. You should be aware of the signs and symptoms of these problems and alert your health care provider immediately if you think you are experiencing any of them.

## Placenta Previa

**Placenta previa** is a condition in which the placenta lies low in the uterus and covers part of the internal opening of the cervix (called the **internal os**). Because it covers this opening, the placenta blocks the baby's exit from the uterus.

Placenta previa occurs in 1 in 200 pregnancies. Although the reasons why placenta previa happens in some women are unknown, it is more common in women with the following conditions:

- Have had more than one child
- Have had a **cesarean delivery**
- Have had surgery on the uterus
- Are carrying twins or triplets

Smoking and cocaine use during pregnancy also may increase the risk of placenta previa.

If placenta previa is not diagnosed and managed, it can lead to serious complications, including *hemorrhage* and infection in the mother. Multiple transfusions may be needed. In some cases, an emergency *hysterectomy* may be necessary to stop bleeding. Placenta previa also poses risks for the baby. Because it may be necessary to deliver the baby early, there is an increased risk that the baby will have problems associated with being born *preterm*, including neurologic problems, respiratory complications, and other potentially long-term disabilities. Fortunately, most cases of placenta previa are diagnosed well before labor begins, so appropriate steps can be taken to reduce these risks.

## Types

Placenta previa is categorized into different types depending on the location of the placenta and how much of the internal os is covered:

* Complete—The placenta completely covers the internal os.
* Partial—The placenta partially covers the internal os.
* Marginal—The placenta reaches the internal os but does not cover it.

A low-lying placenta is one that implants in the lower part of the uterus but does not reach the internal os.

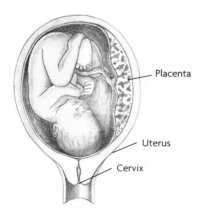 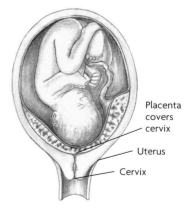

**Normal position of placenta.** The placenta normally attaches high on the uterine wall, away from the cervix.

**Placenta previa.** In this condition, the placenta lies low in the uterus and either partly or completely blocks the cervix.

## Signs and Symptoms

Painless vaginal bleeding is the main sign of placenta previa. The bleeding usually occurs near the end of the second trimester or at the start of the third trimester. Bleeding episodes often are small at first and frequently stop on their own. A more severe bleeding episode may follow. Call your health care provider right away if you have any bleeding in your third trimester. However, not every woman with placenta previa will have bleeding. About one in four women with this condition do not have any bleeding.

## Diagnosis

Most cases of placenta previa are diagnosed during a routine **ultrasound exam** in the first or second trimester, before any bleeding occurs. If you are diagnosed with placenta previa before 21 weeks of pregnancy, you most likely will be monitored with periodic ultrasound exams. Most cases of partial placenta previa and low-lying placenta previa resolve on their own by 32–35 weeks of pregnancy as the lower part of the uterus stretches and thins out. Labor and delivery then can proceed normally.

## Treatment

If placenta previa does not go away by itself, other measures usually are taken. The goal is to prolong the pregnancy as much as possible to give the baby enough time to grow and develop while also monitoring for severe bleeding in the mother. If you have episodes of bleeding, you may need to stay in the hospital, where your condition and the baby's condition can be watched closely. You may need blood **transfusions**. An ultrasound exam will be done to check the position of the placenta within the uterus. You may receive drugs called **corticosteroids** to help the baby's lungs and other organs develop in case of a **preterm** delivery.

If the bleeding stops on its own and you are less than 34 weeks along, it may be possible to monitor your condition on an outpatient basis (you don't have to stay in the hospital). However, you will need to see your health care provider frequently and call him or her immediately if you have any vaginal bleeding. You also need to be able to get to a hospital quickly in case of emergency.

If you have no other complications and the baby also is doing well, a cesarean delivery usually is recommended from 36 and 0/7 weeks to 37 and 6/7 weeks of pregnancy. If you have other medical conditions, fetal complications, or additional problems with the placenta (see "Placenta Accreta"), delivery may take place earlier, from 34 and 0/7 weeks to 35 and 6/7 weeks of pregnancy. Your health care provider may refer you to a *neonatologist*, who can provide information about what to expect when a baby is born preterm.

## Placental Abruption

*Placental abruption* occurs when the placenta separates from the wall of the uterus before or during birth. This often causes vaginal bleeding and severe pain in the abdomen. Placental abruption is a potentially dangerous problem for the woman and her baby. The baby may get less oxygen, and the woman can lose a large amount of blood. Prompt treatment is needed.

Only 1% of pregnant women have this problem, and it usually occurs in the last 12 weeks before birth. Placental abruption happens more often in women who have **high blood pressure**, smoke, or use cocaine or amphetamines during pregnancy. It also is more common in women who

- have already had children
- are older than 35 years
- have had placental abruption before
- have sickle cell disease

### Types

Placental abruption is classified into different types depending on the extent of the abruption and where the separation is located:

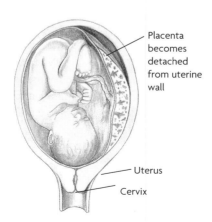

Placenta becomes detached from uterine wall

Uterus

Cervix

**Placental abruption.** The placenta becomes detached from the uterine wall.

- Complete—The entire placenta separates from the wall of the uterus.
- Partial—Part of the placenta separates from the wall of the uterus.

### Signs and Symptoms

The most common signs and symptoms are vaginal bleeding and abdominal or back pain. If the abruption is partial, there may only be bleeding. Some women do not have a lot of bleeding with placental abruption because the blood becomes trapped inside the uterus behind the placenta.

### Treatment

Treatment for placental abruption depends on your condition and how far along you are in your pregnancy. An ultrasound exam may be done, but sometimes it's not possible to identify placental abruption with ultrasound. If you have lost a lot of blood, you may need a blood transfusion. After your condition is stabilized, your health care provider will check the fetal heart rate. You may have to stay in the hospital so doctors can watch your condition closely.

If the abruption is small, and you are near your due date, labor may be induced, or you may have a cesarean delivery if there are other problems. Sometimes bleeding stops on its own. In this case, you will be monitored closely to make sure the abruption does not get worse. If your due date is still far off (you're between 24 weeks and 34 weeks of pregnancy), you may receive drugs called **tocolytics** to help delay delivery and corticosteroids to help the baby's lungs mature. After 34 weeks of pregnancy, the baby usually is delivered. Although there is a risk of the baby having health problems related to prematurity, it is safer to deliver the baby in some cases.

## Placenta Accreta

Placenta accreta is a general term used to describe a condition in which the placenta (or part of the placenta) invades and becomes inseparable from the uterine wall. A major risk factor for this condition is a previous cesarean delivery, with the risk increasing with the number of prior cesarean deliveries. Having had any type of surgery that causes damage to the muscle wall of the uterus, called the **myometrium**, increases the risk. Types of surgery that do this include the surgical removal of **fibroids** that are inside the wall of the uterus, **endometrial ablation** performed with heat, and **uterine artery embolization**. Other risk factors include increasing age and multiple pregnancy.

Placenta accreta occurs in about 1 in 533 pregnancies. This condition can cause severe, life-threatening blood loss during delivery when the placenta separates from the uterus after the birth of the baby.

### Types

When the placenta extends into the muscular wall of the uterus, it is called placenta increta. When the placenta extends through the entire wall of

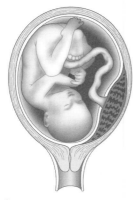

**Placenta accreta.** The placenta invades the wall of the uterus.

the uterus, it is called placenta percreta. In some cases of placenta percreta, the placenta can extend into nearby organs, such as the bladder.

## Signs and Symptoms

Placenta accreta may cause bleeding during the third trimester, and it also commonly occurs with placenta previa. However, there may be no clear warning signs of this condition as there are with placenta previa and placental abruption.

## Diagnosis

Health care providers try to diagnose placenta accreta before delivery so they are prepared for potential hemorrhage and complications. In the past, placenta accreta often was not diagnosed until after the baby was delivered. This still happens, but an ultrasound exam can identify most cases of placenta accreta well before delivery. Your health care provider will have a higher level of suspicion for this condition if you have risk factors. If results of an ultrasound exam are not clear, a procedure called *magnetic resonance imaging* may be done to clarify them.

## Treatment

The recommended treatment for placenta accreta is a planned cesarean delivery followed by a hysterectomy. If placenta accreta is suspected, your health care provider will start to plan when and where you will give birth. You most likely will be cared for by a team of health care providers, including a surgeon and a neonatologist. You may be moved to another hospital with special facilities and staff who are experienced in managing this condition and where blood for transfusion is on hand. Although the goal is a planned cesarean delivery, emergency delivery may be necessary.

When you will have your baby is a decision that will be made between you and your health care provider. A test (*amniocentesis*) can be done to determine whether the fetal lungs are mature, and delivery then can take place. It also may be suggested that delivery be done at 34 weeks without this test. You may be given corticosteroids to help speed the development of the fetal lungs and other organs.

You need to know that you are at risk of life-threatening hemorrhage during delivery, and that a hysterectomy may be necessary to save your life. Blood for transfusion will be ordered so that it is there if it is needed. In some cases, it may be possible to avoid hysterectomy, but there are significant risks with this approach, including heavy bleeding. You may need to have a hysterectomy in any case. However, if you want to have more children, you may want to discuss this option with your health care providers, who can explain the risks to you in more detail.

# RESOURCES

The following resources offer more information about placental conditions:

**Placenta Accreta, Increta, and Percreta**
March of Dimes
www.marchofdimes.org/pregnancy/placental-accreta-increta-and-percreta.aspx
*Offers basic information about these pregnancy complications.*

**Placenta Previa**
Medline Plus/U.S. National Library of Medicine
www.nlm.nih.gov/medlineplus/ency/article/000900.htm
*Covers all aspects of placenta previa, including signs and symptoms, diagnosis, and treatment.*

**Placental Abruption**
Medline Plus/U.S. National Library of Medicine
www.nlm.nih.gov/medlineplus/ency/article/000901.htm
*Provides an overview of placental abruption.*

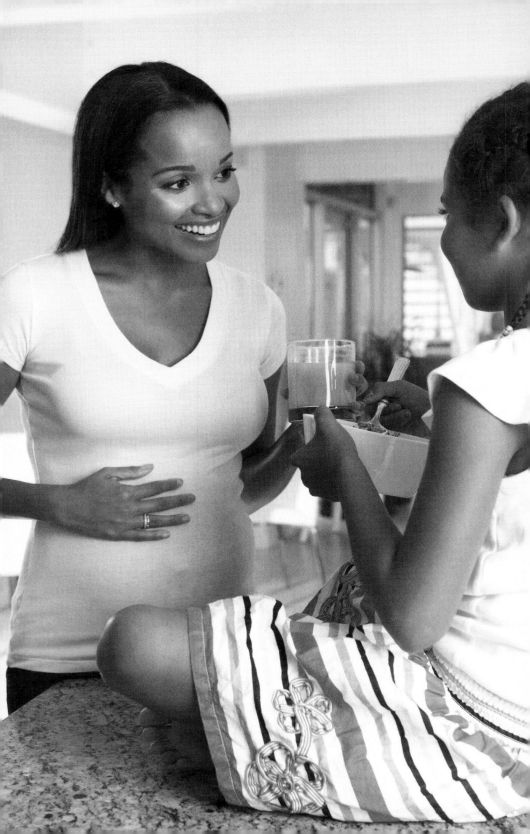

Chapter 30

# Protecting Yourself From Infections

Certain infections can pose risks to you and your unborn baby. Some infections can be passed from you to the baby during pregnancy; others can be transmitted to the baby during childbirth. Many of the tests and exams given during **prenatal care** visits are used to detect these infections. Early diagnosis often is the key to minimizing complications for you and your baby. But by far the best way to reduce your risk of problems caused by infections is prevention (see box "Simple Steps for Preventing Infections").

## What Happens During an Infection

Infections are diseases caused by **pathogens**. Pathogens include **bacteria**, **viruses**, fungi, and parasites. When your body is invaded by one of these organisms, the body's **immune system** swings into action. The immune system is a collection of **cells** and tissues that detect the presence of a pathogen, sound an alarm, and unleash defenses to fight off the infection. To fight some infections, the immune system makes **antibodies**. These special proteins are produced by certain immune cells in response to a pathogen. They "tag" pathogenic cells for destruction by other parts of the immune system.

Antibodies are the basis of some of the blood tests used to detect whether you have a specific infection. These tests can show whether antibodies have formed in your body. If they have, it means you have been exposed to that infection. In many cases, once the body makes antibodies to a disease, you

## Simple Steps for Preventing Infections

- Make sure your vaccines are up to date before you become pregnant.

- Know the symptoms of infections so you can alert your health care provider right away if they occur.

- Do not engage in behavior that increases the risk of infections.

- Use good hygiene, including washing your hands often.

- Avoid contact with people who are sick.

become *immune* to the disease and will not get it in the future. That's because the antibodies made against the infection stay in your body and are prepared to fight off the same infection if you encounter it again.

An infection may not cause any signs or symptoms. For some infections, signs and symptoms only occur as the infection progresses. If you have any unusual signs or symptoms, alert your health care provider right away. Infections caused by bacteria or parasites often can be treated with medications. Some medications are available that can decrease the severity of certain viral infections. The sooner you start treatment, the better.

## Immunizations and Pregnancy

Preventing infections in the first place can help keep you and your baby healthy during pregnancy and after the baby is born. You may think that only babies and children need to have immunizations, but adolescents, adults, and older adults all need certain immunizations at certain times. Pregnant women and women who are thinking about becoming pregnant also need certain vaccines. Two vaccines that are especially important for pregnant women are the flu (*influenza*) vaccine and the **tetanus toxoid, reduced diphtheria toxoid, and acellular pertussis (Tdap) vaccine**. A pregnant woman with the flu has a greater chance of severe illness for herself and serious problems for her unborn baby, including **preterm** labor and delivery, than women who are not pregnant. **Pertussis**, or whooping cough, is highly contagious and can be life threatening for infants because they cannot be vaccinated until they are 2 months of age.

But are vaccines safe for pregnant women? You may be concerned about reports that vaccines containing thimerosal, a mercury-containing preservative added to certain vaccines, including the flu vaccine, can cause **autism**. You may have heard it suggested that vaccines can lead to debilitating side effects or that they can cause the diseases that they are supposed to protect against. Educating yourself is a good first step in allaying these concerns. Here is the most up-to-date information regarding some of these claims:

- There is no scientific evidence showing that thimerosal-containing vaccines cause harmful effects in children born to women who received these vaccines. If you still have concerns about thimerosal, there are versions of the influenza vaccine without thimerosal. It's important to know, though, that experts have not indicated a preference for any particular group— including pregnant women—to get either thimerosal-free or thimerosal-containing vaccines.

- Vaccines are developed with the highest standards of safety. Vaccines approved by the U.S. Food and Drug Administration and recommended by the Advisory Committee on Immunization Practices (which is part of the Centers for Disease Control and Prevention [CDC]) have been thoroughly researched. Vaccines have been used for several decades in pregnant women without any adverse effects. But as with any medication, vaccination can have some risks. Individuals react differently to vaccines, and there is no way to predict how individuals will react to a particular vaccine. Most side effects of vaccines are mild, such as a sore arm or a low fever, and go away within a day or two. Severe side effects and reactions are rare. The CDC monitors side effects and reactions for all vaccines given in the United States. When you receive a vaccine, you also should receive a Vaccine Information Statement that lists the possible side effects and reactions associated with that vaccine (see the "Resources" section in this chapter). If you have concerns about vaccine side effects, talk to your health care provider.

- Most vaccines are made with inactivated or killed versions of a pathogen. Some vaccines are made with parts of the pathogen (like the components that make up the cell wall of a bacterium) or with an inactivated **toxin** made by the pathogen. None of these things can cause the disease itself when given as a vaccine. Certain vaccines do contain live, attenuated viruses. "Attenuated" means that the virus has been weakened so that it cannot cause disease. These include the **live attenuated influenza vaccine** given as a nasal spray; the **measles–mumps–rubella (MMR) vaccine**; and the **varicella (chickenpox)** vaccine. There is a small, theoretical risk that these viruses can transform in the body and recover their disease-causing abilities. There are no documented cases where this has happened. However, to eliminate the risk altogether, it is best to get the MMR and varicella vaccines at least 4 weeks before trying to become pregnant. You should not receive a live, attenuated vaccine while pregnant.

## Vaccine-Preventable Diseases

Vaccine-preventable diseases include *influenza*; *pertussis*; *hepatitis A virus infection*; *hepatitis B virus infection*; *human papillomavirus (HPV)*; *herpes zoster (shingles)*; *tetanus* and *diphtheria*; measles, mumps, and rubella; varicella (chickenpox); *pneumococcal disease*; and *meningococcal disease*. These diseases are discussed below. Recommendations for immunizations during pregnancy can be found in Table 30-1.

### Influenza

Influenza (the flu) is a contagious infection of the **respiratory system**. It is caused by a virus. Signs and symptoms include fever, headache, fatigue, muscle aches, coughing, congestion, runny nose, and sore throat. The flu is much more serious than a cold. It can cause serious complications, such as pneumonia. Pregnant women, their unborn babies, and newborns have a high risk of serious illness and complications from the flu.

The flu vaccine does "double duty" by protecting both you and your baby. Babies can't be vaccinated against the flu until they are 6 months old. When you get a flu shot during pregnancy, the protective antibodies that are made in your body are transferred to your baby. These antibodies will give protection against the flu until your baby can be vaccinated at 6 months of age. All pregnant women should be vaccinated early in the "flu season" (October through May) as soon as the vaccine is available regardless of how far along they are in their pregnancy. Women who haven't been vaccinated early in the flu season still can get the vaccine at any time during flu season as long as the vaccine supply lasts. Women with medical conditions that increase the risk of flu complications should consider getting the vaccine before the flu season starts.

The flu shot is safe for pregnant women. There have been no reports of harmful consequences of the flu shot for either pregnant women or their babies. There is no risk that the flu shot will cause you to get the flu. The flu shot contains an inactivated form of the virus that cannot cause

## Table 30-1 Immunizations and Pregnancy

| Vaccine | Do You Need It? |
|---------|-----------------|
| Influenza | Yes! You need a flu shot every year for your protection and for the protection of others around you. It's safe to get the vaccine during pregnancy. |
| Tetanus, diphtheria, whooping cough (pertussis) (Tdap, Td) | Yes! Women who are pregnant need a dose of Tdap vaccine (adult whooping cough vaccine) during each pregnancy, preferably during the third trimester. After that, you'll need a Td booster dose every 10 years. Talk to your health care provider if you haven't had at least three tetanus- and diphtheria-containing shots sometime in your life or if you have a deep or dirty wound. |
| Varicella (chickenpox) (VAR) | No.* Varicella vaccine is not recommended to be given during pregnancy, but if you inadvertently receive it, this is not a cause for concern. If you haven't been vaccinated or had chickenpox, it's best for you (and any future baby) to be protected with the vaccine before trying to get pregnant. If you were born in the United States in 1980 or later and have never had chickenpox or the vaccine, you need to get two doses 4–8 weeks apart. |
| Hepatitis A (HepA) | Maybe. You need this vaccine if you have a specific risk factor for hepatitis A virus infection* or simply want to be protected from this disease. The vaccine usually is given in two doses over a 6-month period. It's safe to get this vaccine during pregnancy. |
| Hepatitis B (HepB) | Maybe. You need this vaccine if you have a specific risk factor for hepatitis B virus infection* or simply want to be protected from this disease. The vaccine usually is given in three doses over a 6-month period. It's safe to get this vaccine during pregnancy. It's important, too, that your newborn baby gets started on his or her hepatitis B vaccination series before leaving the hospital. |
| Human papillomavirus (HPV) | No. This vaccine is not recommended during pregnancy, but if you inadvertently receive it, this is not a cause for concern. HPV vaccine is recommended for all women 26 years or younger, so make sure you are vaccinated before or after your pregnancy. The vaccine is given in three doses over a 6-month period. |
| Measles, mumps, and rubella (MMR) | No. The MMR vaccine is not recommended during pregnancy, but if you inadvertently receive it, this is not a cause for concern. At least one dose of MMR vaccine is recommended for you if you were born in 1957 or later. (And you may need a second dose.*) It's best for you (and any future baby) to receive the protection vaccination provides before trying to conceive. |
| Meningococcal (MCV4, MPSV4) | Maybe. You need this vaccine if you have one of several health conditions or if you are between the ages of 19–21 years and a first-year college student living in a residence hall and you either have never been vaccinated or were vaccinated before age 16 years.* It's safe to get the vaccine during pregnancy. |
| Pneumococcal (PCV13, PPSV23) | Maybe. You need this vaccine if you have a specific risk factor for pneumococcal disease, such as diabetes. If you're unsure of your risk, talk to your health care provider to find out if you need this vaccine.* It's safe to get the vaccine during pregnancy. |

*Consult your health care provider to determine your level of risk for infection and your need for this vaccine.

the disease. However, pregnant women should not get the intranasal flu vaccine, which is a live, attenuated vaccine and is not approved for use in pregnant women.

## Pertussis

Pertussis (also called whooping cough) is a highly contagious disease that causes severe coughing. People with pertussis may make a "whooping" sound when they try to breathe and are gasping for air. Newborns and infants are at a high risk of severe pertussis infection that sometimes can be life threatening. However, infants cannot be vaccinated against pertussis until they are aged 2 months.

The tetanus toxoid, reduced diphtheria toxoid, and acellular pertussis (Tdap) vaccine prevents three different diseases: tetanus, diphtheria, and pertussis. All pregnant women should receive the Tdap vaccine during each pregnancy, preferably between 27 weeks and 36 weeks of pregnancy. Getting the vaccine between 27 weeks and 36 weeks of pregnancy helps your body make enough antibodies to protect you from the disease and also allow antibodies to be transferred to your baby. Tdap vaccination during pregnancy is an effective and safe way to protect yourself and your baby from serious illness and complications of pertussis. If you do not get Tdap during pregnancy, you should get it immediately after you have your baby.

If you have family members who will be in contact with your baby or who have contact with other infants younger than 12 months, and they have not been vaccinated with Tdap, they also should receive a single dose of Tdap. This dose should be given at least 2 weeks before they have any close contact with an infant.

You can't get tetanus, diphtheria, or pertussis from the Tdap vaccine. Tdap contains inactivated versions of the toxins produced by tetanus and diphtheria bacteria combined with inactivated parts of the bacterial cells that cause pertussis. These are enough to make your body produce antibodies against these illnesses, but they cannot cause the diseases themselves.

## Tetanus and Diphtheria

Tetanus is caused by bacteria that enter the body through a break in the skin. It can lead to paralysis of the breathing muscles and is fatal in 20% of cases. Diphtheria also is caused by bacteria. It can restrict breathing and also can be fatal. Both diseases can be prevented with a combined vaccine (tetanus and diphtheria, or Td, vaccine) or with Tdap. Adults need to get a booster shot of Td every 10 years. At least one of these shots should be Tdap. Pregnant women who are due for a booster shot of Td vaccine (it has been more than 10 years since the last booster with Td) should receive a booster dose with Tdap between 27 weeks and 36 weeks of pregnancy.

If you are pregnant and injure yourself and you need a tetanus booster (it has been more than 5 years since your last tetanus shot), you should be vaccinated with Tdap, no matter what stage of pregnancy you are in. You don't need to be revaccinated with Tdap in the same pregnancy if you received the vaccine in the first or second trimester.

## Varicella

Varicella, also known as chickenpox, is caused by the **varicella zoster virus (VZV)**. In children, varicella usually does not cause serious illness. In adults, varicella may result in severe complications, like pneumonia. A pregnant woman infected with VZV can pass (transmit) the virus to her baby. When this occurs in the first 28 weeks of pregnancy, it can lead to a rare condition called **congenital varicella syndrome**. This syndrome may cause low birth weight, scarring of the skin, small limbs, and brain and eye defects. When transmission occurs later in pregnancy, the baby may develop a painful skin rash known as herpes zoster (shingles) early in life. If a pregnant woman becomes infected 5 days before to 2 days after delivery, the baby may develop severe varicella, which can be fatal if it is not recognized and treated promptly.

If you get varicella during pregnancy, symptoms can be treated with an antiviral medication, but this treatment does not prevent or reduce the severity of congenital varicella syndrome. Pregnant women with varicella are at high risk of pneumonia. You need to seek medical care immediately if you have a high fever, a cough, shaking chills, or shortness of breath. If you are pregnant and have been exposed to someone with varicella, you should contact your health care provider immediately.

The varicella vaccine is given in two doses 4–8 weeks apart. Because it contains a live, attenuated virus, it is not recommended for pregnant women. However, there have been no reports of the baby becoming infected when the vaccine has been given inadvertently during pregnancy. When you get the vaccine, you should avoid pregnancy for 1 month after each dose. If you have never had varicella and have not had the vaccine, you should have the first dose of vaccine before you leave the hospital after you have your baby. If you have had varicella in the past, you do not need to get the vaccine.

Once you've had varicella, VZV never leaves your body. It stays in an inactivated state in certain nerves. The virus can become activated later and cause the painful skin rash known as shingles. A vaccine can be given to prevent shingles and is recommended for adults 60 years and older, but because it contains a live, attenuated virus, it is not recommended for pregnant women.

## Hepatitis Infections

**Hepatitis** is a viral infection that affects the liver. The four common kinds of hepatitis virus that cause infection are hepatitis A virus, hepatitis B virus, hepatitis C virus, and hepatitis D virus. Hepatitis A virus cannot be passed to a baby during pregnancy, and hepatitis D virus is rare. Hepatitis B virus and hepatitis C virus are of the greatest concern during pregnancy because they are most likely to be passed to the baby. Hepatitis A and hepatitis B infections can be prevented with vaccines. There is no vaccine for hepatitis C. Hepatitis C is discussed later in this chapter under "Other Infections."

**Hepatitis B.** Hepatitis B is passed from person to person though contact with body fluids. This can happen during unprotected sex or while sharing needles used to inject ("shoot") drugs. A baby can be infected during birth if the mother has hepatitis B. Hepatitis B often causes no symptoms. Some people have signs and symptoms such as fever, nausea, tiredness, and loss of appetite. In most people, the virus goes away by itself. But in some people, the virus does not go away. These people become carriers of the virus who can infect others. Carriers also may develop chronic hepatitis, which can lead to cirrhosis, liver cancer, and early death.

If no preventive steps are taken, between 70% and 90% of women infected with hepatitis B virus will pass the infection to their babies during pregnancy. Hepatitis may be severe in babies and can be life threatening. Even babies who appear well may be at risk of serious health problems. Infected newborns have a high risk (up to 90%) of becoming carriers of the virus.

The hepatitis B vaccine is a series of three shots and is recommended for everyone through 18 years of age and all adults who want the vaccine or who are at risk of becoming infected with hepatitis B virus. The vaccine consists of a purified protein from the hepatitis B virus. It can be given to pregnant women, postpartum women, and women who are breastfeeding. All infants should receive their first dose of hepatitis B vaccine before leaving the hospital after birth. The second dose is given when the baby is 1–2 months old, and the third dose is given when the baby is 6–18 months old.

All pregnant women are tested for hepatitis B infection early in prenatal care. If you test negative for hepatitis B virus and have risk factors for becoming infected (if you inject illegal drugs, for example), you should be offered the hepatitis B vaccine.

Babies born to infected mothers will receive the first dose of hepatitis B vaccine within 12 hours of birth. They also will receive a medication called **hepatitis B immune globulin (HBIG)** soon after birth. HBIG contains antibodies to the virus and may give additional protection against infection. The rest of the vaccine series then will be given over the next 6 months. With this treatment, the chance of the baby getting the infection is greatly reduced. Women who have hepatitis B infection still can breastfeed their babies.

**Hepatitis A.** Hepatitis A is spread by eating food or drinking water that has the virus or by direct contact with an infected person. Hepatitis A virus infection can cause sudden fever, loss of appetite, nausea, stomachache, dark urine, jaundice, and a general feeling of being unwell. The hepatitis A vaccine is recommended for persons who are at increased risk of infection, such as people traveling to areas where Hepatitis A is common or those with liver disease. The vaccine is safe for women who are pregnant or breastfeeding. A combination vaccine that provides protection against both hepatitis A virus and hepatitis B virus also is available for people 18 years and older.

## Human Papillomavirus

Human papillomavirus is a very common virus that can be passed from person to person. More than 100 types of HPV have been found, and about 30 of these types are spread from person to person through sexual contact. Some types of HPV cause genital warts, while others cause cancer of the *cervix*, anus, vulva, and vagina. Pregnancy can cause an existing HPV infection to worsen. Genital warts can become more numerous and may bleed. Genital warts can be treated during pregnancy by freezing them, removing them with a laser, or taking certain medications. Some of the medications used to treat genital warts should not be used during pregnancy because they may be toxic to the baby.

There is no cure for HPV, so it is best to try to prevent it. Three vaccines are available that can protect against some of these HPV types. One vaccine protects against type 6 and type 11, which cause the most cases of genital warts, and against type 16 and type 18, which cause the most cases of cervical cancer. Another vaccine protects against type 16 and type 18. A third type protects against nine types of HPV.

All three vaccines are given in a series of three shots to females aged 9 years to 26 years. Males in this age group also can get the four-type vaccine and the nine-type vaccine. At this time, the HPV vaccines are not recommended for use during pregnancy. However, they can be given while breastfeeding. It is a good idea to make sure that you have completed the HPV vaccine series before becoming pregnant. If you become pregnant in between doses of the HPV vaccine series, you should complete the series after having your baby.

Another measure that can be taken to help prevent cervical cancer is to have regular cervical cancer screening as recommended for your age and health history. Using condoms with your sexual partner may reduce your risk of HPV infection.

### Measles, Mumps, and Rubella

These three diseases are discussed together because they are prevented with a combination vaccine known as the MMR vaccine:

- Measles (rubeola) infection causes fever, runny nose, cough, and a rash all over the body. In more serious cases, ear infection, seizures, pneumonia, or brain damage can result. Some people who get measles can die.

- Mumps infection starts out with flu-like symptoms including fever, headache, muscle aches, fatigue, and loss of appetite. The salivary glands become swollen and painful. Serious cases of mumps can result in deafness or fertility problems.

- Rubella infection causes a high fever and a rash that last a few days in most people. Rubella is much more serious for some people. Pregnant women who get rubella can pass it to the baby, causing **miscarriage**, fetal death, or **preterm** delivery. In newborns, rubella can cause a very serious disease called congenital rubella syndrome (CRS). Congenital rubella syndrome can cause deafness; serious defects of the eyes, heart, and brain; intellectual disability; and growth problems. Infants with CRS also are highly contagious and can spread the disease to others.

The MMR vaccine is given to children in two doses. Adults 18 years and older who were born after 1956 also should get a dose of MMR unless they can show that they have either been vaccinated or had all three diseases. Because it is a live, attenuated vaccine, pregnant women should wait to get the vaccine until after delivery and then wait at least 1 month to become pregnant again. All pregnant women are tested to see if they are immune to rubella early in their prenatal care. If you are not immune (if you do not have antibodies showing a previous infection or immunization against rubella), it is recommended that you receive the vaccine after delivery.

## Meningococcal Meningitis

Meningitis is an infection of the protective coverings of the brain and spinal cord. It can be caused by different types of pathogens. Meningitis caused by a type of bacteria called meningococcus is very serious. The bacteria multiply quickly and can cause severe illness in just 1 or 2 days. Signs and symptoms include a high fever; headache; stiff neck; small, dark spots on the arms and legs; confusion; nausea; vomiting; and trouble looking into bright lights. This disease can cause death or serious long-term complications in about 25% of people who get the infection.

Getting a vaccine is the best way to prevent meningococcal meningitis infection. Ideally, you should get the meningococcal meningitis vaccine called MenACWY at age 11–12 years. However, if you weren't vaccinated, you can be vaccinated with MenACWY or with another type of vaccine called MPSV4. You may need this vaccination if you have been exposed to someone with meningococcal meningitis, you're traveling to an area where the illness is common, or you have certain medical conditions. Both vaccines are made from parts of the wall that surrounds the meningococcus bacterium. Talk to your health care provider for more information on this vaccine.

## Pneumococcal Pneumonia

Like meningitis, there are different kinds of pneumonia caused by different types of pathogens. One form of pneumonia is caused by a type of bacteria called *Streptococcus pneumoniae*. The bacteria are spread easily among people and can cause lower respiratory tract infections, ear infections, and sinus infections. Infections can be more serious or life threatening in some people. In older adults and in people with long-term illnesses especially, the infection can cause bacteremia (bacteria in the bloodstream), meningitis, and pneumonia. The infection also can cause long-term problems, such as brain damage or hearing loss.

A vaccine is available that prevents pneumococcal pneumonia. The vaccine is made from components of the bacterial cell wall. The vaccine is recommended for people 65 years and older or for younger adults who have risk factors for pneumonia, such as smoking and diabetes. If you are in a high-risk group and could become pregnant, you should get the vaccine before becoming pregnant. If you are already pregnant, talk to your health care provider about whether you should get this vaccine. There have been no reports of any harmful effects when the vaccine has been given during pregnancy.

## Other Infections

Other infections that can affect pregnancy are discussed in the following section. These infections cannot be prevented by vaccines. However, other steps often can be taken to help prevent them.

### *Group B Streptococci*

About 10–30% of pregnant women carry a bacterium known as ***group B streptococci (GBS)***. In women, GBS most often is found in the vagina and rectum. Both men and women can have GBS, and usually the bacteria live in the body without causing any harm—you won't have any symptoms.

Although GBS is fairly common in pregnancy, very few babies actually become sick with group B streptococcal infection. If group B streptococcal bacteria are passed from a woman to her baby, the baby may become infected. This is rare and happens to only 1–2% of babies. The risk of infection is higher in babies who are born before 37 weeks of pregnancy. Babies who do become infected may have early or late infections:

- Early infections—A baby typically gets sick within the first 6 hours after birth or up to the first 7 days. These infections can cause severe problems, such as inflammation of the brain (meningitis), pneumonia, and fever. About 5% of babies with early infections die, even with immediate treatment.

- Late infections—A baby gets sick between a week to a few months after birth. About one half of late infections are passed from the mother to the baby during birth. The rest are from other sources of infection, such as contact with people who have GBS. Late infections are serious and can cause meningitis.

Pregnant women are screened for GBS as part of routine prenatal care. The test for GBS is called a culture. It usually is done between week 35 and week 37 of pregnancy. In this test, a swab is used to take a sample from the vagina and rectum. This procedure is quick and is not painful. The sample then is tested for the group B streptococcal bacteria. If the results show that GBS is present, ***antibiotics*** are given once you go into labor to help prevent the baby from becoming infected. You need to have a GBS test during each pregnancy, regardless of your GBS test results in previous pregnancies. The number of GBS that a person has may change over time. You could have large numbers of GBS and then have low levels months or years later.

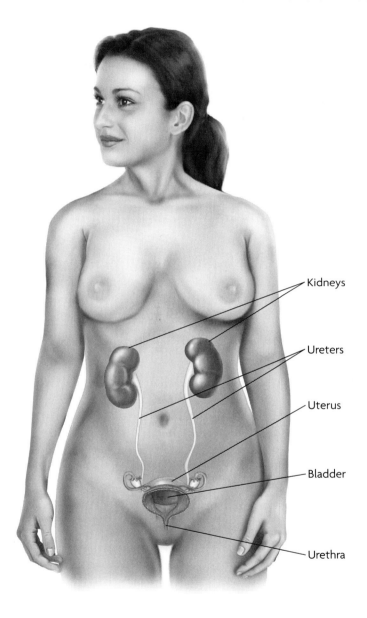

**Female urinary tract.** If not treated, an infection of the bladder can spread to the kidneys.

Some women do not need to be tested for GBS. If you have had a previous child who had a GBS infection, you won't be tested, but you will receive antibiotics during labor. If you have GBS bacteria in your urine at any point during your pregnancy, you also will not be tested and will receive antibiotics during labor. Additionally, you won't be tested if your GBS status is not known when you go into labor and you have one of the following:

- A fever
- You go into labor before 37 weeks of pregnancy
- It has been 18 hours or more since your water broke

If you meet any of these criteria, you will automatically receive antibiotics during labor without being tested.

## Urinary Tract Infections

Urinary tract infections—infections of the **bladder**, **kidney**, or **urethra**—are common in pregnancy. Severe infections can cause problems for both you and the baby, so it is important to treat these infections early. Because some urinary tract infections may not cause any symptoms, you will be tested at your first prenatal visit. If an infection is found, it can be treated easily with antibiotics.

When an infection of the bladder does cause symptoms, you may feel a burning pain when you urinate. Bladder infections also can cause an increased urge to urinate, blood in the urine, and abdominal pain.

If a bladder infection is not treated or is not cured by treatment, it may result in a kidney infection. It is important to finish any medications prescribed for a bladder infection, even after your symptoms go away. A kidney infection can cause symptoms such as chills, fever, back pain, rapid heart rate, and nausea or vomiting. Contact your health care provider right away if you have any of these symptoms so that you can be treated with antibiotics. If left untreated, a kidney infection can lead to premature labor or severe infection.

## Sexually Transmitted Infections

**Sexually transmitted infections (STIs)** are infections that are spread by sexual contact. They can be caused by bacteria, viruses, or parasites. Sexually transmitted infections can cause severe damage to your body if they are not diagnosed and treated. Some STIs can be harmful during pregnancy. Pregnant women receive screening for some STIs as part of their routine prenatal care. It is important to protect yourself against STIs by following these guidelines:

- Limit your sexual partners. The more sexual partners you have, the higher your risk of getting STIs.

- Know your partner. Ask about your partner's sexual history. Ask whether he or she has had STIs. Even if your partner has no symptoms, he or she still may be infected.

- Use a condom. Both male and female condoms are sold over the counter in drug stores. They help protect against STIs.

- Avoid contact with any sores on the genitals.

**Genital Herpes.** *Genital herpes* is an infection that can cause painful sores and blisters on or around the sex organs as well as on the mouth, eyes, and fingers. Other symptoms include swollen glands, fever, chills, muscle aches, fatigue, and nausea. Sometimes, however, there are no symptoms.

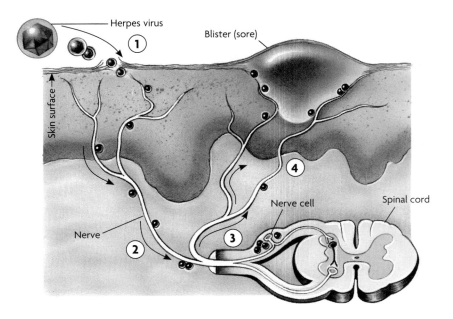

**How herpes reappears after you are infected.** When you are first infected, the herpes virus passes through your skin (*1*). It travels along nerves (*2*) and settles at nerve cells near your spine (*3*). If something triggers the virus, it travels back along the nerves (*4*) to the surface of the skin, and a new outbreak occurs.

The infection is spread by direct contact with a person who has active sores. In some cases, the virus can be passed to others even when the sores have healed. Although the sores heal, the virus stays in your body until some event triggers a new bout and a new outbreak of sores occurs. For most people, these outbreaks are not as painful or severe as the initial outbreak. Some people feel certain symptoms for a few days before an outbreak, such as a tingling or burning sensation. This is called a *prodrome*.

There is no cure for genital herpes. Antiviral medications are available that may prevent some outbreaks or decrease their length or severity. These medications must be taken every day.

In rare cases, newborns can become infected with the herpes virus during birth if the mother has herpes sores at the time of delivery. Newborn herpes infection can cause damage to the nervous system, blindness, intellectual disability, or death. The risk is highest when a woman gets herpes for the first time late in pregnancy (30–50%). The risk is low in women with a recurrent outbreak at the time of delivery (2–3%).

If you have a history of genital herpes, antiviral medication may be recommended during the last 4 weeks of your pregnancy. This treatment has been shown to reduce the recurrence of herpes at delivery. If you have had herpes in the past but have no herpes sores at the time of delivery, the baby can be born vaginally. If there are signs of active infection when you are in labor, you may need to have your baby by cesarean delivery to decrease the chance that he or she will be infected.

If you or your sexual partner has herpes, you should not have sexual contact while sores are present or if you or your partner has prodromal symptoms. You should use condoms during sex (although condoms are only 50% effective in reducing transmission of the herpes virus). In the last 6–8 weeks of pregnancy, you should not have sexual contact if your partner has an outbreak (if your partner has oral herpes, oral–genital contact should be avoided).

If you have genital or oral herpes, a few precautions are needed to avoid infecting your newborn. Wash your hands often and before touching the baby, and avoid putting the baby in contact with anything that may be infectious. You still can breastfeed if there are no herpes sores in the breast area and any other active sores are covered.

**Gonorrhea and Chlamydia.** Both *gonorrhea* and *chlamydia* are caused by bacteria. Women 25 years and younger are at greater risk of both of these infections, although they can occur at any age. They often occur at the same time.

Chlamydia and gonorrhea can cause infections in the mouth, reproductive organs, and rectum. In women, the most common place these infections occur is the cervix. From the cervix, the bacteria can spread into the uterus and fallopian tubes and cause **pelvic inflammatory disease (PID)**. PID is a serious infection that can damage the fallopian tubes, which can lead to infertility. Scarring in the fallopian tubes as a result of the damage caused by PID also increases the risk of **ectopic pregnancy**.

If untreated, both infections can cause problems during pregnancy. A pregnant woman with untreated chlamydia or gonorrhea has an increased risk of **premature rupture of membranes (PROM)**, preterm birth, and fetal growth problems. Gonorrhea also has been linked to miscarriage and infection of the amniotic fluid. Gonorrhea and chlamydia can be passed from the mother to the baby during childbirth. Babies born to infected mothers may have **conjunctivitis** (an infection of the eyes). Chlamydia may cause pneumonia in an infected infant, and gonorrhea may cause infection of the infant's heart, brain, joints, and skin. To prevent conjunctivitis caused by gonorrhea, the eyes of all newborns are treated at birth regardless of whether the mother is infected. If a newborn has signs and symptoms of gonorrhea or chlamydia infection, he or she will receive treatment with antibiotics. The mother and the mother's sex partners also need to be treated.

Women with chlamydia or gonorrhea often have only mild symptoms or no symptoms at all. Symptoms may include the following:

* A discharge from a woman's vagina or a man's penis
* Painful or frequent urination
* Pain in the pelvis or abdomen
* Burning or itching in the vaginal area
* Redness or swelling of the vulva
* Bleeding between periods
* Sore throat with or without fever
* Swollen or enlarged lymph nodes

All pregnant women are tested for chlamydia early in pregnancy, and women with certain risk factors are screened later in pregnancy as well. Women at increased risk of gonorrhea or who have symptoms are tested for this infection early in pregnancy and may be tested again in the third trimester. Both infections can be treated with antibiotics during pregnancy. Sex partners also need to be treated.

**Human Immunodeficiency Virus.** *Human immunodeficiency virus (HIV)* is spread through contact with body fluids—mainly blood or semen—from an infected person. The most common ways that HIV is passed to others are by sexual contact and by sharing needles used to inject drugs.

Once in the body, HIV destroys cells that are part of the immune system—the body's natural defense against disease. This leaves the body open to serious infections, some of which can cause death. When a person with HIV gets one of these infections or has a very low level of these immune system cells, he or she has developed **acquired immunodeficiency syndrome (AIDS)**.

There is no cure for HIV infection. An infected person will have the virus for the rest of his or her life.

In most cases, a person who has been infected with HIV doesn't get sick right away. It can take 5 years or more for some people to start showing the signs and symptoms of AIDS. Some people have a brief illness like the flu around the time they become infected with HIV. Later symptoms can include weight loss, fatigue, swollen lymph nodes, night sweats, fever, diarrhea, and cough.

HIV can be passed from mother to baby during pregnancy, at the time of vaginal delivery, or during breastfeeding. In the United States, an estimated 280,000 women are living with HIV, and as many as 15% do not know it. About 80% of these women are of childbearing age. For this reason, all pregnant women are tested for HIV early in prenatal care. The test may be repeated in the third trimester if a woman is at high risk of HIV infection (for example, if she lives in an area with high rates of HIV).

If a woman finds out she is infected early in pregnancy, she can get medical care that can greatly improve her own health as well as protect the health of her baby. This care includes taking medications and, in some cases, having a cesarean delivery. The baby also will be given medication during the first 6 weeks of life. In the United States, women with HIV should not breastfeed, as breastfeeding may transmit the virus. This program of treatment prevents 99% of infected women from passing the infection to their babies. Without treatment, one in four babies will become infected with HIV.

**Syphilis.** *Syphilis* is caused by bacteria and occurs in stages. It is spread more easily in some stages than in others. If not treated, syphilis can cause heart and brain damage, blindness, paralysis, and death. If found early and treated, syphilis may cause less damage.

Syphilis can be passed from a woman to her baby through the placenta. If this occurs, there is an increased risk of preterm birth, stillbirth, and death. Infants who are born infected and who survive may have serious health problems involving the brain, eyes, teeth, skin, and bones.

Syphilis causes very few signs or symptoms in the early stage of the disease. A small sore may develop at the site of infection. This sore—called a chancre—is painless. It may be in the vagina where it cannot be seen. The chancre heals by itself, but the infection remains. Later symptoms include a rash, sluggishness, or slight fever.

In the very early stages of syphilis, a blood test may or may not find the disease. If a chancre is present, syphilis can be diagnosed by scraping tissue from the chancre. The chancre will go away even without treatment. After the chancre goes away, the only sure way to diagnose syphilis is by a blood test.

All women are tested for syphilis early in pregnancy. The test may be repeated later in pregnancy if a woman lives in an area where syphilis is common. Syphilis infection during pregnancy is treated with antibiotics. Blood tests are needed to ensure that the treatment is working. Babies born to women who have syphilis or have been treated for syphilis during pregnancy are tested for the infection and receive treatment if the infection is present.

**Trichomoniasis.** *Trichomoniasis* is caused by the microscopic parasite *Trichomonas vaginalis*. Women who have trichomoniasis are at an increased risk of infection with other STIs. There is some research that suggests a link between trichomoniasis and certain pregnancy problems, such as PROM, preterm birth, and fetal growth problems.

Signs of trichomoniasis may include a yellow-gray or green vaginal discharge. The discharge may have a fishy odor. There may be burning, irritation, redness, and swelling of the vulva. Sometimes there is pain during urination. Often, a woman has mild or no symptoms. Trichomoniasis can be treated during pregnancy with medication.

### Hepatitis C Infection

The hepatitis C virus is spread by direct contact with infected blood. This can happen while sharing needles or sharing household items that come into contact with blood. A baby can be infected during birth if the mother has a hepatitis C infection. It also can be spread during unprotected sex, but it is harder to spread the virus this way. It is not spread by casual contact or breastfeeding.

Hepatitis C virus infection causes signs and symptoms similar to those of hepatitis B virus infection. It also can cause no symptoms. Unlike hepatitis B virus infection, most adults infected with the hepatitis C virus—75% to 85%—become carriers. Most carriers develop long-term liver disease. A smaller number will develop cirrhosis and other serious, life-threatening liver problems. About 4% of pregnant women who are infected with the hepatitis C virus will pass it to their babies. The risk is related to how much of the virus a woman has and whether she also is infected with HIV.

If you have risk factors for infection, you should be tested for the hepatitis C virus during pregnancy. If you are infected with the hepatitis C virus, your baby will be tested, usually when he or she is at least 18 months of age. Babies who do become infected with the hepatitis C virus will need ongoing medical care. You also will need long-term health care. Various antiviral drugs are used to treat people infected with the hepatitis C virus. Being infected with the hepatitis C virus does not mean that you cannot breastfeed.

## Tuberculosis

*Tuberculosis (TB)* is a disease caused by bacteria that are carried through the air and are passed on to others when an infected person coughs or sneezes. Tuberculosis infection usually occurs in the lungs.

If your health care provider determines that you have risk factors for TB, such as moving from a country that has a high rate of TB infection, you should be tested with a skin test or a blood test during pregnancy. If the test results are positive, you will need a chest X-ray or sputum culture test to confirm the result.

Tuberculosis can be either active or latent. Active TB can cause symptoms such as fever, weight loss, night sweats, a cough, chest pain, and fatigue. Active TB usually shows up on a chest X-ray.

Latent TB, however, usually does not cause any symptoms and will not show up on a chest X-ray. Most people who are infected with TB have latent TB. Their bodies are able to stop the bacteria from growing. The bacteria become inactive but remain alive in the body and can become active later.

In pregnant women with latent TB who have a normal chest X-ray, treatment of latent TB may be delayed until 2–3 months after delivery. Women with latent TB that threatens to become active should receive treatment during pregnancy. Most experts recommend waiting until the second trimester of pregnancy to begin treatment. Although the drug used to treat latent TB is not known to cause birth defects, risks of drug-related problems for the baby are minimized when treatment is started after the first trimester, when most of the major organ systems form. Medication needs to be taken for 2–9 months. It is important to finish the treatment. It is safe to breastfeed while receiving treatment after the baby is born.

For women with active TB, treatment with several different drugs (called multidrug therapy) is given. Therapy lasts at least 6 months. There is no published information about the safety of the drugs used to treat active TB in pregnancy. However, they have been used in pregnant women with no apparent problems for either the woman or the baby.

TB can be passed to the baby before birth through the placenta or after birth if the baby inhales infected body fluids. In the rare cases in which this occurs, the baby will receive treatment after birth.

## Bacterial Vaginosis

An imbalance of the bacteria growing in the vagina can cause **bacterial vaginosis**. It is the most common cause of a vaginal discharge that has a fishy odor. Bacterial vaginosis may cause a thin grayish or white discharge. The odor may be worse after intercourse. Itching around the vagina also may occur. However, 50% of women with bacterial vaginosis do not have any symptoms.

Bacterial vaginosis is not an STI. Some studies suggest that women who have this infection during pregnancy are at greater risk of preterm birth or PROM. If bacterial vaginosis is diagnosed in a pregnant woman who has symptoms, treatment is recommended; treatment is not recommended if symptoms are not present. Treatment involves oral medication or medication inserted into the vagina.

At this time, routine screening of pregnant women without symptoms is not recommended. However, in women with high-risk pregnancies, some research shows that screening for and treating bacterial vaginosis with oral antibiotics may decrease the risk of preterm PROM and preterm delivery; other research shows no such decrease in risk.

## Listeriosis

**Listeriosis** is a serious infection caused by eating food contaminated with the bacterium *Listeria monocytogenes*. Pregnant women are about 20 times more likely than other healthy adults to get listeriosis, and about one third of listeriosis cases happen during pregnancy.

If you become infected during pregnancy, you may have symptoms similar to the flu. The infection is very serious and can lead to miscarriage, stillbirth, preterm delivery, or infection of the baby. Prompt diagnosis and treatment may prevent the baby from becoming infected. Listeriosis is diagnosed with a blood test and is treated with antibiotics.

To decrease your risk of getting listeriosis, take these precautions:

- Thoroughly cook raw food from animal sources, such as beef, pork, or poultry.

- Avoid the following risky foods (foods that are more likely to have the bacteria):
  - Hot dogs, lunch meats, cold cuts (when served chilled or at room temperature; heat to internal temperature of 165°F or steaming hot)

- Refrigerated pâté and meat spreads
- Refrigerated smoked seafood
- Raw (unpasteurized) milk
- Unpasteurized soft cheeses such as feta, queso blanco, queso fresco, Brie, queso panela, Camembert, and blue-veined cheeses

• Wash raw vegetables thoroughly before eating.

• Keep uncooked meats separate from vegetables and from cooked and ready-to-eat foods.

• Wash hands, knives, and cutting boards after handling uncooked foods.

## Cytomegalovirus

**Cytomegalovirus (CMV)** is a common virus. Between 50% and 80% of women in the United States become infected with CMV by age 40 years. About 1–4 in 100 women become infected for the first time during pregnancy. CMV is hard to detect because it rarely causes symptoms. When it does, the symptoms include fever, sore throat, and fatigue. Healthy people generally do not need treatment for CMV infection. Those who are sick with other illnesses may need treatment with antiviral medications.

Women usually become infected through contact with an infected person's body fluids, such as urine, saliva, blood, and semen. Health care workers and people who work with children are most at risk of getting the infection. The virus can be transmitted to the baby through the placenta during pregnancy or after birth to the infant through contact with the mother's infected body fluids. This is more likely to happen if the infection occurs for the first time during pregnancy or if a past infection has been reactivated, especially in the last trimester of pregnancy. Babies who are born at term usually do not get sick if they are infected with CMV during birth or after birth through breast milk. However, preterm babies and low-birthweight babies are likely to get sick if they are infected during birth or through breast milk. Breastfeeding is not recommended if you are currently infected with CMV and your baby is preterm.

CMV infection can cause serious problems in infants, including **jaundice**, neurologic problems, and hearing loss. Cytomegalovirus is the leading cause of hearing loss in children in the United States, accounting for one third of all cases. Developmental delays are common. There is no treatment for CMV, although people who are sick with other diseases often are given antiviral medication if they contract CMV. Infants infected with CMV at birth may be treated with antiviral medication, but this treatment carries significant risks.

If you are concerned about CMV infection, talk with your health care provider about being tested. You can take some simple steps to avoid CMV infection:

* Wash your hands with soap and water after changing diapers, feeding a child, or handling a child's toys.

* Be careful when kissing a child to avoid contact with the child's saliva.

* Do not share eating utensils or toothbrushes with children.

### *Toxoplasmosis*

*Toxoplasmosis* is an infection caused by a parasite that usually is passed to people through undercooked contaminated meat or from animals. Toxoplasmosis may cause no symptoms. When symptoms do appear, they are like flu symptoms, such as fatigue and muscle aches. If you were infected before you were pregnant, you won't pass toxoplasmosis on to your baby. You can, however, pass it on to your baby if you are infected for the first time while you are pregnant.

Although you may not have symptoms, there is a possibility of serious problems for the baby, such as diseases of the nervous system and eyes. If you are infected during pregnancy, medication is available. You and your baby should be monitored closely during your pregnancy and after your baby is born.

Cats that go outside and hunt wild prey play a role in the spread of toxoplasmosis. They become infected by eating infected rodents, birds, or other small animals. The parasite then is passed in the cat's feces. You don't have to get rid of your cat while you are pregnant, but you need to take some precautions. If you own a cat that goes outdoors, avoid changing cat litter if possible. If no one else can do it, wear disposable gloves and wash your hands thoroughly with soap and water afterwards. Change the litter daily. Clean litter is not dangerous. It's only used cat litter that can transmit the infection. Do not adopt or handle stray cats, especially kittens. Do not get a new cat while you're pregnant.

Other steps that you can take to prevent toxoplasmosis include the following:

* Only eat meat that has been thoroughly cooked.

* Wash cutting boards, counters, utensils, and hands with hot soapy water after contact with raw meat, poultry, seafood, or unwashed fruits or vegetables.

- Wear gloves when gardening and during any contact with soil or sand because it might be contaminated with cat feces.

- Wash hands thoroughly after gardening or contact with soil or sand.

### Parvovirus

**Parvovirus** is a contagious infection also known as "fifth disease." It's common among school children, and if you had it during your childhood, you aren't likely to get it again.

Parvovirus can cause cold-like symptoms followed by a rash on the cheeks, arms, and legs. It also often causes pain and swelling in the joints that can last from days to weeks.

If you think you have been exposed to parvovirus or have any of the symptoms, see your health care provider so that you can have a blood test to confirm whether you have been infected. Parvovirus rarely causes problems for pregnant women or for the baby. In a few cases, parvovirus may cause miscarriage. If you have symptoms of parvovirus, see your health care provider. A test can be done to see if you have the infection. If you do, you may need to have ultrasound exams for a few weeks to check the health of the baby.

---

# RESOURCES

These resources offer more information about immunizations and infections during pregnancy:

**Centers for Disease Control and Prevention**
*Site that provides immunization recommendations for all age groups. Some of the relevant information available about vaccines and pregnancy include the following:*
- Influenza and pregnancy: www.cdc.gov/flu/protect/vaccine/pregnant.htm
- Pregnancy and whooping cough: www.cdc.gov/vaccines/adults/rec-vac/pregnant/whooping-cough/index.html
- Vaccine recommendations from the Advisory Committee on Immunization Practices: www.cdc.gov/vaccines/hcp/acip-recs/index.html
- Vaccine Information Statements: www.cdc.gov/vaccines/hcp/vis/

**Food Safety for Moms-To-Be**
U.S. Food and Drug Administration
www.fda.gov/food/resourcesforyou/healtheducators/ucm081785.htm
*U.S. Food and Drug Administration site that gives advice about how to safely prepare, cook, and store food and the special precautions that pregnant women need to take to make sure their food is safe.*

**Immunization for Women**
www.immunizationforwomen.org
*Comprehensive site from the American College of Obstetricians and Gynecologists covering all aspects of immunization for women.*

**Sexually Transmitted Infections**
Centers for Disease Control and Prevention
www.cdc.gov/std/default.htm
*Provides current information about sexually transmitted infections, including signs and symptoms, treatment, and prevention.*

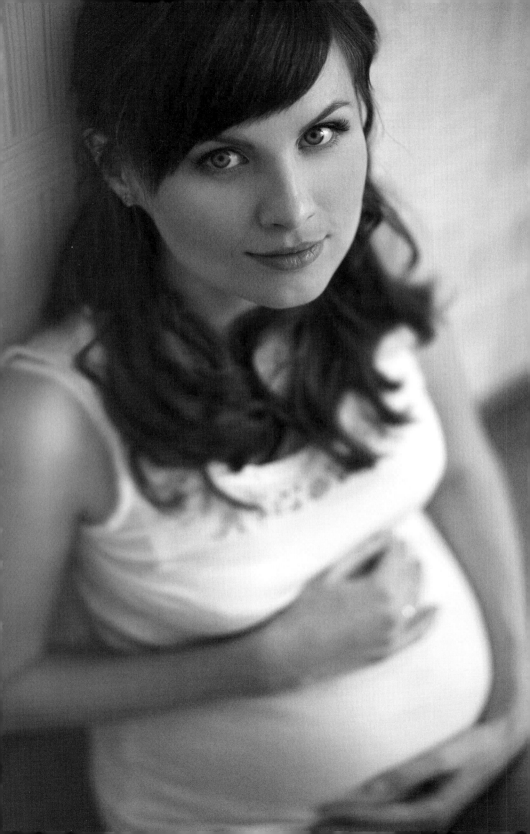

Chapter 31

# Growth Problems

In some pregnancies, the unborn baby does not grow and develop as expected. Some babies are born smaller than average, whereas others are born larger than average. Either situation can cause problems for the woman and her baby. Often, growth problems with the baby are anticipated because the woman has a medical condition or a complication has occurred during pregnancy. Routine monitoring also is done throughout pregnancy to detect growth problems. In many cases, if a problem with the baby's growth is suspected during pregnancy, steps can be taken to minimize further complications.

## Fetal Growth Restriction

When a developing baby is smaller than expected, the health care provider will try to determine whether the baby is healthy and is just not as large as other babies or whether there is a health problem that is preventing the baby from meeting his or her growth potential. The term *fetal growth restriction (FGR)* (formerly referred to as "intrauterine growth restriction") is used to describe babies who are developing in the uterus and whose estimated fetal weight appears to be lower than expected. The term "small for gestational age" (SGA) is used to describe babies who are born at a weight that is below normal. Babies are considered to be SGA when they are born smaller than 9 out of 10 babies who are the same *gestational age*.

Fetal growth restriction significantly increases the risk of serious problems during labor and delivery and health problems for the newborn baby. The more severely a baby is affected by growth restriction, the greater the risk of these problems occurring. A small number of growth-restricted babies also may have health problems later in life.

## Causes

The pregnant woman's health can be one of the main risk factors for FGR. Women with the following chronic (long-lasting) health problems are at increased risk of having a baby affected by FGR:

- **Hypertension (*high blood pressure*)**
- **Kidney disease**
- **Diabetes mellitus**
- Certain heart and lung diseases
- **Antiphospholipid syndrome**
- **Hemoglobinopathies** (such as **sickle cell disease**)

In addition to the health problems themselves, the use of certain drugs to treat some medical conditions, such as hypertension, epilepsy, and blood clots, can increase the risk of FGR. Pregnancy complications, including multiple pregnancy and placental problems, increase the risk of FGR, as does becoming sick with certain infections during pregnancy, such as **cytomegalovirus**, **rubella** (German measles), and **varicella** (**chickenpox**).

Other risk factors for FGR include poor nutrition and unhealthy habits during pregnancy. Smoking, alcohol use, and use of illegal drugs are known risk factors for FGR. A pregnant woman who smokes is three and a half times more likely to have an SGA baby than a nonsmoker. The risk of SGA is increased with only one or two alcoholic drinks per day. Illegal drugs, such as heroin and cocaine, greatly increase the risk of having an SGA baby.

Fetal growth restriction may be a sign of a problem with the baby's health. Fetal growth restriction is associated with certain chromosomal abnormalities, such as **trisomy 13** and **trisomy 18**. Babies who are born with heart defects are more likely to have SGA compared with other babies. **Gastroschisis**, a birth defect that affects the abdominal wall, is commonly associated with fetal growth restriction.

## Diagnosis

There are several ways that FGR is diagnosed during pregnancy. Many of the exams that you have during **prenatal care** visits are designed to find this problem as early as possible:

- Fundal height measurement—Beginning at about 24 weeks of pregnancy, your health care provider will measure the fundal height—the distance from your pubic bone to the top of your uterus—at each prenatal visit. Recording these measurements allows your health care provider to assess your baby's size and growth rate.

- **Ultrasound exam**—Between week 18 and week 22 of pregnancy, most women have an ultrasound exam. During this exam, the baby's measurements are taken and used to estimate his or her weight.

If your health care provider suspects that you have FGR, or if you have risk factors for FGR, you may have more frequent ultrasound exams (usually about every 2–4 weeks) to track the growth of your baby throughout your pregnancy.

As your due date approaches, special tests of fetal health may be done on a weekly basis. These tests may include **Doppler velocimetry** (a special ultrasound exam that measures the blood flow in several of the baby's arteries), **nonstress test**, **contraction stress test**, **biophysical profile**, or **modified biophysical profile**. These tests are discussed in more detail in Chapter 26, "Testing to Monitor Fetal Well-Being."

## Management

Managing FGR depends in part on what's causing it. Your health care provider will try to find out the cause of your baby's FGR. If a medical condition is thought to be the cause, for example, your health care provider will make sure that you are getting the optimal treatment. If a genetic disorder is suspected, you may have tests to find out the type of disorder. But even if the cause is found, there is little that can be done during pregnancy to reverse FGR. Stopping smoking, however, has been shown to be helpful. Women who stop smoking before 16 weeks of pregnancy see the most benefits in improving the birth weight of their babies, but even stopping as late as the seventh month can have a positive effect on the baby's weight.

There is no hard and fast rule about when a baby with FGR should be delivered. In some cases, early delivery may be recommended. This recommendation may be made if results of fetal testing suggest that the baby is having problems or if ultrasound exams show that the baby has stopped growing altogether. In other cases, if results of fetal testing indicate that the baby is doing well, it may be recommended that you deliver the baby at term. If you do deliver the baby early, you may be given medications that help the baby's organs mature and that reduce the risk of cerebral palsy. You also may be transferred to a hospital with a high-level **neonatal intensive care unit** that provides specialized care for **preterm** infants.

### Prevention

You can improve your chances of having a normal-weight baby by practicing healthy eating habits and making sure you're getting all the proper nutrients recommended by your health care provider and in the month-to-month sections of this book. What's even more crucial is giving up any lifestyle habits you have that could be harmful. Do not drink alcohol or smoke while you are pregnant. If you are using illegal drugs, such as heroin or cocaine, get counseling right away to help you stop.

Taking steps to prevent having a baby that is smaller than normal is important. Talk with your health care provider honestly if you are having trouble giving up unhealthy habits so he or she can get you the help you need.

## Macrosomia

When a baby is born larger than expected, he or she often is described as being "large for gestational age (LGA)." Babies are considered LGA when they are born bigger than 9 out of 10 babies born at the same gestational age. Macrosomia is the term that describes a baby that has grown very large—one that weighs more than about 4,000–4,500 grams at birth (between 8 pounds, 13 ounces and 9 pounds, 14 ounces)—regardless of gestational age.

Several risk factors are associated with macrosomia, including gestational and pregestational diabetes mellitus, a prior history of macrosomia, being overweight before pregnancy, excessive weight gain during pregnancy, having had more than one child, and having a male baby.

Diabetes can lead to macrosomia if your blood **glucose** level is high throughout pregnancy. Too much glucose reaches the baby, which can cause the baby to grow too large. Because macrosomia can cause problems during delivery, it is important to manage your diabetes and follow your health care provider's advice closely (see Chapter 23, "Diabetes Mellitus," for more discussion on diabetes during pregnancy).

### Diagnosis

Like SGA, it is difficult to diagnose macrosomia. It can be diagnosed with certainty only after the baby is born. Measuring fundal height and feeling the abdomen, as well as ultrasound exams, may be used to help predict macrosomia. Interestingly, some studies suggest that as you approach your due date, you may be able to estimate the baby's weight just as well as your health care provider can with an ultrasound exam.

## Complications

Macrosomia can cause complications for the woman and her baby. The most common are problems with labor and delivery. Women who have large babies are more likely to have a ***cesarean delivery***. The baby can be affected by a difficult delivery—large babies are at greater risk of low ***Apgar scores*** (see Chapter 16, "The Postpartum Period") and are more likely to need specialized care in a neonatal intensive care unit.

***Shoulder dystocia*** is a problem during labor and delivery and occurs when the baby's shoulders are too big (wide) to fit through the woman's birth canal. Although shoulder dystocia also can occur during delivery of normal-sized babies, it happens more often in cases of macrosomia. It cannot be predicted before labor. It can lead to injury of the baby, including fracture of the collarbone and damage to the brachial plexus. The brachial plexus is a collection of nerves near the shoulder. These nerves can become compressed or stretched, causing weakness or paralysis in the arm and shoulder. This condition often resolves on its own by 1 year of age. Brachial plexus injury is rare, and it also can occur in babies of normal size, during cesarean deliveries, and in the absence of shoulder dystocia.

When a baby's shoulders are having difficulty passing through the birth canal, the health care provider can try to change the woman's position to open the pelvis wider. There are also a number of techniques that can be used to ease the delivery of the baby's shoulders and prevent injury. However, there are some babies for whom these techniques will not be successful even in the hands of a very experienced provider.

Suspected macrosomia by itself is not always an indication for cesarean delivery because predicting macrosomia before birth is so inaccurate and because cesarean deliveries carry more risks for women than vaginal deliveries. Damage to the baby still can occur even when a cesarean delivery is performed. Cesarean delivery may be considered, however, if the baby is estimated to weigh more than 5,000 grams (about 11 pounds) in women without diabetes mellitus. For women with diabetes, health care providers may recommend the option of a planned cesarean delivery if the baby is estimated to weigh 4,500 grams or more.

# RESOURCES

The following resources offer more information about some of the topics discussed in this chapter:

**Fetal Macrosomia**
Mayo Clinic
www.mayoclinic.org/diseases-conditions/fetal-macrosomia/basics/definition/con-20035423
*Provides basic and in-depth explanations of macrosomia including causes, diagnosis, and management.*

**Intrauterine Growth Restriction**
Medline Plus
www.nlm.nih.gov/medlineplus/ency/article/001500.htm
*Offers a basic explanation of FGR and gives links to additional sources of information.*

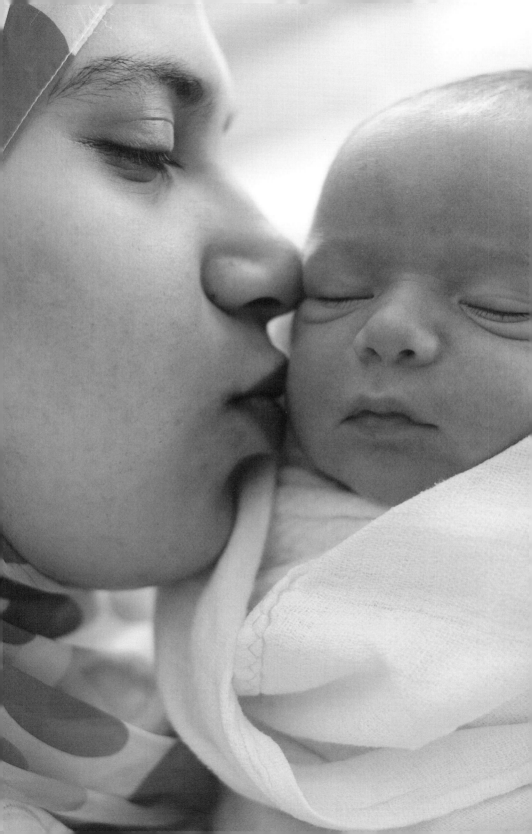

## Chapter 32

# Problems During Labor and Delivery

Although most women go through labor and deliver their babies without difficulty, sometimes problems occur. Some women have risk factors that make these problems more likely. In some cases, problems during labor and delivery can be anticipated, and appropriate actions can be taken beforehand to minimize risks. However, sometimes problems occur even if everything has gone well during pregnancy.

As soon as you arrive at the hospital in labor, your health care team will monitor you and your baby to make sure that all is going well. Ongoing monitoring throughout labor and delivery and after you give birth may help detect any problems early. In many situations, the earlier a problem is found and managed, the better the outcome.

## Abnormal Labor

When labor does not progress as it should, it is referred to as abnormal labor or **labor dystocia**. You also may hear the term "failure to progress" used to describe a labor that is progressing slowly or that has stopped. Dystocia is the main reason why a baby is born by **cesarean delivery** rather than through the vagina.

### Causes

Possible causes of abnormal labor include the following:

- Large baby (**macrosomia**)—Babies weighing more than 8 pounds and 13 ounces (4,000 grams) to 9 pounds and 15 ounces (4,500 grams) are considered larger than average and can make vaginal birth more difficult.

- Baby's position—Sometimes, babies lie in the uterus in unusual positions that make delivery through the vagina difficult (known as ***malpresentation***). For example, in a ***breech presentation***, the baby's buttocks are positioned to come out of the vagina first. In a face presentation, the baby's head is bent back so that it passes through the pelvis face first. In some cases, the baby's hand or foot may be alongside the head in the birth canal during delivery (called compound presentation).

- Problems with the cervix or uterus—If the uterus does not contract at the right time intervals and with enough pressure, labor can take longer and may need to be helped along.

- ***Obesity***—Being obese may increase the risk of macrosomia, which in turn increases the risk of labor problems. Having too much body fat may obstruct the passage of a normal-sized baby through the pelvis.

### Risks

When problems with labor occur, it takes longer to deliver the baby. The main risk with a longer labor is that it can cause ***chorioamnionitis***. This is an infection of the membranes that surround the baby in the uterus. In most cases, ***antibiotics*** are effective in treating the infection. In rare cases, chorioamnionitis can lead to serious complications for both the mother and the baby. For the mother, it can cause a life-threatening condition called ***sepsis***. For the baby, it can cause lung problems, cerebral palsy, developmental disabilities, and, in a few cases, ***stillbirth***. However, the relationship between chorioamnionitis and a longer labor is not clear. Chorioamnionitis may itself cause a longer labor rather than being a consequence of a longer labor.

Another risk of abnormal labor is that it may lead to a cesarean delivery. A cesarean delivery carries several risks for the mother, including heavy blood loss or blood clots in the legs, pelvic organs, or lungs. Infection can occur after a cesarean delivery. With each cesarean delivery, the risk of placental problems occurring in future pregnancies increases.

### Assessment

Labor is divided into three stages. During the first stage, the cervix dilates as the uterus contracts. In the second stage, the woman actively pushes the baby out of the vagina. In the third stage, the ***placenta*** is delivered. Health care providers measure how long each stage of labor takes to determine whether labor is progressing as it should. Many factors can influence how labor progresses. First-time moms usually have longer labors than moms who have given birth before. Whether you have an *epidural block* also is a factor in how long labor lasts. Usually, labor is longer if you have an epidural.

## Management

If the health care team monitoring you observes that your labor is going too slowly or has stopped, there are several options available to help get your labor back on track. The decision of which option or options to use depends on the risks and benefits of each option. Sometimes, the first option that is tried is simply to wait for a while to see if labor progresses on its own. In some situations, *augmentation of labor* may be tried. In labor augmentation, medications or other means are used to stimulate contractions of the uterus:

- *Amniotomy*—If your water has not broken yet, your health care provider may perform an amniotomy, which involves making a small hole in the *amniotic sac* to release the *amniotic fluid*. Amniotomy has been shown to speed up labor in some cases by allowing the fetal head to put more dilating force on the cervix. It also releases *prostaglandins*, which are the body's natural labor stimulants.

- *Oxytocin*—Another intervention that may be tried is the administration of oxytocin. Oxytocin is a hormone that brings on and strengthens labor contractions. Your body naturally produces oxytocin. If your health care provider gives you oxytocin, it will be a synthetic form of the hormone. Oxytocin increases the strength of your contractions. If oxytocin is administered, the fetal heart rate most likely will be monitored continuously.

In some cases, it may be decided to deliver the baby with the help of forceps or vacuum extraction. This is called an *operative vaginal delivery* (see Chapter 14, "Operative Delivery and Breech Presentation"). Your health care provider also may decide that a cesarean delivery is needed.

## Shoulder Dystocia

*Shoulder dystocia* occurs when one of the baby's shoulders doesn't come out of the vagina after the baby's head is delivered. It's caused by the impaction of the baby's shoulder behind the front or back part of the mother's pelvic bones. In some cases, shoulder dystocia is easy to diagnose. In other cases, it is difficult to know that it is happening. Health care providers diagnose shoulder dystocia when gentle downward traction is not successful and additional help is needed to deliver the baby's shoulders.

Diabetes and having a large baby increase the risk of shoulder dystocia. It also tends to recur; if you had shoulder dystocia in a previous delivery, it is more likely to happen again. However, shoulder dystocia also occurs in the absence of any risk factors. For this reason, it is difficult to predict and prevent.

Shoulder dystocia can result in fetal injury, most commonly to the collarbone, arm, and a group of nerves called the brachial plexus. Shoulder dystocia can cause the nerves in the brachial plexus to become stretched or compressed. Damage to the nerves may result in weakness or paralysis in the arm and shoulder. Brachial plexus injury usually resolves on its own in the first year of the baby's life and causes no permanent disability. Women who have deliveries complicated by shoulder dystocia have an increased risk of postpartum **hemorrhage** and serious tears of the **perineum** (the area between the **anus** and the vaginal opening) requiring surgery to repair them.

When shoulder dystocia is recognized, you will be told to stop pushing. Usually, an intervention called the McRoberts maneuver is tried first. This position can help dislodge the baby's shoulders by causing the baby's head to rotate and flattening your spine. Your health care provider may try other maneuvers as well.

If you've had shoulder dystocia during a previous delivery, you and your health care provider may want to think about how you will have your baby in

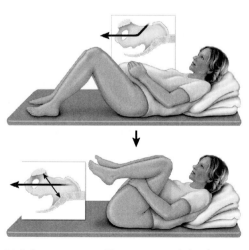

**McRoberts maneuver.** This position may help relieve shoulder dystocia. Reprinted from Beckman RBC, Ling FW, Herbert WNP, Laube DW, Smith RP, Casanova R, et al. Obstetrics and gynecology. 7th ed. Philadelphia (PA): Lippincott Williams & Wilkins.

a subsequent pregnancy. A cesarean delivery does not necessarily prevent injuries to the baby. Also, more often than not, most subsequent deliveries are not complicated by shoulder dystocia. You and your health care provider should consider several factors when making this decision, including the estimated weight of the baby, whether you have been able to control your blood **glucose** level if you had diabetes during pregnancy, and whether your prior baby sustained an injury during delivery.

## Umbilical Cord Compression

During labor, the **umbilical cord** can become compressed if it wraps around parts of the baby (such as the baby's neck) or if the cord becomes tangled or knotted. Compression of the cord can reduce or restrict blood flow to the baby. Cord compression can be detected by changes in the fetal heart rate and steps usually can be taken to prevent it from causing serious complications.

### Risk Factors

Umbilical cord compression is more likely to occur if the level of amniotic fluid is abnormally low (a condition called **oligohydramnios**) or after your water has broken. The amniotic fluid provides a space for the umbilical cord to float freely. After your water breaks, this space is lost, and the umbilical cord can become wrapped around the baby. Sometimes, the uterine contractions during labor compress the umbilical cord.

### Signs and Symptoms

Umbilical cord compression usually causes a change in the fetal heart rate. This change can be detected with fetal monitoring during labor.

### Management

If the fetal heart rate changes during labor in a way that suggests umbilical cord compression, usually the first thing that is done is to change your position. A shift in your position often can relieve the pressure on the umbilical cord. Another intervention that can be done is called amnioinfusion. Fluid is delivered into the uterus through a tube inserted into the uterus through the cervix. This fluid provides a buffering space for the cord and can reduce compression. The tube then is removed before delivery of the baby. If the fetal heart rate changes persist even after these things are tried, a cesarean delivery may be needed.

## Umbilical Cord Prolapse

Although rare, sometimes the baby's umbilical cord comes out of the vagina alongside the baby's head during delivery. If this happens, the umbilical cord can become pinched (or compressed) and the baby may not get enough oxygen. This is known as **umbilical cord prolapse**. It can cause serious harm to the baby or fetal death if it is not managed immediately.

## Risk Factors

Certain pregnancy conditions can increase the risk of umbilical cord prolapse:

- Baby's position (malpresentation)—Although most cases of cord prolapse occur when the baby is in a normal, head-down position (**vertex presentation**), there is a higher risk of cord prolapse with abnormal presentations. A breech presentation (in which the feet or buttocks of the baby are born first) carries the highest risk of cord prolapse.

- Prematurity or low birth weight—Smaller-than-normal babies have an increased risk of cord prolapse.

- Twin pregnancy—The risk of cord prolapse is increased for the second-born twin.

- Rupture of membranes—When the **amniotic membranes** rupture during the normal course of labor (your water breaks), the cord may be carried along in the gush of amniotic fluid as it leaves the uterus. This risk is increased even more if there is a greater-than-normal amount of amniotic fluid (a condition called **polyhydramnios**).

## Signs and Symptoms

The first sign of cord prolapse is a sudden decrease in the baby's heart rate. It may be possible to feel the cord in the vagina.

## Management

Prompt delivery of the baby is needed if cord prolapse is diagnosed or suspected. This most often means a **cesarean birth**. However, if your health care provider believes that a vaginal birth will be safer and quicker, the baby may be delivered through the vagina. In the meantime, the health care provider may try to reduce the pressure on the umbilical cord by inserting a hand into the vagina and lifting the baby's head off the cord. You may be placed in a knee-to-chest position to further alleviate pressure on the cord.

In most cases of cord prolapse, delivery occurs without any problems and the baby is healthy. The time between recognizing that the cord is prolapsed and the time of delivering the baby is a factor in success, but other factors, including how severe the prolapse is and how long it has been present, also play a role.

## Postpartum Hemorrhage

When a woman delivers a baby—either vaginally or by cesarean—and then begins to bleed heavily, it is known as postpartum hemorrhage. Postpartum hemorrhage causes about 140,000 deaths of new mothers around the world each year. The severe blood loss also can cause serious complications for the woman.

Postpartum hemorrhage can happen within the first 24 hours of delivering a baby (called "primary" or early hemorrhage) or between 1 day and 12 weeks after delivery (called "secondary" or late hemorrhage). Primary hemorrhage happens in 4% to 6% of all pregnancies. More than 80% of these hemorrhages are caused by *uterine atony*. Uterine atony occurs when the muscles of the uterus do not contract normally to tighten the blood vessels after the baby and placenta are delivered. Another common cause is a problem with the placenta called *placenta accreta*. In this condition, the placenta grows into the uterine wall and cannot be separated from it. This can cause hemorrhage during the third stage of labor when the placenta is delivered. Placenta accreta can be diagnosed during pregnancy in most cases, and steps can be taken before labor and delivery to help manage postpartum hemorrhage (see Chapter 29, "Placental Problems"). *Uterine rupture* also can cause postpartum hemorrhage. This can occur when a previous cesarean scar tears during labor.

### Risk Factors

Postpartum hemorrhage often happens without warning to women who have no risk factors. However, the following conditions can increase the risk of having excessive blood loss after delivery:

- Long labor
- Augmented labor
- Fast labor
- History of postpartum hemorrhage
- *Episiotomy*
- *Preeclampsia*
- Larger uterus from having a large baby, twins, or too much amniotic fluid
- Cesarean delivery
- Asian or Hispanic ethnicity
- Chorioamnionitis

### Management

Even if you do not show signs of heavy bleeding, it is routine for providers to administer oxytocin soon after delivery to prevent uterine atony and associated bleeding. If heavy bleeding does occur, the health care team will respond quickly to stop the bleeding. When postpartum hemorrhage is caused by uterine atony, one of the first steps is for the health care provider to use his or her hands to massage or apply pressure to the uterus to make it contract. Medications such as oxytocin, prostaglandins, or others also may be used for the initial treatment of uterine atony to make the uterus contract and reduce bleeding.

If these steps do not work, the health care provider may insert a gauze material or a device into the uterus to stop the bleeding. Sometimes, surgery may be needed to stop blood loss. **Uterine artery embolization** is a technique that can be performed without an abdominal incision. It involves inserting a device into an artery to stop bleeding. Other types of surgery require an abdominal incision (**laparotomy**) so that your health care provider can gain access the uterus. Several surgical techniques are available. The arteries to the uterus may be tied off to stop the flow of blood. The uterus may be compressed with different kinds of sutures to stop bleeding. If these techniques do not work, an emergency hysterectomy may need to be done.

Depending on how much blood has been lost, you may need a blood transfusion. Once your condition is stable, your health care provider may recommend that you take extra iron supplements to replace the iron in your body that was lost during heavy bleeding. Taking a prenatal vitamin along with two extra iron tablets (300 mg) may help your body recover faster.

## Endometritis

**Endometritis** is an infection of the **endometrium,** the lining of the uterus. When it happens after childbirth, it is called **postpartum endometritis**. Postpartum infections used to be very common and were caused by unhygienic conditions during childbirth. Endometritis is now rare following a delivery. However, the chance of getting endometritis is up to 10 times higher after a cesarean delivery. For this reason, preventive treatment with antibiotics is given before all cesarean deliveries. Giving **antibiotics** before a cesarean delivery reduces the risk of endometritis by 75%.

### Risk Factors

In addition to cesarean delivery, there are other risk factors for postpartum endometritis. These include prolonged rupture of membranes, a labor that lasts a long time and has required many vaginal exams, and having a fever during labor.

## Signs and Symptoms

Most cases of endometritis are diagnosed within a few days of delivery. Fever is a common early sign of endometritis. Other signs and symptoms include a tender or painful abdomen, tiredness, and just feeling sick. The normal discharge that occurs after childbirth, called *lochia*, may have a foul odor.

## Management

Postpartum endometritis is treated with antibiotics. It usually takes 1–2 days for you to start feeling better and for your fever to go down. If you don't respond to the antibiotics, your health care provider may look for other causes of your infection, such as a wound infection or a retained placenta (when part of the placenta is not expelled from the uterus and is instead retained inside).

Your baby may be affected if you have postpartum endometritis. The baby's health care provider usually is informed about your condition. Steps may be taken to check the baby for signs of infection and to give the appropriate treatment.

---

# RESOURCES

These resources offer more information about problems during labor and delivery:

**Childbirth Problems**
Medline Plus
www.nlm.nih.gov/medlineplus/childbirthproblems.html#cat42
*General information and links about various complications that can occur during and after labor and delivery.*

**Prevention and Management of Postpartum Hemorrhage**
American Family Physician
www.aafp.org/afp/2007/0315/p875.html
*Article written for doctors that describes the diagnosis and treatment of postpartum hemorrhage.*

# Part VIII
# Pregnancy Loss

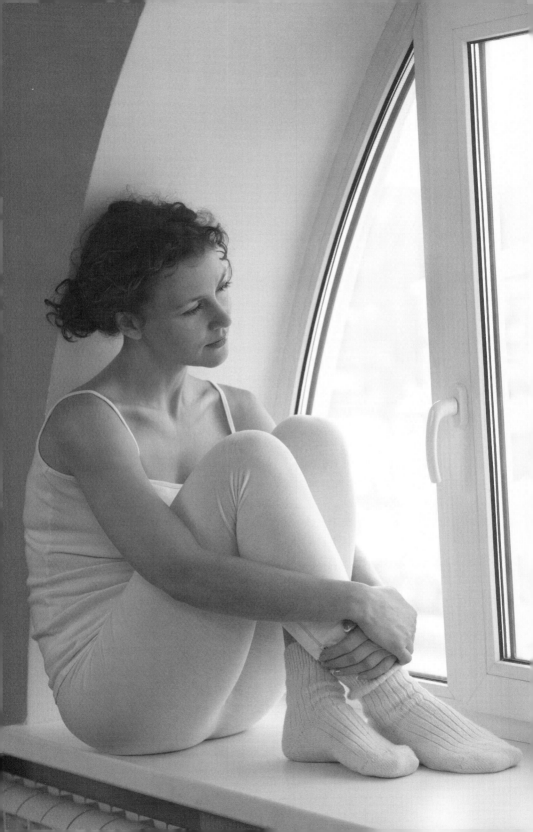

# Chapter 33

# Early Pregnancy Loss
## Miscarriage, Ectopic Pregnancy, and Gestational Trophoblastic Disease

Chances are good that your pregnancy will proceed normally and you will have a healthy baby. But sadly, some problems do occur that cause the loss of the pregnancy. Losing a pregnancy—no matter how early— can cause feelings of sadness and grief. You and your partner will need to heal both physically and emotionally. For most parents, emotional healing takes a good deal longer than physical healing.

## Miscarriage

A normal pregnancy lasts about 40 weeks. The loss of a pregnancy before 13 completed weeks of pregnancy is called early pregnancy loss or **miscarriage**. Miscarriages occur in about 15% of known pregnancies. Some miscarriages take place before a woman misses her menstrual period or is even aware that she is pregnant.

### Causes

It is important for a woman who has had a miscarriage to know that this is something that happened, not something that she caused. She can almost always be reassured that nothing she has done could have caused the miscarriage. Working, exercising, stress, arguments, having sex, or having used birth control pills before getting pregnant do not cause miscarriage. Few medications can result in miscarriage. Morning sickness—the nausea and vomiting that is common in early pregnancy—also does not cause miscarriage. Some women who have had a miscarriage believe that it was caused by a recent fall, blow, or even a fright. In most cases, this is not true. It is simply that these things happened to occur around the same time and are fresh in her memory.

Smoking, alcohol, and caffeine have been studied as causes of miscarriage. Some research suggests that smoking increases the risk of miscarriage, but other research suggests that it does not. Drinking 10 or more alcoholic drinks per week may increase the risk of miscarriage, but the risk with lower levels of drinking is not clear. In any case, it is best to avoid smoking and drinking alcohol during pregnancy. Consuming 200 mg or less of caffeine a day (the amount in two cups of coffee) does not appear to increase the risk of miscarriage.

The majority of miscarriages are caused by a random event in which the **embryo** does not develop, often because it received an abnormal number of **chromosomes**. Chromosomes are in each **cell** of the body and carry the blueprints (**genes**) that direct how we develop and function. Most cells have 23 pairs of chromosomes for a total of 46 chromosomes. **Sperm** and **egg** cells each have 23 chromosomes. During **fertilization**, when the egg and sperm join, the two sets of chromosomes come together. If an egg or sperm has an abnormal number of chromosomes, the embryo also will have an abnormal number and development will not occur normally, sometimes resulting in a miscarriage. The likelihood of this kind of chromosome problem occurring increases as a woman gets older. For women older than 40 years, about one third of pregnancies end in miscarriage, most as a result of this type of chromosome abnormality. There is also some evidence that chromosome abnormalities increase as men get older, although it is not clear at what age this begins.

### Signs and Symptoms

Bleeding is the most common sign of miscarriage. You should call your health care provider if you have any of these signs or symptoms:

- Vaginal spotting or bleeding with or without pain

- A gush of fluid from your vagina, regardless of the presence of pain or bleeding

- Passage of tissue from the vagina

A small amount of bleeding early in pregnancy is common and does not necessarily mean that you will have a miscarriage. If your bleeding is heavy or occurs along with a pain like menstrual cramps, miscarriage is more likely, and you should contact your health care provider right away.

## Diagnosis

If you have bleeding or cramping, your health care provider may do an **ultrasound exam**. This exam can check whether the pregnancy is growing normally. If your pregnancy is advanced enough, the ultrasound exam can detect whether there is a heartbeat. The presence of a heartbeat is reassuring and suggests a much higher chance that the pregnancy will continue. If a heartbeat isn't found, it may mean that it is still too early and the pregnancy too small to detect the heartbeat. However, in some cases, not detecting a heartbeat indicates that the embryo is not developing or has stopped growing. Your health care provider also may do a **pelvic exam** to see if your **cervix** has begun to open (dilate). **Dilation** of the cervix indicates that a miscarriage is more likely.

If your health care provider does not think that a miscarriage has occurred and it appears that your pregnancy is growing normally, there is a good chance that your pregnancy will continue without further problems. You may be advised to rest and to avoid **sexual intercourse**. Although these measures have not been proved to prevent miscarriage, they may help reduce discomfort and make you less anxious.

## Treatment

It is rarely possible to prevent or stop a miscarriage. After a miscarriage occurs, all of the pregnancy tissue may not have been expelled. This is called an incomplete miscarriage. There are several options to remove this tissue. The choice of which option to use depends on many factors, including how large the pregnancy has grown.

If you do not show any signs of an infection, your health care provider may recommend waiting and letting the tissue pass naturally. This usually takes up to 2 weeks, but it may take longer in some cases. Another option is to take medication that helps expel the tissue. With these options, you will have bleeding, some of which can be heavy. Cramping pain, diarrhea, and nausea also can occur. You may pass tissue in addition to bleeding. With an early miscarriage, the pregnancy tissue usually resembles a blood clot that is mixed with grey-white material or a clear, fluid-filled sac.

In some cases, a procedure called vacuum aspiration may be done to remove the remaining tissue. This procedure involves inserting a device into the uterus. It often can be performed in your health care provider's office.

If the pregnancy is large or if you are bleeding heavily, your provider may recommend a procedure called a *dilation and curettage (D&C)*. A D&C usually is performed in an operating room. The cervix is dilated and an instrument is used to remove the remaining tissue. Risks of both of these procedures include bleeding, infection, and injury to internal organs. Before having any procedure, your health care provider will discuss with you how the procedure is done as well as the risks and benefits. If your blood type is Rh negative, you will receive a shot of *Rh immunoglobulin* to prevent problems in a future pregnancy. See Chapter 28, "Blood Type Incompatibility," for more information about this issue.

### Recovery

After a miscarriage, you may be advised not to put anything into your vagina (such as using tampons or having sexual intercourse), usually for 2 weeks. This is to help prevent infection. You should see your health care provider for a follow-up visit a few weeks after your miscarriage. Call your health care provider right away if you have any of the following signs or symptoms:

• Heavy bleeding
• Fever
• Chills
• Severe pain

### Trying Again

You can ovulate and become pregnant as soon as 2 weeks after an early miscarriage. If you do not wish to become pregnant again right away, be sure to use birth control. If you do wish to become pregnant, you do not have to wait to begin trying again. You may want to wait until after you have had several regular menstrual periods so that calculating the due date of your next pregnancy is easier. You should take all the time you need to recover from a miscarriage before attempting to become pregnant again. There is no single answer as to the best length of time to wait, as this will vary between couples.

You may be concerned about your ability to have another baby after a miscarriage. Miscarriage usually does not predict what will happen in a future pregnancy, and most women who have a miscarriage will go on to have successful pregnancies. Repeated miscarriages are rare. Testing and evaluation can be done to try to find a cause if you have several miscarriages. Even if no cause is found, most couples will have successful pregnancies after repeated miscarriages.

## Ectopic Pregnancy

In a normal pregnancy, a fertilized egg moves through the *fallopian tube* and implants in the lining of the uterus, where it starts to grow. When a fertilized egg grows outside of the uterus, it is called an *ectopic pregnancy*. About 2% of pregnancies are ectopic. Most ectopic pregnancies occur in the fallopian tube. Because it is outside of the uterus, an ectopic pregnancy cannot grow to produce a healthy baby, and it can threaten the mother's health because of internal bleeding. An ectopic pregnancy cannot move or be moved to the "right place." For these reasons, an ectopic pregnancy must be ended either by surgery or with medical treatment.

### Risk Factors

Any sexually active woman of childbearing age is at risk of ectopic pregnancy. However, women who have had the following conditions or procedures are at higher risk:

- Previous ectopic pregnancy
- Prior tubal surgery (such as *tubal sterilization*)
- Previous pelvic or abdominal surgery
- Certain *sexually transmitted infections*
- *Pelvic inflammatory disease*
- *Endometriosis*

Some of these conditions produce scar tissue in the tubes. This may keep a fertilized egg from reaching the uterus.

Other factors that increase a woman's risk of ectopic pregnancy include smoking and the use of *assisted reproductive technology*, such as *in vitro fertilization*, to become pregnant.

### Signs and Symptoms

The symptoms of ectopic pregnancy sometimes include the symptoms of normal pregnancy, such as tender breasts or an upset stomach. Some women may have no symptoms at all and may not even know they are pregnant. If you have an ectopic pregnancy, you may have any or all of the following symptoms:

- Vaginal bleeding that is not at the time of your normal menstrual period
- Sudden, sharp pain in your abdomen or pelvic area
- Shoulder pain
- Weakness, dizziness, or fainting

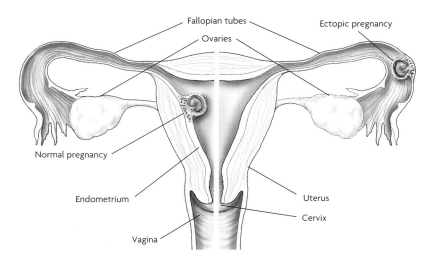

**Ectopic pregnancy.** In a normal pregnancy (*left*), the fertilized egg or fetus grows in the uterus. In an ectopic pregnancy (*right*), the fertilized egg or fetus grows in the fallopian tube or other abdominal organ.

These symptoms can occur before you even suspect you are pregnant. If you have these symptoms, call your health care provider right away. If you have vaginal bleeding with abdominal or shoulder pain or weakness, dizziness, or fainting, you should go to the hospital for evaluation.

## Diagnosis

If your health care provider thinks you may have an ectopic pregnancy, he or she will do a urine pregnancy test or give you a blood test to check your levels of **human chorionic gonadotropin (hCG)**—the hormone that is produced when a woman is pregnant. You also will have an ultrasound exam performed to see where the pregnancy is developing. If the diagnosis is unclear, the hCG test may be repeated a couple of days later to see if the levels of hCG in your blood have increased appropriately. If the levels are the same or lower, and a pregnancy is not seen growing in the uterus, an ectopic pregnancy or miscarriage is the most likely diagnosis.

Tests to find ectopic pregnancy take time. Results may not be clear right away. However, if your health care provider suspects that you have internal bleeding or a ruptured fallopian tube, this is an emergency that will require surgery. If the pregnancy is still in the early stages and the fallopian tube is not in danger of rupture, medical treatment may be an option.

## Treatment

There are two methods used to treat an ectopic pregnancy: medication and surgery. If your health care provider decides medication is the best choice, you will be given a drug called methotrexate. It will end the pregnancy by stopping the growth of the pregnancy. The ectopic pregnancy then is absorbed by the body.

**Taking Methotrexate.** There are many factors that go into the decision to use methotrexate. It cannot be used for women who are breastfeeding or who have certain health problems. The advantage of methotrexate treatment is that it preserves your fallopian tube and may help you to avoid surgery. The disadvantage is that it takes time for the ectopic pregnancy to be absorbed. Methotrexate also can cause unpleasant side effects. It is important to weigh the benefits and risks of this treatment carefully.

Methotrexate often is given in either one or two doses. In some cases, it may be given in many doses over several days. After treatment, it takes about 4–6 weeks for the pregnancy to be absorbed.

Before you take methotrexate, your health care provider will take a sample of your blood to check the functions of certain organs as well as the levels of the pregnancy hormone hCG. After receiving the methotrexate, you will have more blood tests for several days to check if the levels of hCG are decreasing as they should. If levels haven't decreased enough, surgery or another dose of methotrexate may be recommended.

While you are taking methotrexate, you will be monitored closely. During and after treatment, you should avoid the following:

- Alcohol
- Vitamins containing *folic acid*
- Exposure to sunlight
- Nonsteroidal antiinflammatory drugs, such as ibuprofen
- Sex

Your health care provider will tell you when you can safely resume these activities.

Medical treatment of an ectopic pregnancy can have some side effects. Most women have abdominal pain. Vaginal bleeding or spotting also may occur. Other side effects from the drug may include the following:

- Nausea
- Vomiting
- Diarrhea
- Dizziness

During methotrexate treatment, the risk of fallopian tube rupture still is present. Alert your health care provider if you have any of the following signs or symptoms of tubal rupture:

- Sharp abdominal pain
- Shoulder pain
- Fainting, dizziness, or weakness.

After your treatment is complete, careful follow-up over time (about 30 days) is needed until hCG is no longer found in your blood.

**Surgery.** In some cases, the ectopic pregnancy can be removed through a small cut made in the tube during a *laparoscopy*. In this procedure, an instrument called a *laparoscope* is inserted through a small opening in your abdomen. A larger incision in the abdomen may be needed if the pregnancy is large, if rupture of the fallopian tube is suspected, or if significant blood loss is a concern. With either of these approaches, some or all of the tube may need to be removed.

It is important that all of the ectopic pregnancy is removed. If any tissue is retained, it may cause internal bleeding. Blood tests for hCG may be needed for a few weeks after surgery to ensure that the pregnancy has been removed completely.

If you have had surgery and your fallopian tube has been left in place, there is a good chance that you can have a normal pregnancy in the future. However, once you have had an ectopic pregnancy, you are at higher risk of having another one. During future pregnancies, you may want to be alert for signs and symptoms of ectopic pregnancy until your health care provider confirms that the pregnancy is growing in the right place.

## Gestational Trophoblastic Disease

*Gestational trophoblastic disease (GTD)* is a rare group of disorders in which abnormal tissue forms from the placenta. The most common form of GTD is "molar pregnancy," which also is called a *hydatidiform mole*. A hydatidiform mole results when a sperm fertilizes an egg that does not contain any genetic material. The part of the placenta that grows into the wall of the uterus— known as *villi*—become swollen with fluid and resemble a cluster of grapes. A complete hydatidiform mole contains no fetal tissue. A partial hydatidiform mole contains some fetal tissue, but it is not able to grow or survive because it has abnormal genetic material.

### Signs, Symptoms, and Diagnosis

Most cases of GTD cause symptoms that signal a problem. The most common symptom is vaginal bleeding during the first trimester. Other signs of molar pregnancy, such as a uterus that is too large for the stage of the pregnancy, may be found by your health care provider. If your health care provider suspects a molar pregnancy, he or she may order an ultrasound exam and an hCG test. An abnormally high level of hCG for the stage of pregnancy suggests molar pregnancy, but high levels are not always present. Your health care provider will perform an ultrasound exam to determine if you have a molar pregnancy. If a molar pregnancy is found, a series of tests will be done to check for other medical problems that sometimes occur along with it. These problems include **high blood pressure**, **anemia**, and **hyperthyroidism** (overactive thyroid gland). Many of these problems go away when the molar pregnancy is removed.

### Treatment

If you have GTD, the tissue must be removed. This usually is done with a D&C in a similar fashion to the procedure that is sometimes performed for a miscarriage (see the explanation under "Miscarriage" earlier in this chapter). About 90% of women whose molar pregnancies are removed require no further treatment. However, careful follow-up is needed and regularly scheduled tests of hCG levels are done for at least 6 months and up to 1 year. After the pregnancy has been removed, abnormal cells may remain. This is called persistent GTD. It is indicated by hCG levels that increase or stay the same. Persistent GTD also can occur after a normal pregnancy. Some forms of persistent GTD are **malignant** (cancerous), and in a small number of women, malignant cells travel to other parts of the body. Persistent GTD is treated with medication and sometimes **hysterectomy** (removal of the uterus). Treatment is completely successful in most cases.

If you have had a molar pregnancy, your health care provider may advise you to wait 6 months to 1 year before trying to become pregnant again. It is safe to use birth control pills during this time. The chances of having another molar pregnancy are low (about 1%).

## Coping With the Loss

After the loss of a pregnancy, you need to heal both physically and emotionally. For many women, emotional healing takes a good deal longer than physical healing. The feelings of loss can be intense. Even if the pregnancy ended very early, the sense of bonding between a woman and her pregnancy can be strong. The loss of a pregnancy—no matter how early—can cause feelings of sadness and grief.

Grief can involve a wide range of feelings. You may find yourself searching for the reason your pregnancy ended. You may wrongly blame yourself. You may have headaches, lose your appetite, feel tired, or have trouble concentrating or sleeping. Sometimes, *depression* requiring treatment can occur. Your feelings of grief may differ from those of your partner. You are the one who has felt the physical changes of pregnancy. Your partner also may grieve but may not express feelings in the same way you do. This may create tension between the two of you when you need each other the most.

If either of you is having trouble handling the feelings that go along with this loss, talk to your health care provider. You also may find it helps to talk with a counselor.

# RESOURCES

The following resources offer more information about pregnancy loss:

**Ectopic Pregnancy**
Medline Plus
www.nlm.nih.gov/medlineplus/ency/article/000895.htm
*Discusses causes, risk factors, and treatment of ectopic pregnancy.*

**Gestational Trophoblastic Disease**
Medline Plus
www.nlm.nih.gov/medlineplus/ency/article/007333.htm
*Provides basic information about GTD and links to additional resources.*

**Recurrent Pregnancy Loss**
American Society for Reproductive Medicine
www.reproductivefacts.org/FACTSHEET_Recurrent_Pregnancy_Loss
*Expert discussion about recurrent pregnancy loss, including possible causes. Also explains how recurrent pregnancy loss may be evaluated and the chances of successful pregnancy after recurrent pregnancy losses.*

**SHARE: Pregnancy and Infant Loss Support, Inc.**
www.nationalshare.org
*Organization that provides support for families who have lost a baby through miscarriage, stillbirth, or newborn death.*

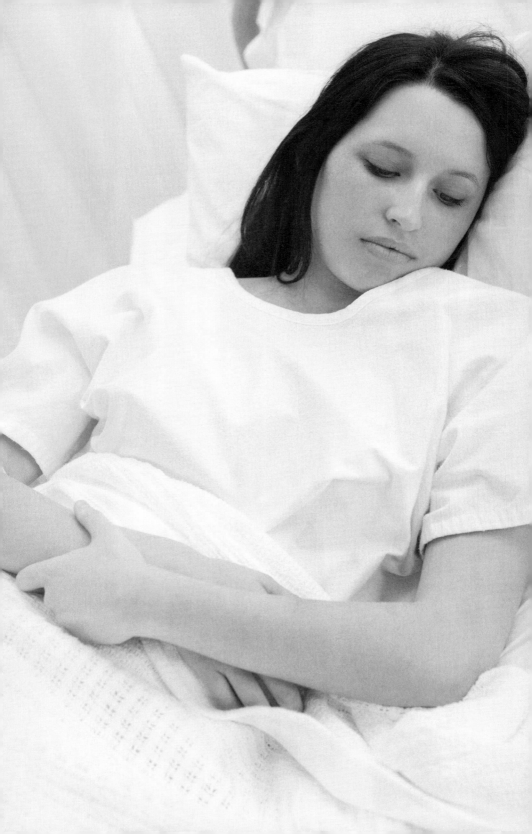

Chapter 34

# Late Pregnancy Loss
## Stillbirth

When a baby dies inside the womb after 20 weeks of pregnancy, it is called a *stillbirth*. The loss of a baby is tragic, and you will be faced with intense feelings of sadness and shock. It will help to grieve for however long you need and to have the support of your partner and loved ones during this difficult time. It may help to understand what went wrong, but sometimes it isn't possible to find a complete answer to this question.

## How Stillbirth Is Diagnosed

In many cases of stillbirth, a problem is suspected before the baby is born. The mother may notice that the baby has stopped moving. Stillbirth may be diagnosed during labor if the fetal heartbeat cannot be found with a fetal monitor. Sometimes, a health care provider is unable to hear the baby's heartbeat at a prenatal visit.

If there are concerns about the baby, an *ultrasound exam* may be done to check that the baby's heart is beating. If a heartbeat cannot be found, then the baby has died in the uterus. Your health care provider will talk with you about the best options for delivery. In the second trimester, a procedure called *dilation and evacuation* can be considered. After the second trimester, labor may be induced. The decision depends on your health and the stage of your pregnancy.

## What Went Wrong?

Perhaps the most difficult question for your health care provider to answer is what happened. Unfortunately, the reasons for most stillbirths are unknown. The death may be caused by a **birth defect**. Sometimes the baby will have trouble growing in the uterus because of problems with the **placenta** or the mother's circulation. Certain infections can cause mild illnesses or go unnoticed in the mother but can seriously affect the baby or result in stillbirth. Examples include certain viral infections, such as a **genital herpes** infection contracted for the first time during pregnancy, **cytomegalovirus** infections, and **parvovirus**. Other types of infections, such as **syphilis** and **toxoplasmosis**, also can increase the risk of stillbirth (see Chapter 30, "Protecting Yourself From Infection"). Problems with **chromosomes**, such as an abnormal number of chromosomes, are found in about 1 in 10 stillbirths. Medical conditions that affect the mother, such as **high blood pressure**, **kidney disease**, or **diabetes mellitus**, also can be a factor in stillbirth. Complications during labor and delivery, such as problems with the placenta or **umbilical cord**, infection, or lack of **oxygen**, can cause a baby's death, but these problems are unlikely if labor is monitored closely. Stillbirth almost never occurs because of something a woman has done or because of a medication she has taken.

## Tests and Evaluations

After a stillbirth, results from exams and tests usually are gathered to try to find out the most likely cause. A team of health care professionals may be involved, including your health care provider and others with special expertise. A physician with expertise in genetics (**geneticist**), a pediatrician, or a **neonatologist** may evaluate the baby after birth to look for signs of an inheritable genetic condition or a syndrome. A **pathologist** may perform certain tests to look for evidence of birth defects, abnormal placental development, or infections.

Your health care provider will take a careful history of the course of your pregnancy and document problems or illnesses that you had, if this hasn't already been done. A family history also may be taken to look for possible inherited disorders. Photographs may be taken of the baby to use during the evaluation, and the baby's measurements and weight will be recorded.

If your health care provider suspects that the cause of stillbirth is related to a genetic problem or infection of the baby, **amniocentesis** may be recommended before delivery. It is easier to grow **cells** obtained through amniocentesis than to grow cells taken from a stillborn baby after birth. To perform amniocentesis, a thin needle is guided through the woman's abdomen and uterus. A small sample of **amniotic fluid** is withdrawn. This fluid contains cells from the baby. The cells are grown in a special culture and the chromosomes in the cells then can be counted and analyzed. Sometimes blood tests from the mother also can be helpful if infection is suspected.

In some cases, an autopsy may be recommended. During an autopsy, an exam of the baby's organs is performed to look for birth defects or abnormalities in the baby's development. Tests to look for infection may be performed on the baby or the placenta. If you do not want an autopsy, other exams and tests may be available. These include a physical exam of the baby and the placenta, X-rays, taking samples of tissue for tests, and **magnetic resonance imaging**. With these alternatives, the baby's organs are left intact. Although the exact reason why your baby died may not be found, an autopsy or these other tests may help answer questions about what happened. This information could be useful to you and your health care provider in planning future pregnancies.

## Grieving

The death of a baby is a profoundly painful event. Grief is a normal, natural response to the loss of a baby. Mourn your loss for as long as you need (see box "Honoring Your Loss"). It's best to go through the complete grieving period to help you cope and move ahead. Remember that each parent grieves in a different way. It is important to talk with your partner or another person whom you trust about what you are feeling.

## The Stages of Grief

Grieving includes a wide range of feelings. Just as each pregnancy is unique, ways to react to a pregnancy loss also are unique. The process you follow will be affected by the culture you were raised in, your role in the family, your experiences with death, and what you think others expect of you.

Your grief may last for weeks, months, or years. The grieving process involves certain stages that can overlap and repeat. However, the process often seems to follow a pattern, and progress through shock, numbness, and disbelief; searching and yearning; anger or rage; depression and loneliness; and acceptance.

## Honoring Your Loss

Grieving your loss will take time. There are a few things that may make dealing with the pain a little easier:

- Saying good-bye—Right after your baby is born, it is often helpful to hold your baby to say good-bye. The hospital staff may take pictures of your baby or give you keepsakes, such as the baby's cap, a handprint or footprint, an identification bracelet, or a crib card from your baby. If these things are not offered to you, ask for them.

- Express yourself—Talk about your feelings with your partner, family, and friends. It often helps to write down your thoughts in a journal or in letters to the baby and others.

- Reach out—Tell your family and friends what they can do to help you and your partner, whether it's cooking a meal, doing house chores, running errands, or just spending time with you.

- Take care of yourself—Eat healthy, try to get enough sleep every night, and stay physically active. Avoid using alcohol or drugs to cope with the grief.

- Choose a name—Naming the baby helps give him or her an identity. A name allows you, your friends, and your family to refer to a specific child, not just "the baby you lost." You may want to use the name you first chose or pick another one.

- Plan a funeral or memorial service—For many parents, it's a great comfort to have family and friends acknowledge the life and death of their baby and to express their sorrow at a special service. You may wish to contact a funeral home for burial or cremation.

### Shock, Numbness, and Disbelief

When faced with news of their baby's death, parents often think that it is not really happening or that it can't be true. You may have trouble grasping the news or feel nothing at all. You may deny that the loss has occurred. Even though you and your partner may be together physically, you each may feel a very private sense of being alone or empty.

## Searching and Yearning

These feelings tend to overlap with the initial shock and get stronger over time. You may start looking for a reason for your baby's death—who or what caused him or her to die. It is common during this stage to feel guilty. You may think that you somehow brought about your baby's death and blame yourself for things you did or did not do. You may have dreams about the baby and yearn for what might have been.

## Anger or Rage

"What did I do to deserve this?" and "How could this happen to me?" are common questions after losing a baby. In this stage of grief, you may direct your anger at your partner, the doctors or health care providers, the hospital staff, or even other women whose babies were born healthy. Many parents feel angry if the cause of the stillbirth cannot be determined. Test results can take weeks or months to arrive, which can add to your frustration and anger. It's good to accept your anger, express it, and try to get it out of your system. If you or your partner feel angry toward each other, it may be hard for you to comfort each other. Anger becomes unhealthy if you turn it inward and direct it toward yourself.

## Depression and Loneliness

In this stage, the reality sinks in that you have lost your baby. You may feel tired, sad, and helpless. You may have trouble getting back into your normal routine. The support from friends and family that you received during the early weeks of your loss may not be as intense as it once was, even though you still need comfort and kindness. Slowly, you will start to get back on your feet and work through your loss.

## Acceptance

In this final stage of grieving, you come to terms with what has happened. Your baby's death no longer rules your thoughts. You start to have renewed energy. Although you will never forget your baby, you begin to think of him or her less often and with less pain. You pick up your normal daily routine and social life. You make plans for the future.

As you come to terms with your baby's death, you may feel guilty about moving through the worst of your grief. However, it's okay to accept what has happened. A normal part of life is planning for the future. Moving on does not mean that you will forget your baby; it just means that you are healing and are ready to accept what life has to offer.

## You and Your Partner

Your relationship with your partner may be affected by the stress of the loss of your child. You may have trouble getting your thoughts and feelings across to each other. One or both of you may feel hostile toward the other. You may find it hard to have sex again or do other things together that you used to enjoy. This is normal. Try to be patient with each other. Let your partner know what your needs are and what you are feeling. Take time to be tender, caring, and close. Make an extra effort to be open and honest.

Throughout the grieving process, your partner may not respond in the same way as you do. Your partner may feel differently from you and may be able to move on before you are ready. Your partner may not want to talk about the loss when you do. Each person should be allowed to grieve in his or her own way. Try to understand and respond to your partner's needs as well as your own.

## Seeking Support

Surround yourself with your partner, family, and friends for support during the coming months. Know that you are not alone. A number of people have the knowledge and skills to help you. Ask your health care provider to direct you to support systems in your community. These can include childbirth educators, self-help groups, social workers, and clergy. Take time to find one that suits you best (see the "Resources" section in this chapter).

Many grieving parents find it helpful to get involved with groups of parents who have gone through the same loss. Members of such support groups respect your feelings, understand your stresses and fears, and have a good sense of the kindness you need.

Professional counseling also can help to relieve your pain, guilt, and depression. Talking with a trained counselor can help you understand and accept what has happened. You may wish to get counseling for only yourself, for you and your partner, or for your entire family.

## Another Pregnancy

In time, you may feel ready to start planning your next pregnancy. You can plan your next pregnancy when you and your partner are physically and emotionally ready to do so. Before thinking about getting pregnant again, allow time for you and your partner to work through your feelings. After losing a baby, some couples feel a need to have another baby right away. They think it will fill the empty feeling or take away the pain. A new baby cannot replace the baby that was lost. If you have another baby too soon after your loss, you may find it hard to think of the new child as a separate and special person.

Should you choose to have another pregnancy, keep in mind that the chances of losing another baby are very small in most cases. If the cause of the stillbirth is not known, and you do not have a medical condition such as diabetes, the chance of stillbirth happening again is less than 1%. Even so, you may be anxious and worried during your next pregnancy. There may be things that you can do to get in the best health possible before pregnancy, such as weight loss if you are obese, genetic counseling if a genetic disorder is suspected, and tests and evaluations if you have a history of a medical condition. During pregnancy, ultrasound exams and other tests may be used to monitor fetal health. Anniversary days of your due date, when you lost your baby, or the baby's birthday will likely be sad times for many years and can be particularly stressful during a future pregnancy. Throughout your pregnancy, emotional support and reassurance are vital. Your health care provider may be able to recommend appropriate counseling or a support group if you feel this would be helpful to you.

## The Future

The pain of losing your baby will never vanish completely, but it will not always be the main focus in your life and thoughts. At some point, you will be able to talk and think about the baby more easily and with less pain. One day you'll find yourself doing more of the things you used to do, such as enjoying favorite activities, renewing friendships, and looking forward to the future.

# RESOURCES

The following resources offer more information about stillbirth:

**CLIMB: Center for Loss in Multiple Birth, Inc.**

www.climb-support.org

*Gives support for families who have experienced loss during a multiple pregnancy or during infancy and childhood.*

**The Compassionate Friends**

www.compassionatefriends.org/home.aspx

*Offers support for families experiencing grief following the death of a child of any age.*

**SHARE: Pregnancy and Infant Loss Support, Inc.**

www.nationalshare.org

*Organization that provides support for families who have lost a baby through miscarriage, stillbirth, or newborn death.*

# Part IX
# Looking Ahead

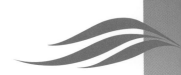

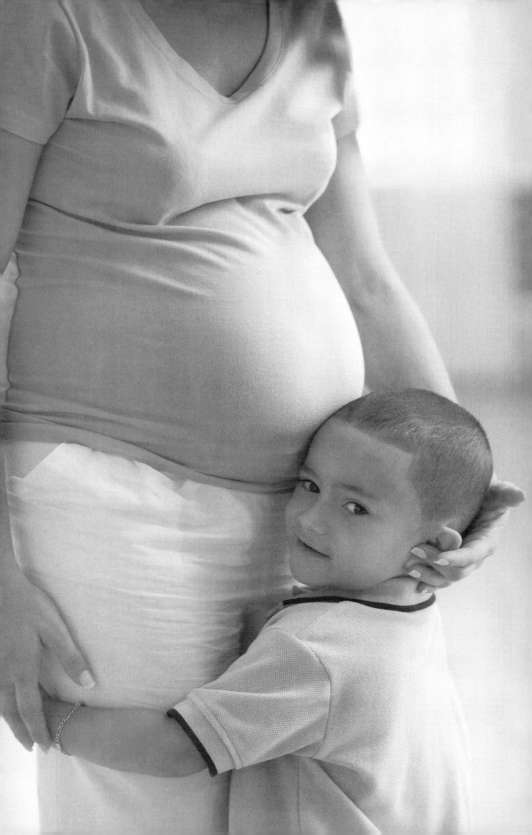

Chapter 35

# Having Another Baby

## What to Expect the Second Time Around

Now that you've been through pregnancy and childbirth, you already know a lot about what to expect if you become pregnant again. It is important to remember, however, that every pregnancy is different. Whether you are just thinking about having another child or you are already pregnant, there are a few things you and your partner should consider.

## Planning Another Baby

Some couples feel having siblings close together in age is better. Others think having the first child near school age before having another baby fits their lifestyle best.

The timing of when to plan your next pregnancy is a decision for both you and your partner. Only you two can decide what you are ready to handle— physically, emotionally, and financially (see box "The Cost of Raising a Child"). However, there are some medical issues that you should keep in mind when deciding when to have another baby.

### How Long Should You Wait?

When you decide to become pregnant again, schedule a **preconception** checkup with your health care provider to discuss your plans. It's recommended that women wait at least 18 months after having a baby before trying to get pregnant again in order to have the best health outcomes for both mom

## The Cost of Raising a Child

When trying to decide on how many children they want, many couples consider the financial expense. To raise a child from birth to age 18 years will cost a middle-income couple about $241,000, according to a report by the U.S. Department of Agriculture. This figure includes expenses such as housing, transportation, food, health care, clothing, and childcare. But it doesn't include the cost of college. The amount of money you spend can change depending on where you live, your marital status, and how many children you already have. To get an estimate of how much it would cost you to raise a child, access the calculator on the U.S. Department of Agriculture's web site at www.cnpp.usda.gov/calculatorintro.htm.

Data from U.S. Department of Agriculture. Expenditures on children by families. USDA Center for Nutrition Policy and Promotion, 2012.

and baby. Some studies report a greater risk of certain complications, including **preterm** birth and lower-than-average birth weight, when the time between pregnancies is 18 months or less. There are a few theories about why these problems may occur. Some experts believe having children too close together doesn't give you enough time to replenish your body's nutrients. Other theories suggest that a woman's body needs sufficient time to heal from childbirth before attempting another pregnancy. Infections also may play a role.

This is not to say that all women need to wait 18 months between pregnancies. For example, women who are older than 35 years also need to be aware of their declining fertility as they think about adding to their families. If you are older than 35 years, an interval of 12 months between pregnancies may be acceptable. It is a good idea to discuss your individual situation with your health care provider, including your age, family history, and medical history, when deciding how to space your children.

It also is helpful to await the return of regular menstrual cycles. Having a regular menstrual cycle will help you detect pregnancy earlier and can assist your health care provider in estimating your due date.

### Is Your Body Ready?

Think about whether you have the energy to be a mom to another baby. One thing that is almost always true of a later pregnancy is that you will be more tired than your first time. There are a few reasons for this. First, you will be older than you were during your first pregnancy. You may not have had a chance to get back in shape after giving birth. Second, you'll have another child (or children) to take care of, which can be tiring even when you aren't pregnant.

During your preconception visit, your health care provider will make sure you are as healthy as possible and are sticking to a healthy diet and lifestyle. For example, if you haven't had much success getting back to your prepregnancy weight since having your first baby, your health care provider may tell you that now is the time to try harder. Results of some studies show that gaining too much weight between pregnancies may lead to complications, such as **high blood pressure** and **gestational diabetes mellitus**.

You also will be reminded to start (or continue) taking a daily vitamin supplement that contains 400 micrograms of **folic acid** to help prevent **neural tube defects**. In addition, your health care provider will make sure any immunizations you need are up to date.

Overall, as you plan your next pregnancy, be sure to follow the same healthy habits you did the first time around. Start by reviewing the suggestions in Chapter 1, "Getting Ready for Pregnancy."

## You're Pregnant Already

What will your second pregnancy be like? While every pregnancy is different, there are a few things that you can expect. The changes your body will experience during pregnancy won't be such a surprise this time around. You may even find that you don't have the roller coaster of emotions that you did with your first pregnancy. But keep in mind that no two pregnancies progress in exactly the same way. It's best to be prepared for some things to be different.

### How Will It Be Different?

There are some stages of pregnancy that tend to change after your first time. No two pregnancies are alike, so here are a few things likely to be different this time around:

- You'll show earlier—In fact, you may need to start wearing maternity clothes before your fourth month. That's because your abdominal muscles were stretched by your prior pregnancy and they may not have regained their former strength. As a result, these muscles won't hold the growing uterus in or up as well as they did during the first pregnancy.

- You'll feel the baby move sooner—You may feel this baby move a few weeks earlier than you felt your first baby move. The baby isn't really moving sooner. You just know what it first feels like this time.

- You'll notice **Braxton Hicks contractions** sooner—Braxton Hicks contractions may show up during the second trimester rather than the third trimester, for instance.

- Your breast changes are different—They may not be as tender or grow as much as they did before. If you breastfed your first baby, your breasts may begin to leak earlier in pregnancy, too.

### Possible Problems

Although every pregnancy is different, you'll likely have at least some of the same discomforts you had the first time. Knowing this can help motivate you to take steps to lessen or possibly prevent them altogether. For example, if you had constipation or hemorrhoids last time, you can try to prevent these problems early on by eating plenty of fiber or taking a fiber supplement, drinking plenty of water, and exercising regularly.

Besides these normal pregnancy symptoms, if you're a healthy woman and had no serious problems the first time around, your risk of complications now is low. If, however, you have certain medical conditions, such as high blood pressure or diabetes, they can cause problems during pregnancy. Your health care provider will want to be sure these conditions are under control as this pregnancy progresses.

If you had any serious complications during your first pregnancy, such as preterm birth, **postpartum depression**, or gestational diabetes mellitus, you may be at higher risk of these problems happening again. Make a visit with your health care provider as soon as you know you're pregnant if you had one of the following complications. You can find out how to recognize any symptoms earlier, and there also may be steps you can take to reduce your risks:

- Preterm birth—Women who've had a preterm birth are almost two times more likely to have another one. Your health care provider may tell you to avoid strenuous physical activity and watch for the signs and symptoms of infection. Additional testing, such as an **ultrasound exam** to measure cervical length, may be offered, and you may receive certain treatments, depending on your situation.

- **Preterm premature rupture of membranes (PROM)**—The risk of preterm PROM happening in another pregnancy is increased if you have had it before. However, preterm PROM can happen even when there are no known risk factors. Your health care provider may recommend certain treatments and monitoring if you have a history of preterm PROM.

- Postpartum depression—Talk to your health care provider about what steps you can take to decrease your risk of developing postpartum depression this time around, ideally before you become pregnant. It may be recommended that you begin treatment with an antidepressant right after you give birth to prevent postpartum depression. If you were taking antidepressants before pregnancy, your health care provider can assess your situation and help you decide whether to continue taking medication during your pregnancy. If you do continue taking medication, changes may be made to the type or dosage.

- Gestational diabetes—If you had gestational diabetes in your first pregnancy, you are more likely to have it again. In addition, because up to 50% of women with gestational diabetes develop diabetes later in life, you should expect to have your blood glucose level tested beginning 6–12 weeks after giving birth and then at least once every 3 years. Your health care provider also will discuss ways to lower your risk through diet, exercise, and possibly medication.

- *Preeclampsia*—If you had preeclampsia or eclampsia in a prior pregnancy, you have an increased risk of having it again in a subsequent pregnancy. For this reason, you should see your health care provider early in pregnancy, and ideally before pregnancy, to discuss and address whether you have additional risk factors (such as obesity, high blood pressure, or type 2 diabetes), have certain baseline tests, and get advice about how to optimize your health. Other tests and interventions may be recommended during pregnancy. You also should be familiar with the signs and symptoms of preeclampsia and know how to reach your health care provider right away if you have any of them.

- *Fetal growth restriction*—Women who previously have given birth to a smaller-than-normal infant are more at risk of this condition in their next pregnancy. Your health care provider may order serial ultrasound exams during your second pregnancy to monitor your baby's growth.

## Telling Your Other Children

You may wonder when the best time is to tell your other children that you're going to have another baby. You know your children best, so it's really your decision when to tell them. It depends on how old your children are and how you think they will handle the news.

Some experts suggest that you should wait until sometime after your first trimester, when the risk of miscarriage decreases. You may want to wait until after a healthy pregnancy is confirmed by listening for the baby's heartbeat or by ultrasound exam. With very young children, it may be a good idea to wait until you're starting to show. Your children may have a hard time imagining there's a baby growing inside you if your body still looks the same. It can be easier to explain once you have a little bump.

Whenever you do give the news, be sure to remind your children that you love them and that the new baby won't change that. To prevent your children from feeling left out, involve them in your pregnancy as much as you can. The relationship between siblings is one of the longest and most important ones in life. These tips can help promote the bond right from the start:

- Involve them in picking out the baby's name.

- Tell your children about the role they can play in helping you with the new baby.

- Read books together about pregnancy and on being a big brother or sister.

- Show your children their own baby pictures.

- Take your children shopping and let them pick out items for their new baby brother or sister.

You may want to set up the baby's room early. If you need to move your children out of a crib or into a different room, do it as early as possible so that they don't feel displaced by the new baby. You can ask them to help decorate the room or even suggest that they pick a few of their old toys to give to the baby.

Remember that welcoming another baby into the family likely will bring both happiness and anxiety for your other children. Just do your best to plan ahead for the new arrival to help make the transition as easy as possible.

# RESOURCES

The following resources offer more information about some of the topics discussed in this chapter:

**Having Another Baby**

www.havinganotherbaby.com

*Web site created by a child psychologist that explores issues such as birth order, sibling rivalry, and preparing children for a sibling, as well as lots of information on stepfamilies.*

**Preconception Health and Health Care**

www.cdc.gov/preconception/planning.html

*Useful preconception care information from the Centers for Disease Control and Prevention that's relevant to all moms-to-be, whether they're having their first baby or their second and beyond.*

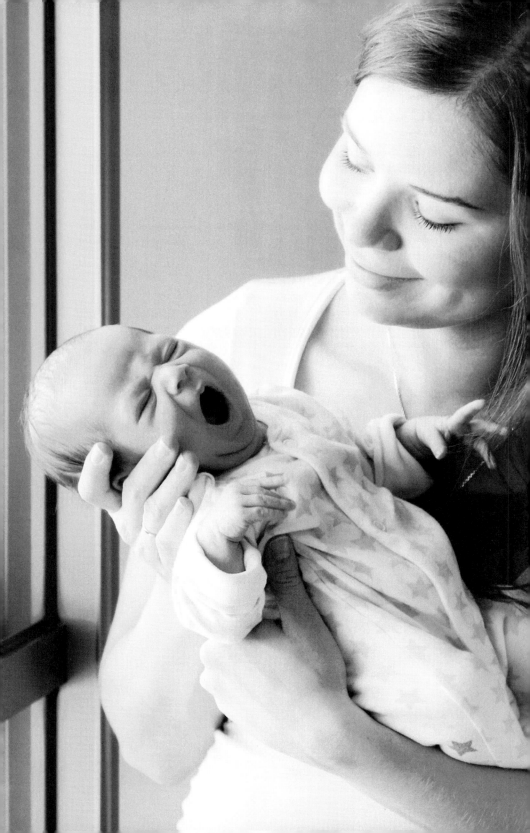

# Glossary

*Acceleration:* An increase in the fetal heart rate.

*Acquired Immunodeficiency Syndrome (AIDS):* A group of signs and symptoms, usually of severe infections, occurring in a person whose immune system has been damaged by infection with human immunodeficiency virus (HIV).

*Allele:* The alternative form of a single gene.

*Alveoli:* The small sacs in the lungs that allow oxygen to be transferred from the lungs to the blood.

*Amniocentesis:* A procedure in which a needle is used to withdraw and test a small amount of amniotic fluid and cells from the sac surrounding the fetus.

*Amnionicity:* In a multiple pregnancy, the determination of whether the babies share an amniotic sac or have their own amniotic sacs.

*Amniotic Fluid:* Water in the sac surrounding the fetus in the mother's uterus.

*Amniotic Membranes:* Another term for the amniotic sac; the fluid-filled sac in the mother's uterus in which the fetus develops.

*Amniotic Sac:* Fluid-filled sac in the mother's uterus in which the fetus develops.

*Amniotomy:* Artificial rupture of the amniotic sac.

*Analgesic:* A drug that relieves pain without causing loss of consciousness.

*Anemia:* Abnormally low levels of blood or red blood cells in the bloodstream. Most cases are caused by iron deficiency, or lack of iron.

*Anencephaly:* A type of neural tube defect that occurs when the fetus's head and brain do not develop normally.

*Anesthesia:* Relief of pain by loss of sensation.

*Anesthesiologist:* A doctor who is an expert in pain relief.

*Anesthetic:* A drug used to relieve pain.

*Aneuploidy:* Having an abnormal number of chromosomes.

*Anorexia Nervosa:* An eating disorder in which distorted body image leads a person to diet excessively.

*Antibiotics:* Drugs that treat certain types of infections.

*Antibody:* A protein in the blood produced in reaction to foreign substances, such as bacteria and viruses that cause infection.

*Antidepressants:* Medications that are used to treat depression.

*Antigen:* A substance, such as an organism causing infection or a protein found on the surface of blood cells, that can induce an immune response and cause the production of an antibody.

*Antiphospholipid Syndrome (APS):* A disorder in which proteins called antibodies are mistakenly made against certain substances in the blood involved in normal blood clotting. It can lead to abnormal blood clotting and pregnancy complications, including pregnancy loss.

*Anus:* The opening of the digestive tract through which bowel movements leave the body.

*Apgar Score:* A measurement of a baby's response to birth and life on its own, taken 1 and 5 minutes after birth.

*Assisted Reproductive Technology:* A group of infertility treatments in which an egg is fertilized with a sperm outside the body; the fertilized egg then is transferred to the uterus.

*Augmentation of Labor:* The use of medications or other means to stimulate contractions of the uterus during labor.

*Autism:* A group of developmental disorders that range from mild to severe and that result in communication problems, problems interacting with others, behavioral difficulties, and repetitive behaviors.

*Autoimmune Disorder:* A condition in which the body attacks its own tissues.

*Autosomal Dominant:* A genetic disorder caused by one defective gene; the defective gene is located on one of the 22 chromosomes that are not the sex chromosomes.

*Autosomal Recessive:* A genetic disorder caused by two defective genes, one inherited from each parent; the defective genes are located on one of the 22 chromosomes that are not the sex chromosomes.

*Autosomes:* Any of the chromosomes that are not the sex chromosomes; in humans, there are 22 pairs of autosomes.

*Bacteria:* One-celled organisms that can cause infections in the human body.

*Bacterial Vaginosis:* A type of vaginal infection caused by the overgrowth of a number of organisms that are normally found in the vagina.

*Bariatric Surgery:* Surgical procedures that cause weight loss for the treatment of obesity.

*Basal Body Temperature:* The temperature of the body at rest.

*Bilirubin:* A yellow substance that is formed from the breakdown of red blood cells. High levels of bilirubin in the blood may result in jaundice in newborns.

*Biophysical Profile (BPP):* An assessment of fetal heart rate by electronic fetal monitoring and assessment of fetal breathing, body movement, muscle tone, and the amount of amniotic fluid by ultrasound. The biophysical profile can be modified to include only some of these tests.

*Birth Defect:* A physical problem or intellectual disability that is present at birth.

*Bladder:* A muscular organ in which urine is stored.

*Blastocyst:* The cluster of cells formed 4–5 days after fertilization

*Bloom Syndrome:* An autosomal recessive inherited disorder of short stature that causes sensitivity to light, increased risk for some forms of cancer, and other health problems.

*Body Mass Index (BMI):* A number calculated from height and weight that is used to determine whether a person is underweight, normal weight, overweight, or obese.

*Braxton Hicks Contractions:* False labor pains.

*Breech Presentation:* A position in which the feet or buttocks of the fetus would be born first.

*Bulimia Nervosa:* An eating disorder in which a person binges on food and then forces vomiting or abuses laxatives.

*Calorie:* A unit of heat used to express the fuel or energy value of food.

*Canavan Disease:* An inherited disorder that causes progressive damage to brain cells.

*Carpal Tunnel Syndrome:* A condition caused by compression of the median nerve in the carpal tunnel of the wrist; symptoms include pain and burning or tingling in the fingers and hand, sometimes extending up to the elbow.

*Carrier:* [genetics] A person who shows no signs of a particular disorder but could pass the gene on to his or her children.

*Carrier:* [infections] A person who is infected with the organism of a disease without showing symptoms and who can transmit the disease to another person.

*Catheter:* A tube used to drain fluid from or administer fluid to the body.

*Cell:* The smallest unit of a structure in the body; the building blocks for all parts of the body.

*Cell-Free DNA:* DNA from the fetus that circulates freely in a pregnant woman's blood. It is the basis of a noninvasive prenatal screening test.

*Cephalopelvic Disproportion:* A condition in which a baby is too large to pass safely through the mother's pelvis during delivery.

*Cerclage:* A procedure in which the cervical opening is closed with stitches in order to prevent or delay preterm birth.

*Cerebral Palsy:* A long-term disability of the nervous system that affects young children in which control of movement or posture is abnormal and is not the result of a recognized disease.

*Cervical Ripening:* The process by which the cervix softens in preparation for labor.

*Cervix:* The lower, narrow end of the uterus at the top of the vagina.

*Cesarean Birth:* Birth of a baby through surgical incisions made in the mother's abdomen and uterus.

*Cesarean Delivery:* Delivery of a baby through surgical incisions made in the mother's abdomen and uterus.

*Chickenpox:* Also called varicella; a contagious disease caused by a virus that results in small, fluid-filled blisters on the skin.

*Chlamydia:* A sexually transmitted infection caused by bacteria that can lead to pelvic inflammatory disease and infertility.

*Chloasma:* The darkening of areas of skin on the face during pregnancy.

*Cholesterol:* A natural substance that serves as a building block for cells and hormones and helps to carry fat through the blood vessels for use or storage in other parts of the body.

*Chorioamnionitis:* Inflammation or infection of the membrane surrounding the fetus.

*Chorion:* The outer membrane that surrounds the fetus.

*Chorionicity:* In a multiple pregnancy, the determination of whether the babies share a chorion or have their own chorions.

*Chorionic Villi:* Microscopic, fingerlike projections that make up the placenta.

*Chorionic Villus Sampling (CVS):* A procedure in which a small sample of cells is taken from the placenta and tested.

*Chromosomes:* Structures that are located inside each cell in the body and contain the genes that determine a person's physical makeup.

*Chronic Hypertension:* High blood pressure that was diagnosed before the current pregnancy.

*Color Blindness:* An inherited deficiency in the ability to see certain colors that usually affects males.

*Colostrum:* A fluid secreted in the breasts at the beginning of milk production.

*Combined Spinal–Epidural (CSE) Block:* A form of regional anesthesia or analgesia in which pain medications are administered into the spinal fluid (spinal block) as well as through a thin tube into the epidural space (epidural block).

*Complete Blood Count (CBC):* A blood test that describes the size, shape, appearance, and amount of different cell types in the blood, such as white blood cells, red blood cells, and platelets. It also includes the hematocrit (the percentage of blood that is made up of red blood cells) and measurement of the level of hemoglobin (the protein that carries oxygen in red blood cells).

*Congenital Rubella Syndrome (CRS):* A condition that can be present in the newborn after a fetus has been infected with the rubella virus (also known as German measles) during the first trimester of pregnancy. Long-term complications can include heart and eye problems, deafness, and intellectual disability.

*Congenital Varicella Syndrome:* A condition that can be present in the newborn after a fetus has been infected with varicella (chickenpox) usually during the first or second trimester of pregnancy. Long-term complications can include eye abnormalities, brain damage, and limb abnormalities.

*Conjunctivitis:* Inflammation of the tissue that covers the inside of the eyelids and the outer surface of the eye.

*Contraction Stress Test (CST):* A test in which mild contractions of the mother's uterus are induced and the fetus's heart rate in response to the contractions is recorded using an electronic fetal monitor.

*Contrast Agent:* A substance that is injected into the body (usually into the veins or arteries) during certain X-ray procedures that allows specific structures or tissues to be seen.

*Corticosteroids:* Hormones given to help fetal lungs mature, for arthritis, or for other medical conditions.

*Crowning:* The phase in Stage 2 of childbirth when a large part of the baby's scalp is visible at the vaginal opening.

*Cystic Fibrosis:* An inherited disorder that causes problems in digestion and breathing.

*Cytomegalovirus (CMV):* A virus that can be transmitted to a fetus if a woman becomes infected during pregnancy. It can cause hearing loss, intellectual disability, and vision problems in infected infants.

*Deep Vein Thrombosis (DVT):* A condition in which a blood clot forms in veins in the leg or other areas of the body.

*Depression:* Feelings of sadness for periods of at least 2 weeks.

*Diabetes Mellitus:* A condition in which the levels of sugar in the blood are too high.

*Diagnostic Tests:* Tests that look for a disease or cause of a disease in people who are believed to have or who have an increased risk of a disease.

**Diamniotic–Dichorionic:** Describes twin embryos in which each twin has its own gestational sac surrounded by a complete layer of membranes (the inner amnion and the outer chorion) and separate placentas. These twins are usually fraternal (non-identical, with different genetic material), but sometimes can be identical (have the same genetic material).

**Diamniotic–Monochorionic:** Describes twin embryos formed from the same egg in which each twin has its own gestational sac surrounded by its own inner layer of membranes (the amnion), but a single outer layer of membranes (the chorion) surrounds both sacs together. These twins share a single placenta and are identical (have the same genetic material).

**Diastolic Blood Pressure:** The force of the blood in the arteries when the heart is relaxed; the lower blood pressure reading.

**Dietary Fiber:** The part of whole grains, vegetables, fruits, and nuts that is not digested in the digestive tract.

**Dilation:** Widening the opening of the cervix.

**Dilation and Curettage (D&C):** A procedure in which the cervix is opened and tissue is gently scraped or suctioned from the inside of the uterus.

**Dilation and Evacuation:** A procedure performed after 12 weeks of pregnancy in which the cervix is dilated and the contents of the uterus are removed.

**Diphtheria:** A bacterial infection in which a membrane forms in the throat that can block the flow of air; a toxin produced by the bacteria can also damage the heart and nerves.

**Discordant:** A large difference in the size of fetuses in a multiple pregnancy.

**DNA:** The genetic material that is passed down from parents to offspring. DNA is packaged in structures called chromosomes.

**Doppler Velocimetry:** A test that measures the flow of blood in a blood vessel. It can be used to measure the blood flow in the umbilical artery of the fetus to assess the blood flow through the placenta. It often is used to evaluate fetal growth restriction.

**Doula:** A birth coach or aide who gives continual emotional and physical support to a woman during labor and childbirth.

**Down Syndrome:** A genetic disorder caused by the presence of an extra chromosome and characterized by intellectual disability, abnormal features of the face, and medical problems such as heart defects. Many children with Down syndrome live to adulthood.

**Early Term:** The period from 37 and 0/7 weeks through 38 and 6/7 weeks of pregnancy.

**Eclampsia:** Seizures occurring in pregnancy and linked to high blood pressure.

**Ectopic Pregnancy:** A pregnancy in which the fertilized egg begins to grow in a place other than inside the uterus, usually in one of the fallopian tubes.

*Edema:* Swelling caused by fluid retention.

*Effacement:* Thinning out of the cervix.

*Egg:* The female reproductive cell produced in and released from the ovaries; also called the ovum.

*Elective Delivery:* A delivery that is done for a nonmedical reason.

*Electronic Fetal Monitoring:* A method in which electronic instruments are used to record the heartbeat of the fetus and contractions of the mother's uterus.

*Embryo:* The developing organism from the time it implants in the uterus up to 8 completed weeks of pregnancy.

*Endometrial Ablation:* A minor surgical procedure in which the lining of the uterus is destroyed to stop or reduce menstrual bleeding.

*Endometriosis:* A condition in which tissue that lines the uterus is found outside of the uterus, usually on the ovaries, fallopian tubes, and other pelvic structures.

*Endometritis:* Infection of the lining of the uterus.

*Endometrium:* The lining of the uterus.

*Epidural Block:* A type of regional anesthesia or analgesia in which pain medications are given through a tube placed in the space at the base of the spine.

*Episiotomy:* A surgical incision made into the perineum (the region between the vagina and the anus) to widen the vaginal opening for delivery.

*Estimated Due Date (EDD):* The estimated date that a baby will be born.

*Estrogen:* A female hormone produced in the ovaries.

*Exclusive Breastfeeding:* A type of feeding in which human milk is the only food provided to the baby.

*Expanded Carrier Screening:* A carrier screening technology that allows a large number of disorders to be screened for simultaneously.

*External Cephalic Version:* A technique, performed late in pregnancy, in which the doctor manually attempts to move a breech baby into the head-down position.

*Factor V Leiden:* The name of a specific genetic change that can result in an increased chance of developing blood clots.

*Fallopian Tubes:* Tubes through which an egg travels from the ovary to the uterus.

*Familial Dysautonomia:* An inherited autosomal recessive disease of childhood that affects the nervous system and can affect the perception of pain and temperature as well as digestion and movements.

*Fanconi Anemia Group C:* A inherited recessive disorder that causes a decrease in bone marrow function, physical abnormalities, and an increased risk of certain types of cancer.

*Fertilization:* Joining of the egg and sperm.

*Fetal Alcohol Syndrome:* The most severe disorder resulting from alcohol use during pregnancy. It can cause abnormalities in brain development, physical growth, and facial features.

*Fetal Blood Sampling:* A procedure in which a sample of blood is taken from the umbilical cord and tested.

*Fetal Fibronectin:* A protein that helps the amniotic sac stay connected to the inside of the uterus.

*Fetal Growth Restriction:* An abnormally small fetus whose estimated weight is less than 9 out of 10 fetuses of the same gestational age.

*Fetus:* The developing organism in the uterus from the ninth week of pregnancy until the end of pregnancy.

*Fibroids:* Benign growths that form in the muscle of the uterus.

*Fluorescence in Situ Hybridization:* A laboratory technique that is used to screen for common chromosome problems, such as trisomy 21, in cells obtained by amniocentesis or chorionic villus sampling. Results are available fairly quickly because the cells do not need to be grown in a culture prior to testing.

*Folic Acid:* A vitamin that has been shown to reduce the risk of certain birth defects when taken in sufficient amounts before and during pregnancy.

*Follicle-Stimulating Hormone (FSH):* A hormone produced by the pituitary gland that helps an egg to mature.

*Forceps:* Special instruments placed around the baby's head to help guide it out of the birth canal during delivery.

*Fraternal Twins:* Twins that have developed from two fertilized eggs that are not genetically identical.

*Full Term:* The period from 39 and 0/7 weeks through 40 and 6/7 weeks of gestation.

*Gastroschisis:* A birth defect in which a hole is formed in the abdominal wall of the fetus through which the bowel can stick out. It can be can be diagnosed prenatally with ultrasound and is treated with surgery after birth.

*Gaucher Disease:* An inherited genetic disorder in which a substance called glucosylceramidase builds up in cells of the liver, spleen, lymph nodes, lungs, and bone marrow and causes impairment of the liver and the nervous system. The signs and symptoms vary widely and range from mild to severe.

*Gene:* A segment of DNA that contains instructions for the development of a person's physical traits and control of the processes in the body. It is the basic unit of heredity and can be passed down from parent to offspring.

*General Anesthesia:* The use of drugs that produce a sleep-like state to prevent pain during surgery.

*Genetic Counselor:* A health care professional with special training in genetics and counseling who can provide expert advice about genetic disorders and prenatal testing.

*Genetic Disorder:* A term for a disorder caused by a change in genes or chromosomes.

*Geneticist:* A specialist in genetics.

*Genital Herpes:* A sexually transmitted infection caused by a virus that produces painful, highly infectious sores on or around the sex organs.

*Gestational Age:* The age of a pregnancy calculated from the number of weeks that have elapsed from the first day of the last normal menstrual period.

*Gestational Diabetes Mellitus:* Diabetes that arises during pregnancy.

*Gestational Hypertension:* New-onset high blood pressure that occurs after 20 weeks of pregnancy.

*Gestational Trophoblastic Disease (GTD):* A rare disorder of pregnancy in which cells from the placenta grow abnormally and form a mass in the uterus.

*Gingivitis:* Inflammation of the gums.

*Glucose:* A sugar that is present in the blood and is the body's main source of fuel.

*Gonorrhea:* A sexually transmitted infection that may lead to pelvic inflammatory disease, infertility, and arthritis.

*Group B Streptococci (GBS):* A type of bacteria that normally lives in the digestive and reproductive tracts of men and women and that can be passed to a woman's baby during labor and delivery if she has the bacteria late in her pregnancy. GBS can cause serious infection in some newborns. Antibiotics can be given during labor and delivery to women at risk of passing the bacteria to their babies in order to prevent newborn infection.

*HELLP Syndrome:* A severe type of preeclampsia; HELLP stands for hemolysis, elevated liver enzymes, and low platelet count.

*Hemoglobinopathies:* Any inherited disorder caused by changes in the structure of hemoglobin, a substance found in red blood cells that carries oxygen. Examples include sickle cell anemia, sickle cell disease, and the different forms of thalassemia.

*Hemolytic Disease of the Newborn (HDN):* A type of anemia that can affect a fetus or newborn that results from the breakdown of red blood cells by antibodies in the mother's blood.

*Hemophilia:* A disorder caused by a mutated gene on the X chromosome. Affected individuals are usually males who lack a substance in the blood that helps it clot and are at risk of severe bleeding from even minor injuries.

*Hemorrhage:* Heavy bleeding.

*Hepatitis:* Inflammation of the liver.

*Hepatitis A Virus:* The virus that causes hepatitis A.

*Hepatitis B Immune Globulin:* A substance given to provide temporary protection against infection with hepatitis B virus.

*Hepatitis B Virus (HBV):* The virus that causes hepatitis B.

*Hepatitis C Virus:* The virus that causes hepatitis C.

*Herpes Zoster (Shingles):* A disease caused by reactivation of the varicella zoster virus in those who have previously had varicella (chickenpox). It causes a painful rash and blisters.

*High Blood Pressure:* Blood pressure that is elevated above the normal level; also called hypertension.

*Hormones:* Substances made in the body by cells or organs that control the function of cells or organs. An example is estrogen, which controls the function of female reproductive organs.

*Human Chorionic Gonadotropin (hCG):* A hormone produced during pregnancy; its detection is the basis for most pregnancy tests.

*Human Immunodeficiency Virus (HIV):* A virus that attacks certain cells of the body's immune system and causes acquired immunodeficiency syndrome (AIDS).

*Human Papillomavirus (HPV):* The name for a group of related viruses, some of which cause genital warts and some of which are linked to cervical changes and cancer of the cervix, vulva, vagina, penis, anus, and throat.

*Hydatidiform Mole:* Also known as molar pregnancy; a form of gestational trophoblastic disease that results when a sperm fertilizes an egg that does not contain any genetic material. A complete hydatidiform mole contains no fetal tissue. A partial mole contains some fetal tissue, but it is not able to grow or survive.

*Hydramnios:* A condition in which there is an excess amount of amniotic fluid in the sac surrounding the fetus.

*Hyperemesis Gravidarum:* Severe nausea and vomiting during pregnancy that can lead to loss of weight and body fluids.

*Hypertension:* High blood pressure.

*Hyperthyroidism:* A condition in which the thyroid gland makes too much thyroid hormone.

*Hypothyroidism:* A condition in which the thyroid gland makes too little thyroid hormone.

*Hysterectomy:* Removal of the uterus.

*Hysterosalpingogram:* An X-ray procedure with contract material used to view the inside of the uterus and fallopian tubes.

*Hysteroscopic Sterilization:* A sterilization procedure in which the opening of each fallopian tube is blocked with scar tissue formed by the insertion of small implants, preventing sperm from entering the fallopian tubes to fertilize an egg.

*Identical Twins:* Twins that have developed from a single fertilized egg that are usually genetically identical.

*Immune:* Protected against infectious disease.

*Immune System:* The body's natural defense system against foreign substances and invading organisms, such as bacteria that cause disease.

*Incontinence:* Inability to control bodily functions such as urination.

*Induced Abortion:* The planned termination of a pregnancy before the fetus can survive outside the uterus.

*Influenza:* An infection with the influenza virus that most commonly affects the respiratory tract. Symptoms include fever, headache, muscle aches, cough, nasal congestion, and extreme fatigue. Complications can occur in severe cases, such as pneumonia and bronchitis. There are a number of different influenza virus types, including A, B, and C, and different strains, including 18 H types and 11 N types, e.g. H1N1 or "swine flu."

*Insulin:* A hormone that lowers the levels of glucose (sugar) in the blood.

*Internal Os:* The internal opening of the cervix into the uterus.

*Intrauterine Device (IUD):* A small device that is inserted and left inside the uterus to prevent pregnancy.

*Intravenous (IV) Line:* A tube inserted into a vein that is used to deliver medication or fluids.

*In Vitro Fertilization:* A procedure in which an egg is removed from a woman's ovary, fertilized in a laboratory with the man's sperm, and then transferred to the woman's uterus to achieve a pregnancy.

*Isotretinoin:* A prescription medication used to treat acne that can cause severe birth defects if taken during pregnancy.

*Jaundice:* A buildup of bilirubin that causes a yellowish appearance.

*Karyotype:* An image of a person's chromosomes, arranged in order of size.

*Kidney:* One of two organs that cleanse the blood, removing liquid wastes.

*Kidney Disease:* A general term for any disease that affects how the kidneys function.

*Labor:* The process by which the fetus, umbilical cord, and placenta are expelled from the uterus.

*Labor Dystocia:* Abnormal labor.

*Laborist:* An obstetrician–gynecologist who is employed by a hospital or physician group and whose primary role is to care for laboring patients and to manage obstetric emergencies.

*Lactational Amenorrhea Method (LAM):* A temporary method of birth control that is based on the natural way the body prevents ovulation when a woman is breast-feeding. The method may be up to 98% effective if used correctly.

*Lactose Intolerant:* Being unable to digest lactose, a sugar found in many dairy products.

*Laminaria:* Slender rods made of natural or synthetic material that expands when it absorbs water; they are inserted into the opening of the cervix to widen it.

*Lanugo:* The fine hair on the body of the fetus.

*Laparoscope:* An instrument that is inserted into the abdominal cavity through a small incision to view internal organs or to perform surgery.

*Laparoscopic Sterilization:* Sterilization that is performed by laparoscopy, a type of surgery that uses slender instruments inserted through small incisions in the abdomen.

*Laparoscopy:* A surgical procedure in which an instrument called a laparoscope is inserted into the pelvic cavity through a small incision. The laparoscope is used to view the pelvic organs. Other instruments can be used with it to perform surgery.

*Laparotomy:* A surgical procedure in which an incision is made in the abdomen.

*Last Menstrual Period (LMP):* The date of the first day of the last menstrual period before pregnancy that is used to estimate the date of delivery.

*Late-Term Pregnancy:* The period from 41 and 0/7 weeks through 41 and 6/7 weeks of pregnancy.

*Laxative:* A product that is used to empty the bowels.

*Linea Nigra:* A line running from the navel to pubic hair that darkens during pregnancy.

*Listeriosis:* A type of food-borne illness caused by bacteria that is found in unpasteurized milk, hot dogs, luncheon meats, and smoked seafood.

*Live, Attenuated Influenza Vaccine:* An influenza vaccine containing live viruses that have been altered to not cause disease. It is given as a nasal spray. It is not recommended for pregnant women.

*Local Anesthesia:* The use of drugs that prevent pain in a part of the body.

*Lochia:* Vaginal discharge that occurs after delivery.

*Low Birth Weight:* Weighing less than 5 ½ pounds at birth.

*Lupus:* An autoimmune disorder that causes changes in the joints, skin, kidneys, lungs, heart, or brain.

*Luteinizing Hormone (LH):* A hormone produced by the pituitary gland that helps an egg to mature and be released.

*Macrosomia:* A condition in which a fetus grows very large.

*Magnesium Sulfate:* A drug that may help prevent cerebral palsy when it is given to women in preterm labor who are at risk of delivery before 32 weeks of pregnancy.

*Magnetic Resonance Imaging (MRI):* A method of viewing internal organs and structures by using a strong magnetic field and sound waves.

*Malignant:* A term used to describe cells or tumors that are able to invade tissue and spread to other parts of the body.

*Malpresentation:* A condition in which a fetus is in a head-down position with the head flexed prior to birth.

*Mastitis:* Infection of the breast tissue that can occur during breastfeeding.

*Maternal–Fetal Medicine Subspecialist:* An obstetrician-gynecologist with additional training in caring for women with high-risk pregnancies; also called a perinatologist.

*Measles–Mumps–Rubella (MMR) Vaccine:* A vaccine against measles, mumps, and rubella that contains live viruses that have been altered to not cause disease. It is not recommended for pregnant women.

*Meconium:* A greenish substance that builds up in the bowels of a growing fetus.

*Melanin:* A dark pigment that gives color to the skin and hair.

*Melasma:* A common skin problem that causes brown to gray-brown patches on the face. Also known as "chloasma" or "mask of pregnancy."

*Meningococcal Disease:* Inflammation of the coverings of the brain and spinal cord (meninges) caused by a bacterium called meningococcus.

*Metabolism:* The physical and chemical processes in the body that maintain life.

*Microarray:* A technology that examines all of a person's genes to look for certain genetic disorders or abnormalities. Microarray technology can find very small genetic variations that have gone undetected by conventional genetic tests.

*Miscarriage:* Loss of a pregnancy that occurs before 20 weeks of pregnancy.

*Modified Biophysical Profile:* A modified version of the biophysical profile that is used to monitor fetal well-being; it usually includes a fetal heart rate assessment and assessment of the amount of amniotic fluid.

*Monoamniotic–Monochorionic:* Describes twin embryos formed from the same egg that develop within a single gestational sac surrounded by an inner layer (the amnion) and outer layer (the chorion) of membranes. These twins share a single placenta and are identical (have the same genetic material).

*Monosomy:* A condition in which there is a missing chromosome.

*Mucolipidosis IV:* Also known as Morquio syndrome, an inherited autosomal recessive disorder that mainly affects the bones and skeletal development and also causes visual impairment. It is caused by a change in a protein that helps transport substances into and out of cells.

*Multifetal Pregnancy Reduction:* A first-trimester or early second-trimester procedure for reducing by one or more the total number of fetuses in a multifetal pregnancy.

*Multiple Pregnancy:* A pregnancy in which there are two or more fetuses.

*Mutation:* A permanent change in a gene that can be passed on from parent to child.

*Myometrium:* The muscular layer of the uterus.

*Narcotics:* Drugs that cause insensibility or stupor.

*Neonatal Intensive Care Unit (NICU):* A specialized area of a hospital in which ill newborns receive complex medical care.

*Neonatologist:* A doctor who specializes in the diagnosis and treatment of disorders that affect newborn infants.

*Neural Tube Defect (NTD):* A birth defect that results from incomplete development of the brain, spinal cord, or their coverings.

*Neurofibromatosis:* An autosomal dominant disorder that causes changes in the nervous system, muscles, bones, and skin and tumors called neurofibromas.

*Niemann–Pick Disease Type A:* An inherited disorder that affects fat metabolism and transport through the body. It causes harmful amounts of a substance called sphingomyelin to accumulate in cells of the liver, spleen, lungs, bone marrow, and brain. Children born with this disorder die by age 4 years.

*Nonstress Test (NST):* A test in which changes in the fetal heart rate are recorded using an electronic fetal monitor.

*Nuchal Translucency Screening:* A test in which the size of a collection of fluid at the back of fetal neck is measured by ultrasound to screen for certain birth defects, such as Down syndrome, trisomy 18, or heart defects.

*Nutrients:* Nourishing substances supplied through food, such as vitamins and minerals.

*Obesity:* A condition characterized by excessive body fat.

*Obstetrician–Gynecologist:* A physician with special skills, training, and education in women's health.

*Oligohydramnios:* Low levels of amniotic fluid.

*Operative Vaginal Delivery:* Vaginal delivery of a baby performed with the use of forceps or a vacuum.

*Orgasm:* The climax of sexual excitement.

*Ovaries:* A pair of organs in the female reproductive system that contain the eggs released at ovulation and produce hormones.

*Ovulation:* The release of an egg from one of the ovaries.

*Oxygen:* A gas that is necessary to sustain life.

*Oxytocin:* A hormone made in a part of the brain called the hypothalamus that causes the uterus to contract and milk to be released into the milk ducts of the breast during breastfeeding. A synthetic form of oxytocin can be given as a drug to induce labor contractions or make them stronger.

*Parvovirus:* A virus that can be passed to the fetus during pregnancy. In rare cases, the infection can cause severe anemia that can result in heart failure and fetal death.

*Pathogen:* Any disease-producing agent, such as a bacterium, fungus, protozoon, or virus.

*Pathologist:* A specialist in pathology; a physician who examines tissues and performs or interprets the results of lab tests.

*Pelvic Exam:* A physical examination of a woman's reproductive organs.

*Pelvic Inflammatory Disease:* An infection of the uterus, fallopian tubes, and nearby pelvic structures.

*Pelvic Organ Prolapse:* A condition in which pelvic organs, such as the uterus or bladder, drop downward. It is caused by weakening of the muscles and tissues that support these organs.

*Perineum:* The area between the vagina and the anus.

*Periodontal Disease:* A group of conditions that affect the surrounding and supporting tissues of the teeth.

*Pertussis:* Also known as whooping cough; a highly contagious infection of the respiratory system that causes a severe cough and can result in difficulty breathing. A vaccine called tetanus toxoid, reduced diphtheria toxoid, and acellular pertussis (Tdap) can be given to prevent pertussis.

*Pica:* The urge to eat nonfood items.

*Placenta:* Tissue that provides nourishment to and takes waste away from the fetus.

*Placenta Accreta:* A condition in which part or all of the placenta attaches abnormally to and is inseparable from the uterine wall.

*Placental Abruption:* A condition in which the placenta has begun to separate from the inner wall of the uterus before the baby is born.

*Placenta Previa:* A condition in which the placenta lies very low in the uterus, so that the opening of the uterus is partially or completely covered.

*Pneumococcal Disease:* Diseases that cause pneumonia, an infection of the lungs.

*Polyhydramnios:* An abnormally high amount of amniotic fluid.

*Postpartum Depression:* Intense feelings of sadness, anxiety, or despair after childbirth that interfere with a new mother's ability to function and that do not go away after 2 weeks.

*Postpartum Endometritis:* Infection of the lining of the uterus following childbirth.

*Postpartum Hemorrhage:* Heavy bleeding that occurs after delivery of a baby and placenta.

*Postpartum Sterilization:* A permanent procedure that prevents a woman from becoming pregnant, performed soon after the birth of a child.

*Postterm Pregnancy:* A pregnancy that has reached or extends beyond 42 and 0/7 weeks.

*Preconception:* Before pregnancy.

*Preconception Care:* Medical care that is given before pregnancy to improve the chances of a healthy pregnancy; it includes a physical exam; counseling about nutrition, exercise, and medications; and treatment of certain medical conditions.

*Preeclampsia:* A disorder that can occur during pregnancy or after childbirth in which there is high blood pressure and other signs of organ injury, such as an abnormal amount of protein in the urine, a low number of platelets, abnormal kidney or liver function, pain over the upper abdomen, fluid in the lungs, or a severe headache or changes in vision.

*Preimplantation Genetic Diagnosis:* A type of genetic testing that can be done during in vitro fertilization. Tests are performed on the fertilized egg before it is transferred to the uterus.

*Premature Rupture of Membranes (PROM):* A condition in which the membranes that hold the amniotic fluid rupture before labor.

*Prenatal Care:* A program of care for a pregnant woman before the birth of her baby.

*Presentation:* A term that describes the part of the fetus that is lowest in the vagina during labor.

*Preterm:* Born before 37 weeks of pregnancy.

*Preterm Premature Rupture of Membranes (Preterm PROM):* Rupture of the amniotic membranes that occurs before 37 weeks of pregnancy and before the onset of labor.

*Prodrome:* A symptom that precedes the onset of a disease.

*Progesterone:* A female hormone that is produced in the ovaries and that prepares the lining of the uterus for pregnancy.

*Prostaglandins:* Chemicals that are made by the body that have many effects, including causing the muscle of the uterus to contract, usually causing cramps.

*Proteinuria:* The presence of an abnormal amount of protein in the urine.

*Quickening:* The mother's first feeling of movement of the fetus.

*Rectum:* The last part of the digestive tract.

*Respiratory Distress Syndrome (RDS):* A condition of some babies in which the lungs are not mature and causes breathing difficulties.

*Respiratory System:* The body system that allows oxygen to be absorbed into the bloodstream and carbon dioxide to be removed from the body. The main organs of the respiratory system are the nose, larynx (voice box), trachea (windpipe), and lungs.

*Rh Factor:* A protein that can be present on the surface of red blood cells.

*Rh Immunoglobulin (RhIg):* A substance given to prevent an Rh-negative person's antibody response to Rh-positive blood cells.

*Rh Sensitization:* The presence of Rh antibodies in the bloodstream of an Rh-negative person. It happens when an Rh-negative person's blood comes into contact with Rh-positive blood.

*Rubella:* A virus that can be passed to the fetus if a woman becomes infected during pregnancy and that can cause miscarriage or severe birth defects.

*Sciatica:* Pain or numbness anywhere along the course of the sciatic nerve, typically occurring from the buttock down the back of the leg. It sometimes is associated with weakness of the leg muscles that are controlled by the sciatic nerve.

*Screening Tests:* Tests that looks for possible signs of disease in people who do not have symptoms.

*Sedative:* A drug that eases nervousness or tension.

*Seizure Disorders:* Any condition that causes seizures, in which abnormal brain nerve cell electrical activity results in a change in movement, consciousness, mood, or emotions. Epilepsy is one kind of seizure disorder.

*Sepsis:* A condition in which pathogens are present in the blood. It is a serious condition that can be life threatening.

*Sex-Linked Disorder:* A genetic disorder caused by a change in a gene or genes that are located on the sex chromosomes.

*Sexual Intercourse:* The act of the penis of the male entering the vagina of the female (also called "having sex" or "making love").

*Sexually Transmitted Infection (STI):* An infection that is spread by sexual contact, including chlamydia, gonorrhea, human papillomavirus infection, herpes, syphilis, and infection with human immunodeficiency virus (HIV, the cause of acquired immunodeficiency syndrome [AIDS]).

*Shoulder Dystocia:* A situation during childbirth in which one or both of the baby's shoulders does not deliver easily after delivery of the head.

*Sickle Cell Disease:* An inherited disorder in which red blood cells have a crescent shape, causing chronic anemia and episodes of pain. It occurs most often in African Americans.

*Sperm:* A cell produced in the male testes that can fertilize a female egg.

*Spina Bifida:* A neural tube defect that results from incomplete closure of the fetal spine.

*Spinal Block:* A type of regional anesthesia or analgesia in which pain medications are administered into the spinal fluid.

*Station:* A measurement in numbers that describes the location of the presenting part of the fetus relative to a part of the mother's pelvis called the ischial spines.

*Stem Cells:* Cells with the ability to become (differentiate into) specialized cells.

*Sterilization:* A permanent method of birth control.

*Stillbirth:* Delivery of a dead baby.

*Sudden Infant Death Syndrome (SIDS):* The unexpected death of an infant and in which the cause is unknown.

*Surfactant:* A substance produced by cells in the respiratory system that contributes to the elasticity of the lungs and keeps them from collapsing.

*Syphilis:* A sexually transmitted infection that is caused by an organism called *Treponema pallidum*; it may cause major health problems or death in its later stages.

*Systemic Lupus Erythematosus:* An autoimmune disorder that affects the connective tissues in the body and can cause arthritis, kidney disease, heart disease, and blood disorders and complications during pregnancy.

*Systolic Blood Pressure:* The force of the blood in the arteries when the heart is contracting; the higher blood pressure reading.

*Tay–Sachs Disease:* An inherited birth defect that causes intellectual disability, blindness, seizures, and death, usually by age 5 years. It most commonly affects people of Eastern European Jewish (Ashkenazi Jews), Cajun, and French Canadian descent.

*Teratogens:* Agents that can cause birth defects when a woman is exposed to them during pregnancy.

*Testes:* Two male organs that produce sperm and the male sex hormone testosterone.

*Testosterone:* A hormone produced by the testes in men and in smaller amounts by the ovaries and other tissues in women that is responsible for male sex characteristics such as hair growth, muscle development, and a lower voice.

*Tetanus:* A disease caused by bacteria that can enter the body through a puncture wound such as from a metal nail, wood splinter, or insect bite. The bacteria produce a toxin that can paralyze the breathing muscles. A vaccine is available that protects against tetanus.

*Tetanus Toxoid, Reduced Diphtheria Toxoid, and Acellular Pertussis (Tdap) Vaccine:* A vaccine that includes a combination of tetanus toxoid, diphtheria toxoid, and acellular pertussis.

*Thalassemia:* A group of inherited anemias caused by the decreased production of one or more component of hemoglobin, the molecule that carries oxygen in red blood cells.

*Thyroid Hormone:* The hormone that is made by the thyroid gland.

*Tocolytic:* A drug used to slow contractions of the uterus.

*Toxin:* A substance produced by bacteria that is toxic to other living organisms.

*Toxoplasmosis:* An infection caused by *Toxoplasma gondii,* an organism that may be found in raw and rare meat, garden soil, and cat feces and can be harmful to the fetus.

*Transabdominal Ultrasound Exam:* A type of ultrasound exam in which a device is moved across the abdomen.

*Transducer:* A device that emits sound waves and translates the echoes into electrical signals.

*Transfusion:* Direct injection of blood, plasma, or platelets into the bloodstream.

*Transvaginal Ultrasound Exam:* A type of ultrasound exam in which a device specially designed to be placed in the vagina is used.

*Trial of Labor After Cesarean Delivery (TOLAC):* Labor in a woman who has had a previous cesarean delivery with a goal of having a vaginal birth after cesarean delivery (VBAC).

*Trichomoniasis:* A type of vaginal infection caused by a one-celled organism that is usually transmitted through sex.

*Trimester:* Any of the three 3-month periods into which pregnancy is divided.

*Trisomy:* A condition in which there is an extra chromosome.

*Trisomy 13 (Patau syndrome):* A chromosomal disorder that causes serious problems with the brain and heart as well as extra fingers and toes, cleft palate and lip, and other defects. Most infants with trisomy 13 die within the first year of life.

*Trisomy 18 (Edwards syndrome):* A chromosomal disorder that causes severe intellectual disability and serious physical problems such as a small head, heart defects, and deafness. Most infants with trisomy 18 die before birth or within the first month of life.

*Trisomy 21 (Down syndrome):* A genetic disorder in which abnormal features of the face and body, medical problems such as heart defects, and intellectual disability occur. Many children with Down syndrome live to adulthood.

*Tubal Sterilization:* A method of female sterilization in which the fallopian tubes are tied, banded, clipped, sealed with electric current, or blocked by scar tissue formed by the insertion of small implants.

*Tuberculosis:* A disease caused by bacteria that usually affects the lungs but also can affect other organs in the body. If not treated, it can be fatal.

*Turner Syndrome:* A condition affecting females in which there is a missing or damaged X chromosome. It causes a webbed neck, short height, and heart problems but does not usually cause developmental delays.

*Twin–Twin Transfusion Syndrome (TTTS):* A condition of identical twin fetuses when the blood passes from one twin to the other through a shared placenta.

*Ultrasound Exam:* A test in which sound waves are used to examine internal structures. During pregnancy, it can be used to examine the fetus.

*Umbilical Cord:* A cord-like structure containing blood vessels that connects the fetus to the placenta.

*Umbilical Cord Prolapse:* An emergency situation in which the umbilical cord comes out of the vagina before delivery of the baby.

*Urethra:* A tube-like structure through which urine flows from the bladder to the outside of the body.

*Uterine Artery Embolization:* A procedure in which the blood vessels to the uterus are blocked. It is used to treat postpartum hemorrhage and other problems that cause uterine bleeding.

*Uterine Atony:* A condition in which the muscles of the uterus do not contract normally after the baby and placenta are delivered; it is a common cause of postpartum hemorrhage.

*Uterine Rupture:* A condition in which the uterus tears during labor.

*Uterus:* A muscular organ located in the female pelvis that contains and nourishes the developing fetus during pregnancy.

*Vacuum Extraction:* The use of a special instrument attached to the baby's head to help guide it out of the birth canal during delivery.

*Vacuum Extractor:* A metal or plastic cup that is applied to the fetus' head with suction to assist delivery.

*Vagina:* A tube-like structure surrounded by muscles leading from the uterus to the outside of the body.

*Vaginal Birth After Cesarean Delivery (VBAC):* Giving birth vaginally after having a previous cesarean delivery.

*Varicella:* Also called chickenpox; a contagious disease caused by a virus that results in fluid-filled blisters on the skin.

*Varicella Zoster Virus (VZV):* Virus that causes chickenpox and shingles.

*Vasectomy:* A method of male sterilization in which a portion of the vas deferens is removed.

*Ventilator:* A machine that blows air into the lungs to help a person breathe.

*Vernix:* The greasy, whitish coating of a newborn.

*Vertex Presentation:* A normal position assumed by a fetus in which the head is positioned down ready to be born first.

*Villi:* Finger-like projections containing blood vessels that attach the placenta to the mother's uterine wall.

*Virus:* An agent that causes certain types of infections.

*Vulva:* The external female genital area.

*Yeast Infection:* Infection caused by one-celled organisms called yeast.

To calculate your body mass index, find your height in inches in the left column. Then look across the line to find your weight in pounds. The number at the top of that column is your body mass index (BMI).

## Body Mass Index Table

| | NORMAL | | | | | | OVERWEIGHT | | | | | OBESE | | | | | |
|---|---|---|---|---|---|---|---|---|---|---|---|---|---|---|---|---|---|
| **BMI** | 19 | 20 | 21 | 22 | 23 | 24 | 25 | 26 | 27 | 28 | 29 | 30 | 31 | 32 | 33 | 34 | 35 |
| **HEIGHT (Inches)** | **BODY WEIGHT (Pounds)** | | | | | | | | | | | | | | | | |
| 58 | 91 | 96 | 100 | 105 | 110 | 115 | 119 | 124 | 129 | 134 | 138 | 143 | 148 | 153 | 158 | 162 | 167 |
| 59 | 94 | 99 | 104 | 109 | 114 | 119 | 124 | 128 | 133 | 138 | 143 | 148 | 153 | 158 | 163 | 168 | 173 |
| 60 | 97 | 102 | 107 | 112 | 118 | 123 | 128 | 133 | 138 | 143 | 148 | 153 | 158 | 163 | 168 | 174 | 179 |
| 61 | 100 | 106 | 111 | 116 | 122 | 127 | 132 | 137 | 143 | 148 | 153 | 158 | 164 | 169 | 174 | 180 | 185 |
| 62 | 104 | 109 | 115 | 120 | 126 | 131 | 136 | 142 | 147 | 153 | 158 | 164 | 169 | 175 | 180 | 186 | 191 |
| 63 | 107 | 113 | 118 | 124 | 130 | 135 | 141 | 146 | 152 | 158 | 163 | 169 | 175 | 180 | 186 | 191 | 197 |
| 64 | 110 | 116 | 122 | 128 | 134 | 140 | 145 | 151 | 157 | 163 | 169 | 174 | 180 | 186 | 192 | 197 | 204 |
| 65 | 114 | 120 | 126 | 132 | 138 | 144 | 150 | 156 | 162 | 168 | 174 | 180 | 186 | 192 | 198 | 204 | 210 |
| 66 | 118 | 124 | 130 | 136 | 142 | 148 | 155 | 161 | 167 | 173 | 179 | 186 | 192 | 198 | 204 | 210 | 216 |
| 67 | 121 | 127 | 134 | 140 | 146 | 153 | 159 | 166 | 172 | 178 | 185 | 191 | 198 | 204 | 211 | 217 | 223 |
| 68 | 125 | 131 | 138 | 144 | 151 | 158 | 164 | 171 | 177 | 184 | 190 | 197 | 203 | 210 | 216 | 223 | 230 |
| 69 | 128 | 135 | 142 | 149 | 155 | 162 | 169 | 176 | 182 | 189 | 196 | 203 | 209 | 216 | 223 | 230 | 236 |
| 70 | 132 | 139 | 146 | 153 | 160 | 167 | 174 | 181 | 188 | 195 | 202 | 209 | 216 | 222 | 229 | 236 | 243 |
| 71 | 136 | 143 | 150 | 157 | 165 | 172 | 179 | 186 | 193 | 200 | 208 | 215 | 222 | 229 | 236 | 243 | 250 |
| 72 | 140 | 147 | 154 | 162 | 169 | 177 | 184 | 191 | 199 | 206 | 213 | 221 | 228 | 235 | 242 | 250 | 258 |
| 73 | 144 | 151 | 159 | 166 | 174 | 182 | 189 | 197 | 204 | 212 | 219 | 227 | 235 | 242 | 250 | 257 | 265 |
| 74 | 148 | 155 | 163 | 171 | 179 | 186 | 194 | 202 | 210 | 218 | 225 | 233 | 241 | 249 | 256 | 264 | 272 |
| 75 | 152 | 160 | 168 | 176 | 184 | 192 | 200 | 208 | 216 | 224 | 232 | 240 | 248 | 256 | 264 | 272 | 279 |
| 76 | 156 | 164 | 172 | 180 | 189 | 197 | 205 | 213 | 221 | 230 | 238 | 246 | 254 | 263 | 271 | 279 | 287 |

*Source: National Heart, Lung, and Blood Institute. Clinical guidelines on the identification, evaluation, and treatment of overweight and obesity in adults. U.S. Department of Health and Human Services, 1998 June: 139*

# Appendix A
# Body Mass Index Chart

| | | | | EXTREME OBESITY | | | | | | | | | | | | | | |
|---|---|---|---|---|---|---|---|---|---|---|---|---|---|---|---|---|---|---|
| 36 | 37 | 38 | 39 | 40 | 41 | 42 | 43 | 44 | 45 | 46 | 47 | 48 | 49 | 50 | 51 | 52 | 53 | 54 |
| 172 | 177 | 181 | 186 | 191 | 196 | 201 | 205 | 210 | 215 | 220 | 224 | 229 | 234 | 239 | 244 | 248 | 253 | 258 |
| 178 | 183 | 188 | 193 | 198 | 203 | 208 | 212 | 217 | 222 | 227 | 232 | 237 | 242 | 247 | 252 | 257 | 262 | 267 |
| 184 | 189 | 194 | 199 | 204 | 209 | 215 | 220 | 225 | 230 | 235 | 240 | 245 | 250 | 255 | 261 | 266 | 271 | 276 |
| 190 | 195 | 201 | 206 | 211 | 217 | 222 | 227 | 232 | 238 | 243 | 248 | 254 | 259 | 264 | 269 | 275 | 280 | 285 |
| 196 | 202 | 207 | 213 | 218 | 224 | 229 | 235 | 240 | 246 | 251 | 256 | 262 | 267 | 273 | 278 | 284 | 289 | 295 |
| 203 | 208 | 214 | 220 | 225 | 231 | 237 | 242 | 248 | 254 | 259 | 265 | 270 | 278 | 282 | 287 | 293 | 299 | 304 |
| 209 | 215 | 221 | 227 | 232 | 238 | 244 | 250 | 256 | 262 | 267 | 273 | 279 | 285 | 291 | 296 | 302 | 308 | 314 |
| 216 | 222 | 228 | 234 | 240 | 246 | 252 | 258 | 264 | 270 | 276 | 282 | 288 | 294 | 300 | 306 | 312 | 318 | 324 |
| 223 | 229 | 235 | 241 | 247 | 253 | 260 | 266 | 272 | 278 | 284 | 291 | 297 | 303 | 309 | 315 | 322 | 328 | 334 |
| 230 | 236 | 242 | 249 | 255 | 261 | 268 | 274 | 280 | 287 | 293 | 299 | 306 | 312 | 319 | 325 | 331 | 338 | 344 |
| 236 | 243 | 249 | 256 | 262 | 269 | 276 | 282 | 289 | 295 | 302 | 308 | 315 | 322 | 328 | 335 | 341 | 348 | 354 |
| 243 | 250 | 257 | 263 | 270 | 277 | 284 | 291 | 297 | 304 | 311 | 318 | 324 | 331 | 338 | 345 | 351 | 358 | 365 |
| 250 | 257 | 264 | 271 | 278 | 285 | 292 | 299 | 306 | 313 | 320 | 327 | 334 | 341 | 348 | 355 | 362 | 369 | 376 |
| 257 | 265 | 272 | 279 | 286 | 293 | 301 | 308 | 315 | 322 | 329 | 338 | 343 | 351 | 358 | 365 | 372 | 379 | 386 |
| 265 | 272 | 279 | 287 | 294 | 302 | 309 | 316 | 324 | 331 | 338 | 346 | 353 | 361 | 368 | 375 | 383 | 390 | 397 |
| 272 | 280 | 288 | 295 | 302 | 310 | 318 | 325 | 333 | 340 | 348 | 355 | 363 | 371 | 378 | 386 | 393 | 401 | 408 |
| 280 | 287 | 295 | 303 | 311 | 319 | 326 | 334 | 342 | 350 | 358 | 365 | 373 | 381 | 389 | 396 | 404 | 412 | 420 |
| 287 | 295 | 303 | 311 | 319 | 327 | 335 | 343 | 351 | 359 | 367 | 375 | 383 | 391 | 399 | 407 | 415 | 423 | 431 |
| 295 | 304 | 312 | 320 | 328 | 336 | 344 | 353 | 361 | 369 | 377 | 385 | 394 | 402 | 410 | 418 | 426 | 435 | 443 |

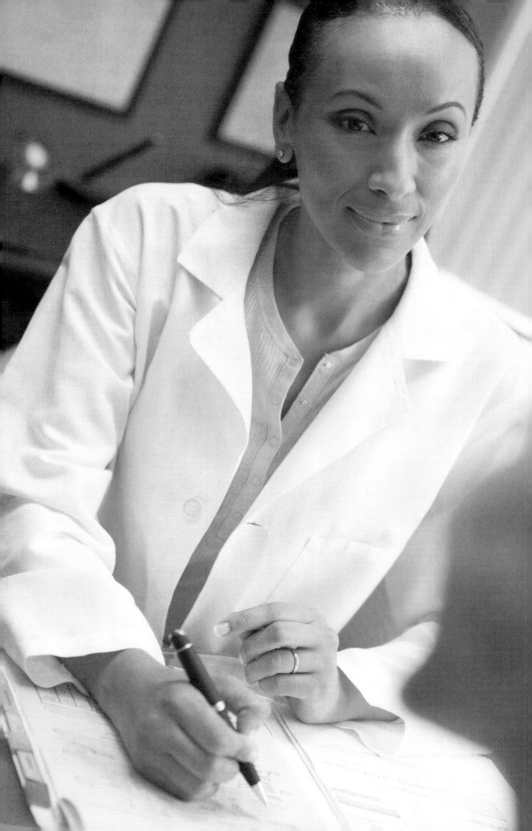

# Health Questions for
# Your First Prenatal Care Visit

Before your first prenatal care visit, make sure that you know the answers to these questions. You can fill out this form if you'd like, but be aware that your health care provider may have his or her own form for you to complete.

---

What was the date of your last menstrual period? _____

Was it a normal period in terms of length and amount? _____

What symptoms have you had since your last menstrual period? _____

**Past Pregnancies**

Total number of pregnancies:

*Number of pregnancies that were:*

Full term _____

Premature _____

Miscarriages _____

Induced abortions _____

Ectopic pregnancies _____

Multiple births _____

Number of living children _____

## Fill in the following information for each of your past live births:

| Date of Birth | Gestational Age at Birth (Weeks) | Length of Labor (Hours) | Birth Weight | Sex | Type of Delivery | Anesthesia | Place of Delivery | Complications, Including Preterm Labor |
|---|---|---|---|---|---|---|---|---|
| | | | | | | | | |
| | | | | | | | | |
| | | | | | | | | |
| | | | | | | | | |
| | | | | | | | | |
| | | | | | | | | |

## Your Medical History

*Please check off whether you have or have had any of the following conditions:*

Drug allergies/reactions _____

Latex allergy/reaction _____

Food/seasonal/environmental allergies_____

Neurologic disease or epilepsy_____

Thyroid dysfunction_____

Breast disease_____

Lung disease, such as asthma_____

Heart disease_____

High blood pressure (hypertension) _____

Cancer_____

Hematologic disorders_____

Anemia____

Gastrointestinal disorders_____

Hepatitis or liver disease_____

Kidney disease or urinary tract infection_____

Varicose veins or blood clots in the legs_____

Diabetes mellitus (type 1 or type 2)_____

Gestational diabetes mellitus_____

Autoimmune disorders (lupus, multiple sclerosis, inflammatory bowel disease)_____

Dermatologic disorders_____

Operations/hospitalizations_____

Gynecologic surgery_____

Anesthetic complications_____

History of blood transfusions_____

Infertility_____

Assisted reproductive technology treatment_____

Uterine abnormalities_____

History of abnormal Pap test result_____

History of sexually transmitted infections_____

Psychiatric illness_____

Depression, including postpartum depression_____

Trauma or violence_____

## Lifestyle Issues

### Smoking
Did you smoke before pregnancy? ❑ Y ❑ N   If yes, how much?_____
Do you currently smoke? ❑ Y ❑ N   If yes, how much?_____

### Alcohol
Did you drink alcohol before pregnancy? ❑ Y ❑ N   If yes, how much?_____
Do you drink alcohol now? ❑ Y ❑ N   If yes, how much?_____

### Illegal Drugs
Did you use illegal drugs before pregnancy? ❑ Y ❑ N   If yes, what type and how much?

_____

Do you use illegal drugs now? ❑ Y ❑ N   If yes, what type and how much?

_____

### Your Home Life
Do you feel safe in your current living situation? ❑ Y ❑ N
Do you feel safe with your current partner? ❑ Y ❑ N
If you answered "No" to either of these questions, please exercise caution and do not leave this form where your partner may see it. Both you and your baby may be at risk in this situation. It is important that you protect yourself and your baby by finding a safe place.

### Genetic Background

*Please indicate whether you, your baby's father, or anyone in either family has had any of the following conditions:*

| Condition | Y | N |
|---|---|---|
| Thalassemia (Italian, Greek, Mediterranean, or Asian background) | | |
| Neural tube defect (spina bifida, meningomyelocele, anencephaly) | | |
| Congenital heart defect | | |
| Down syndrome | | |
| Tay–Sachs disease (Ashkenazi Jewish, Cajun, French Canadian) | | |
| Canavan disease (Ashkenazi Jewish) | | |
| Familial dysautonomia (Ashkenazi Jewish) | | |
| Sickle cell disease or trait (African) | | |
| Hemophilia or other blood disorders | | |
| Muscular dystrophy | | |
| Cystic fibrosis | | |
| Huntington chorea | | |
| Intellectual disability/autism including Fragile X | | |
| Other inherited genetic or chromosomal disorder | | |
| Maternal metabolic disorder (eg, type 1 diabetes, phenylketonuria) | | |
| Birth defects not listed above | | |
| Recurrent pregnancy loss or a stillbirth | | |

Have you or your baby's father had a child with a birth defect not listed above? ❏ Y ❏ N
If yes, what type?

*Please list all medications you have taken since your last menstrual period (include supplements, vitamins, herbs, and over-the-counter drugs). Please include the strength and dosage.*

| Drug | Strength (eg, milligrams) | Dosage |
|---|---|---|
| | | |
| | | |
| | | |
| | | |
| | | |
| | | |

## Infection History

Do you live with someone with tuberculosis or have you been exposed to tuberculosis?
❏ Y ❏ N

Do you or your sexual partner have oral or genital herpes? ❏ Y ❏ N

Have you had a rash or viral illness since your last menstrual period? ❏ Y ❏ N

Have you had a previous child with Group B streptococcal infection? ❏ Y ❏ N

Have you ever had a sexually transmitted infection, such as gonorrhea, chlamydia, human immunodeficiency virus (HIV) infection, syphilis, or human papillomavirus (HPV) infection? *Circle all that apply.* ❏ Y ❏ N

Do you have hepatitis B virus or hepatitis C virus infection? ❏ Y ❏ N

## Immunization History

| Immunization | Yes (month/year) | No | If no, postpartum vaccine indicated? |
|---|---|---|---|
| Tdap or Td | | | |
| Influenza* | | | |
| Varicella* | | | |
| MMR* | | | |
| Hepatitis A | | | |
| Hepatitis B | | | |
| Meningococcal | | | |
| Pneumococcal | | | |

*Live vaccines should not be given during pregnancy. Live vaccines include the live intranasal influenza, varicella, and MMR vaccines. All women who will be pregnant during influenza season (October through May) should receive inactivated influenza vaccine at any point during pregnancy. MMR and varicella should be given after pregnancy if needed.

Abbreviations: Td, tetanus–diphtheria; Tdap, tetanus toxoid, reduced diphtheria toxoid, and accellular pertussis; MMR, measels–mumps–rubella.

## Your Questions

*Please list any questions that you would like to ask your pregnancy health care provider.*

_____

_____

_____

_____

_____

_____

_____

_____

_____

_____

_____

_____

_____

_____

_____

_____

_____

_____

_____

_____

_____

_____

_____

_____

_____

_____

_____

_____

*Adapted from The American College of Obstetricians and Gynecologists. ACOG Antepartum Record. Version 6. ACOG: Washington, DC; 2007.*

# Index

Page numbers followed by italicized letters *b, f,* and *t* indicate boxes, figures, and tables, respectively.

4-point kneeling, 73*b*

**A**

Abdomen
 implantation in, 61
 postpartum exercises for, 283
Abdominal pain
 lower, 91
 lower postpartum, 288
 placental abruption and, 510
Abdominal wall defects, 104, 391*b*
Abnormal labor
 assessment of, 550–551
 causes of, 549–550
 management of, 551
 overview of, 549
 risks of, 550
ABO incompatibility, 503
Accelerations, fetal heart rate, 480
Accidental bowel leakage, 286
Accreditation Association for Ambulatory Health Care, 98
Aches, 132. *See also* Backaches; Headache
Acne, 68–69
Acquired immunodeficiency syndrome
  (AIDS), 82, 177, 532
Active labor
 process of, 246*f*
 signs of, 247

Active labor (*continued*)
 what happens during, 249
 what you can do during, 249–250
Active tuberculosis, 534
Advisory Committee on Immunization
  Practices, 517
AEDs. *See* Antiepileptic drugs
Affordable Care Act, 308, 351, 356
AIDS. *See* Acquired immunodeficiency
  syndrome
Air travel, 118–121
ALA. *See* Alpha-linolenic acid
Alpha-linolenic acid (ALA), 322–323
Albuterol, 432*b*, 433
Alcohol, as teratogen, 389, 390
Alcohol drinking
 avoiding during pregnancy, 52–53,
  53*b*
 birth defects and, 391*b*
 breastfeeding and, 53*b*, 345
 fetal growth restriction and, 542
 formula-feeding and, 354
 methotrexate and, 567
 miscarriage and, 562
 during pregnancy, 13–14,
  397–398
Allergy remedies, 55, 104, 391*b*
Allogenic transplantation, 155
American Academy of Pediatrics, 98, 196

American Association of Birth Centers, 98
American College of Nurse-Midwives Division of Accreditation, 56
American Dental Association, 92
American Society for Reproductive Medicine, 362*b*
Amniocentesis
    for baby's blood type, 503
    as diagnostic test, 75, 83, 371, 459
    placenta accreta and, 512
    prenatal care and, 101, 123
    procedure for, 468–469, 469*f*
    Rh immunoglobulin after, 502
    Rh sensitization and, 501
    stillbirth evaluation and, 574–575
    timing of, 460*f*
    ultrasound guidance and, 479
Amnioinfusion, 553
Amnionicity, 364
Amniotic fluid
    amniotomy and, 551
    baby's body temperature and, 171, 276
    biophysical profile of, 482
    breech presentation and, 258
    development of, 35
    diagnostic tests of, 75
    in discordant twins, 369
    fetal swallowing of, 89
    gestational diabetes mellitus and, 421
    fetal well-being testing and, 476
    late-term or postterm pregnancy and, 216
    leaking, amniocentesis or chorionic villus sampling and, 469
    preeclampsia and, 413
    pregestational diabetes mellitus and, 423
    premature rupture of membranes and, 493
    stillbirth evaluation and, 574–575
    ultrasound exam of, 122, 479
    umbilical cord compression and, 553
    in vagina, premature rupture of membranes and, 492
    water and formation of, 152*b*

Amniotic membranes, 238
Amniotic sac. *See also* Premature rupture of membranes; Rupture of membranes; The bag of waters
    amniotomy of, 551
    fetal fibronectin and, 489–490
    formation of, 35
    multiple pregnancy and, 364
    pregestational diabetes mellitus and, 423
    stripping membranes, 238, 238*f*
Amniotomy, 238–239, 551
Amphetamines, 510
Analgesics, 182, 223–224
Anal sphincter, perineal tear and, 282
Anemia
    celiac disease and, 436
    delayed cord clamping and, 184
    gestational trophoblastic disease and, 569
    iron supplements for, 319
    testing for, 79, 164
Anencephaly, 44*b*
Anesthesia. *See also* General anesthesia
    birth plan on, 156*b*
    for cesarean delivery, 265
    consent form for, 249
    for dental procedures, 92
    food and liquid intake guidelines for, 209
    during labor, questions on, 57
    obesity during childbirth and, 379
    options for, 180
    for pain relief during childbirth, 223–227
    problems, cesarean delivery and, 138, 239–240
Anesthesiologists, 182, 225, 265, 381
Anesthetics, 265, 268, 280
Aneuploidy, 455, 456, 459, 465–468, 465*t*
Angiotensin-converting enzyme inhibitors, 395, 430
Angiotensin II receptor blockers, 430
Anorexia nervosa, 384
Antacids, 132

Antibiotics
  on baby's eyes, 279
  for bacterial vaginosis, 103
  for cesarean delivery, 266, 556
  for chlamydia or gonorrhea, 531
  for chorioamnionitis, 550
  for Group B streptococci during
    labor, 200, 492, 526
  for listeriosis, 134, 325
  for mastitis, 342
  obesity during cesarean delivery and,
    381
  for postpartum endometritis, 557
  preterm premature rupture of mem-
    branes and, 493
  for syphilis, 533
  for urinary tract infection, 81
Antibodies
  antiphospholipid syndrome and, 436
  breastfeeding and, 195
  in colostrum, 70
  delayed cord clamping and, 184
  in human milk, 330
  immunity and, 516
  infections and, 515–516
  Rh factor and, 81, 501
  Rh sensitization and, 500–501,
    500–501f
Antidepressants, 162, 290, 396
Antiepilepsy drugs (AEDs), 440
Antigens, 279, 331b, 499
Antihistamines, 104
Antiinflammatory medications, 438
Antiphospholipid syndrome (APS),
    436–437, 542
Antithrombin deficiency, 439
Antiviral medications, 77, 521, 530,
    534, 536
Anxiety, 159, 162
Anxiety disorders, 442
Apgar score, 275–276, 276t, 545
APS. See Antiphospholipid syndrome
ART. See Assisted reproductive
    technologies
Asian ethnicity, 555
Aspirin, 132, 415, 436, 437
Assisted reproductive technologies
    (ART), 8, 362b, 565

Asthma, 291, 396, 431–433, 431f, 432b,
    444
Augmentation of labor, 551, 555
Autism, 517
Autoimmune disorders, 435–438
Autologous transplantation, 155
Autopsy, 575
Autosomal dominant gene disorders,
    453
Autosomal recessive gene disorders,
    453–454
Autosomes, 451

**B**
Baby
  appearance of, at birth, 277–278
  behavior of, at birth, 278
  care plan, 157b
  feeding cues by, 343
  hepatitis B vaccine for, 522, 523
  safe sleep position for, 162–163, 169
  weight gain by, 46b
Baby blues, 289, 373–374
Baby Friendly hospitals, 332, 333b
Baby-led latch, 337
Baby's age, lactational amenorrhea and,
    303–304
Baby's clothes, 208b
Baby's movement. See also Fetal
    movement counts; Kick counts
  assessment of, 125–126
  biophysical profile and, 482
  changes in, 215
  counts, 478
  exercise during pregnancy and, 48b
  fetal heart rate and, 480
  reduced, 213, 476
  subsequent pregnancy and, 588
  ultrasound exams and, 479
Baby's weight
  at birth, 277
  ultrasound exams and, 479
  vaginal birth after cesarean delivery
    success and, 272
Backaches. See also Aches; Headache
  exercise and, 47
  lower, 109, 110, 149, 150f
  preterm labor and, 489b

Back labor, 144
Bacteremia, pneumococcal, 525
Bacteria
   infections caused by, 515
   *Salmonella*, 134
   in sushi and raw fish, 126
   urinalysis of, 81
   vaccines made with, 4
Bacterial vaginosis, 102–103, 535
Balance, 48, 135, 438
Balanced translocations, in chromo-
      somes, 456–457
Ball shoulder stretch, 136*b*
Ball wall squat, 153*b*
Bariatric surgery, 13, 382–383
Barrier birth control methods, 301–303
Basal body temperature, 20; 20*f*
Beclomethasone dipropionate, 105
Bed rest, 182, 372
Best for Babes, 332
Bilirubin, 503
Biophysical profile (BPP)
   fetal growth testing and, 543
   gestational diabetes mellitus and, 421
   late-term or postterm pregnancy and,
      216
   modified, 482
   multiple pregnancy and, 371
   overview, 481–482
Bipolar disorder, 442
Birth. *See* Childbirth; Delivery
Birth control
   bariatric surgery and, 383
   implant, 167, 296–297*t*, 298–299
   injection, 296–297*t*, 299
   methods, 296–297*t*, 298–304
   miscarriage and, 564
   obesity during pregnancy and,
      382
   overview, 295
   permanent, 304–308
   pills, 296–297*t*, 299–300, 300*f*,
      561–562
   postpartum, 166–167, 288, 426
   stopping, pregnancy and, 20–21
Birth defects
   alcohol and, 397–398
   antidepressants and, 162

Birth defects (*continued*)
   aspirin or nonsteroidal antiinflamma-
      tory drugs and, 132
   background risk, 386
   breech presentation and, 258
   choline and, 133*b*
   definition of, 449
   elevated core body temperature and, 402
   environmental exposure history, 392,
      393–394*t*, 394
   environmental toxins, 398–401
   folic acid and, 319
   infections as cause of, 3
   medications and, 395–397
   multiple pregnancy and, 370–371
   obesity during pregnancy and, 379
   overview, 389–390
   planning another baby and, 587
   pregestational diabetes mellitus and, 423
   questions for health care provider on,
      402
   resources, 402–403, 472
   risk reducing checklist, 390–391*b*
   seizure disorders and, 441
   stillbirth and, 574
   substance abuse and, 54
   teratogens, pregnancy and, 392
   testing for, 40, 73, 79, 101
   ultrasound exams and, 480
   X-rays and, 401–402
Birthing ball, 156*b*, 192, 229, 230*f*
Birthing bed, 192, 229, 230*f*
Birthing chair, 156*b*, 192, 229, 230*f*
Birthing pool or tub, 192
Birthing stool, 156*b*, 192, 229, 230*f*
Birth places, 98
Birth plan, 154, 156–157*b*
Bishop score, 237–238
Bisphenol-A (BPA), 355
Bladder
   active labor and, 250
   catheter in, cesarean delivery and, 266
   cesarean delivery and injury to, 74,
      138, 268
   infections of, 527*f*, 528
   Kegel exercises and, 50*b*
   pregnancy and, 38
   pressure during birth on, 282

Blastocyst, 33

Bleeding. *See also* Vaginal bleeding
after delivery, hypothyroidism and, 433
after miscarriage, 564
in brain, early preterm birth and, 139
in brain, preterm multiple birth and, 365
internal, ectopic pregnancy and, 566, 568
in second or third trimester, premature rupture of membranes and, 492
von Willebrand disease and, 440

Bloating, 38, 47, 435–436

Blood clots or clotting. *See also* Deep vein thrombosis
antiphospholipid syndrome and, 436–437
bed rest with multiple pregnancy and, 372
HELLP syndrome and, 411
hemophilia and, 7*t*
platelets and, 79
postpartum combined hormonal birth control and, 299
thrombophilias and, 438–440
vaginal birth after cesarean delivery and, 271
von Willebrand factor and, 440

Blood disorders, testing for, 476

Blood in stools, breastfeeding and, 344–345

Blood patch, 225

Blood pressure. *See also* High blood pressure; Hypertension; Preeclampsia
epidural block and, 225
measuring, 407–408
monitoring, hypertension and, 410
overview, 407
prenatal care and, 60, 101

Blood tests
for antiepilepsy drug levels, 442
in early pregnancy, 79, 81–82
for genetic disorders, 75
for glucose levels, 418–419
for hemolytic disease of the newborn, 503
for lead exposure, 125

Blood tests (*continued*)
for newborns, 279, 280
for pregnancy, 39
for Rh factor, 501

Blood transfusion
cesarean delivery and, 268
delayed cord clamping and, 184
hemolytic disease of the newborn and, 503
placenta accreta and, 513
placental abruption and, 166, 511
placenta previa and, 166, 508–509
postpartum hemorrhage and, 556
Rh immunoglobulin and, 502

Blood types
ABO incompatibility and, 503
Rh factor and, 499
Rh incompatibility and, 499–503, 500–501*f*
testing for, 79, 81, 252

Blood volume, pregnancy and, 430

Bloom syndrome, 6, 463

Blunt trauma, Rh sensitization and, 501

BMI. *See* Body mass index

Body image, pregnancy and, 139, 386

Body mass index (BMI)
calories during pregnancy and, 313
cesarean delivery on request and, 138
low, premature rupture of membranes and, 492
obesity and, 377–378
during pregnancy, 12–13
weight gain and, 45–46

Bottle-feeding, 195–196, 350–351*b*.
*See also* Formula-feeding

Bottles, 355

BPA. *See* Bisphenol-A

BPP. *See* Biophysical profile

Brachial plexus injury, 545, 552

Bradley method, 180–181, 227, 232

Brain development, 133*b*, 171, 209*b*

Bras
hands-free pumping, 349
nursing, 196
during postpartum period, 287
pregnancy and, 69–70

BRATT diet, 42, 208

Braxton Hicks contractions
  characteristics, 151
  preterm labor versus, 165, 183
  subsequent pregnancy and, 588
  third trimester and, 149
  true labor versus, 189–190, 213–214,
    213*t*
Breastfeeding. *See also* Breast milk;
  Feeding your baby
  after childbirth, 202, 334–335, 335*f*
  antidepressants and, 290
  baby care plan on, 157*b*
  baby latching on, 335, 336*b*, 337
  benefits, 329–331
  as best for baby, 167
  birth control injection and, 299
  blood pressure medications and, 410
  breast care and, 286–287
  challenges, 338–342
  checking baby's technique for, 337
  combined hormonal birth control
    and, 299
  common questions about, 342–349
  decision on, 193, 195–196
  delayed milk production and,
    339–340
  on demand, 337–338, 340
  engorgement and, 286–287, 339
  exclusive, 343
  gestational diabetes mellitus and, 422
  herpes infection and, 530
  human papillomavirus vaccines and,
    524
  lactational amenorrhea method and,
    303–304
  low milk supply, 340
  mastitis and, 341–342
  menstrual period return and, 288
  multiple pregnancy and, 373
  nicotine and, 291
  obesity and, 381
  pain and, 334, 337, 338–339
  planning for, 137, 332
  pregestational diabetes mellitus and,
    426
  resources, 202, 356–357
  sore nipples and, 338–339
  teratogen exposure during, 392

Breastfeeding (*continued*)
  twins, 346, 347*b*
  vaginal dryness and, 293–294
  vitamin D supplement to, 338
  weaning baby from, 342–343
  who shouldn't, 331–332, 331*b*
  working and, 349–353
Breast implants, 346
Breast milk. *See also* Breastfeeding
  delayed production of, 339–340
  expressing, 339, 349, 350–351*b*, 351
  low supply of, 340
  storing, 349, 353*b*
Breast pumps. *See also* Expressing milk
  flat nipples and, 341
  maintenance, 351*b*
  types, 352
  use of, 352–353
  use of, at work, 349
Breasts. *See also* Nipples
  blocked ducts in, 341, 341*f*
  changes in, 69–70, 70*f*
  milk production and firmness or
    softness of, 343
  painful lumps in, 288
  postpartum engorgement, 286–287
  red streaks on, 288, 341
  subsequent pregnancy and, 588
  surgery on, breastfeeding and, 346
  tenderness and swelling, 38
  weight gain and, 46*b*
Breathing difficulty
  in later weeks of pregnancy, 173
  postpartum chest pain and, 288
  preeclampsia and, 142, 412*b*
  systemic analgesics and, 224
Breathing support, preterm births and,
  494
Breathing techniques
  during early labor, 247
  paced breathing exercise, 210*b*
  pain during childbirth and, 223
  in transition to stage 2 of labor,
    251
Breech presentation
  abnormal labor and, 550
  cesarean delivery and, 264
  delivery options, 260–261

Breech presentation (*continued*)
  manual rotation, Rh sensitization
    and, 501
  overview, 201, 257–258, 259*f*
  premature rupture of membranes
    and, 492
  resources, 261
  turning the baby, 258–260, 259*f*
  types of, 245*f*
  umbilical cord prolapse and, 554
Bulimia nervosa, 384–385

**C**
Caffeine, 61–62, 143, 323, 562. *See also*
    Coffee
Calcium
  bariatric surgery and, 383
  breastfeeding and, 344
  focus on, 175*b*
  lactose intolerance and, 184–185
  recommendations, 318*t*, 319–320
Calculator, preterm birth, 495
Calf pain or swelling, 48*b*, 149, 174,
    190. *See also* Leg pain, swelling, or
    tenderness
Calories
  breastfeeding and, 167, 330, 344,
    346
  breastfeeding with diabetes and, 426
  empty, 320
  intake during pregnancy, 10–11,
    313
  multiple pregnancy and, 369
  obesity and weight loss during
    pregnancy and, 382
  in sugar and sugar substitutes, 71
  weight gain and, 12, 45–46
Campylobacteriosis, 134
Canavan disease, 6, 463
Carbamazepine, 395
Cardiovascular disease, 411–412. *See
    also* Heart disease
Carpal tunnel syndrome, 190
Carriers
  of autosomal recessive gene
    disorders, 453–454, 455*f*
  of hepatitis B virus, 522
  of hepatitis C virus, 533

Carrier screening
  about, 459
  available types of, 6–7*t*
  deciding to undergo, 461–462
  important considerations with, 464
  procedure, 462–463
  recommendations, 6, 8
  results, 463
  timing of, 460*f*, 464
Car seat, infant, 180, 197–199, 198*b*,
    203
Car travel, 117–118
CBC. *See* Complete blood count
Celiac disease, 324, 436, 445
Cell-free DNA test, 371, 465*t*, 466*b*
Centering Pregnancy, 57
Cephalopelvic disproportion, 264
Cerclage, preterm labor and, 491
Cerebral palsy, 139, 365, 488, 550
Certified midwives (CMs), 56
Certified nurse–midwives (CNMs),
    56
Certified professional midwives
    (CPMs), 56
Cervical cap, 296–297*t*, 302, 302*f*
Cervical length, 488*b*, 489–490
Cervical mucus, 18, 212, 492. *See also*
    Mucus plug
Cervical ripening, 216, 237–238, 244
Cervix. *See also* Dilation
  abnormal labor and, 549–550
  Braxton Hicks contractions and, 151
  breech presentation and, 260
  cancer screening, 79
  chorionic villus sampling through,
    469–470, 470*f*
  human papillomavirus and cancer of,
    523–524
  labor and delivery and, 216–217
  multiple pregnancy assessment of,
    371
  opening, prelabor contractions and,
    190
  placenta and, 507
  postpartum checkup of, 293
  prenatal care in eighth month, 182
  preterm labor and, 487, 489
  surgery, preterm births and, 488*b*

Cesarean delivery. *See also* Delivery; Labor and delivery problems; Pregnancy; Surgery; Vaginal birth after cesarean delivery
  abnormal labor and, 550
  afterbirth, 267
  anesthesia for, 265
  asthma and, 431
  breastfeeding after, 334, 336*b*
  breech presentation and, 201, 260
  chronic hypertension and, 409
  combined hormonal birth control and, 299
  consent form for, 249
  continuous labor support and, 232
  external cephalic version and, 259
  failed induction and, 239–240
  failure to progress and, 263–264
  fasting before, 209
  genital herpes and, 530
  gestational diabetes mellitus and, 378, 418
  human immunodeficiency virus and, 532
  at home after, 269
  incisions for, 266–267, 267*f*
  labor induction and, 239
  labor slowing or stopping and, 255
  macrosomia and, 545
  for monochorionic–monoamniotic babies, 368
  multiple pregnancy and, 372
  obesity during pregnancy and, 391*b*
  overview, 263
  placenta accreta and, 511–512
  placenta in subsequent pregnancies and, 240
  placenta previa and, 166, 507, 509
  placental abruption and, 166, 511
  postpartum exercise and, 290
  postpartum hemorrhage and, 555
  postpartum sterilization and, 305
  preeclampsia and, 413
  premature rupture of membranes, baby's position and, 492
  preparing for, 265–266
  prostaglandins after, 238
  questions for health care provider on, 57

Cesarean delivery (*continued*)
  reasons for, 251, 263–265
  recovery, 268–269
  resources, 272
  risks, 268
  rooming in after, 278
  shoulder dystocia and, 552
  spinal block for, 226
  subsequent pregnancy after, 73–74
  umbilical cord compression and, 553
  umbilical cord prolapse and, 554
Cesarean delivery on request, 136, 137–138, 265
Cetirizine, 104
Chancre, 532–533
Chemicals, 15, 58, 86, 389, 392
Chest pain, postpartum, 288
Chickenpox. *See* Varicella
Chickenpox vaccine. *See* Varicella vaccine
Childbirth
  baby care plan after, 157*b*
  obesity risks during, 379
  preparation methods, 180–181, 185, 227–228, 374
  procedures after, 253
  resources, 253
  Rh sensitization and, 501
  sexual intercourse after, 293–295
  stage 1, active labor, 246*f*, 247–250
  stage 1, early labor, 244–247, 246*f*
  stage 2, 246*f*, 251–252
  stage 3, 246*f*, 252–253
  transition to stage 2 of, 250–251
Childbirth educators, 56
Child care, 99, 177–178, 179–180*b*, 180. *See also* Children
Children. *See also* Child care
  cost of raising, 100*b*, 586*b*
  in the delivery room, 212
  with diabetes, obesity and, 422
  other, involving in pregnancy, 140–141, 144, 589–591
  previous, placental abruption and, 510
  spacing, 295, 488*b*, 585–586
Child Tax Credit, 99
Chilling, in food handling, 326
Chills, miscarriage and, 564

Chlamydia, 4–5, 83, 200, 530–531
Chloasma, 76
Chlorpheniramine, 104
Cholesterol, 315
Choline, 132–133, 133*b*
Chorioamnionitis, 331*b*, 550, 555
Chorion, 366
Chorionicity, 364
Chorionic villi, 34, 34*f*
Chorionic villus sampling (CVS)
    as diagnostic test, 75, 371, 459, 460*f*
    procedure for, 469–470
    Rh immunoglobulin after, 502
    Rh sensitization and, 501
    timing for, 83
    ultrasound exam and, 479
Chromosomal disorders, 74–75,
    455–457
Chromosomes. *See also* Genetic
    disorders
    birth defects and, 449
    characteristics, 451–453, 452*f*
    miscarriage and, 562
    problems, miscarriage and, 61
    problems, stillbirth and, 574
Chronic hypertension. *See also* Hyper-
    tension
    definition of, 407
    risks, 408–409, 409*f*
    treatment, 410
Circumcision, 178*f*
    arranging for, 280
    baby care plan on, 157*b*
    considerations about, 177
    decisions about, 136
    resources, 185
    von Willebrand disease and, 440
Cleanliness, food handling, 325
Cleft lip, 441
Cleft palate, 441, 454
Clindamycin, 103
Clomiphene citrate, 362*b*
CMs. *See* Certified midwives
CMV. *See* Cytomegalovirus
CNMs. *See* Certified nurse–midwives
Cocaine, 507, 510
Coffee, 61–62, 323. *See also* Caffeine
Cold remedies, 55, 391*b*

Colds, 77, 397
Cold sores, 331*b*, 332. *See also* Genital
    herpes
Color blindness, 449, 451*t*, 454
Colostrum, 70, 334
Combined first-trimester screening,
    465*t*, 466
Combined hormonal birth control
    methods, 296–297*t*, 299–300
Combined spinal–epidural (CSE) block,
    226, 265
Coming in, breast milk, 334
Complete blood count (CBC), 79
Complete breech presentation, 257*f*
Complete placental abruption, 510
Complete placenta previa, 508
Complex carbohydrates, 314
Compound presentation, 550
Condoms
    birth control using, 294, 296–297*t*,
        301–302, 301*f*
    genital herpes and, 530
    hepatitis B virus risk and, 524
    sexually transmitted infections and,
        5, 529
Congenital heart disease, 279, 429–430
Congenital rubella syndrome (CRS),
    524
Congenital varicella syndrome, 521
Congestion, 109–110
Conjunctivitis, 531
Consent forms, 248–249
Constipation
    celiac disease and, 436
    exercise and, 47
    fiber intake and, 315
    iron level in vitamin supplements
        and, 71*b*
    irritable bowel syndrome and, 435
    pregnancy and, 70, 150–151
Contact sports, 50
Continuous labor support, 232
Contraception. *See* Birth control
Contractions
    during active labor, 247, 249–250
    delivery of placenta and, 252–253
    during early labor, 244, 246
    exercise during pregnancy and, 48*b*

Contractions (*continued*)
  experience of, 213
  induced labor, 240
  preterm labor in multiple pregnancy
    and, 365
  preterm labor and, 489*b*
  stage 2 of childbirth and, 251
Contraction stress test (CST), 216, 421,
  476*b*, 483, 543
Contrast agents, 401–402
Cooking, in food handling, 326
Copper intrauterine device, 20–21,
  298
Cord blood
  banking, 155, 158, 168, 184
  blood typing using, 252
Corticosteroids
  for asthma, 432*b*, 433
  for asthma during pregnancy, 396
  nasal spray, 105
  placenta accreta and, 512
  placental abruption and, 511
  placenta previa and, 509
  preeclampsia and, 414
  preterm labor in multiple pregnancy
    and, 365
  premature rupture of membranes
    and, 493
  preterm labor and, 490
CPMs. *See* Certified professional
  midwives
Cradle hold, for breastfeeding, 336*b*
Cramps
  abdominal, labor in preterm multiple
    pregnancy and, 366
  abdominal, preterm labor and, 489*b*
  amniocentesis and, 469
  irritable bowel syndrome and, 435
  leg, 174
Cri du chat syndrome, 457
Criss-cross hold, for breastfeeding
  twins, 347*b*
Crohn disease, 435, 444
Cromolyn, 432*b*
Cross-cradle hold, for breastfeeding,
  336*b*
Crowning, 244
Crown–rump length, 60
CRS. *See* Congenital rubella syndrome

CSE. *See* Combined spinal–epidural
  anesthesia
CST. *See* Contraction stress test
CVS. *See* Chorionic villus sampling
Cycling, for exercise, 49
Cystic fibrosis
  as autosomal recessive gene disorder,
    454
  characteristics, 451*t*
  resources, 472
  screening test, 6, 6*t*, 74, 459, 463
Cytomegalovirus (CMV) infection,
  331*b*, 391*b*, 536–537, 542,
  574

**D**

D&C. *See* Dilation and curettage
Dads, future, 14*b*, 60, 75
Death of baby. *See* Stillbirth
Deep vein thrombosis (DVT). *See also*
  Blood clots
  antiphospholipid syndrome and,
    436–437
  bed rest with multiple pregnancy and,
    372
  cesarean delivery and, 266, 268
  combined hormonal birth control
    and, 299
  lupus and, 437
  obesity during childbirth and, 379,
    381
  travel and, 117, 119*b*
Dehydration, 43, 121
Delayed cord clamping, 184
Delayed lactogenesis, 339–340
Deletion, in chromosomes, 456
Delivery. *See also* Cesarean delivery;
    Labor and delivery problems; Preg-
    nancy; Surgery; Vaginal birth after
    Cesarean delivery
  before 39 weeks, 211
  birth plan on, 154–155
  common terms, 243–244
  fetal growth restriction and, 541–542
  gestational diabetes mellitus and, 422
  getting ready for, 178, 180
  multiple pregnancy and, 372
  obesity during pregnancy and, 381
  options to consider, 74, 136–137

Delivery (*continued*)
  positions for, 192–193
  pregestational diabetes mellitus and, 426
  preparing for changes in, 272
  questions for health care provider on, 57
  resources, 253
  settings for, 98, 137
Delivery room, children in, 212
Dental caries (cavities), 42, 92
Dental X-rays, 104
Depot medroxyprogesterone acetate (DMPA), 299
Depression
  eating disorders and, 385
  postpartum, 289–290
  postpartum, multiple pregnancy and, 373–374
  postpartum, subsequent pregnancy and, 588, 589
  as preexisting health condition, 8–9
  during pregnancy, 159, 162
  pregnancy and medication for, 396, 442–443
  pregnancy loss and, 570
  screening test, 160–161*b*
  stillbirth and, 577
Desloratadine, 104
Developmental disabilities, 457, 472, 493–494, 550
DHA. *See* Docosahexaenoic acid
Diabetes educators, 420
Diabetes mellitus. *See also* Gestational diabetes mellitus; Pregestational diabetes mellitus; Glucose
  anesthesia and, 209
  control of, before pregnancy, 415
  fetal growth restriction and, 542
  fetal well-being testing and, 475
  gestational diabetes mellitus and, 422
  labor induction and, 235
  macrosomia and, 545
  multifactorial gene disorders and, 454
  obesity during pregnancy and, 381
  overview, 417
  pneumococcal pneumonia and, 525

Diabetes mellitus (*continued*)
  preeclampsia and, 411
  pregestational, 8–9, 330, 417, 422–426
  screening test, 81
  shoulder dystocia and, 552
  stillbirth and, 574
  uncontrolled, as teratogen, 389, 390
  type 1 diabetes mellitus, 417, 422–426
  type 2 diabetes mellitus, 330, 417, 422–426
Diagnostic tests
  deciding to undergo, 461–462
  definition of, 449
  for genetic disorders, 8, 74, 459, 460*f*
  positive carrier results and, 464
Diamniotic–dichorionic twins, 366, 367*f*
Diamniotic–monochorionic twins, 367, 367*f*
Diaphragm, 296–297*t*, 302, 302*f*
Diarrhea
  celiac disease and, 436
  on cruise ships, 121
  food poisoning and, 324
  infections and, 134–135
  inflammatory bowel disease and, 435
  irritable bowel syndrome and, 435
  methotrexate and, 567
  miscarriage and, 563
  during pregnancy, 78
  preterm labor and, 142, 165, 366, 489*b*
Diastolic blood pressure, 408
Dick-Read, Grantly, 227
Dietary fiber, 11
Dietitians, 420
DiGeorge syndrome, 457
Digestive diseases, 434–436, 444–445
Dilation. *See also* Cervix
  abnormal labor and, 549
  during active labor, 247
  cervical ripening and, 217, 237–238, 244
  definition of, 243
  labor and, 245*f*
  labor issues, cesarean delivery and, 263–264
  miscarriage diagnosis and, 563
  preterm labor and, 487

Dilation and curettage (D&C), 564, 569
Dilation and evacuation, 573
Diphtheria, 164, 518, 520–521
Discordant twins, 369
Diuretics, 384
Diving, 50
Dizziness. *See also* Faintness
  ectopic pregnancy and, 565–568
  exercise during pregnancy and, 48*b*,
    115
  regional anesthesia and, 225
  in second trimester, 110–111
DMPA. *See* Depot medroxyprogesterone
  acetate
DNA, 451–453, 452*f*
Docosahexaenoic acid (DHA), 209*b*,
  322–323
Domestic violence, 83–85, 86
Dominant genetic disorders, 450*t*, 453,
  455*f*
DONA International, 154
Doppler auscultation device, 65, 67*f*
Doppler ultrasound exam, 479
Doppler velocimetry, 543
Double breast pumps, 349, 352
Double-clutch hold, for breastfeeding,
  347*b*
Double-cradle hold, for breastfeeding,
  347*b*
Douching, 62
Doulas, 137, 138, 153–154, 232
Downhill snow skiing, 49
Down syndrome. *See also* Trisomy 21
  cell-free DNA test for, 466*b*
  as chromosomal disorder, 456
  multiple pregnancy and, 371
  quad screen for, 467
  resources, 472
  screening tests, 74–75, 459, 465*t*
Doxylamine, 42
Dreams, unusual or strange, 92
Drinking fluids
  breastfeeding and, 344
  morning sickness and, 42
  working during early pregnancy and,
    59
Drinking problems, 53*b*. *See also*
  Alcohol drinking

Drugs. *See* Illegal drugs; Medications
Duchenne muscular dystrophy, 451*t*
Due date, estimating, 40–41, 40*b*, 60
Duplication, in chromosomes, 456
DVT. *See* Deep vein thrombosis
Dwarfism, 433
Dysautonomia, familial, 6, 463

**E**

Early labor, 244–247, 246*f*
Early-onset preeclampsia, 411
Early preterm birth, 139
Early term, 205, 493–494
Eating disorders
  getting help for, 385
  harm of, 385
  overview, 384
  past, pregnancy and symptoms of, 386
  resources, 386
  types of, 384–385
Eclampsia, 236, 368, 411
*E. coli.* See *Escherichia coli*
Ectopic pregnancy
  early pregnancy loss due to, 61
  normal pregnancy versus, 566*f*
  pelvic inflammatory disease and, 531
  resources, 570
  Rh immunoglobulin after, 502
  Rh sensitization and, 501
  risk factors, 565–566
  treatment, 567–568
ECV. *See* External cephalic version
Eczema, breastfeeding and, 344–345
EDD. *See* Estimated due date
Edema, 109
Edinburgh Postnatal Depression scale,
  160–161
Edwards syndrome, 456. *See also*
  Trisomy 18
EEOC. *See* Equal Employment
  Opportunity Commission
Effacement, of cervix, 217, 243, 245*f*,
  487
Eggs
  abnormal number of chromosomes
    in, 562
  assisted reproductive technologies
    and, 362*b*

Eggs (*continued*)
  chromosomes in, 451
  female sterilization and, 304–305
  fertilization of, 33
  formation of, 107
  hysteroscopic sterilization and, 167
  life span of, 17
  pregnancy and, 15–16, 16*f*
Eicosapentaenoic acid (EPA), 322–323
Elective delivery, 211
Elective induction, 236
Electronic fetal monitoring, 248
Embryo
  development, 34–35
  development, miscarriage and, 562
  fertility treatments and, 362*b*
  identical twins and, 363, 363*f*
  multiple pregnancy and, 361
  preimplantation genetic diagnosis of,
    470–471
Emergency contraception, 304
Emergency delivery, 512
Emetics, 384
Emotional abuse, 83, 84
Emotional changes, during pregnancy,
  76
Endometrial ablation, 511
Endometriosis, 565
Endometritis, 331*b*, 556–557
Endometrium, 15, 16*f*, 556
Engorgement, 286–287, 339
Environmental exposure history, 392,
    393–394*t*, 394. *See also* Family
    health history
Environmental toxins
  avoiding during pregnancy,
    399–401
  birth defects and, 391*b*
  multifactorial gene disorders and,
    454
  overview, 398
  as teratogens, 389–390
  in the workplace, 398–399
EPA. *See* Eicosapentaenoic acid
Epidural block
  abnormal labor and, 551
  for cesarean delivery, 265
  external cephalic version and, 259
  induced labor and, 240

Epidural block (*continued*)
  for pain relief during labor, 182, 225
  postpartum sterilization and, 305
  pushing and delivery and, 251
  von Willebrand disease and, 440
Epilepsy, 440, 445
Episiotomy
  characteristics and need for, 218
  postpartum hemorrhage and, 555
  postpartum pain and, 288
  questions for health care provider on,
    57
  redness or discharge from, 288
  repair of, 252
Equal Employment Opportunity
    Commission (EEOC), 96, 105
*Escherichia coli* (*E. coli*), 134–135
Estimated due date (EDD), 40–41, 40*b*, 60
Estrogen
  in birth control pills, 166
  changes in levels of, 37
  fetal production of, 89
  pregnancy and, 15, 16, 33
  sex after childbirth and, 294–295
Ethnicity, carrier screening and, 6, 6–7*t*,
    8, 463
*Eunice Kennedy Shriver* National Institute
    of Child Health and Human
    Development, 495
Exclusive breastfeeding, 343, 346
Exercise
  anorexia nervosa and, 384
  gestational diabetes mellitus and, 421
  miscarriage and, 561
  in month 3, 72–73, 73*b*
  in month 4, 95, 95*b*
  in month 5, 113–115, 114*b*
  in month 6, 136*b*
  in month 7, 153*b*
  in month 8, 176–177
  in month 9, 191–192, 191*b*
  in month 10, 210, 210*b*
  in months 1 & 2, 46–50, 50*b*
  multiple pregnancy and, 370
  obesity and weight loss during
    pregnancy and, 382
  obesity during pregnancy and, 380
  preconception recommendations for, 11
  postpartum, 283, 284–285*f*, 290–291

Exercise (*continued*)
  pregestational diabetes mellitus and,
    425
  pregnancy-related stress and, 103
  warning signs to stop, 48–49, 48*b*
  weight gain and, 12–13, 322
Expanded carrier screening, 8, 463
Expected due date. *See* Estimated due
  date
Expenditures on Children by Families,
  100*b*
Expressing milk, 339, 346, 349,
  350–351*b*, 351. *See also* Breast
  pumps
External cephalic version (ECV)
  breech presentation and, 201, 255
  offer of, 199
  options for birth, 260–261
  procedure for, 258–260, 259*f*
Eyesight. *See* Vision problems

**F**
Face, swelling of, preeclampsia and,
  142, 412*b*
Face presentation, 550
Factor V Leiden, 439
Failed induction, 239
Failure to progress, 263–264, 549
Faintness. *See also* Dizziness
  ectopic pregnancy and, 565–568
  exercise during pregnancy and, 48*b*
Fallopian tubes
  ectopic pregnancy and, 565, 566*f*
  fertilization in, 33
  implantation in, 61
  menstrual cycle and, 15, 16*f*
  rupture, 566
  sterilization and, 166–167, 304–305
False labor. *See* Braxton Hicks
  contractions
False-negative results
  consequences of, 467–468
  fetal well-being testing and, 477
  pregnancy tests, 39
  in screening versus diagnostic tests, 461
False-positive results
  consequences of, 467–468
  fetal well-being testing and, 477

False-positive results (*continued*)
  pregnancy tests, 39
  in screening versus diagnostic tests,
    461
  sequential screening and, 467
Familial dysautonomia, 6, 463
Family and Medical Leave Act (FMLA),
  97–98, 105, 308
Family health history, 5, 21, 60, 75,
  574. *See also* Environmental
  exposure history
Family physicians, 55–56
Fanconi anemia group C, 6, 463
FAS. *See* Fetal alcohol syndrome
Fathers, future
  chromosome problem and, 562
  health history of, 60, 75
  tips for, 14*b*
Fatigue. *See also* Tiredness
  celiac disease and, 436
  in later weeks of pregnancy, 175
  managing, 43, 68
  multiple pregnancy and, 373
  multiple sclerosis and, 438
  planning another baby and, 586–587
  postpartum, 287
  as pregnancy sign, 38
  sex after childbirth and, 294
  working during early pregnancy and, 59
FDA. *See* U.S. Food and Drug Administration
Fecal incontinence, 286
Feeding your baby. *See also* Breastfeeding
  baby care plan on, 157*b*
  decision on, 193, 195
  overview, 329
  resources, 356–357
  shared, bottle-feeding and, 350–351*b*,
    354
Feet
  increasing size of, 109
  swelling or pain or numbness or tin-
    gling in, 149, 190
Female condom, 5, 301–302, 301*f*
Female sterilization, 304–307
Fertility
  awareness of, 17–18
  bariatric surgery and, 383

Fertility (*continued*)
  charting, 18*f*
  eating disorders and, 385
  future dads and, 14*b*
  timing of, 17
  treatments, multiple pregnancy and,
    361, 362*b*
Fertilization, 33, 298, 452–453, 453*f*,
  562
Fetal alcohol spectrum disorders, 52, 398
Fetal alcohol syndrome (FAS), 52, 398
Fetal blood sampling, 459
Fetal death, 54, 524
Fetal development
  month 3, 24*f*, 65, 66–67*f*
  month 4, 25*f*, 89–90, 90*f*
  month 5, 26*f*, 107–108
  month 6, 27*f*, 129, 130*f*
  month 7, 28*f*, 147, 148*f*
  month 8, 29*f*, 171, 172*f*
  month 9, 30*f*, 187, 188*f*
  month 10, 31*f*, 205, 206*f*
  months 1 & 2, 23*f*, 33–35, 34*f*, 36*f*
  ultrasound exams and, 479
Fetal fibronectin, 489–490
Fetal growth problems
  antiphospholipid syndrome and, 437
  asthma during pregnancy and, 396
  chlamydia or gonorrhea and, 531
  eating disorders and, 385
  fetal growth restriction, 541–544
  fetal well-being testing and, 476
  lupus and, 437
  macrosomia, 544–545
  multiple pregnancy and, 369
  overview, 541
  preterm birth and, 396
  resources, 546
  trichomoniasis and, 533
  ultrasound exam and, 479
Fetal growth restriction (FGR)
  asthma and, 431
  causes, 542
  diagnosis, 542–543
  high blood pressure and, 408
  management, 543
  overview, 541–542
  prevention, 544

Fetal growth restriction (FGR) (*continued*)
  resources, 546
  subsequent pregnancy and, 589
Fetal heart beat. *See also* Heartbeat
  elective induction and, 236
  listening to, 23*f*, 35, 64, 67*f*, 101
  miscarriage diagnosis and, 563
  multiple pregnancy and, 364
  stillbirth diagnosis and, 573
  ultrasound exam of, 79
Fetal heart rate. *See also* Heart rate
  abnormal, cesarean delivery and, 264
  biophysical profile and, 481–482
  contraction stress test and, 483
  electronic monitoring, 480–481, 481*f*
  external cephalic version and, 259, 260
  monitor, 248
  obesity during labor and, 379
  placental abruption and, 511
  ultrasound exams and, 60, 479
  umbilical cord compression and, 553
  umbilical cord prolapse and, 554
Fetal movement counts, 478. *See also*
    Baby's movement; Kick counts
Fetal position, 277
Fetal scalp electrode, 440
Fetal scalp sampling, 440
Fetal well-being testing
  biophysical profile, 481–482
  contraction stress test, 483
  fetal movement counts, 482
  frequently asked questions on, 476*b*
  interpreting results, 477
  modified biophysical profile, 482
  nonstress test, 480–481, 481*f*
  overview, 475
  resources, 483
  timing for, 477
  types, 478–483
  ultrasound exams, 478–480
  why it may be done, 475–478
Fetus
  biophysical profile and, 482
  diagnostic tests for birth defects, 74
  infections and, 3–4
  keepsake ultrasound exam of, 141,
    143, 479
  teratogen exposure and, 392

Fever
  blocked milk ducts and, 341
  engorgement and, 339
  epidural block and, 225
  during labor, endometritis and, 557
  mastitis and, 342
  miscarriage and, 564
  postpartum, 288
Fexofenadine, 104
FGR. See Fetal growth restriction
Fiber, 152*b*, 315
Fibroids, 258, 511
Fifth disease, 538
Financial issues, 99
Fish
  brain development and, 209*b*
  breastfeeding and, 344
  omega-3 fatty acids and, 322–323
  precautions, 111–112, 127, 327
5p syndrome, 457
Flat nipples, 340–341
Flu, 77–78, 78*b*, 518
Flu nasal spray vaccine, 4, 517–518, 520
Flu vaccine, 4, 516–518, 519*t*
Fluconazole, 103
Fluids, drinking
  breastfeeding and, 344
  exercise and, 114
  morning sickness and, 42
  working during early pregnancy and, 59
Fluorescence in situ hybridization, 471
Fluticasone propionate, 105
FMLA. See Family and Medical Leave Act
Foley bulb, 238
Folic acid
  antiepilepsy drugs and, 441
  bariatric surgery and, 383
  birth defects and, 390–391*b*
  breastfeeding and, 344
  facts on, 44*b*, 318*t*, 319
  form to take, 397
  methotrexate and, 567
  multiple pregnancy and, 369–370
  neural tube defects and, 455
  planning another baby and, 587
  pregestational diabetes mellitus and, 424
  pregnancy and, 12, 318

Follicle-stimulating hormone (FSH), 37
Food allergies, breastfeeding and, 344–345
Food cravings, 93–94
Food groups, 316–317, 317*t*
Food poisoning, 134–135
Food safety, 144, 324–327, 539
Football hold
  for breastfeeding, 336*b*
  for breastfeeding twins, 347*b*
Footling breech presentation, 257*f*
Forceps. See also Operative vaginal delivery
  about, 218
  continuous labor support and, 232
  procedure, 256, 256*f*
  reasons for, 255
  resources, 261
Foremilk, 334
Formula-feeding, 353–355. See also Bottle-feeding
Formulas, types, 354
4p deletion syndrome, 457
4-point kneeling, 284*f*
Fragile X syndrome, 7*t*
Frank breech presentation, 257*f*
Fraternal twins, 363, 363*f*
Front V-hold, for breastfeeding twins, 347*b*
FSH. See Follicle-stimulating hormone
Full term, 205, 236, 258, 277
Fundal height, 122–123, 125*f*, 199, 542–544

**G**
Gastric band surgery, 383
Gastroschisis, 542
Gaucher disease, 6, 463
GBS. See Group B streptococci.
General anesthesia, 92, 182, 226–227, 265, 305. See also Anesthesia
Genes. See also Genetic Disorders
  autoimmune disorders and, 436
  birth defects and, 449
  definition, 451–453, 452*f*
  in chromosomes, 562
  cord blood banking and, 158
  Rh factor in, 499

Genetic counselors
  expanded carrier screening and, 463
  expertise of, 5, 457
  risk assessment by, 75
  testing options and, 450
  test results and, 462, 468
Genetic disorders. *See also*
    Chromosomes; Genes
  birth defect risk and, 390*b*
  carrier screening, 6, 6–7*t*, 8, 462–464
  chromosomal, 455–457
  common types, 465*t*
  cord blood banking and, 158
  deciding to undergo, 461–462
  diagnostic tests, 468–471
  first trimester, 83
  inherited, 452–455, 453*f*, 455*f*
  in multiple pregnancy, 370
  overview, 74–75, 449–450
  resources, 87, 472–473
  risk of, 457, 458*b*, 459
  screening tests, 464–468, 466*b*
  testing for, 8, 74–75, 449–451,
    459–461, 460*f*
  timing of, 460*f*
  types, 459, 460*f*
Geneticist, 574
Genital herpes. *See also* Cold sores
  breastfeeding and, 331*b*, 332
  cesarean delivery and, 264
  labor induction and, 237
  management, 83
  pregnancy and, 529–530
  transmission of, 4
Genital warts, 523
German measles, 82, 391*b*. *See also*
    Rubella
Gestational age
  biophysical profile and, 482
  calculation of, 60
  elective induction and, 236
  estimated due date and, 40
  fetal growth restriction and, 541
  fetal well-being test results and, 475
  multiple pregnancy and, 365*t*
  premature rupture of membranes
    and, 492
  preterm labor and, 489, 490

Gestational age (*continued*)
  ultrasound exams and, 79, 479
Gestational diabetes mellitus. *See also*
    Diabetes mellitus; Glucose
  care after pregnancy, 422
  controlling, 419–421
  fetal well-being testing and, 476
  macrosomia and, 544
  multifetal pregnancy reduction and,
    362*b*
  multiple pregnancy and, 368
  obesity during pregnancy and, 378,
    381, 391*b*
  overview, 417–418
  postpartum checkup of, 293
  resources, 427
  risks, 418
  screening test, 164
  special tests, 421–422
  subsequent pregnancy and, 10,
    588–589
  testing, malabsorptive bariatric sur-
    gery and, 383
  testing for, 418–419
  weight gain and, 322
  weight gain between pregnancies
    and, 587
Gestational hypertension
  definition of, 407
  fetal well-being testing and, 476
  labor induction and, 236
  obesity during pregnancy and, 378
  overview, 410
Gestational trophoblastic disease (GTD),
    568–569, 570
Ginger, morning sickness and, 42
Gingivitis, 91–92
Glucose
  carbohydrates and, 94, 314
  challenge testing for gestational
    diabetes and, 164, 619
  fiber and, 315
  levels of, in gestational diabetes,
    378, 417, 419, 420–421
  levels of, in newborn, 334
  levels of, in pregestational diabetes,
    423–424
  overview, 417

Glucose (*continued*)
macrosomia and, 418, 544
postpartum testing of, 293, 381, 422, 425
urine testing and, 81, 101
Gluten. *See* Celiac disease
Glycemic index, 94*b*
Gonadotropin-releasing hormone (GnRH), 37
Gonadotropins, 362*b*
Gonorrhea, 4, 5, 83, 200, 530–531
Granuloma gravidarum, 92
Graves disease, 401
Grieving, stages of, 575–578
Group B streptococci (GBS), 102, 199–200, 203, 492, 526, 528
Group health care practices, 56
Group prenatal care, 57
Growth problems. *See* Fetal growth problems
GTD. *See* Gestational trophoblastic disease
Gum disease, 91–92
Gymnastics, 49

**H**

Hair dye safety, 86
Hand-expressing breast milk, 351
HBIG. *See* Hepatitis B immune globulin
HBV. *See* Hepatitis B Virus
hCG. *See* Human chorionic gonadotropin
HDN. *See* Hemolytic disease of the newborn
Headache. *See also* Aches; Backaches
epidural block and, 225
exercise during pregnancy and, 48*b*
preeclampsia and, 142, 412*b*
Health care costs, 373, 462
Health care providers. *See also specific types*
choosing, 55–57, 116, 127
expanded carrier screening and, 463
pediatric subspecialists among, 471
test results and, 462, 468
types for pregnancy care, 55–56
Health Hazard Evaluation, 96
Health history. *See* Environmental exposure history; Family health history

Health insurance, 99–101, 105
HealthyChildren.Org, 185
Hearing loss, cytomegalovirus infection and, 536
Hearing test for newborns, 279–280
Heartbeat, fast or racing, in mother, 143. *See also* Fetal heartbeat.
Heartburn, 131
Heart defects
fetal growth restriction and, 542
as multifactorial gene disorder, 454
obesity during pregnancy and, 379, 391*b*
seizure disorders and, 441
Heart disease. *See also* Cardiovascular disease
breastfeeding and, 330
chronic hypertension and, 408
exercise during pregnancy and, 47
fetal well-being testing and, 476
preeclampsia and, 368, 411–412
pregestational diabetes mellitus and, 423
pregnancy and, 429–430
resources, 444
Heart murmur, 429–430
Heel touches, 285*f*
HELLP syndrome, 411
Hematopoietic stem cells, 155
Hemoglobin A1C, 424
Hemoglobinopathies, 542
Hemolytic disease of the newborn (HDN), 500–501, 503–504
Hemophilia, 7*t*, 449, 451*t*
Hemorrhage
cesarean delivery and, 138, 239–240, 268
placenta accreta and, 512–513
placenta previa and, 508
postpartum, 253, 555–556
postpartum, resources, 557
postpartum, shoulder dystocia and, 552
von Willebrand disease and, 440
Hemorrhoids, 173–174, 283
Heparin, 156*b*, 437, 439
Hepatitis, 522
Hepatitis A virus, 518, 519*t*, 522–523

Hepatitis B immune globulin (HBIG), 279, 331*b*, 523
Hepatitis B virus (HBV)
    breastfeeding and, 331*b*
    immunization against, 279, 519*t*
    pregnancy and, 522–523
    screening test, 82
    transmission of, 4
    as vaccine preventable infection, 518
    workplace exposure to, 398–399
Hepatitis C virus, 82, 331*b*, 522, 533–534
Hepatitis D virus, 522
Herbal supplements, 9, 54–55, 391*b*, 397
Heroin, 54
Herpes simplex virus infection. *See also* Genital herpes
    breastfeeding and, 331*b*, 332
    reappearance of, 529–530, 529*f*
    stillbirth and, 574
Herpes zoster, 518, 521–522
Hiccups, baby's, 129, 478
High blood pressure. *See also* Blood pressure; Hypertension; Preeclampsia
    bed rest and, 182
    breastfeeding and, 330
    exercise during pregnancy and, 47
    fetal growth restriction and, 542
    fetal well-being testing and, 475
    gestational diabetes mellitus and, 418–419
    gestational trophoblastic disease and, 569
    kidney disease and, 430
    labor induction and, 235
    multiple pregnancy and, 368
    obesity during pregnancy and, 378
    overview, 407
    placental abruption and, 510
    as preexisting health condition, 8–9
    pregestational diabetes mellitus and, 423
    resources, 415
    stillbirth and, 574
    subsequent pregnancy and, 10
    types of, 407
High blood pressure (*continued*)
    weight gain and, 322
    weight gain between pregnancies and, 587
High-glycemic foods, 93, 94*b*
High-risk obstetricians, 55–56, 365*b*. *See also* Maternal–fetal medicine subspecialists
High-risk thrombophilias, 439
HIV. *See* Human immunodeficiency virus
HMBANA. *See* Human Milk Banking Association of North America
Home, giving birth at, 98
Hormonal intrauterine devices, 298
Horseback riding, 49
Hospital
    admission to, 248–249
    baby friendliness, 332, 333*b*
    baby's stay in, 193
    bed rest with multiple pregnancy in, 372
    as birth centers, 98
    breastfeeding in, 334–335
    discharge from, 280
    health care provider affiliations with, 57
    packing for, 193, 194*b*
    registering at, 178
    tour of, 181
    trial of labor after cesarean delivery and, 270–271
    when to go to, 211, 246–247
Hot flashes, 132
Hot tubs, safety of, 85–86, 402
HPV. *See* Human papillomavirus
Human chorionic gonadotropin (hCG), 33, 37, 39, 566, 569
Human immunodeficiency virus (HIV)
    breastfeeding and, 167, 331
    circumcision and, 177
    preconception testing for, 5
    pregnancy and, 531–532
    screening newborns for, 280
    screening test, 82, 200
    transmission of, 4
    workplace exposure to, 398
Human Milk Banking Association of North America (HMBANA), 348

Human papillomavirus (HPV), 4, 518,
519t, 523–524
Hydatidiform mole, 568
Hydramnios, 423
Hyperemesis gravidarum, 42–43
Hyperglycemia, 425
Hypertension. *See also* Blood pressure;
High blood pressure; Preeclampsia
chronic, 408–410
multifetal pregnancy reduction and,
362b
overview, 407
resources, 415
Hyperthyroidism, 433, 476, 569
Hypnobirthing, 228, 232
Hypoglycemia, 424
Hypothyroidism, 433
Hysterectomy
cesarean delivery and, 74, 138, 268
persistent gestational trophoblastic
disease and, 569
placenta accreta and, 512, 513
placenta previa and, 508
postpartum hemorrhage and, 556
Hysterosalpingogram, 167, 307
Hysteroscope, 307
Hysteroscopic sterilization, 167,
306–307, 307f
Hysteroscopy, 305

**I**

IBCLCs. *See* International board-certified lactation consultants
IBD. *See* Inflammatory bowel disease
IBS. *See* Irritable bowel syndrome
Ibuprofen, 132, 567
Identical twins, 363, 363f
Illegal drugs. *See also* Medications
avoiding during pregnancy, 13–14,
53–54
fetal growth restriction and, 542
intravenous, hepatitis B virus and, 522
as teratogens, 389
Immunity, 82, 334, 516
Immunizations. *See also* Infections;
Vaccines
preconception care and, 3–5
pregnancy and, 516–518, 519t
resources, 21, 538–539

Implant, birth control, 167, 296–297t,
298–299
Implantation, 33, 61
Implantation bleeding, 37
Income taxes, 99
Incomplete miscarriage, 563
Incontinence
fecal, 286
postpartum, 282
vacuum extraction and, 257
vaginal delivery and, 137
Indicated preterm birth, 487
Indirect Coombs test, 501
Induced abortion, 501
Infant car seat, 180, 197–199, 198b, 203
Infantile myxedema, 433
Infants. *See* Newborns
Infections. *See also* Immunizations,
Pathogens; Sexually transmitted
infections
after childbirth, 253
amniocentesis or chorionic villus
sampling and, 469
bacterial vaginosis, 535
birth defects and, 391b
breastfeeding with, 331–332, 331b
cesarean delivery and, 74, 138,
239–240, 268
cytomegalovirus, 536–537
fetus and, 3–4
food poisoning and, 134–135
group B streptococci, 526, 528
hepatitis C virus, 533–534
labor and delivery in water and, 137
labor induction and, 239
listeriosis, 535–536
mastitis, 341–342
in mother, placenta previa and, 508
obesity during pregnancy and, 391b
overview, 515
parvovirus, 538
pedicures and, 202
during pregnancy, preterm births and,
488b
premature rupture of membranes
and, 492–493
prevention, 516b
resources, 538–539
sexually transmitted, 528–533

Infections (*continued*)
    stillbirth and, 574
    toxoplasmosis, 537–538
    tuberculosis, 534–535
    uterine, labor induction and, 236
    uterine, premature rupture of
        membranes and, 491–492
    vaccine-preventable, 518, 519t,
        520–525
    vaccines, pregnancy and, 516–518
Inflammatory bowel disease (IBD), 435
Influenza, 77–78, 78b, 518
Influenza vaccine, 516, 517–518, 519t
Injection, birth control, 296–297t, 299
Institute of Medicine, 168, 380
Insulin, 417, 421, 425
Insulin pump, 425–426
Insulin resistance, 422
Integrated screening, 465t, 467
Intellectual disabilities
    alcohol drinking and, 391, 398
    aneuploidy and, 456
    birth defects and, 7t, 449, 450t,
        458b
    chromosomal disorders and, 457
    congenital rubella syndrome, 524
    infantile myxedema and, 433
    newborn herpes infection and, 530
Intermediate kidney disease, 430–431
Internal os, 507
International Association for Medical
    Assistance to Travelers, 118b
International board-certified lactation
    consultants (IBCLCs), 332, 337,
    340
International Childbirth Education
    Association, 185, 232
International travel, 118b
Intimate partner violence, 83–85
Intrauterine devices (IUDs), 20–21,
    167, 296–297t, 298
Intrauterine growth restriction. *See*
    Fetal growth restriction
Inverted nipples, 202, 340–341
In vitro fertilization
    ectopic pregnancy and, 565
    estimated due date and, 40
    positive carrier results and, 464
    preeclampsia and, 411

In vitro fertilization (*continued*)
    preimplantation genetic diagnosis and,
        470–471
    sterilization and, 304
Iodine, 131, 401–402, 433
Iron
    bariatric surgery and, 383
    delayed cord clamping and, 184
    form to take in pregnancy, 397
    need in pregnancy for, 318, 318t, 319
Iron supplements
    constipation and, 150
    multiple pregnancy and, 369–370
    need in pregnancy for, 71b
    postpartum hemorrhage and, 556
Irritable bowel syndrome (IBS), 435, 444
Isotretinoin, 9, 69, 395
Itching, 76, 175
IUDs. *See* Intrauterine devices

**J**
Jaundice, newborn, 184, 257, 418, 503,
    536
Joint pain, 48

**K**
Karyotype, 470–471
Keepsake ultrasound exam, 141, 143, 479
Kegel exercises, 50b, 282
Kick counts, 215, 216, 421, 478. *See also*
    Baby's movement; Fetal movement
    counts
Kidney disease
    chronic hypertension and, 408
    fetal growth restriction and, 542
    fetal well-being testing and, 476
    preeclampsia and, 412
    pregestational diabetes mellitus and, 423
    pregnancy and, 430–431
    resources, 444
    stillbirth and, 574
Kidneys
    chronic hypertension and, 408
    diabetes mellitus and, 417
    infections of, 527f, 528
    preeclampsia and, 142, 368, 378
    pregnancy and, 38
    problems, labor induction and, 235
    urine production in fetus by, 89

Kneeling heel touch, 176*b*
Knee raises, 284–285*f*

**L**
Labia, 278
Labor. *See also* Labor and delivery
    problems; Labor coach; Labor
    induction; Pregnancy; Preterm labor
    birth plan on, 154–155, 156*b*
    Braxton Hicks contractions and, 189
    common terms, 243–244
    continuous support for, 232
    doulas and, 154
    early, 244–247
    eating and drinking during, 209
    failure to progress, cesarean delivery
        and, 263–264
    false versus true, 213*t*
    fetal growth restriction and, 541–542
    gestational diabetes mellitus and, 422
    getting ready for, 177, 178
    hemorrhoids after, 283
    knowing when you're in, 212–213
    multiple pregnancy and, 372
    nausea and start of, 208
    obesity during pregnancy and, 381
    old wives' tales on starting, 217
    options to consider, 136–137
    overview, 243
    pain expected during, 223
    pain relief during, 181–182
    positions for, 192–193
    pregestational diabetes mellitus and, 426
    preterm, signs and symptoms of, 366
    preterm multiple pregnancy and,
        365–366
    resources, 253
    rupture of membranes and, 183
    Rh sensitization and, 501
    slowing or stopping, 255
    stillbirth diagnosis during, 573
    vaginal birth after cesarean delivery
        after, 74
    in water, 137
Labor and delivery problems. *See also*
    Cesarean delivery; Delivery; Labor;
    Labor and delivery problems; Vagi-
    nal birth after cesarean delivery
    abnormal labor, 549–551

Labor and delivery problems (*continued*)
    endometritis, 556–557
    overview, 549
    postpartum hemorrhage, 555–556
    resources, 557
    shoulder dystocia, 551–552, 552*f*
    umbilical cord compression, 553
    umbilical cord prolapse, 553–555
Labor coach. *See also* Labor
    doula as, 154
    help during labor and delivery by, 247,
        250–252
Labor dystocia, 549–551
Labor induction. *See also* Labor
    decision on, 216–217
    method for, 237–239
    overview, 235
    placental abruption and, 511
    reasons for, 235–236
    resources, 219, 240
    risks, 239–240
    stillbirth and, 573
    when not to, 237
Laborists, 56
Lab tests. *See* Blood tests;
    Diagnostic tests; Genetic disorder
    screens and tests; Pregnancy tests;
    Screening tests
Lactational amenorrhea method (LAM),
    303–304, 331
Lactation consultants, 332, 337, 340
LactMed, 348
Lactose intolerance, 184–185, 324, 344
La Leche League International, 196, 202,
    332, 357
LAM. *See* Lactational amenorrhea method
Lamaze, Fernand, 227
Lamaze method, 180–181, 227, 232
Laminaria, 217, 238
Lanugo, 107, 108*f,* 171, 205
Laparoscope, 306, 568
Laparoscopic sterilization, 167
Laparoscopy, 306
Laparotomy, 556
Large for gestational age (LGA). *See*
    Macrosomia
Last menstrual period (LMP), 40–41,
    277. *See also* Menstrual period
Latching on, 335, 336*b,* 337, 339

LATCH system, for car seats, 198*b*
Late deceleration, 483
Late hemorrhage, 555
Latent labor, 244. *See also* Early labor
Latent tuberculosis, 534–535
Late preterm babies, 493–494
Late-term pregnancy, 216, 476
Laxatives, 55, 384, 391*b*
Lead exposure
    avoiding during pregnancy, 399–400
    birth defects and, 391*b*
    pregnancy and, 392, 403
    prenatal, 123, 125
Leg cramps, 174
Leg extensions, 285*f*
Leg pain, swelling, or tenderness, 190,
    288. *See also* Calf pain or swelling
Leg slides, 284*f*
Let-down reflex, 334, 335*f*, 340, 351
Leukotriene receptor antagonist, 432*b*
LGA. *See* Large for gestational age
LH. *See* Luteinizing hormone
Licensed midwives, 56
Linea nigra, 76
*Listeria monocytogenes*, 535
Listeriosis, 134–135, 324–325, 535–536
Live, attenuated viruses, vaccines and,
    4, 517–518, 522
Liver damage or disease, 368, 533
Live viruses, vaccines and, 82
LMP. *See* Last menstrual period
Local anesthesia, 224, 306
Lochia, 281, 557
Loop electrosurgical excision procedure,
    488*b*
Loratadine, 104
Low back pain, 109, 110, 149, 150*f*
Low birth weight baby
    anemia and, 319
    bacterial vaginosis and, 102
    coffee drinking and, 61–62
    domestic violence and, 84
    eating disorders and, 385
    lead exposure and, 125
    secondhand smoke and, 52
    smoking and, 51
    spacing pregnancies and, 586
    umbilical cord prolapse and, 554
Low-glycemic foods, 93, 94*b*, 315

Low-risk thrombophilias, 439
Lubricants, for vaginal dryness, 293–294
Lung disease, 47
Lung function, 432, 494
Lupus. *See* Systemic lupus erythemetosus
Luteinizing hormone (LH), 18, 37

**M**
Macrosomia
    abnormal labor and, 449
    cesarean delivery and, 264
    gestational diabetes mellitus and, 418
    obesity during pregnancy and, 379
    overview and diagnosis, 544
    postpartum hemorrhage and, 555
    pregestational diabetes mellitus and,
        423, 426
    resources, 546
    weight gain and, 322
Magnesium sulfate, 366, 490
Magnetic resonance imaging (MRI), 401,
    512, 575
Malabsorptive bariatric surgery, 382, 383
Malaria, 118*b*
Male condom, 301–302, 301*f*
Male infertility, 14*b*
Male sterilization, 307–308, 308*f*
Malpresentation, 550, 554
Marketplace health insurance plans,
    99–100
Mask of pregnancy, 76
Massage, 126, 132, 228, 247
Mastitis, 331*b*, 341–342, 350*b*
Maternal–fetal medicine subspecialists,
    55–56, 365*b*, 429, 437
Maternal serum alpha fetoprotein
    (MSFAP), 460*f*, 466–467
Maternity bras, 69–70
Maternity leave, 58, 99, 178
McRoberts maneuver, 552, 552*f*
MCV4 vaccine, 519*t*
Measles, 518
Measles–mumps–rubella (MMR)
    vaccine, 4, 517–518, 519*t*, 524
Meconium, 107–108
Medicaid, 100, 101
Medical problems during pregnancy
    asthma, 431–433, 431*f*
    autoimmune diseases, 435–438

Medical problems during pregnancy
(*continued*)
diabetes mellitus, 417–427
digestive diseases, 434–436
heart disease, 429–430
hypertension and preeclampsia,
407–415
kidney disease, 430–431
mental illness, 442–443
physical disability, 443
resources, 444–445
seizure disorders, 440–442
thrombophilias, 438–440
thyroid disease, 433–434, 434*f*
von Willebrand disease, 440
Medications. *See also* Illegal drugs
after delivery of placenta, 252–253
antiepilepsy, 441–442
antiinflammatory, 438
for asthma during pregnancy,
432–433, 432*b*
avoiding during pregnancy, 54–55
bariatric surgery and, 383
birth defects and, 391*b*
bladder infection, 528
for blood pressure, 410, 414
during breastfeeding, 332, 348–349,
357
for cervical ripening, 217, 238
for ectopic pregnancy, 567–568
fetal growth restriction and, 543
formula-feeding and, 354
for gestational diabetes mellitus, 421
for human immunodeficiency virus,
532
inflammatory bowel disease and, 435
irritable bowel syndrome and, 435
kidney disease and, 430
for lupus during pregnancy, 438
for mental illness, 442–443
miscarriage and, 562
for miscarriage treatment, 563
obesity and weight loss during
pregnancy and, 382
for pain relief during childbirth,
223–227, 249–250
placenta and, 34
pregestational diabetes mellitus and,
425

Medications (*continued*)
pregnancy and, 9, 394–397
prescription, 9, 54–55, 60, 395–397
reaction to, cesarean delivery and, 268
as teratogens, 389–390
tuberculosis, 534
Melanin, 76, 147
Melasma, 76
MenACWY (vaccine), 525
Meningitis, 525
Meningococcal disease, 518, 519*t*, 525
Menstrual calendar, 19*f*
Menstrual cycle, 15–16, 16*f*, 17–18, 18*f*
Menstrual period. *See also* Last menstrual
period
anorexia nervosa and, 384
definition of, 16
estimated due date and, 40–41
heavier postpartum bleeding during,
288
lactational amenorrhea method and,
303–304
postpartum return of, 288
stopping of, 33
Mental illness, 442–443, 445
Mercury
avoiding during pregnancy, 400
birth defects and, 391*b*
in fish, 111–112, 168, 209, 323
as teratogen, 389
Methimazole, 433
Methotrexate, 567–568
Metronidazole, 103
Microarray analysis, 471
Microwave
baby's bottles and, 355–356
breast milk and, 353*b*
for sterilizing breast pump, 352
Midwives, 56, 232
Milk banks, human, 348, 356
Miscarriage
amniocentesis or chorionic villus
sampling and, 469
antiphospholipid syndrome and, 437
causes, 561–562
coffee drinking and, 61–62
diagnosis, 563
domestic violence and, 84
eating disorders and, 385

Miscarriage (*continued*)
    fetal tissue, passed, 61, 562
    kidney disease and, 430
    lead exposure and, 125
    listeriosis and, 324, 535
    lupus and, 437
    overview, 561
    pregestational diabetes mellitus and, 423
    recovery, 564
    resources, 570, 580
    Rh immunoglobulin after, 502
    Rh sensitization and, 501
    risk of, 57, 91
    rubella and, 524
    *Salmonella* and, 134
    signs and symptoms, 60–61, 562–563
    subsequent pregnancy and, 10
    thrombophilias and, 439
    treatment, 563–564
    trying again, 564
    unbalanced translocations and, 457
    von Willebrand disease and, 440
MMR. *See* Measles–mumps–rubella vaccine
Modified biophysical profile, 482, 543
Molar pregnancy, 568–569
Monoamniotic–monochorionic twins, 367, 367*f*
Monochorionic–monoamniotic babies, 367*f*, 368
Monosodium glutamate, 133
Monosomy, 456
Morning sickness, 41–43, 46, 63, 364
Mouth, changes in, 91–92
MPSV4 vaccine, 519*t*, 525
MRI. *See* Magnetic resonance imaging
MSFAP. *See* Maternal serum alpha fetoprotein
Mucolipidosis IV, 6, 463
Mucus plug, 212. *See also* Cervical mucus
Multifactorial gene disorders, 454–455
Multifetal pregnancy reduction, 362*b*
Multiple pregnancy. *See also* Triplets; Twins
    bed rest and, 182
    breech presentation and, 258
    cesarean delivery of, 264
    delivery, 372

Multiple pregnancy (*continued*)
    duration of, 365*t*
    exercise and, 47
    fertility treatments and, 362*b*
    fetal growth restriction and, 542
    fetal well-being testing and, 477
    fraternal or identical, 363, 363*f*
    getting ready for, 373–374
    hyperemesis gravidarum and, 42–43
    loss in, resources, 580
    overview, 361
    placenta accreta and, 511
    preterm births and, 488*b*
    process of, 361
    resources, 374
    risks, 364–369
    signs of, 364
    ultrasound exam of, 79, 479
    what to expect, 369–372
Multiple sclerosis, 438, 445
Multivitamins, 41, 44*b*, 45, 383, 424. *See also* Vitamins; Vitamin supplements
Mumps, 518, 524
Muscle control, multiple sclerosis and, 438
Mutations, 452–453, 471
Myometrium, 511
MyPlate food-planning guide, 11, 316, 321*f*, 326
Myxedema, 433

**N**
Narcotics, 224
National Cancer Institute's Smoking Quitline, 13, 51
National Domestic Violence Hotline, 85–86
National Institute for Occupational Safety and Health (NIOSH), 58, 96, 105
National Marrow Donor Program, 158, 168
Nausea
    active labor and, 249
    ectopic pregnancy and, 567
    morning sickness and, 41–43
    postpartum, 288
    preeclampsia and, 142, 412*b*
    pregnancy, gastric band surgery and, 383
    as pregnancy sign, 38
    start of labor and, 208

Neonatal intensive care units (NICUs), 350b, 414, 494, 543
Neonatologists
infant medical disorders and, 471
neonatal intensive care units and, 494
placenta accreta and, 512
placenta previa and, 509–510
preterm births and, 495
stillbirth evaluation and, 574
Nervous system development, 112b
Nesting instinct, 214
Neural tube, development of, 35
Neural tube defects (NTDs)
folic acid and, 44b, 319, 391b
as multifactorial gene disorder, 454–455
obesity during pregnancy and, 379
screening tests, 74–75, 459, 465–468, 465t
second trimester screens for, 466–467
seizure disorders and, 441
Neurofibromatosis, 450t, 453
Newborns
early cesarean delivery and, 138
feeding, decision on, 193, 195
jaundice and, 184, 257
screening tests, 279–280
sleep by, 278
Nicotine replacement products, 51–52
NICUs. See Neonatal intensive care units
Niemann–Pick disease type A, 6, 463
NIOSH. See National Institute for Occupational Safety and Health
Nipples. See also Breasts
breastfeeding and repositioning surgery for, 346
breastfeeding and tenderness of, 338–339
for formula-feeding, 355
inverted, breastfeeding and, 202, 340–341
Nipple shields, 341
Nonsteroidal antiinflammatory drugs (NSAIDs), 132, 567
Nonstress test (NST)
biophysical profile and, 481–482
fetal growth testing and, 543

Nonstress test (NST) (continued)
gestational diabetes mellitus and, 421
late-term or postterm pregnancy and, 216
mild gestational hypertension and, 413
multiple pregnancy and, 371
overview, 480–481
preeclampsia without severe features and, 413
Nosebleeds, 109–110
NSAIDs. See Nonsteroidal antiinflammatory drugs
NST. See Nonstress test
NTDs. See Neural tube defects
Nuchal translucency screening, 74–75, 466
Nurse practitioners, 56
Nursery, hospital, 157b, 193
Nurses, continuous labor support by, 232
Nursing. See Breastfeeding
Nursing bra, 196
Nutrition
balancing your diet, 314–316
five food groups, 316–317
in month 3, 71–72, 72f
in month 4, 93–94
in month 5, 111–113
in month 6, 132–135
in month 7, 151–152, 152b
in month 8, 175, 175b
in month 9, 191, 191b
in month 10, 208–209
in months 1 & 2, 44–46, 46t
multiple pregnancy and, 369–370
obesity during pregnancy and, 380
overview, 313
planning healthy meals, 316, 320–321
postpartum, 287, 291, 309
resources, 326–327
special concerns, 322–326
vitamins and minerals, 318–320
weight gain during pregnancy and, 321–322, 322t
Nutritional supplements, 9. See also Vitamin supplements
Nutritionists, 420

## O

Obesity
abnormal labor and, 550
anesthesia and, 209
birth defects and, 391*b*
body mass index and, 12
breastfeeding and, 330
children with diabetes and, 422
combined hormonal birth control
and, 299
defining, 377–378
diabetes testing and, 419
exercise program and, 13
managing, during pregnancy,
379–381
multiple pregnancy and, 370, 370*t*
overview, 377
preeclampsia and, 411
pregnancy and, 377–383
resources, 386
risks during pregnancy, 378–379
vaginal birth after cesarean delivery
success and, 272
weight gain during pregnancy and,
47*t*, 321, 322*t*
weight-loss surgery for, 13
Ob-gyns. *See* Obstetrician–gynecologists
Obsessive–compulsive disorder, 162, 442
Obstetrician–gynecologists (ob-gyns),
55, 280, 365*b*
Occupational Safety and Health Act,
96–97, 398–399
Occupational Safety and Health
Administration (OSHA), 58, 96,
105, 398–399
Oligohydramnios, 553
Omega-3 fatty acids, 112*b*, 209*b*, 315,
322–323, 400
Operative vaginal delivery. *See also*
Forceps; Vacuum extraction
abnormal labor and, 551
about, 218
questions for health care provider on,
57
reasons for, 251, 255–256
risks, 257
types of, 256
von Willebrand disease and, 440
Opioids, 54

Oral herpes, 530
Organization of Teratology Information
Specialists (OTIS), 395
Organ systems, development of, 9, 89
Orgasms, 140, 307
OSHA. *See* Occupational Safety and
Health Administration
OTIS. *See* Organization of Teratology
Information Specialists
Ovarian cancer, breastfeeding and,
330–331
Ovaries
egg release from, 15, 33
formation of, 107
monitoring developing eggs in,
362*b*
postpartum release of, 288
ultrasound exam of, 79
Over-the-counter drugs
for acne during pregnancy, 68–69
avoiding during pregnancy, 54–55
birth defects and, 391*b*
for constipation, 151
for heartburn, 132
pregnancy and, 9, 397
prenatal care and, 60
Overweight
body mass index and, 12
children, diabetes and, 422
chronic hypertension and, 415
exercise program and, 13
gestational diabetes mellitus and,
418
macrosomia and, 544
multiple pregnancy and, 370, 370*t*
resources, 386
weight gain during pregnancy and,
47*t*, 321, 322, 322*t*
Ovulation
basal body temperature and, 20, 20*f*
breastfeeding and, 295, 331
charting fertility and, 18*f*
induced, multiple pregnancy and,
362*b*
miscarriage and, 564
pregnancy and, 15–17, 17*f*
pregnancy tests and, 39
Ovulation predictor kits, 18
Oxycodone, 13, 54

Oxytocin
  abnormal labor and, 551
  contraction stress test and, 483
  during active labor, 250
  breastfeeding and, 167, 330
  labor induction and, 239
  postpartum hemorrhage and, 556
  premature rupture of membranes
    and, 492

**P**

Paced breathing exercise, 210b
Pacifiers, 163, 333b, 345
Pain relief during childbirth
  childbirth preparation methods,
    227–228
  considerations in eighth month,
    181–182
  decisions, 136
  medications, 223–227
  overview, 223
  resources, 232
  techniques, 229–231
Pain relievers, over-the-counter, 55,
  391b
Panic disorder, 442
Parallel hold, for breastfeeding twins,
  347b
Partial hydatidiform mole, 568
Parvovirus, 538, 574
Past pregnancies. See also Subsequent
  pregnancy
  breech presentation and, 258
  labor and, 246
  preconception care, 9–10
  premature rupture of membranes
    and, 492
  prenatal care and, 60
Patau syndrome, 456. See also Trisomy 13
Patch, birth control, 299–300, 300f
Pathogens, 398, 515. See also Infections
Pathologists, 574
Patient-controlled epidural analgesia,
  225
PCV13 vaccine, 519t
PE. See Pulmonary embolism
Peak Day, for cervical mucus, 18
Pedicures, 202
Pelvic bone pain, 150

Pelvic exam
  during labor, breech presentation and,
    258
  miscarriage diagnosis and, 563
  postpartum, 293
  prelabor contractions and, 190
  prenatal care visit, 60, 79
  preterm labor and, 489
Pelvic inflammatory disease (PID), 531,
  565
Pelvic organ prolapse, 257
Pelvic pressure, 190, 366, 489b
Perinatologists, 55–56, 365b
Perineal tear, 281–282, 288, 552
Perineum, 252, 257
Periodontal disease, 92
Permanent birth control, 304–308
Pertussis, 164, 516, 518, 520
Pesticides, 400–401
Phenylephrine, 104
Phenylpropanolamine, 104
Phospholipids, 436
Physical abuse, 83–84
Physical disabilities
  pregnancy and, 443
  preterm birth and, 493–494
Physician assistants, 56
Physicians, choosing, 55, 116, 127
Pica, 94, 125
PID. See Pelvic inflammatory disease
Pilates, 114
Pituitary gland, 37
Placenta
  abnormal labor and, 550–551
  banking blood from, 155, 158
  bisphenol-A and, 355
  B vitamins and, 133b
  cell-free DNA test from, 466b
  characteristics, 507
  delivery of, 244, 252–253
  development of, 34, 34f
  growth of, 33
  high blood pressure and blood flow to,
    408
  insulin and, 421
  late-term or postterm pregnancy and,
    216
  lead exposure and, 123
  multiple pregnancy and, 364

Placenta (*continued*)
oxygen received through, 34, 143, 276
preeclampsia and, 378
problems, 507–513, 542, 574
retained, 557
Rh sensitization and blood from, 501
teratogens passed through to, 392
ultrasound exams and position of, 479
weight gain and, 46*b*
Placenta accreta, 268, 511–513, 555
Placenta increta, 511, 513
Placental abruption
chronic hypertension and, 409
external cephalic version and, 259, 260
fetal well-being testing and, 477
labor induction and, 235
premature rupture of membranes
and, 492
thrombophilias and, 439
types, signs, and treatment, 510–511
vaginal bleeding and, 165–166
Placenta percreta, 511–512, 513
Placenta previa
breech presentation and, 258
cesarean delivery and, 264, 268
diagnosis of, 509
external cephalic version and, 259
labor induction and, 237
overview, 507–508
resources, 513
signs and symptoms, 509
treatment, 509–510
types of, 508, 508*f*
vaginal bleeding and, 165–166
Pneumococcal disease, 518, 519*t*, 525
Pneumonia, 521, 525
Polydactyly, 450*t*
Polyhydramnios, 554
Positions
alternative birthing, 57
of baby, abnormal labor and, 550
of baby, breech presentation and, 258
for breastfeeding, 336*b*, 338–339
changing, during early labor, 247
for delivery, 251–252
for labor and delivery, 192–193,
229–230
safe, for baby sleeping, 162–163
for sex after childbirth, 294

Positions (*continued*)
sleeping, 122
umbilical cord compression and, 553
umbilical cord prolapse and, 554
Postpartum depression, 289–290, 443,
588–589
Postpartum endometritis, 556
Postpartum hemorrhage, 138, 555–556
Postpartum period
birth control, 295–304
checkup, 292–293
exercises for, 284–285*b*, 290–291
first 3 months, 286–289
first week, 280–283, 286
glucose testing, 422
lifestyle changes, 291
life with your new baby, 292
nutrition, 291
permanent birth control, 304–308
preeclampsia and, 411
problem signs and symptoms, 288–289
resources, 309–310
returning to work, 308–309
right after birth, 275–280
Postpartum sterilization, 305–306, 305*f*, 502
Postpartum thyroiditis, 434
Postterm pregnancy, 216, 236, 477
PPSV23 vaccine, 519*t*
Preconception care
carrier screening, 6, 6–7*t*, 8, 459
chronic hypertension and, 414–415
family health history, 5
infections and immunizations, 3–5
kidney disease and, 430
medications and supplements, 9
overview, 3
past pregnancies, 9–10
physical disabilities and, 443
planning another baby and, 585–586
preexisting health conditions, 8–9
pregestational diabetes mellitus and,
423–424
reducing birth defect risk and, 390*b*
resources, 21
Preeclampsia. *See also* Blood pressure;
High blood pressure; Hypertension;
Preeclampsia
antiphospholipid syndrome and, 437
chronic hypertension and, 409

Preeclampsia (*continued*)
concerns regarding, 141
diagnosis, 412–413
eating disorders and, 385
exercise during pregnancy and, 47
fetal well-being testing and, 476
gestational diabetes mellitus and,
418–419
hyperthyroidism and, 433
kidney disease and, 430
labor induction and, 236
lupus and, 437
multiple pregnancy and, 368
obesity during pregnancy and, 378,
391*b*
overview, 411
postpartum hemorrhage and, 555
pregestational diabetes mellitus and,
423
prevention, 414–415
resources, 144, 415
risks, 411–412
screening test, 81
signs and symptoms, 142–143, 201,
214–215, 412, 412*b*
subsequent pregnancy and, 10, 589
treatment, 413–414
vaginal birth after cesarean delivery
success and, 272
Preexisting health conditions, 8–9
Pregestational diabetes mellitus. *See also*
Diabetes mellitus
breastfeeding and, 330
controlling, 424–425
macrosomia and, 544
overview, 422
postpartum care, 426
preconception care for, 423–424
preconception questions on, 8–9
resources, 427
risks to pregnancy, 423
special tests, 425–426
Pregnancy. *See also* Delivery; Labor;
Subsequent pregnancy; *specific
medical conditions*
autoimmune disorders and, 436
basal body temperature and, 20, 20*f*
birth control and, 20–21
body changes and, 37–41

Pregnancy (*continued*)
fertility awareness and, 17–18, 18*f*
fetal development during, 22, 23–31*f*
flu shot during, 518
immunizations and, 516–518
length of, vaginal birth after cesarean
delivery success and, 272
menstrual calendar and, 19*f*
menstrual cycle and, 15–17, 17*f*
Peak Day and, 18
pregestational diabetes mellitus and, 423
Rh sensitization and, 501
Pregnancy Discrimination Act, 96
Pregnancy exposure registries, 396–397,
402
Pregnancy loss
coping with, 569–570
early, 561–570
ectopic pregnancy, 565–568, 566*f*
gestational trophoblastic disease,
568–569
grieving, 575–578
late, 573–580
resources, 570
Pregnancy tests, 37, 39, 236
Preimplantation genetic diagnosis, 464,
470–471
Prelabor contractions, 189–190. *See also*
Braxton Hicks contractions
Premature delivery. *See* Preterm births
Premature rupture of membranes
(PROM). *See also* Amniotic sac;
Rupture of membranes; The bag of
waters
bacterial vaginosis and, 103, 535
chlamydia or gonorrhea and, 531
exercise during pregnancy and, 47
external cephalic version and, 260
labor induction and, 236
overview, 487, 491–492
risks, 492
signs and symptoms, 183
subsequent pregnancy and, 588–589
trichomoniasis and, 533
Premenstrual dysphoric disorder, 290
Premenstrual syndrome, 290
Prenatal care
blood type incompatibility testing, 499
childbirth partner and, 137

Prenatal care (*continued*)
  delivery planning during, 74
  for depression, 159
  fetal growth testing during, 542–543
  future dads and, 14*b*
  gestational diabetes mellitus and, 420
  hepatitis B virus and, 522
  infection detection during, 515
  in month 3, 78–79
  in month 4, 101
  in month 5, 122–123
  in month 6, 141
  in month 7, 164
  in month 8, 182
  in month 9, 199–201
  in month 10, 214
  in months 1 & 2, 59–60
  multiple pregnancy and, 364
  multiple pregnancy monitoring,
    371–372
  multivitamin monitoring, 45
  for numbness in legs or feet, 190
  before traveling, 117
  weight check during, 322
Prescription medications, 9, 54–55, 60,
  395–397
Presentation, definition of, 244
Preterm birth. *See also* Preterm labor
  bottle-feeding after, 350*b*
  breastfeeding and, 330
  breech presentation among, 258
  cesarean delivery and, 267
  chlamydia or gonorrhea and, 531
  chronic hypertension and, 409, 410
  diagnosing, 141
  early, 139
  evaluation of baby after, 253
  fetal growth problems and, 396
  fetal growth restriction and, 543
  low milk supply and, 340
  multifetal pregnancy reduction and,
    362*b*
  multiple pregnancy and, 364–366
  neonatal intensive care units and,
    494
  obesity during pregnancy and, 379
  overview, 493–494
  placenta previa and, 508–509
  resources, 496

Preterm birth (*continued*)
  spacing pregnancies and, 586
  special care for, 495
  subsequent pregnancy and, 10, 588
  substance abuse and, 54
  surfactant replacement therapy for, 494
  umbilical cord prolapse and, 554
Preterm labor. *See also* Labor; Preterm
    birth
  bed rest and, 182
  exercise during pregnancy and, 47
  management, 489–490
  overview, 487–488
  pregestational diabetes mellitus and, 423
  prevention, 491
  resources, 496
  risk factors, 488–489
  sexually transmitted infections and, 83
  signs and symptoms, 165, 183, 489
  signs of, 142
  ultrasound exam and, 479
Preterm premature rupture of
    membranes, 183, 487, 491, 492, 493
Preterm PROM. *See also* Preterm prema-
    ture rupture of membranes.
Previous pregnancies. *See* Past
    pregnancies
Private cord blood banks, 158
Progesterone
  changes in levels of, 37
  constipation and, 150
  pregnancy and, 15, 16, 33
  shots, preterm labor and, 491
Progestin, 298–299
Progestin-only birth-control pills,
    296–297*t*, 301
Prolapsed cord, 260
PROM. *See* Premature rupture of
    membranes
Propylthiouracil, 433
Prostaglandins, 140, 217, 238, 551, 556
Proteinuria, 412
Pseudoephedrine, 104
Psychotherapy, 443
Pubic symphysis, 150, 150*f*
Public cord blood banks, 155, 158
Pulmonary embolism (PE), 119*b*, 437
Pulse oximetry test, 279
Pumps. *See* Breast pumps

## Q

Quadruplets, 365*t*
Quickening, 109
Quitline, National Cancer Institute's
    Smoking, 13, 51

## R

Race, carrier screening and, 6, 6–7*t*, 8
Racquet sports, 50
Radiation, 104, 119, 391*b*, 401
Radioactive iodine, 433
Radioisotopes, 401
Raw foods, 325
Read method, 180–181, 227
Recessive genetic disorders, 450*t*, 451*t*,
    453–454, 455*f*
Rectal bleeding, 435
Rectum
    constipation in pregnancy and, 150
    perineal tear and, 282
    postpartum accidental bowel leakage,
      286
    in transition to stage 2 of labor, 251
    varicose veins near, 174
Red blood cells, 79, 81
Red streaks on breasts, 288, 341
Refrigeration, of bottles and nipples, 356
Regional anesthesia, 182, 224–226, 253,
    305
Relaxation techniques, 176–177, 176*b*,
    223
Relaxin, 149
Remission, in autoimmune disorders,
    435, 438
Respiratory distress syndrome, 139, 423,
    494
Respiratory system, 224, 518
Resuscitation, preterm births and, 494
Rh antibody screening, 164
Rheumatic fever, 429–430
Rheumatoid arthritis, 438
Rh factor, 81, 499
RhIg. *See* Rh immunoglobulin
Rh immunoglobulin (RhIg), 81, 164,
    502–503, 564
Rh incompatibility, 499, 500–501, 504
Rh sensitization, 477, 500–501,
    500–501*f*, 501–502

Rooming in, 157*b*, 193, 278
Rooting reflex, 335
Rubella, 82, 518, 524, 542. *See also*
    German measles
Rubeola. *See* Measles
Rupture of membranes. *See also*
    Amniotic sac; Premature rupture
    of membranes
    during active labor, 250
    labor in preterm multiple pregnancy
      and, 366
    preterm labor and, 489*b*
    process of, 212–213, 215
    prolonged, endometritis and, 556–557
    umbilical cord prolapse and, 554

## S

Sacroiliac ligaments, 149, 150*f*
Salivation, excessive, 93
Salmeterol, 432*b*
Salmonellosis, 134
Salt, in foods, 133
Saturated fats, 315
Saunas, safety of, 85–86, 402
SCHIP. *See* State Children's Health
    Insurance Program
Schizophrenia, 442
Sciatica, 149
Sciatic nerve, 150*f*
Screening tests
    for birth defects, 101
    of cord blood, 158
    deciding to undergo, 461–462
    definition of, 449
    for genetic disorders, 6, 74–75, 459,
      460*f*, 465–468
    in last month of pregnancy, 200–201
    for newborns, 279–280, 309
Screen negative results, 468
Screen positive results, 468
Scuba diving, 50
Seat belts, 118, 120*b*, 121
Seated ball balance, 95*b*
Seated side stretch, 153*b*
Secondary hemorrhage, 555
Secondhand smoke, 13–14, 52
Sedatives, 224
Seizure disorders, 8–9, 440–442, 445

Selective serotonin reuptake inhibitors, 162
Sepsis, 550
Sequential screening, 465*t*, 467
Sex chromosomes, 451, 452, 452*f*, 466*b*
Sex-linked disorders, 454
Sexual abuse, 83–84
Sexual intercourse
    after childbirth, 293–295
    Braxton Hicks contractions and, 151
    miscarriage and, 561, 563
    during pregnancy, 140, 182, 213–214
Sexually transmitted infections (STIs)
    birth control methods and, 296–297*t*
    chlamydia, 530–531
    circumcision and, 177
    ectopic pregnancy and, 565
    future dads and, 14*b*
    genital herpes, 529–530, 529*f*
    gonorrhea, 530–531
    human immunodeficiency virus, 531–532
    preconception care for, 4–5
    protection against, 528–529
    resources, 539
    screening tests, 78
    syphilis, 532–533
    trichomoniasis, 533
SGA. *See* Small for gestational age
Shellfish, 209*b*, 322–323, 344
Shingles. *See* Herpes zoster
Ship, travel by, 121
Shortness of breath, 48*b*, 173
Shoulder dystocia, 545, 551–552, 552*f*
Showing, of pregnancy, 91, 587
Sickle cell anemia, 450*t*
Sickle cell disease
    as autosomal recessive gene disorder, 454
    fetal growth restriction and, 542
    folic acid and, 44*b*
    placental abruption and, 510
    resources, 473
    screening test, 6, 6*t*, 74, 463
Side-lying position, for breastfeeding, 336*b*
SIDS. *See* Sudden infant death syndrome
Sitz bath, perineal tear and, 282

Skating, in-line, 49
Skiing, downhill snow, 49
Skin changes, 76, 87, 384
Skin treatments, 55, 391*b*
Sleep
    comfortable position for, 122
    exercise and, 47
    by newborn babies, 278
    pregnancy-related stress and, 104
    rapid eye movement, 129, 147
    safe position for baby, 162–163, 169
    snoring during, 207
    suggestions for, 68
    trouble, in ninth month, 190
SMA. *See* Spinal muscular atrophy
Small for gestational age (SGA), 541
Smells, morning sickness and, 42
Smoking
    avoiding during pregnancy, 51–52
    breastfeeding and, 345
    chronic hypertension and, 414–415
    fetal growth restriction and, 542–543
    future dads and, 14*b*
    miscarriage and, 562
    placental abruption and, 510
    placenta previa and, 507
    pneumococcal pneumonia and, 525
    postpartum, 291
    during pregnancy, 13–14
    premature rupture of membranes and, 492
    preterm births and, 488*b*
    resources, 63
Snacks, 42, 59, 112–113, 321
Snoring, 207
Snow skiing, 49
Somites, 35
Sophrology, 228
Spacing children, 295, 488*b*, 585–586
Sperm
    abnormal number of chromosomes in, 562
    chromosomes in, 451
    ejaculation of, 17
    fertilization and, 33
    fraternal twins and, 363, 363*f*
    intrauterine devices and, 298
    unhealthy substances and, 13–14

Spermicides, 296–297*t*, 303, 303*f*
Spider veins, 93
Spina bifida, 44*b*, 74
Spinal block, 182, 226, 240, 265, 440
Spinal muscular atrophy (SMA), 7*t*
Sponge, birth control, 296–297*t*, 302, 303*f*
Spoons hold, for breastfeeding twins, 347*b*
Spotting. *See* Vaginal spotting
Squat bar, 156*b*, 192, 230*f*
Squatting during labor, 229, 252
Standing back bend, 191*b*
State Children's Health Insurance Program (SCHIP), 101
State Health Insurance Exchanges, 99–100
Station, 244, 245*f*
Stem cells, 155, 184
Sterilization
   for birth control, 166, 296–297*t*
   of bottles and nipples, 356
   female, 304–307, 305*f*
   intrauterine device effectiveness vs., 298
   male, 307–308, 308*f*
   postpartum, Rh immunoglobulin and, 502
Stillbirth
   chorioamnionitis and, 550
   diagnosis, 573
Stillbirth
   fetal well-being testing and risk of, 475
   overview, 573
   planning next pregnancy after, 579
   reasons for, 574
   resources, 570, 580
   subsequent pregnancy and, 10
   tests and evaluations after, 574–575
STIs. *See* Sexually transmitted infections
Storing milk, 349, 353*b*
*Streptococcus pneumoniae*, 525
Stress
   irritable bowel syndrome and, 435
   mental illness and, 442
   miscarriage and, 561
   multiple pregnancy and, 373
   of parenting, 292

Stress (*continued*)
   postpartum depression and, 290
   pregnancy-related, 103–104, 162
   sex after childbirth and, 294
Stretches
   before exercise, 115
   seated side, 153*b*
Stretch marks, 76, 77*f*
Stroke, 378, 408, 412
Structural chromosomal disorders, 456–457
Subclinical hypothyroidism, 434
Subsequent pregnancy. *See also* Past pregnancy; Pregnancy
   cesarean delivery decision and, 73–74
   planning, 585–587
   possible problems with, 588–589
   previous pregnancy vs., 587–588
   previous problems and, 10
   resources, 591
   Rh incompatibility and, 499–501
   stillbirth and, 579
Substance abuse
   avoiding during pregnancy, 53–54
   breastfeeding and, 332
   future dads and, 14*b*
   during pregnancy, 13–14
   preterm births and, 488*b*
   resources, 62
Sucking reflex, 107, 108*f*
Sudden infant death syndrome (SIDS)
   breastfeeding and, 195, 330
   secondhand smoke and, 13–14, 291
   sleep position and, 162–163, 163*f*
   smoking and, 51
Sugar substitutes, 71–72
SuperTracker program, 316
Supplements. *See* Herbal supplements; Vitamin supplements
Surfactant, 147, 494
Surfing, 50
Surgery. *See also* Cesarean delivery; Delivery; Labor and delivery problems; Pregnancy; Vaginal birth after cesarean birth
   bariatric, 13, 382–383
   on breasts, breastfeeding and, 346

Surgery (*continued*)
  for ectopic pregnancy, 567, 568
  for postpartum hemorrhage, 556
  during pregnancy, 104
  sterilization, 304–306
Sushi, eating, 126
Sweating, postpartum, 288
Swimming, 49, 113–114, 153*b*, 291,
  380
Syphilis, 4, 83, 200, 532–533, 574
Systemic analgesics, 224
Systemic lupus erythematosus, 411,
  437–438, 445, 475
Systolic blood pressure, 408

**T**

Tachysystole, uterine, 239
Tai chi, 114
Tay–Sachs disease
  as genetic disorder, 6, 7*t*, 449, 450*t*,
    454
  resources, 473
  screening test, 74, 463
TB. *See* Tuberculosis.
Tdap. *See* Tetanus toxoid, reduced
    diphtheria toxoid, and acellular
    pertussis vaccine
Teeth, loosening or erosion of, 92
Temperature, baby's, maintaining,
  276–277. *See also* Basal body
    temperature
Teratogens, 389, 392
Term premature rupture of membranes,
  491
Testes, 107
Testosterone, 89
Tetanus, 164, 518, 520–521
Tetanus toxoid, reduced diphtheria
    toxoid, and acellular pertussis
    (Tdap) vaccine, 4, 164, 516
  pregnancy and, 519*t*, 520
Thalassemias
  characteristics, 7*t*, 450*t*
  screening test, 6, 8, 74, 463
The American College of Obstetricians
    and Gynecologists
  on birth settings, 98
  on breastfeeding, 167
  on breastfeeding duration, 342

The American College of Obstetricians
    and Gynecologists (*continued*)
  on cell-free DNA test, 466*b*
  on eating and drinking during labor,
    209
  on episiotomies, 218
  on finding physicians, 55, 127
  on hepatitis B virus risk during
    pregnancy, 399
  on labor in water, 137
  on ultrasound exams for sex determi-
    nation, 115
The bag of waters, 238. *See also*
    Amniotic sac; Premature rupture of
    membranes; Rupture of membranes
The Joint Commission, 98
Theophylline, 432*b*
Thimerosal-containing vaccines, 517
Three-dimensional ultrasound exams,
  143, 479
Thrombophilias, 411, 438–440
Thyroid disease, 433–434
Thyroid gland, 434*f*
Thyroid hormone, 433
Thyroxine, 433
Timing of contractions, 189, 211, 213*t*, 247
Timing of screening and diagnostic tests,
  460*f*, 461–462
Tiredness. *See also* Fatigue
  endometritis and, 557
Tocolytics, 366, 490, 511
TOLAC. *See* Trial of labor after cesarean
    delivery
Tooth decay, 42, 92
Toxins, 4, 51, 389, 517
Toxoplasmosis, 86, 280, 391*b*, 537–538,
  574
Transabdominal chorionic villus
    sampling, 469
Transabdominal ultrasound, 79, 80*f*, 480
Transcervical chorionic villus sampling,
  469–470, 470*f*
Transducer, 60, 79, 480
Transfusion. *See* Blood transfusion
Translocation, in chromosomes, 456–457
Transplantation, autologous or allogenic,
  155
Transvaginal ultrasound, 79, 80*f*, 480,
  488*b*, 489

Transverse incision, 266–267, 267f, 270
Transverse lie, labor induction and, 237
Travel, 116–121, 118b, 119b, 120b, 435
Trial of labor after cesarean delivery (TOLAC), 263, 264, 270
*Trichomonas vaginalis*, 533
Trichomoniasis, 4, 533
Trimesters, weeks of pregnancy divided into, 40
Tripelennamine, 104
Triplets. *See also* Multiple pregnancy
average gestational age at delivery of, 365t
breastfeeding, 346
fertility treatments and, 362b
formation process, 363–364
placenta, amniotic sac, and chorion for, 367
placenta previa and, 507
statistics on, 361
Trisomies, 456, 459
Trisomy 13, 456, 465t, 466b, 542
Trisomy 18, 456, 465t, 466b, 467, 542
Trisomy 21, 456. *See also* Down syndrome
TTTS. *See* Twin–twin transfusion syndrome
Tubal sterilization, 166–167, 305, 565
Tuberculosis (TB), 82, 332, 534–535
Turner syndrome, 456
22q11.2 deletion syndrome, 457
Twins. *See also* Multiple pregnancy
average gestational age at delivery of, 365t
breastfeeding, 346, 347b
fertility treatments and, 362b
fraternal or identical, 363, 363f
placenta previa and, 507
postpartum hemorrhage and, 555
resources, 374
statistics on, 361
types of, 366–368, 367f
umbilical cord prolapse and, 554
weight gain during pregnancy and, 322t
Twin–twin transfusion syndrome (TTTS), 367–368

**U**
Ulcerative colitis, 435
Ultrasound exam
for amniotic fluid problems, 166
antiphospholipid syndrome and, 437
biophysical profile and, 481–482
chronic hypertension and, 410
confirm breech presentation, 258
detect heartbeat, 35
of developing eggs, 362b
elective induction and, 236
estimated due date and, 40
external cephalic version and, 260
fetal growth testing and, 543
keepsake, 141, 143, 479
for genetic disorders, 74–75
gestational trophoblastic disease and, 569
macrosomia and, 544
mild gestational hypertension and, 413
miscarriage diagnosis and, 563
multiple pregnancy and, 371
nuchal translucency screening, 74–75, 466
obesity during pregnancy and, 379
placenta accreta and, 512
placental abruption and, 511
for placenta previa, 509
prenatal care and, 60
preterm labor, 489
procedure for, 480
resources, 483
Rh incompatibility and, 503
safety, 476b
stillbirth diagnosis and, 573
timing for, 477
transabdominal, 80f
transvaginal, 80f
why it is done, 78–79, 478–479
Umbilical cord
banking blood from, 155, 158
breech presentation and, 260
compression, 553
cutting, 252
delayed clamping of, 184
formation of, 34, 34f
late-term or postterm pregnancy and, 216

Umbilical cord (*continued*)
in monochorionic–monoamniotic
babies, 368
problems, fetal well-being testing and,
477
problems, premature rupture of
membranes and, 491
problems, stillbirth and, 574
prolapse, 237, 553–555
Unbalanced translocations, in
chromosomes, 456, 457
Undercooked foods, 325
Underweight mother, 12, 47*t*, 322*t*, 370*t*
Unsatisfactory result, in contraction
stress test, 483
Unsaturated fats, 315
Urethra, 282, 527*f*, 528
Urinalysis, 81, 101, 412–413
Urinary tract infections, 81, 101–102,
527*f*, 528
Urination
frequency, 38, 189, 207
hyperemesis gravidarum and, 43
painful postpartum, 282, 288
Urine culture, 81
Urine leakage, 492
Urine test for pregnancy, 39
U.S. Department of Agriculture
on cost of raising a child, 100*b*, 586*b*
MyPlate food-planning guide, 11,
316, 321*f*, 326
U.S. Department of Labor, 96–97,
398–399
U.S. Food and Drug Administration
(FDA), 133, 209*b*, 355, 395, 517
Uterine artery embolization, 511, 556
Uterine atony, 555, 556
Uterine rupture, 138, 238–239, 270,
555
Uterine tachysystole, 239
Uterus
abnormal labor and, 550
before and after birth, 283*f*
breastfeeding and contraction of, 195
changes in size of, 125*f*
fertilization and, 33
increased size of, 91
infection, labor induction and, 236
menstrual cycle and, 15–16, 16*f*

Uterus (*continued*)
multiple pregnancy and, 364
placenta accreta and, 511–513
placenta attachment to, 507
postpartum checkup of, 293
shape of, breech presentation and, 258
shrinking after delivery, 252–253, 281
sperm in, 17
surgery, labor induction and, 237
surgery, placenta previa and, 507
surgery, preterm births and, 488*b*
ultrasound exam of, 79
weight gain and, 46*b*

**V**
Vaccine Information Statement, 517
Vaccines. *See also* Immunizations
for hepatitis B virus risk during
pregnancy, 399, 523–524
in preconception care, 3–4
pregnancy and, 516–518, 519*t*
preventing infections with, 516*b*
resources, 538–539
Vacuum aspiration, 563–564
Vacuum extraction, 218, 255–256, 256*f*,
261. *See also* Operative vaginal
delivery
Vacuum extractor, 256
Vagina
exercise and fluid gushing or leaking
from, 48*b*
menstrual cycle and, 16*f*
postpartum checkup of, 293
prenatal care in 8th month, 182
vacuum extraction and, 257
varicose veins near, 174
Vaginal birth
breech presentation and, 260–261
preeclampsia and, 413
umbilical cord prolapse and, 554–555
Vaginal birth after cesarean delivery
(VBAC). *See also* Cesarean delivery;
Delivery; Labor and delivery
problems; Pregnancy;
Surgery
about, 74
benefits, 271
best chances for success with, 272
factors to consider, 270–271

Vaginal birth after cesarean delivery (*continued*)
  overview, 263, 269–270
  preparing for changes with, 272
  resources, 273
  risks, 271
Vaginal bleeding. *See also* Bleeding
  amniocentesis or chorionic villus sampling and, 469
  domestic violence and, 84
  ectopic pregnancy and, 565–566
  exercise during pregnancy and, 47, 48*b*
  gestational trophoblastic disease and, 569
  miscarriage and, 60–61, 562
  placenta accreta and, 512
  placental abruption and, 510
  placenta previa and, 509
  postpartum, 281
  during pregnancy, preterm births and, 488*b*
  premature rupture of membranes diagnosis and, 492
  seeking medical help for, 213
  smoking and, 51
  in third trimester, 165–166
  ultrasound exam and, 479
Vaginal discharge
  bacterial vaginosis and, 535
  labor in preterm multiple pregnancy and, 366
  postpartum, bad-smelling, 289, 557
  pregnancy-related changes and, 102–103
  premature rupture of membranes and, 492
  preterm labor and, 489*b*
Vaginal dryness
  breastfeeding and, 293–294
  estrogen cream for, 294–295
Vaginal progesterone, 491
Vaginal ring, 299–300, 300*f*
Vaginal spotting
  after sex, 140
  ectopic pregnancy and, 567
  implantation and, 37
  miscarriage and, 61, 562
  start of labor and, 214, 215

Vaginal transducer, 480
Valproic acid, 395
Varicella, 144, 332, 389, 518, 542
Varicella vaccine, 4, 144, 517–518, 519*t*, 521–522
Varicella zoster virus (VZV), 521
Varicose veins, 174
Vas deferens, 308*f*
Vasectomy, 167, 307–308, 308*f*
VBAC. *See* Vaginal birth after cesarean delivery
Vegetarian diets, 323–324
Ventilators, 494
Vernix, 107, 108*f*
Vertex presentation, 201, 244, 245*f*, 257–258, 554
Vertical incision, 266–267, 267*f*
Vertical pocket measurement, of amniotic fluid, 482
Villi, 568
Viruses
  infections caused by, 515
  live, vaccines made with, 4, 82, 517–518, 522
  placenta and, 34
  travel by ship and, 121
Vision problems
  diabetes mellitus and, 417
  early preterm birth and, 139
  multiple sclerosis and, 438
  preeclampsia and, 142, 412*b*
  pregestational diabetes mellitus and, 423
Vitamin A, 9, 315, 318*t*, 383, 389
Vitamin B, 132–133, 133*b*
Vitamin B$_6$, 42, 318*t*
Vitamin B$_{12}$, 318*t*, 383
Vitamin C, 191*b*, 318*t*
Vitamin D
  bariatric surgery and, 383
  deficiency, 168
  fats and, 315
  formula-feeding and, 353
  sources and effects of, 318*t*, 320
  supplement to breastfeeding, 338
Vitamin E, fats and, 315
Vitamin K
  fats and, 315
  shot, 279

Vitamin supplements. *See also*
   Multivitamins; Nutritional
   supplements
   avoiding during pregnancy, 55
   birth defects and, 391*b*
   constipation and iron level in, 71*b*
   with folic acid and iron, 320
   pregnancy and, 9, 397
Vitamins. *See also* Multivitamins
   digestive diseases and, 435
   inflammatory bowel disease and, 435
Vomiting
   morning sickness and, 41–43
   postpartum, 288
   preeclampsia and, 142, 412*b*
   pregnancy, gastric band surgery and,
      383
   as pregnancy sign, 38
Von Willebrand disease, 440
Von Willebrand factor (vWF), 440
Vulva, 174
vWF. *See* Von Willebrand factor
VZV. See Varicella zoster virus

**W**

Wage and Hour Division (WHD),
      Department of Labor, 97
Walking
   alternatives to, 113–114
   as exercise during pregnancy, 49, 95
   during labor, 247, 250
   obesity during pregnancy and, 380
   pain relief during childbirth and, 231
   for postpartum exercise, 291
   warning signs to stop, 48*b*
Walking epidural, 226
Warfarin, 389, 395, 439
Water breaking, 212–213, 215, 249
Water skiing, 50
Weakness, ectopic pregnancy and,
      565–568
Weaning, 342–343
Weight, prepregnancy, preterm births
      and, 488*b*
Weight gain
   by baby, 46*b*, 90, 129, 147
   between pregnancies, 587
   body mass index and, 12–13

Weight gain (*continued*)
   breastfeeding baby and, 344
   eating and, 10–11
   eating disorders and, 385
   excessive, macrosomia and, 544
   exercise and, 47
   gluten-free diet and, 436
   hyperemesis gravidarum and, 43
   in month 3, 71, 72*f*
   in month 4, 93–94
   in month 5, 113
   in month 6, 135
   in month 7, 151–152
   in months 1 & 2, 45–46, 47*t*
   multiple pregnancy and, 364, 370, 370*t*
   obesity during pregnancy and,
      380–381
   recommendations, 321–322, 322*t*, 380*t*
   resources, 386
   sudden, preeclampsia and, 142, 412*b*
Weight loss, 46, 382, 414, 422, 424
Weight-loss surgery, 13
WHD. *See* Wage and Hour Division
White blood cells, 79, 81, 195
Whooping cough, 164, 520
Witch-hazel compresses, cold, 282, 283
Wolf-Hirschhorn syndrome, 457
Working
   breastfeeding and, 349–353
   discrimination issues, 58, 105
   during early pregnancy, 58–59
   miscarriage and, 561
   return to, 308–309
Workplace safety considerations, 58, 105
World Health Organization, 333*b*

**X**

X chromosome, 451
X-linked genetic disorders, 451*t*, 455*f*
X-rays, 104, 401–402, 575

**Y**

Y chromosome, 451
Yeast infections, 103
Yoga, 103, 113, 191, 228

**Z**

Zygote, 33